NURSING TODAY

Transition and Trends

JoAnn Zerwekh, EdD, RN, FNP, CS
University of Phoenix Online Campus
Phoenix, Arizona
Capella University
Minneapolis, Minnesota
Executive Director
Nursing Education Consultants
Dallas, Texas

Jo Carol Claborn, MS, RN, CNS
Executive Director
Nursing Education Consultants
Dallas, Texas

SAUNDERS
An Imprint of Elsevier Science

SAUNDERS
An Imprint of Elsevier Science

11830 Westline Industrial Drive
St. Louis, Missouri 63146

NURSING TODAY: TRANSITION AND TRENDS   ISBN 0-7216-9692-9
Copyright © 2003, Elsevier Science (USA). All rights reserved.

Previous editions copyrighted 1994, 1997, 2000.

Library of Congress Cataloging-in-Publication Data

Nursing today: transitions and trends/[edited by] Joann Zerwekh,
Jo Carol Claborn.—4th ed.
        p. cm.
    Includes bibliographical references and index.
    ISBN 0-7216-9692-9
      1. Nursing—Vocational guidance. 2, Nursing—Social aspects.
    I. Zerwekh, JoAnn Graham. II. Claborn, Jo Carol.

    RT82.N874 2002
    610.73′06′9—dc21

                                    2002030914

Acquisitions Editor: Tom Wilhelm
Developmental Editor: Eric Ham
Publishing Services Manager: Deborah L. Vogel
Design Manager: Bill Drone
Cover and Interior Designer: Lee Goldstein

GW/QWF

Printed in the United States of America.

Last digit is the print number: 9   8   7   6   5   4   3   2   1

NURSING TODAY

Transition and Trends

CONGRATULATIONS
You now have access to Saunders' "Get Connected" Bonus Package!

Here's what's included to help you "Get Connected"

sign on at:

www.wbsaunders.com/MERLIN/Zerwekh/nsgtoday/

A website just for you as you learn leadership and management skills with the new 4th edition of **Nursing Today: Transition and Trends.**

what you will receive:

Whether you're a student or an instructor, you'll find information just for you, including
- Passcode-protected faculty resources
- Key book features and descriptions
- Links to related products
- Author information

Plus:

WebLinks

An exciting new program that allows you to directly access hundreds of active websites keyed specifically to the content of this book. The WebLinks are continually updated, with new ones added as they develop.

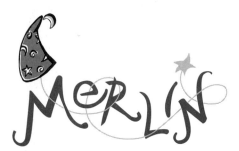

SAUNDERS
An Imprint of Elsevier Science

To Charles Graham, Hazel Cooper, and Lucy Claborn
for providing wisdom and support that can only come from parents.

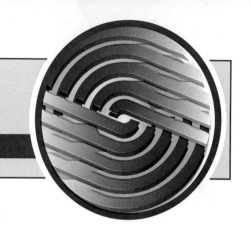

Contributors

Linda T. Anglin, DA, RNC
Associate Professor Emeriti
Bradley University Department of Nursing
Peoria, Illinois
Historical Perspectives: Influences of the Past

Jo Carol Claborn, MS, RN, CNS
Executive Director
Nursing Education Consultants
Dallas, Texas
*Reality Shock; Employment Considerations:
Opportunities and Résumés; NCLEX-RN
and the New Graduate*

Gail M. Collier, RN
Senior Nurse Recruiter
Children's Medical Center of Dallas
Dallas, Texas
*Employment Considerations: Opportunities and
Résumés*

Sharon Decker, RN, CS, MSN, CCRN
Professor and Director of Clinical Simulations
Texas Tech University Health Sciences Center
Lubbock, Texas
Time Management

Mary E. Foley, RN, MS
Immediate Past—President
American Nurses Association
Washington, DC
A Collective Voice in the Workplace

Mitzi A. Forbes, PhD, RN
Assistant Professor
University of Wisconsin—Milwaukee
School of Nursing
Milwaukee, Wisconsin
Instructor
University of Phoenix—Online
*Complementary and Alternative Therapies in
Nursing and Health Care*

Tom Gaglione, RN, MN
Adjunct Faculty
Nursing Education Consultants
Dallas, Texas
Adjunct Faculty
Group Process and Team Building

Ruth Hansten PhD, MBA, BSN, FACHE
Principal, Hansten Healthcare
Port Ludlow, Washington
Delegation in the Clinical Setting

Lynette W. Jack, PhD, RN, CARN
Associate Professor
University of Pittsburgh School of Nursing
Pittsburgh, Pennsylvania
Effective Communication

Marilynn Jackson, PhD, MA, BSN
Principal, Intuitive Options
Tyler, Texas
Delegation in the Clinical Setting

Ela-Joy Lehrman, MS, MAEd, PhD, RN, CNM
Professor and Chair
College of Nursing and Health Sciences
Southern Arizona Campus
University of Phoenix
Tucson, Arizona
Using Nursing Research in Practice

Isela Luna, PhD, RN, CLNC
Manager, Carondelet Community Trust
Carondelet Health Network
Tucson, Arizona
Health in Community: Nursing's Role

Janet M. McLellan, RN, MSN, BC, NSA
Nursing Online Faculty, University of Phoenix
Healthcare Consultant, Healthlink
Houston, Texas
Nursing Informatics

Barbara J. Michaels, EdD, LMFT, RN
Faculty (retired)
El Centro College Dallas
Texas Marriage and Family Therapist Private
  Practice
Dallas, Texas
Self-Care Strategies

Nellie Nelson, MSN, RN, CARN
Chairperson for Health Science Division
Scottsdale Community College
Scottsdale, Arizona
Image of Nursing: Influences of the Present

Alice B. Pappas, PhD, RN
Associate Professor and Associate Dean
Louise Herrington School of Nursing
Baylor University
Dallas, Texas
Interviewing for Employment; Ethical Issues

Robin L. Perin, RN, BS, JD
General Counsel for University Physicians, Inc.
Tucson, AZ
Legal Issues

Carol Singer, EdD, RN
Associate Dean, Health Sciences
Manatee Community College
Bradenton, Florida
Challenges of Nursing Management

Betty J. Skaggs, PhD, RN
Assistant Professor of Clinical Nursing
  and Director, Learning Center
The University of Texas at Austin
School of Nursing
Austin, Texas
Political Action in Nursing

Susan Sportsman, RN, PhD
Dean, College of Health Sciences and
  Human Services
Midwestern State University
Wichita Falls, Texas
*The Health Care Organization and Patterns of
  Nursing Care Delivery*

Gayle Varnell, PhD, RN, CPNP
Associate Professor and Assistant Dean
  for Advanced Practice
The University of Texas at Tyler College
  of Nursing and Health Sciences
Tyler, Texas
Nursing Education

JoAnn Zerwekh, EdD, RN, FNP, CS
University of Phoenix Online Campus
Phoenix, Arizona
Capella University
Minneapolis, Minnesota
Executive Director
Nursing Education Consultants
Dallas, Texas
*Reality Shock; Conflict Management; Trends and
  Economics in the Health Care Delivery System*

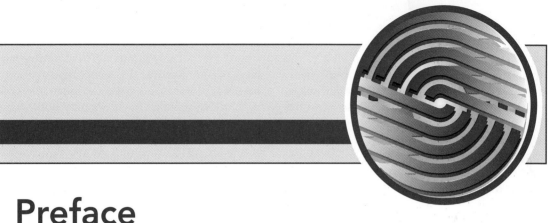

Preface

Nursing Today: Transition and Trends evolved out of the author's experiences with the nursing student in his or her final semester and the student's transition into the realities of nursing practice. There is a need for the graduating nurse to become aware of the transition process *before* graduation. Nursing education and the transition process is experiencing a tremendous impact from changes in the health care delivery system. We have responded to these changes by adding information in areas that nursing faculty specifically requested. In this fourth edition, we have continued to provide the graduate nurse with information on delegation and management, plus we have added a new chapter on nursing informatics. We kept the same easy reading style to present timely information along with information on nursing management and leadership in both hospital and community settings. It is our belief that the graduating nurse can benefit from practical guidelines regarding the transition from student to effective practice at entry level.

The experience of other nursing faculty, Marlene Kramer's research on reality shock, and Patricia Benner's work on performance characteristics of beginning and expert nurses continues to impact the need for transition courses in the school curriculum. These courses focus on trends and issues to assist the new graduate to be better prepared to practice nursing in today's world. With the increased demands and realities of the health care system, it is necessary for the new graduate to make the transition to an independent role more rapidly. We have written this book to be used in these transition type courses and by the individual student to assist them to anticipate the encounters in a rapidly changing, technologically-oriented work environment.

We have revised and updated each chapter regarding the changes in the health care delivery system along with presenting more information about nursing management. There is an increased focus on the use of the Internet as a resource for the transitioning graduate. All *cartoons* have been redesigned and redrawn by C.J. Miller, RN, to provide an updated look. Each chapter begins with *student objectives* and a *quote* as an introduction to the content of the chapter. As you read a chapter, you will find practical application to the concepts discussed. *Critical Thinking Boxes* in the text highlight information to facilitate the critical thinking process. Using a *question approach*, material is presented in a logical, easy-to-read manner. There are also opportunities to respond to *thought-provoking questions* and *student exercises* to facilitate self-evaluation.

The student is given an overall view of the nursing profession from past historical events that influenced nursing to the present day image, the legal, ethical, political, and on-the-job issues confronting today's nurse. Communication in the workplace, time management, how to write an effective résumé, interviewing tips, employee benefits, and self-care strategies are among the sound career advancement tools provided.

For Nursing Faculty:

Our key goal in developing this book has been timely information that is applicable to current practice and fun to read. An *Instructor's Manual*, which is web-based, is available from the publisher to assist faculty in planning and promoting a positive transition experience. This valuable web site contains suggestions for classroom and clinical-based student activities.

At the request of nursing faculty using our book, we have provided a secure, updated web-based Test Bank and have expanded the web page, which supports the textbook. Another new feature available on the faculty web page is a PowerPoint presentation for each chapter. The web page will continue to provide updated information as new trends and issues affect the practice of nursing.

Please consult your local Elsevier (Mosby-Saunders) representative for more details.

JoAnn Zerwekh, EdD, RN, FNP, CS
Jo Carol Claborn, MS, RN, CNS

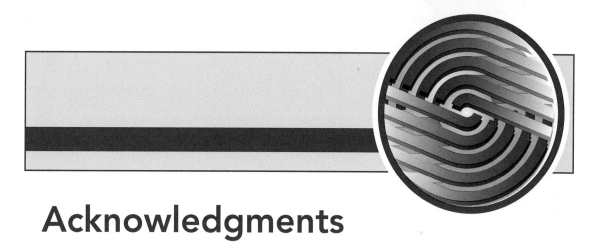

Acknowledgments

The success of previous editions of this book is due to the contributions and efforts of our chapter contributors who provided their expertise and knowledge. This new edition is no exception. We thank the staff at Elsevier Health Sciences: Michael Ledbetter, Senior Nursing Editor, for his expertise and advice and Eric Ham, Developmental Editor, who we have worked most closely with in this revision process. His creativity and guidance have provided a new look for this fourth edition, and we are grateful to Eric for his ability to quickly smooth out the wrinkles that often occur in the production of a book.

Last, but certainly not least, we want to thank our adult children for their continued support in our writing endeavors—Tyler, Ashley, Jaelyn, Mike, and Kimberley. We thank our parents, Charles Graham and Hazel Cooper, who have been there for us since the beginning and have encouraged our continued growth. We also thank Tom Gaglione and Robert Claborn for their unending support, patience, and sense of humor. We love you all!

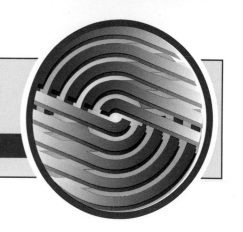

Contents

Unit III
NURSING MANAGEMENT

Unit IV
HEALTH CARE DELIVERY SYSTEM

UNIT V
ETHICAL AND LEGAL ISSUES IN NURSING

UNIT VI
IN SEARCH OF EMPLOYMENT: FINDING YOUR NICHE IN THE WORLD

UNIT I

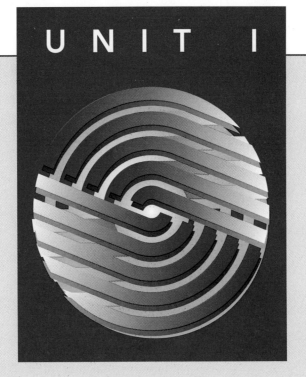

ROLE
TRANSITIONS

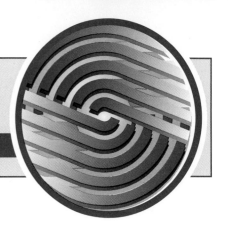

Reality Shock

JOANN ZERWEKH, EdD, RN, FNP, CS
JO CAROL CLABORN, MS, RN, CNS

If only dreams and reality were not so far apart.

— *Miguel de Cervantes*

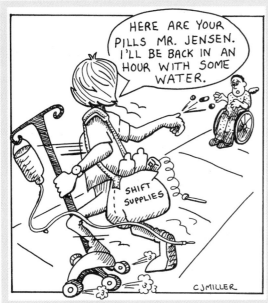

Role transition can be a complex experience.

After completing this chapter, you should be able to:

■ Discuss the concept of reality shock.

■ Identify the characteristics of reality shock.

■ Compare and contrast the phases of reality shock.

■ Identify times in your life when you have experienced a reality shock or role transition.

■ Describe four possible resolutions for reality shock.

WELCOME TO THE WORLD OF NURSING. We have written this book for YOU. That's right—you, student-almost-graduate nurse. Our goal is to help make your life easier during the transition period when you adjust both personally and professionally to graduation from nursing school and the beginning of your first job as a professional nurse. We have designed this book to help you keep your feet on the ground and your head out of the clouds as well as to boost your spirits when the going gets rough. We offer many down-to-earth tips that will save you time and energy.

As you thumb through this book, you will notice that there are cartoons and critical-thinking questions that encourage your participation. Don't be alarmed; we know you have been overloaded with "critical thinking" during nursing school! These critical-thinking questions are not meant to be graded; instead, their purpose is to encourage you to begin thinking about your transition into nursing practice and to guide you through the book in a practical, participative manner. Our intention is to add a little humor here and there while giving information on topics such as reality shock, the image of nursing, the job search, politics in nursing, nursing education programs, nursing management skills, effective communication, ethical and legal issues, career planning, and burnout prevention, just to name a few. We want you to be informed about the controversial issues affecting nursing today. After all, the future of nursing rests with **you!**

Are you ready to begin? Then let's start with the real stuff. You are beginning to see the light at the end of the tunnel. It has been a long struggle, but you are almost there. Nursing is one of the most rewarding professions you can pursue. However, it can also be one of the most frustrating. As with marriage, raising children, and the pursuit of happiness, there are ups and downs. We seldom find the world or our specific situation the exact way we thought it would or should be. Often your fantasy of what nursing should be is not what you will find nursing to be.

> You will cry, but you will also laugh.
>
> You will share with people their darkest hours of pain and suffering, but
>
> You will also share with them their hope, healing, and recovery.
>
> You will be there as life begins and ends.
>
> You will experience great challenges that lead to success.
>
> You will experience failure and disappointment.
>
> You will never cease to be amazed at the resilience of the human body and spirit.

TRANSITIONS

The paradox of nursing will become obvious to you early in your career. This realization usually occurs during the first six months of your first job. Your control over the basic conditions of your work life is usually limited, but your ability and skill in creating the experiences of your work life can be unlimited. Therein is the key to your successful role transition. Transitions are a part of nursing.

WHAT ARE TRANSITIONS?

Transitions are passages or changes from one situation, condition, or state to another that occur over time. They have been classified into the following four major types: developmental (e.g., becoming a parent, midlife crisis), situational (graduating from a nursing program, career change, divorce), health-illness (e.g., dealing with a chronic illness), and organizational (e.g., change in leadership, new staffing patterns) (Schumacher and Meleis, 1994).

 Transitions are complex processes, and a lot of transitions occur at the same time.

WHAT ARE IMPORTANT FACTORS INFLUENCING TRANSITIONS?

Understanding the transition experience from the perspective of the person who is experiencing it is important because the *meaning* of the experience may be positive, negative, or neutral. The transition may be desired (e.g., starting school, successfully finishing school, and passing NCLEX) or undesirable (e.g., the death of a family member, after which you have to assume a new role in your family). *Expectation* about the transition process may or may not be realistic. Often, when you know what to expect, the stress associated with the change or transition is reduced. Another factor in the transition process is the new *level of knowledge and skill* required, as is the availability of needed resources within the *environment*.

The role-transition process from student to graduate nurse does not take place automatically. Having the optimal experience during role transition requires lots of attention, planning, and determination on your part. How you perceive and handle the transition will determine how well you progress through the process. It is important that you keep a positive attitude. Emotions and work situations are going to be up and down, but that is okay. It is expected, and you are going to be able to deal with it effectively. The wide range of emotions experienced during the transition process can often affect your *emotional and physical well-being*.

So, let's get started. Reality shock may be one of the first hurdles of transition to conquer in your new role as a graduate nurse or registered nurse (RN—real nurse☺).

REALITY SHOCK

WHAT IS REALITY SHOCK?

Reality shock is a term often used to describe the reaction experienced when one moves into the work force after several years of educational preparation. The recent graduate is caught in the situation of moving from a familiar, comfortable educational environment into a new role in the work force in which the expectations are not clearly defined or may not even be realistic. For example, as a student you were taught to consider the patient in a holistic framework, but in practice you often do not have the time to consider the psychosocial or teaching needs of the patient, even though they must be attended to and documented.

The recent graduate in the workplace is expected to be a capable, competent nurse. That sounds fine. However, sometimes there is a hidden expectation that graduate nurses function as though they have five years of nursing experience. This has even greater impact considering that there may be no "buffer time" after graduation. Today, with the computerized examination (NCLEX), the time from graduation to beginning work as an RN may be as short as two weeks. This situation may leave the graduate with feelings of powerlessness, depression, and insecurity because of an apparent lack of effectiveness in the work environment. The process of reality shock and transition is not unique to nursing. It is present in many professions as the graduate moves from the world of academia to the world of work and begins to adjust to the expectations and values of the work force.

WHAT ARE THE PHASES OF REALITY SHOCK?

Kramer (1974) described the process of reality shock as it applies to nursing (Table 1-1). Adjustments begin to take place as the graduate nurse adapts to the reality of the practice of nursing. The first phase of adjustment is the honeymoon phase (Fig. 1-1). The recent graduate is thrilled with completing school and accepting a first job. Life is a bed of roses because everyone knows nursing school is much harder than nursing practice. There is no more writing nursing care plans deep into the night. No one is watching over your shoulder while you insert a catheter or give an intravenous medication. You're not a "student" anymore—now you're a nurse! During this exciting phase, your perception of the situation may feel unreal and distorted, and you may not be able to understand the overall picture.

TABLE 1-1

Phases of Reality Shock

Honeymoon	Shock and Rejection	Recovery
Sees the world of nursing looking quite rosy Often fascinated with the thrill of "arriving" in the profession	Has excessive mistrust Experiences increased concern over minor pains and illness Experiences decrease in energy and feels excessive fatigue Fells like a failure and blames self for every mistake Bands together and depends on people who hold the same values Has a hypercritical attitude Feels moral outrage	Beginning sense of humor is the first sign Decrease in tension Increase in ability to objectivity

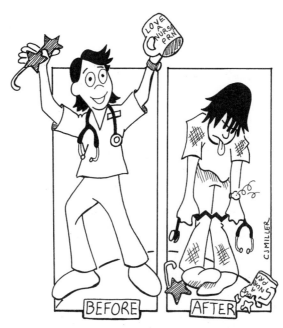

FIGURE 1-1
Reality Shock. The honeymoon's over.

I just can't believe how wonderful everything is! Imagine getting a paycheck—money, at last! It's all great. Really, it is.

The honeymoon phase is frequently short-lived as the graduate begins to identify the conflicts between the way she or he was taught and the reality of what is done. Every graduate nurse will have a unique way of coping with the situations; however, some common responses have been identified. The graduate may cope with this conflict by withdrawing or rejecting the values learned during nursing school. This may mark the end of the honeymoon phase of transition. The phrase "going native" was used by Kramer and Schmalenberg (1977) to describe recent graduates as they begin to cope and identify with the reality of the situation by rejecting the values from nursing school and beginning to function like everyone else does.

Mary was assigned 10 patients for the morning. There were numerous medications to be administered. It was difficult to carry all of the medication administration records to each room for patient identification. Because she "knew the patients," and the other experienced nurses did not check identification, she decided she no longer needed to check a patient's identification before administering medication. Later in the day, she gave insulin to Mrs. James, a patient she "knew"; unfortunately, the insulin was for Mrs. Phillips, another patient she "knew."

With experiences such as this during transition, the graduate begins to feel like a failure, taking the blame for every mistake. The graduate may become morally outraged at having been put in such a position. When the bad days begin to outnumber the good days, the graduate nurse may experience frustration, fatigue, and anger and may consequently develop a hypercritical attitude toward nursing. Some graduates become very disillusioned and drop out of nursing altogether. This is the period of shock and rejection.

> I had just completed orientation in the hospital where I had wanted to work since I started nursing school. I immediately discovered that the care there was so bad that I did not want to be a part of it. At night I went home very frustrated that the care I had given was not as I was taught to do it. I cried every night and hated to go to work in the morning. I did not like anyone with whom I was working. My stomach hurt, my head throbbed, and I had difficulty sleeping. It was hard not to work a double shift because I was worried about who would take care of those patients if I was not there.

A successfully managed transition period begins when the graduate nurse is able to evaluate the work situation objectively and effectively predict the actions and reactions of the staff. Nurturing the ability to see humor in a situation may be the first step. As the graduate begins to laugh at some of the situations encountered, the tension decreases and the perception increases. It is during this critical period of recovery that conflict resolution occurs. If this resolution occurs in a positive manner, it enables the graduate nurse to grow more fully as a person. This growth also enables the graduate to meet the work expectations to a greater degree and to see that she or he has the capacity to change a situation. If the conflict is resolved in a less-positive manner, however, the graduate's potential to learn and grow is limited.

Kramer (1974) described four groups of graduate nurses and the steps they took to resolve reality shock. The graduates who were considered to be most successful at adaptation were those who "made a lot of waves" within both their job setting and their professional organizations. Accordingly, they were not content with the present state of nursing but worked to affect a better system. This group of graduates was able to take worthwhile values learned during school and integrate them into the work setting. Often they returned to school—but not too quickly.

> I am really glad that I became a nurse. Sure, there are plenty of hassles, but the opportunities are there. Now that I am more confident of my skills, I am willing to take risks to improve patient care. Why, last week my head nurse, who often says jokingly, "You're a thorn in my side," appointed me to the Nursing Standards Committee. I feel really good about this recognition.

Another group limited their involvement with nursing by just putting in the usual 8-hour day. Persons in this group seldom belonged to professional organizations and cited as their reasons for working "to provide for my family," "to buy extra things for the house," and "to support myself." Typically, this type of conflict resolution leads to burnout, during which time the conflict would be turned inward, leading to constant griping and complaining about the work setting.

> I was so happy, at first. Gee, I was able to buy my son all those toys he wanted. Things here always seem to be the same—too many patients, not enough help. I get so upset with the staff, especially the nursing assistants, and the care that is given to patients. I wonder whether I will ever get the opportunity to practice nursing as I was taught. Well, I'll hang on 'till my husband finishes graduate school, then I'll quit this awful job!

Another group of graduates seemed to have found their niche and were content within the hospital setting. However, their positive attitude toward the job did not extend to nursing as a profession; in fact, it was the opposite. Rather than leave the organization during conflict, these "organization nurses" would change units or shifts—anything to avoid increasing demands for professional performance.

> During those first few months as I was just getting started, I sure had a tough time.
> It was difficult learning how to delegate tasks to the aides and practical nurses.
> But now that I have started working for Dr. Travis, everything is under my control.
> I just might go back to school someday.

The last group of graduates frequently changed jobs. After a short-lived career in hospital nursing, this group would pirouette off to graduate school, where they could "do something else in nursing" (i.e., "I can't nurse the way I've been taught, so I might as well teach others how to do things right."). Achieving a high profile in professional nursing organizations was common for these graduates, along with seeking a safer, more idealistically structured environment in which the values learned in school prevail.

> Finally, I got so frustrated with my head nurse that I just resigned. What did she expect
> from a recent graduate?! I couldn't do everything! Cost containment; early discharge;
> no time for teaching; rush, rush, rush, all the time. Well, I've made up my mind to look
> into going back to school to further my career.

The job expectations of the hospital administration or the employing community agency and the educational preparation of the graduate nurse are not always the same. This discrepancy, according to Schempp and Rompre (1986), is the basis of reality shock. Relationships among the staff, nurse professionalism, job satisfaction, and employee alienation were studied by Ahmadi, Speedling, and Kuhn-Weissman (1987). What is of interest in this study—as well as in those of Myrick (1988), Wolfgang (1988), Lund (1988), Horsburgh (1989), and Godinez et al (1999)—is that the issues of reality shock and role transition described by Kramer in the early 1970s are still around. We (nursing) have entered the twenty-first century with many of the same issues we had in the twentieth century. Much of this problem may be related to the fact that clinical instructors often focus on the needs of the patient rather than the needs of the student (Polifroni et al, 1995). We need to search for a way out of this situation (Critical Thinking Box 1-1).

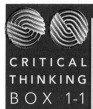

CRITICAL THINKING BOX 1-1

THINK ABOUT...

What is your greatest concern about your transition from school to practice?

It might seem to you right now, after reading all of this information, that reality shock is a life-threatening situation. Be assured, it is not. You may, however, experience a number of physical and psychological symptoms in varying degrees of intensity. For example, you may feel stressed out or have headaches, insomnia, gastrointestinal upset, or a bout of poststudent blues. Just remember that it takes time to adjust to a new routine and that sometimes, even after you've gotten used to it, you still may feel overwhelmed, confused, or anxious. The good news is there are various ways to get through this critical phase of your career while establishing a firm foundation for future professional growth and career mobility. Try the assessment exercise in Critical Thinking Box 1-2.

CRITICAL THINKING BOX 1-2

REALITY SHOCK INVENTORY

All students as well as new graduates, experience reality shock to some extent or another. The purpose of this exercise is to make you aware of how you feel about yourself and your particular life situation.

Directions: To evaluate your views and determine your self-evaluation of your particular life situation, respond to the statements with the appropriate number.

1 Strongly agree	4 Slightly agree
2 Agree	5 Disagree
3 Slightly agree	6 Strongly disagree

1. ❑ I am still finding new challenges and interests in my work.
2. ❑ I think often about what I want from life.
3. ❑ My own personal future seems promising.
4. ❑ Nursing school and/or my work has brought stresses for which I was unprepared.
5. ❑ I would like the opportunity to start anew knowing what I know now.
6. ❑ I drink more than I should.
7. ❑ I often feel that I still belong in the place where I grew up.
8. ❑ Much of the time my mind is not as clear as it used to be.
9. ❑ There's no sense of regret concerning my major life decision of becoming a nurse.
10. ❑ My views on nursing are as positive as they ever were.
11. ❑ I have a strong sense of my own worth.
12. ❑ I am experiencing what would be called a crisis in my personal or work setting.
13. ❑ I can't see myself as a nurse.
14. ❑ I must remain loyal to commitments even if they have not proven as rewarding as I has expected.
15. ❑ I wish I were different in many ways.
16. ❑ The way I present myself to the world is not the way I really am.

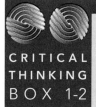

REALITY SHOCK INVENTORY (Cont'd)

17. ❑ I often feel agitated or restless.
18. ❑ I have become more aware of my inadequacies and faults.
19. ❑ My sex life is as satisfactory as it has ever been.
20. ❑ I often think about student and/or friends who have dropped out of school or work.

To compute your score, reverse the number you assigned to statements 1, 3, 9, 10, 11, and 19. For example, 1 would become a 6, 2 would become a 5, 3 would become a 4, 4 would become a 3, 5 would become a 2, and 6 would become at 1. Total the number. The higher the score, the better your attitude. The range is 20–120.

Modified from White, E (1986, April 23): Doctoral dissertation. *Chronicle of Higher Education*. p. 28, with permission.

ROLE TRANSFORMATION

Remember when you first started nursing school? The war stories everybody told you? The changes that occurred in your family as a result of your starting nursing school? Seems like a long time ago, doesn't it? Believe it or not, you have already experienced a role transition—to student nurse. Now, as you draw nearer to the successful completion of that experience, you are ready to embark on a new one. Take a minute to read the thoughts of one of your peers about her transition into nursing (Critical Thinking Box 1-3). (I'm sure you will smile at her satire.)

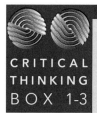

SURVIVAL TECHNIQUES FROM ONE WHO HAS SURVIVED

❑ You finally did it, you have decided nursing is what you want to do for the rest of your life. After all, who would go through all this anguish if you only wanted to do this as a pasttime? If you are taking this like everyone else, you are probably going to do this by trial and error, "war" stories, or by helpful hints from the nursing staff.

❑ You need to prioritize your time. This is a familiar and much used term which you will hear often. It is also easier said than done. If you are single, you have an advantage—maybe. You can decide right now that single is "where it's at" and stay that way for the duration. Of course this means literally living the "single" life. There are no "dinners-for-two," no telephone conversations, no movies at the cinema (rarely any TV)—in other words, no physical contact with the opposite sex. I know you weren't thinking about it anyway, but in case you are studying anatomy and physiology, and hormonal thoughts pervade your consciousness, dismiss them.

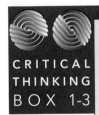

SURVIVAL TECHNIQUES FROM ONE WHO HAS SURVIVED
(Cont'd)

❑ If you are married, I am not suggesting divorce, just abstinence. Hopefully, you kissed your spouse goodbye when you came to school for your first day of class because your next chance will be on your breaks or when you graduate.

❑ If you happen to be a parent, do as I did. I put pictures of myself in all rooms of my house when I started to school so that kids wouldn't forget me. My children, in return, helped me by plastering their faces in my fridge (they know I'll look there) or on my mirror (another sure spot). I have acquired a son-in-law, a daughter-in-law, and five grandchildren in the past two and a half years, and I usually don't recognize them if I run into them on the rare occasions when I go to the store for essentials (like food) or out to pay our utility bills. Christmas is fun though because each year I get to spend a few days getting to know the family again. But we all must wear name tags for the first day!

❑ If your children are small, buy them the Fisher Price Kitchen and teach them how to "cook" nourishing "hot" cereal on the stove that doesn't heat up. For the infant, hang a TPN (hint: Total Parental Nutrition) of Similac with iron at 40 cc/hr that the baby can control by sound! Crying should do it! Instead of a needle, use a nipple....

❑ Diapers—what would we do without those disposable diapers that stay dry for two weeks at a time? You can even buy the kind that you touch the waistband, and Mickey Mouse and his friends jump off to entertain your baby.

❑ Some of you may feel guilty about not fixing those delicious meals your family once enjoyed. Don't! We get two "breaks" a year, and during that time fix barrels of nourishing liquid (you can add a few veggies). When your family gets hungry, just take out enough to keep fluids and lytes balanced. Remind them that this is only going to last another year or two.

❑ Have I covered everything? Oh I forgot dust. . . . Dust used to bother me, but not anymore. I use it to write notes to my 17-year-old, to let him know what time I am going to be in the house, so he won't mistake me for a burglar, and to say *I Love You.*

❑ On a serious note, each semester you will get regrouped with new classmates. They will become your family, your support group. You will form a chain, and everyone is a strong link. This is a group effort. These are people who will laugh with you and cry with you. You will form friendships that will last a lifetime. Take advantage of these opportunities.

❑ On a closing note—do not listen to all the "war stories" that go around— just to the credible ones . . . like mine!

From Beagle, B. (1990). Survival techniques. *AD Clinical Care*, May/June, p. 17, with permission.

Give yourself a well-deserved pat on the back for what you have accomplished thus far. It is important to learn early in your practice of nursing to take time to reflect on your accomplishments. Now, back to the present. Let's look at the current role-transition process at hand, from student to graduate nurse RN (real nurse).

TABLE 1-2

From Novice to Expert

Stage	Characteristics
Novice Nursing student Experienced nurse in a new setting	• No clinical experience in situation expected to perform • Needs rules to guide performance • Experiences difficulty in applying theoretical concepts to patient care
Advanced Beginner Last-semester nursing student Graduate nurse	• Demonstrates ability to deliver marginally acceptable care • Requires prior experience in actual situation to recognize it • Begins to understand the principles that dictate nursing interventions • Continues to concentrate on the rules, and takes in minimum information regarding a situation
Competent 2–3 years clinical experience	• Conscientious, deliberate planning • Begins to see nursing actions in light of clients' long-term plans • Demonstrates ability to cope with and manage different and unexpected situations that occur
Proficient Nurse clinicians Nursing faculty	• Ability to recognize and understand the situation as a whole • Demonstrates ability to anticipate events in a given situation • Holistic understanding enhances decision making
Expert Advanced practice nurse clinicians and faculty	• Demonstrates an understanding of the situation and is able to focus on the specific area of the problem • Operates from an in-depth understanding of the total situation • Demonstrates highly skilled analytical ability in problem solving, performance becomes

Modified from "The Dreyfus Model of Skill Acquisition Applied to Nursing" from *From Novice to Expert* by Patrician Benner. Copyright © 1984 by Addison-Wesley Publishing Company. Reprinted by permission.

WHEN DOES THE ROLE TRANSITION TO GRADUATE NURSE BEGIN?

Does the transition begin at graduation? No. It started when you began to move into the novice role while in your first nursing course (Table 1-2). According to Benner (1984, p. 20),

> Beginners have no experience of the situation in which they are expected to perform. To get them into these situations and allow them to gain experience also necessary for skill development, they are taught about the situation in terms of objective attributes, such as weight, intake/output, temperature, blood pressure, pulse, and other objectifiable, measurable parameters of a patient's conditions—features of the task world that can be recognized without situational experience.

For example, the instructor will give the novice or student nurse specific directions on how to listen for bowel sounds. There will be specific rules on how to guide their actions—rules that are very limited and fairly inflexible. Remember your first clinical nursing experiences? Your nursing instructor was your shadow for patient care. As nursing students enter a clinical area as novices, they have little understanding of the meaning and application of recently learned textbook terms and concepts. Students are not the only novices; any nurse may assume the novice role on entering a clinical setting in which he or she is not comfortable functioning or has no practical experience.

By graduation, most nursing students are at the level of advanced beginner. According to Benner (1984, p. 22),

> Advanced beginners are ones who can demonstrate marginally accepted performance, ones who have coped with enough real situations to note (or to have pointed out to them by a mentor) the recurring meaningful situation components. . . .

To be able to recognize characteristics that can be identified only through experience is the signifying trait of the advanced beginner. Thus, when directed to perform the procedure of checking bowel sounds, the students at this level are learning how to discriminate bowel sounds and understand their meaning. They do not need to be told specifically how to perform the procedure.

Let's look at what you and your nursing instructors can do to promote your well-being and success during the role-transition experience. These activities reinforce your progress and movement along the continuum from advanced beginner to competent nurse.

No more "mama management." It's time to have your nursing instructor cut the umbilical cord and allow you to function more independently during the last semester of clinical training.

More realistic patient-care assignments. Start taking care of increasing numbers of patients to help you with time management and work organization. Evaluate the nursing staff's assignments to determine what is a realistic workload for a recent graduate.

Increased opportunities for follow-up care in the home or community setting. Obtain experience in various community and home-care settings.

Clinical hours that represent realistic shift hours. Obtain experience in receiving shift reports, closing charts, completing patient care, and communicating with the oncoming staff. As a recent graduate, you will be in for a rude awakening if you have never had the opportunity to work a full shift.

Perform nursing procedures instead of observing. Take an inventory of your nursing skills. If there are nursing skills you lack or procedures you are uncomfortable with, take this opportunity while you are still in school to gain the experience. Identify your clinical objectives to meet your personal needs. Request opportunities to practice from your instructor and staff nurses.

More truth about the real work-setting experience. Identify resource people to objectively discuss with you the dilemmas of the workplace. Talk to graduates: Ask them what they know now that they wish they had known the last semester of school.

Look for opportunities to problem-solve and to practice critical thinking. No more "spoon-feeding" from instructors who tell you what to do and how to do it. Now is the time to stand on your own two feet while there is still a backup—your instructor—available.

Request constructive feedback from staff and instructors. Stop avoiding evaluation and constructive criticism. Find out now how you can improve your nursing care. Evaluate your progress on a periodic basis. The consequences may be less severe now than later with your new employer.

HOW CAN I PREPARE MYSELF FOR THIS TRANSITION PROCESS?

Attitude is the latitude between success and failure.

Think positively! Be prepared for the reality of the workplace environment, including both its positives and negatives. You may have encountered by now the "ol' battle-ax" who has a grudge against new nursing graduates.

> I don't know why you ever decided to be a nurse. Nobody respects you. It's all work, low pay. I guess as long as you've got a good back and strong legs, you'll make it.
> Boy, do you have a lot to learn! I wouldn't do it over again for anything!

When you find these nurses, tune them out and steer out of their way! They have their own agenda, and it doesn't include providing supportive assistance to you. Eventually, you will learn how to work with this type of individual (see Chapter 8), but for now, you should concentrate on identifying nurses who share your philosophy and are still smiling.

Surround yourself with nurses who have a positive attitude.

Another way to keep a positive perspective is to focus on the good things that have happened during the shift rather than on the frustrating events. When you feel yourself climbing onto the proverbial "pity pot," ask yourself "Who's driving this bus?" and turn it around! Review the job duties of the nurse from the year 1887 (Fig. 1-2)— and be grateful!

Duties of the Floor Nurse
Circa 1887

In addition to caring for your 60 patients, each nurse will follow these regulations:

1. Daily sweep and mop the floors of your ward, dust the patient's furniture and window sills.

2. Maintain an even temperature in your ward by bringing in a scuttle of coal for the day's business.

3. Light is important to observe the patient's condition, therefore, each day fill kerosene lamps, clean chimneys, and trim wicks. Wash the windows once a week.

4. The nurse's notes are important in aiding the physician's work. Make your pens carefully, you may whittle nibs to your individual taste.

5. Each nurse on day duty will report every day at 7am and will leave at 8pm, except on the Sabbath on which day you will be off from 12 noon to 2pm.

6. Graduate nurses in good standing with the Director of Nurses will be given an evening off each week if you go regularly to church.

7. Each nurse should lay aside from each pay day a good sum of her earnings for her benefits during her declining years, so that she will not become a burden. For example, if you earn $20 a month you should set aside $10.

8. Any nurse who smokes, uses liquor in any form, gets her hair done at a beauty shop, or frequents dance halls will have given the Director of Nurses good reason to suspect her worth, intentions, and integrity.

9. The nurse who performs her labors, serves her patients and doctors faithfully and without fault for a period of 5 years will be given an increase by the hospital administration of 5 cents a day providing there are no hospital debts that are outstanding.

FIGURE 1-2
The duties of a floor nurse, 1887.

Anticipate small irritations and disappointments, and keep them in perspective. Don't let them mushroom into major problems. Turn disappointments and unpleasant situations into learning experiences. Once you have encountered an unpleasant situation, the next time it occurs you will recognize it sooner, anticipate the chain of events, and be better able to handle it.

Don't major in a minor activity.

Be flexible! Procedures, policies, and nursing supervisors are not going to be the same as those experienced in school. Be prepared to do things differently than you learned as a student. You do not have to give up all the values you learned in school, but you will need to reexamine them in light of the reality of the workplace setting.

> **School-learned ideal: Never prepare a medication ahead of time; always prepare it immediately before administration.**

Workplace reality: Staff nurses set up medications for the entire 3 PM to 11 PM shift at 4 PM.

Compromise: Your value system does not allow you to feel comfortable about setting up medications this early in the shift. However, your time organization skills tell you the necessity of planning ahead to complete medications on time. Therefore, in light of the reality of the workplace, you compromise by preparing medications at 3:30 PM for the 4 PM and 6 PM medications and at 7:30 PM for the 8 PM and 10 PM medications. Your primary objective is to administer medications according to the Five Rights. You have appropriately and effectively adapted your value system to meet the challenges of the workplace without losing sight of your values.

School-learned ideal: Sit down with the patient before surgery and provide preoperative teaching.

Workplace reality: One of your home-care patients is receiving daily wound care for an extensive burn. You receive a page message that the patient has been scheduled for grafting in the outpatient surgery department and is to be a direct admit at 6 AM the next morning. You have two more home visits to make—one to hang an intravenous preparation of vancomycin and the other a new hospice admission, which you know will take considerable time.

Compromise: You delegate to one of the home-care practical nurses to take the preoperative teaching and admission instructions to your patient. Later on, you make a telephone call to your preoperative patient and go over the preoperative-care teaching information from the home-care practical nurse. You make arrangements to meet this patient at home immediately after the grafting procedure is complete.

Get organized! Does your personal life seem organized or chaotic, calm, or frantic? Sit back and take a quick inventory of your personal life. How do you expect to get your professional life in order when your personal life is in turmoil? For some helpful tips on organizing your personal life, review the 10 suggestions for getting organized in Figure 1-3. How many do you currently use? Check out the time management chapter (Chapter 9).

Stay healthy! Have you become a "couch potato" while in school? Are you too tired, or do you lack the time to exercise when you get home from work? Candy bars during breaks . . . pepperoni pizza at midnight . . . Twinkies PRN. . . .? How have your eating habits changed during your time in school? Your routine should include exercise, relaxation, and good nutrition. Becoming aware of the negative habits that

1. Start an ongoing list of "Things to Do". It feels so good to cross off the task as you complete it.

2. If you don't already have a file-folder system, then start one immediately. If you can't keep up with magazine and journal articles, or if you don't have time to put your notes together—file them. Get to them when you can.

3. Post a large calendar on the refrigerator door. It is a great way to keep track of a busy family's schedule. Assign each person to write down his or her meetings, practices, etc. in a different colored ink.

4. Keep a shopping list posted on your refrigerator. When you run out of something, write it down right away. This will eliminate extra trips to the grocery store for forgotten items, and it will keep your cabinets fully stocked.

5. Don't spend a lot of time in card shops searching for birthday and anniversary cards. Keep a supply of attractive blank cards on hand for those last minute greetings to be made. Or, buy a bunch of greeting cards and keep them in a letter holder with dividers indicating month and day that cards should be mailed.

6. Set a food timer or alarm clock—and make time for yourself. Tell the children that this is your time to read, watch TV, relax.

7. Neighborhood teenagers are often willing to run errands, mow lawns, wash cars, or clean house. Call on them.

8. Check to see if your cleaner, drug store, or grocer has free delivery—and use it.

9. Do your shopping by mail, TV, or phone. Make use of the numerous catalogs around; get on a mailing list and do your buying from your armchair, or by watching Home Shopping on TV or Internet.

10. Learn to say "NO". Remember, "No" is a complete sentence! It's so easy to get involved in too many activities. Set priorities and do just one to two activities that please you—say "No" to the rest.

FIGURE 1-3
Ten suggestions for organizing yourself.

can have detrimental effects on your state of mind and overall physical health is important in developing a healthy lifestyle.

Find a mentor! Negotiating this critical transition as you begin your nursing career should not be done in isolation. Today the evidence suggests that close support relationships are a key, if not essential, ingredient in the career development of a successful, happy recent graduate (Campbell-Heider, 1986). In addition to your family and close nursing-school friends, it will be important to develop professional support relationships. Keep in touch with nurse recruiters. Recruiters will know where all the recent graduates are in the hospital; maybe they can put you in touch with another recent graduate or with someone who would be a great mentor. Finding a mentor will be an important step in taking care of yourself during your transition process.

A mentor is an established professional (selected by you) who takes a long-term personal interest in your nursing career. The mentor not only serves as a role model or counselor for you but actively advises, guides, and promotes you in your career. A mentor can be any successful, experienced nurse who is committed to a professional career and to being a key figure in your life for a number of years. Mentors should have your best interest at heart and bolster your self-confidence. Mentors should be able to give criticism in a highly constructive, supportive atmosphere. As a result, trust and caring are hallmarks of the bonding that occurs between mentor and graduate. In short, a mentor is "a wise and trusted adviser."

A mentoring relationship is an evolving, personal experience for both mentor and graduate. It involves a personal investment of the mentor in the direction of the graduate's professional development. The mentor also benefits from the association by gaining an awareness and perspective of the recent graduate's role in nursing. Take note of the following characteristics of successful mentors:

- Have experienced role transition and maintained a positive attitude
- Are trustworthy
- Are sincere
- Show mutual respect
- Are not in a position of authority over the graduate
- Promote an easy, give-and-take relationship
- Are experienced
- Have values and goals compatible with those of the graduate
- Are nurturing
- Have a good sense of humor and enjoy nursing!

Many relationships that have value to the graduate may not be classified as mentor-type relationships because of their short duration. The preceptor is most often assigned by the institution to orient the graduate and to be available as a resource in the nursing unit. Preceptor relationships and extended orientation periods are even more important in today's employment settings because of early licensure for recent graduates resulting from the computerization of the NCLEX. Here is one final note about mentorship: There is a short anecdotal story about "Everybody, Somebody, Anybody, and Nobody" that has become part of Internet lore. I think you will understand that *Everybody* has to realize the importance of advancing the field of nursing through mentorship; your task will be to find that *Somebody* willing to extend a hand to guide you through the process.

> There was an important job to be done, and *Everybody* was sure that *Somebody* would do it. *Anybody* could have done it, but *Nobody* did it. *Somebody* got angry about that, because it was *Everybody's* job. *Everybody* thought *Anybody* could do it, but *Nobody* realized that *Everybody* wouldn't do it. It ended up that *Everybody* blamed *Somebody*, when *Nobody* did what *Anybody* could have.

Have some fun! Do something that makes you feel good. This is life, not a funeral service! Nursing has opportunities for laughter and for sharing life's humorous events with patients and co-workers. Surround yourself with people and friends who are lighthearted and merry and who bring those feelings out in you. Remember, the return of humor is one of the first signs of a healthy role transition. Loosen up a little bit. Go ahead, have some fun!

Know what to expect! Plan ahead. How can you expect to do a job correctly if you don't know what the expectations are? Learn the "rules of the road" early. This may be in the hospital, doctor's office, or community setting. While still in school, you may find it helpful to interview nurse managers to determine their perspectives on the role of the graduate nurse during their first 6 months of employment. This will give you a base of reference when you interview for your first job. How do you measure up to some of the common expectations nurse managers may be looking for in a graduate nurse? Are you as follows:

- Excited and sincere about nursing?
- Open-minded and willing to learn new ideas and skills?
- Comfortable with your basic nursing skills?
- Able to keep a good sense of humor?
- Receptive to constructive criticism?
- Able to express your thoughts and feelings?
- Able to evaluate your performance and request assistance?
- Comfortable talking with your patients regarding their individual needs?

WHAT ARE THE "RULES OF THE ROAD" FOR TRANSITION?

To summarize, the role-transition process can be likened to a stoplight. There is the *green light* for *GO*—move ahead, you are going in the right direction. The *yellow light* denotes *CAUTION*—proceed slowly, be sure to look around (CYA—cover your actions—nursing and otherwise; Milazzo, 1990, p. 12). The *red light* means *STOP*—do not proceed, your career direction may need to come to a screeching halt.

The following are helpful tips (i.e., "rules of the road"; Fig. 1-4) contributed by graduates who have successfully made the transition.

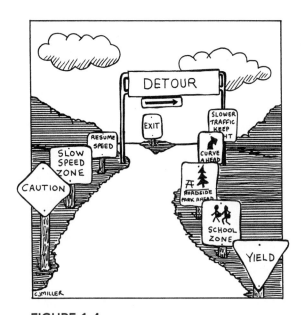

FIGURE 1-4
"Rules of the road" for transition

Stop. Take care of yourself. Take time to plan your transition. Get involved with other recent graduates; they can help you. Don't be afraid to ask questions.

Detour. You will make mistakes: Recognize them, learn from them, and put them in the past as you move forward. Regardless of how well you plan for change, there are always detours ahead. Detours take you on an alternate route. They can be scenic, swampy, or desolate, or they can bog you down in heavy traffic. Don't forget to look for the positive aspects—the detour may open your eyes to new horizons and new career directions.

Curve ahead. Get your personal life in order. Anticipate changes in your schedule. Be adaptable, because the transition process is not predictable.

Yield. You don't always have to be right. Consider alternatives and make compromises within your value system.

Resume speed. Maintain a positive attitude. As you gain experience, you will become better organized and begin to really enjoy nursing. Be aware; sometimes as you resume speed, you may be experiencing another role transition as your career moves in a different direction.

Exit. Pay attention to your road signs; don't take an exit you don't really want. Before you exit your job, critically evaluate the job situation. "Look before you leap": Make sure the change will improve your work situation.

Slower traffic, keep right. You may be more comfortable in the slower-traffic lane with respect to your career direction. Take all the time you need—it's okay for each person to travel at a different speed. Don't get run over in the fast lane.

School zone. Plan for continuing education, whether it be an advanced degree program or one to maintain your clinical skills or license. Allow yourself sufficient time in your new job before you jump back into the role of full-time student.

Slow-speed zone. Take time to get organized before you resume full speed! Have a daily organizational sheet that fits your needs and works for you both in your job and your personal life.

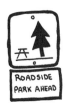

Caution. Don't commit to anything with which you are not professionally or personally comfortable. Think before you act. Don't react. Don't panic. If in doubt, check with another nurse.

Roadside park ahead. Take a break—whether it's 15 minutes or 30 minutes a day to indulge yourself or a week to do something you really want to do.

 Look for the humor in each day, and take time to laugh. You will be surprised by how good it makes you feel!

REFERENCES

Ahmadi KS, Speedling EJ, Kuhn-Weissman G: The newly hired hospital staff nurse's professionalism, satisfaction and alienation, *Int J Nurs Stud* 24(2):107-121, 1987.

Benner P: *From novice to expert*, Menlo Park, Calif, 1984, Addison-Wesley.

Campbell-Heider N: Do nurses need mentors? *Image* 18(3):110-113, 1984.

Godinez G et al: Role transition from graduate to staff nurse: a qualitative analysis, *J Nurse Staff Dev* 15(3):97-110, 1999.

Horsburgh M: Graduate nurses' adjustment to initial employment: natural field work, *J Adv Nurs* 14(8):610-617, 1989.

Kramer M: *Reality shock*, St Louis, 1974, C. V. Mosby.

Kramer M, Schmalenberg C: *Path to biculturalism*, Rockville, Md, 1977, Aspen.

Lund PZ: *Role concepts and role discrepancies of senior baccalaureate nursing students following selected summer work experiences*, New York, 1988, Columbia University Teachers College.

Milazzo V: *How to easily avoid lawyers' traps*, Houston, 1990, Medical-Legal Consulting Institute.

Myrick F: Preceptorship: a viable alternative clinical teaching strategy, *J Adv Nurs* 13(5):588-591, 1988.

Polifroni C et al: Activities and interaction of baccalaureate nursing students in clinical practice, *J Prof Nurs* 11(3):161-169, 1995.

Schempp CM, Rompre RM: Transition programs for new graduates: how effective are they? *J Nurs Staff Dev* 2(4):150-156, 1986.

Schumacher KL, Meleis AI: Transitions: a central concept in nursing, *Image* 26(2):119-127, 1994.

Wolfgang AP: Job stress in the health professions: a study of physicians, nurses, and pharmacists, *J Human Stress* 14(1):43-47, 1988.

ADDITIONAL READINGS

Anderson SL: Preceptor teaching strategies: behaviors that facilitate role transition in senior nursing students, *J Nurs Staff Dev* 7(4):171-175, 1991.

Blanchard SL: The discontinuity between school and practice, *Nurs Manage* 14(4):41-43, 1983.

Bygrave D: The shock of transition, *Nurs Times* 81(2):32-33, 1985.

Carroll TL: Role deprivation in baccalaureate nursing students pre and post curriculum revision, *J Nurs Educ* 28(3):134-139, 1989.

Charron DC: Save the new graduate, *Nurs Manage* 13(11):45-46, 1982.

Gambacorta S: Head nurses face reality shock, too! *Nurs Manage* 14(7):46-48, 1983.

Glennon TK: An additive model to promote biculturism . . . resolves the conflicts between the worlds of academy and clinic, *Nurs Manage* 14(8):28-31, 1983.

Goldfarb S: Reality shock for new OR nurses, *Todays OR Nurse* 8(6):21-23, 1986.

Johnson S: Bridging the gap: a new graduate nurse program that works, *J Nurs Staff Dev* 2(4):166-168, 1986.

Locasto LW, Kockanek D: Reality shock in the nurse educator, *J Nurs Educ* 28(2):79-81, 1989.

Maben J, Clark J: Making the transition from student to staff nurse, *Nurs Times* 92(44):28-31, 1996.

Medendorp SJ: A new grad wonders: can I handle nursing? *J Christ Nurs* 7(3):32-34, 1990.

Naughton TJ: Effect of experience on adjustment to a new job situation, part 2, *Psychol Rep* 60(3):1267-1272, 1987.

Nordgren J, Richardson SJ, Laurella VB: A collaborative preceptor model for clinical teaching of beginning nursing students, *Nurse Educ* 23(3): 27-32, 1998.

Sayeed NA: You may feel wonderfully free . . . problems facing newly qualified staff nurses. *Nurs Times* 79(4):56-58, 1983.

Swayne M: Why we work side by side with student nurses, *RN* 8(6):44-45, 1986.

Tradewell G: Rites of passage: adaptation of nursing graduates to a hospital setting, *J Nurs Staff Dev* 12(4):183-189, 1996.

Vance C: Is there a mentor in your career future? *Imprint* 36(5):41-42, 1989.

INTERNET RESOURCES

Information and Tutorials About Web Browsers and the Internet

http://www.learnthenet.com/english/html/00start.html

General Search Engines

Search engines can be used to search the Internet for references found in subsequent chapters.

AllTheWeb.com (FAST Search)

http://www.alltheweb.com

AllTheWeb.com (also known as FAST Search) is one of the largest indexes of the Web. It offers large multimedia and mobile/wireless Web indexes.

AltaVista

http://www.altavista.com

AltaVista is one of the oldest crawler-based search engines on the Web. It has a large index of Web pages and a large range of power searching commands. In addition, it also offers news search, shopping search, and multimedia search.

AOL Search

http://search.aol.com/

AOL Search allows its members to search across the Web and AOL's own content from one place. The "external" version, listed above, does not list AOL content.

Ask Jeeves

http://www.askjeeves.com

Ask Jeeves is a human-powered search service that attempts to direct you to the exact page that answers your question.

Direct Hit

http://www.directhit.com

Direct Hit measures what people click on in the search results presented at its own site and at its partner sites, such as HotBot. Sites that get clicked on more than others rise higher in Direct Hit's rankings—hence, the nickname of "popularity engine." Aside from running its own Web site, Direct Hit provides the main results that appear at HotBot and is available as an option to searchers at MSN Search. Direct Hit is owned by AskJeeves.com.

Google

http://www.google.com

Google is a top choice of Web-searchers. It offers the largest collection of Web pages of any crawler-based search engine. Google makes heavy use of link analysis as a primary way to rank these pages. This can be especially helpful in finding good sites in response to general search terms such as "cars" and "travel" because users across the Web have, in essence, voted for good sites by linking to them. The system works so well that Google has gained widespread praise for its high relevancy. Google provides Web page search results to a variety of partners, including Yahoo! and Netscape Search. Google also provides the ability to search for images through Usenet discussions and its own version of the Open Directory.

LookSmart

http://www.looksmart.com

LookSmart is a human-compiled directory of Web sites. In addition to being a standalone service, LookSmart provides directory results to MSN Search, Excite, and many other partners.

Lycos

http://www.lycos.com

Lycos started out as a search engine, depending on listings that came from spidering the Web. Its primary listings come from AllTheWeb.com. Lycos acquired the competing HotBot search service, which continues to be run separately.

MSN Search

http://search.msn.com

Microsoft's MSN Search service is a LookSmart-powered directory of Web sites, with secondary results that come from Inktomi. Direct Hit data are also made available.

Yahoo!

http://www.yahoo.com

Yahoo! is the Web's most popular search service and has a well-deserved reputation for helping people find information easily. (Do you Yahoo!?) It is the largest human-compiled guide to the Web, employing approximately 150 editors in an effort to categorize the Web. Yahoo! has well over 1 million sites listed. Yahoo! is the oldest major Web site directory—launched in 1994 (not too old, eh?).

Specialized Search Engines (Medical)

MedHunt

http://www.hon.ch/MedHunt

MedHunt uses both humans and a Web-crawler to build its index of medical information. Searches can be narrowed by region, and a French interface is available.

9-11.com

http://www.9-11.com

Directory and crawler-based medical search engine aimed at general consumers, as well as medical practitioners and researchers.

New Wind Publishing

http://newwindpub.com

Through the Medical Internet textbook link at this site, one can find numerous medical/nursing journals and sites.

UNIT II

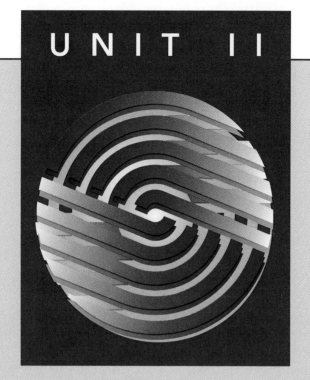

NURSING: A DEVELOPING PROFESSION

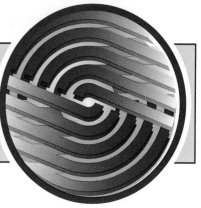

CHAPTER TWO

Historical Perspectives: Influences of the Past

LINDA T. ANGLIN, DA, RNC

History repeats itself because each generation refuses to read the minutes of the last meeting.

— *Anonymous*

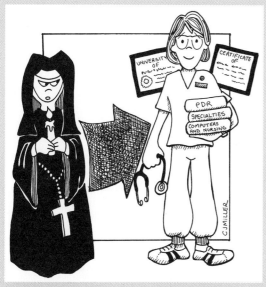

Nursing has come a long way—it is not what it used to be.

After completing this chapter, you should be able to:

▨ Explain the early European contributions to nursing.

▨ Explain the forces that affected the roles of American nurses.

▨ Discuss what nurses do.

29

So you have to study the history of nursing. Generally, the topic is considered boring. Well, be prepared for a different approach to the topic. Knowing the history of our profession guides our understanding of why we do what we do today. This understanding can be useful to us as we set our professional goals. Threads of nursing history can be found throughout the book. Chapters 3 and 4 on the Image of Nursing and Nursing Education contain brief historical reviews of these areas. Understanding the history can often help in deciding what changes are needed, what changes are helpful, and what changes may be unnecessary. Let's begin with a look at where nursing began.

NURSING HISTORY: PEOPLE AND PLACES

WHERE DID IT ALL BEGIN?

Most nursing historians agree that nursing, or the care of the ill and injured, has been done since the beginning of human life and has generally been a woman's role. A mother caring for a child in a cave and someone caring for another ill adult by boiling willow bark to relieve fever both are examples of nursing. The word *nurse* actually is derived from the Latin word *nutricius*, meaning *nourishing*. Roman mythological figures included the goddess Fortuna, who was usually recognized as being responsible for one's fate and who also served as Jupiter's nurse (Dolan, 1969).

Even before Greek and Roman times, ancient Egyptian physicians and nurses assembled voluminous pharmacopoeia with more than 700 remedies for numerous health problems. Great emphasis was placed on the use of animal parts in concoctions that were generally drunk or applied to the body. The physician prescribed and provided the treatments and usually had an assistant who provided the nursing care (Kalisch and Kalisch, 1986). Some ancient medicine was based on driving out the evil spirit rather than curing or treating the malady. The treatments were often very foul and many times included fecal material. By now you may be thinking of the saying, "The treatment was successful, but the patient died."

Advancement of medical knowledge halted abruptly when the Roman Empire was conquered. Any medical and health care knowledge that survived these dark times did so only through the efforts of Jewish physicians who were able to translate the Greek and Roman works (Kalisch and Kalisch, 1986). One bright spot was in Salerno when a school of medicine and health was established for physicians and women to assist in childbirth. In fact, a midwife named Trotula wrote what may be considered the first nursing textbook on the cure of diseases of women (Dalton, 1900). Generally, nursing was performed by designated priestesses and was associated with some type of temple worship. Little information has survived about this early period. Historians have assumed that Hippocrates was assisted by women, but there is little information to support that. From these roots, nursing began to develop as a recognized and valued service to society (Jamieson and Sewall, 1949).

WHY DEACONS, WIDOWS, AND VIRGINS?

Paralleling the fall of the Roman Empire was the rise of Christianity. The early organization of the young Christian church, which was directly affected by the vision of Paul, included a governing bishop and seven appointed deacons. These individuals assisted the apostles in the work of the Church (the word *deacon* means *servant*). The deacon was directly responsible for distributing all the goods and property that apostles relinquished to the Church before they "took up the cross and followed." The apostles were required to give up all material resources to achieve full status in the Church.

Women sympathetic to the Christian cause of aiding the poor were encouraged in this work by the bishops and deacons. Eventually, the deacons relinquished aiding the poor to women and established the position of deaconess for that purpose. To maintain a pure heart, these women were required by the Church to be either virgins or widows. The stipulation for widows, however, was that they had been married only once (Jamieson and Sewall, 1949). The deaconesses carried nursing forward as they ministered to the sick and injured in their homes. Phoebe, a friend of Paul's and the very first deaconess in the young Christian church, has been called the first visiting nurse (Dana, 1936).

Treatments continued to be a mixture of scientific fact, home remedies, and magic. Eventually, an order of widows evolved that was composed of women who were free from home responsibilities and thus were able to give a total commitment to work among the poor. The widows, although not ordained, continued to do the same work as the deaconesses. This was soon followed by the creation of the Order of Virgins as the Church began placing greater value on purity of body. Even though deaconess orders were abolished in the Mediterranean countries, they thrived in other European countries. The traditional commitment to care for the poor and sick became invaluable in a society that generally had neither the time nor the inclination to aid them. Eventually, these women became known as *nuns* (*non nuptae*, not married).

During this time, tremendous upheavals were constantly occurring in the world. Wars, invasions, and battles were constant, and as a result of these encounters the number of widows was significant. Society during this time did not have the sophistication or the means to deal with the dependents of the soldiers killed in battle. As a means of survival, women joined the nuns as a form of protection from starvation and poverty. This was a dark and dreary time in which superstition, witchcraft, and folklore were predominant influences. Because of the need for physical protection, convents were built to shelter these women (Jamieson and Sewall, 1949). The convents became havens to which women could withdraw from ignorance and evil and be nurtured in traditional Christian beliefs (Donahue, 1985). The deaconesses, widows, and virgins continued to minister to and nurse the ill within the safety of the convent.

HOW DID KNIGHTHOOD CONTRIBUTE TO NURSING?

The Holy Wars furthered the development of nursing in a rather interesting way. Because many Christian crusaders became ill while in Jerusalem, a hospital known as the Hospital of St. John was built to accommodate them. Those who fought in these Holy Wars were known as *knights*—men who had taken oaths of chivalry, justice, and piety. They often had men trained in the healing arts accompany them into battle to care for them should they be stricken. These male nurses usually wore a red cross emblazoned on their tunics so that in the heat of battle they could be easily identified and avoid injury or death (Bullough and Bullough, 1978).

The Hospital of St. John gave excellent nursing care. Many of the nurses who survived stayed to work with the hospital organizers. As the battles in the Holy Land continued, the nurses and knights organized a fighting force with a code of rules and a uniform consisting of a black robe with a white Maltese cross, the symbol of poverty, humility, and chastity. They ventured out to rescue the sick and wounded and transported them to the hospital for care, and thus they became known as the *Hospitalers* (Kalisch and Kalisch, 1986). Male nurses dominated these orders. Other orders that emulated the Hospitalers developed in Europe, and more hospitals were opened that used the Hospital of St. John as a model (Donahue, 1985).

The altruistic spirit of nursing was also seen in the craftsmen's guilds. Although their primary purpose was to provide training and jobs through the practice of apprenticeship, the guilds provided care and aid for their members when they became old and could no longer work at their trade. The guilds also assisted members and their families in times of illness and injury. The apprenticeship system—in which experience is gained on the job but no formal education is given—once served as a model for the training of nurses (Donahue, 1985). It is no longer used, however, and is now considered to have been detrimental to the evolution of nursing.

What nursing gained during this period of history was status. The altruistic ideal of providing care as a service performed out of humility and love became the foundation for nursing. The recognition of the value of hospitals grew; all across Europe, cities were building their own hospitals. A general resurgence in the demand for trained doctors and nurses contributed to the building of medical schools and the development of university programs in the art and science of healing.

WHAT ABOUT REVOLTS AND NURSING?

Revolts—not the kind that incurred battles, but revolts of a social nature—were common. There were battles, too; however, the social revolts had a more direct impact on nursing. The revolution of the spirit, more commonly known as the Renaissance, ushered in new concepts of the world—the discovery of the laws of nature by Newton, the exploration of unknown lands, and the growth of secular interests (humanism) over spiritual ones. In this era emerged several outstanding humanists who were to become saints (Donahue, 1985). Interestingly, in depictions of these saints, they are shown as needing nursing care or as giving care to a wounded or injured person.

In Europe, the Protestant Reformation began primarily as a religious reform movement but ended with revolt within the Church. Many hospitals in Protestant countries were forced to close, and those loyal to the Church that operated them were driven out of the country, which resulted in a significant shortage of nurses (mostly nuns) to care for the ill and injured. The poor and ill were considered a burden to society, and those hospitals that remained operational in the Protestant countries became known as "pest houses." To fill the need for nurses, women, many of whom were alcoholics and former prostitutes, were recruited. Generally, a nurse was a woman serving time in a hospital rather than a prison (Donahue, 1985; Jamieson and Sewall, 1949).

The industrial and intellectual revolutions that followed the Reformation all had a significant impact on nursing. During the Industrial Revolution, as production of much-needed goods was streamlined through industrial innovation, craftsmen left the rural life to work in factories. The intellectual contributions of scientists—many of whom were physicians—combined with the inventions of the microscope, thermometer, and pendulum clock, advanced our knowledge and understanding of the world. The invention of the printing press allowed for easier sharing of information, which further contributed to experimentation. Finally, a disease that was feared worldwide was conquered when Edward Jenner (1749-1823) proved the effectiveness of the smallpox vaccination.

Throughout these revolutions, however, the maternal and infant death rates continued to be high. In fact, before his pioneering work in antisepsis in obstetrics, Ignaz Phillipp Semmelweis (1818-1865) observed that patients giving birth in hospitals under the care of educated physicians had significantly higher death rates than women giving birth at home or at clinics with the assistance of midwives.

Despite all of the knowledge gained during this time of revolution, society was generally callous to the plight of children. Children were abandoned without apparent remorse, and infanticide was practiced by poor families desperate to reduce the number of mouths to feed. They had no reliable form of birth control except abstinence. Because it was common practice for the woman hired as a wet nurse to sleep with the infant, many infants were inadvertently suffocated. Donahue (1985) reported that, during this period, 75% of all children baptized were dead before they reached the age of 5 years. Because of the persistence of these sad conditions, children and foundlings' hospitals were established. Eventually, laws were enacted to aid these unfortunate victims (Donahue, 1985).

Existing health care conditions for the ill and injured continued to contribute to high mortality rates. Some sources reported hospital mortality rates as high as 90%. Conditions in the armies were no better. In any military action, mortality rates were high. Reports from the battlefront during the Crimean War suggested that battles were postponed because there were too few able-bodied soldiers to fight. Dysentery and typhoid were the military's nemeses. If a soldier was wounded, infection invariably resulted. Hospitals generally offered no guarantee of survival. In any event, these occurrences had a serious effect on military strategies. If men are ill or injured, battles cannot be won.

Upon this scene entered Florence Nightingale.

FLORENCE NIGHTINGALE: THE LEGEND AND THE LADY

First let's discuss the legend. Published works about Florence Nightingale before the 1960s generally presented the legend. Most authors agreed that she was beautiful, intelligent, wealthy, socially successful, and educated. She certainly had an ability to influence people and used every Victorian secret to accomplish her desires. Although Nightingale believed it improper for her to accept payment for her services, she did demand financial support for materials, goods, and staff to accomplish her programs and goals. Some historians believe that it was through Nightingale's influence that Jean Henri Dunant, a Swiss gentleman, provided the aid to the wounded that lay the foundation for the organization of the International Red Cross (Bullough, Bullough, and Stanton, 1990; Dodge, 1989).

Regardless of what actually happened between Dunant and her, Nightingale's interest and ambition lay in becoming a nurse. Her family was in an uproar over this decision. After all, hospitals were terrible places to go, and nurses were, in most cases, the dregs of society. Hospitals were certainly not places for women of proper social upbringing. Although she was forbidden to, Nightingale studied nursing (in secret). After a fortuitous meeting, a relationship developed between Nightingale and Sidney and Elizabeth Herbert, an influential couple who were interested in hospital reform. Impressed with Nightingale's analytical mind and her ability to apply nursing knowledge to the critical situation in the hospitals (Bullough and Bullough, 1978; Bullough, Bullough, and Stanton, 1990), they encouraged her to study nursing at Kaiserswerth School, run by Lutheran deaconesses (Dolan, 1969). Her family, of course, was very unhappy. In fact, Dodge (1989) reported that the event precipitated a family crisis because they threatened to withdraw financial support.

Nightingale accepted a position as administrator of a nursing home for women, the Institution for the Care of Sick Gentlewomen in Distressed Circumstances. She hired her own chaperon and went to work at reforming the way things were done. Nightingale's interest in hospital reform was insatiable. She visited hospitals and took copious notes on nursing care, treatments, and procedures. She sent reports on hospital conditions to Sidney Herbert, the British secretary of war, while he visited New York. Secretary Herbert then assigned her other hospitals to review. The reviews always included recommendations for improving nursing care. From this early background of experiences, Nightingale was now ready for her greatest mission, the Crimean War. The legend was on the way (Bullough, Bullough, and Stanton, 1990).

In 1854, soldiers were dying, more from common diseases than from bullets. Bullough, Bullough, and Stanton (1990) reported that the Crimean War was a series of mistakes. No plan was made for supplying the troops, no plan was in place to maintain the environment in camps, and no provisions were available to care for the injured after the battle. When Herbert appointed Nightingale as head of a group of nurses to go to Crimea, she had already developed a plan of action. In fact, some historians believe that she was already planning to go in an unofficial capacity. The announcement caused a sensation, and when Nightingale began a rigorous selection process for accepting nurses, many volunteered but few were chosen. She cleaned up the kitchens, the wards, the patients, and the mess. From there the legend grew.

She was clever; after demonstrating the effectiveness of her methods, she withdrew her services. Naturally, all that she had accomplished was done under the scrutiny, skepticism, suspicion, and anger of the physicians. Without the services of the nurses, the abominable conditions quickly returned, and finally the physicians begged her to do whatever she wished—just help! Nightingale responded to the pleading. The actual number of soldiers who benefited from the care of her nurses was immeasurable.

The nurses made rounds day and night, and the legend of the lady with the lamp was born.

Nightingale's great success prompted her to begin developing schools of nursing based on her knowledge of what was effective nursing. Eventually, many schools in Europe and America used the Nightingale model for nursing education. The program was generally 1 year in length, and classes were small. Many women wanted to become nurses; however, only 15 to 20 applicants were accepted for each class. The goals of her programs included training hospital nurses, training nurses to train others, and training nurses to work in the district with the sick poor (Dolan, 1969). In any event, Nightingale had changed society's view of the nurse to one of dignity and value and worthy of respect.

In any legend, the truth is often mixed with myth. The stories surrounding Florence Nightingale are many. What is interesting is that, before the 1970s, authors tended to deify Nightingale or establish her as a saintly person. These myths make for interesting reading. Early nurse historians also contributed to these myths by their interpretations of Nightingale's work. But myths have a purpose. They can be used to explain world views of groups of people or professions at a given time, and they provide explanations for practice beliefs or natural phenomena. Myths tend to maintain a degree of accuracy when the truth is lost. The trick is to separate myth from fact and story from legend and to draw conclusions regarding the occurrences. This is no easy task when one studies Florence Nightingale. Therefore, it is important to read a variety of studies across several time periods before drawing conclusions about the legend and the lady, Florence Nightingale.

In summary, Florence Nightingale had certain characteristics that assisted her in becoming successful during the strict Victorian times in which she lived. She was extremely well educated for her time. She had traveled throughout the world and had the advantage of personal wealth and a gift for establishing relationships with persons of influence and philanthropic spirit. Most portraits depict her as an attractive woman with pleasant features. Contemporary historians agree she had tremendous compassion for all who suffered. She was very strong-willed, a characteristic that carried her through the period of the Crimean War. She had the ability to analyze data and draw relevant conclusions, on which she based her recommendations. Her students of nursing received better preparation than most physicians. She was 36 at the end of the war, and when she returned home, she became a virtual recluse until she died at age 90. She did have some physical ailments: Crimean fever, sciatica, rheumatism, and dilation of the heart, each of which could have crippling side effects and contributed to her becoming bedfast (Bullough, Bullough, and Stanton, 1990). In any event, the legend and the lady had a significant effect on American nursing as we know it today (Dodge, 1989; Dolan, 1969; Bullough and Bullough, 1978; Bullough, Bullough, and Stanton, 1990).

AMERICAN NURSING: CRITICAL FACTORS

WHAT WAS IT LIKE IN COLONIAL TIMES?

In colonial times, nursing responsibilities were shared by all able-bodied persons; however, if there was a choice, women were preferred to do the nursing. Early colonial historians described care for the ill and house chores as the responsibilities of nurses. Although most women of this era were considered dainty (Bradford, 1898), nurses were usually depicted as willing to do hard work. Some colonies had organized nursing services that sought out the sick and provided comfort to those who were ill with smallpox and other diseases (Bullough and Bullough, 1978). There were few trained nurses, however, and most of the individuals who delivered nursing care in the five largest hospitals were men (Dolan, 1969). Eventually, women were hired at the command of George Washington to serve meals and care for the wounded and ill. The era ended with the enactment of the first legislation to improve health and medical treatment and to provide for formal education for society as a whole (Dolan, 1969).

WHAT HAPPENED TO NURSING DURING THE U.S. CIVIL WAR?

The period of the U.S. Civil War witnessed an improvement in patient care through control of the environment in which the patient recovered. The greatest problems for the Army stemmed from the poor sanitary conditions in the camps, which bred diseases such as smallpox and dysentery. The results were many deaths from inadequate nutrition, impure water, and a general lack of cleanliness.

Nurses who had some formal training were recognized as being major contributors to the relative success of hospital treatments. It was in this era that the value of primary prevention, or the prevention of the occurrence of disease by measures such as immunization and the provision of a pure water supply, became understood. Volunteer nurses, mostly women, served in hospitals caring for those wounded soldiers fortunate enough to have survived the trip from the battlefield. Their patients were nursed in a clean environment and were provided with adequate nutrition. The likelihood of their recovering was significantly improved. Astute physicians observed that patients cared for by nurses generally recovered well enough to return to the battlefield. Families, too, saw that when nurses had control over the environment, their ill or injured loved one was more likely to recover—and return home.

As the United States moved into the industrial age of the early 1900s, Victorian values began to permeate the middle and upper-middle classes. Social concerns focused on protecting families from the diseases of the crowded urban areas, and the demand for improved health care increased.

HOW DID THE ROLES OF NURSES AND WIVES COMPARE DURING THE VICTORIAN ERA?

The Victorian era had a significant effect on nurses primarily because they were women. The parallelism between the idealized Victorian woman and the traditional nurse is stunning. The effect of many of the values and beliefs of this era, some historians report, is still felt by women today.

The typical upper-class Victorian household consisted of a husband, who earned a living outside of the home and maintained total control of the family finances, and his wife, who maintained harmony within the home and raised their children. Women's work was generally restricted to philanthropic and voluntary work; they attended teas and other social functions to raise money for organizations and people in need.

Most women were considered fragile and dainty. They were often ill. It has been suggested that their illnesses and frailty were used as a form of birth control to prevent the numerous pregnancies that most women experienced. Some historians concluded that it was through their weaknesses that women gained control and attention. If the wife was ill or frail, maids or servants were hired, but if the wife was healthy, the husband would expect more from her. The Victorian wife was expected to "be good." She was esteemed by her husband but had limited power within the confines of the home and society. She was expected to be hard-working and able to maintain harmony while at the same time being submissive to the demands of her husband. Generally, this fostered dependence on the dominant male figure—the Victorian husband (Rybczynski, 1986).

Let's examine nursing during this same time, especially within the hospital organization. Nurses generally were women who wanted to avoid the drudgery of a Victorian marriage. They were required to be single to make a complete commitment to their vocation. Schooled in submission, women were expected to be equally accommodating within the hospital organization. A good nurse worked for harmony within the hospital. She was expected to be hard-working and submissive. The doctor and the hospital administrator were frequently the same person, usually a man, who expected position and power to go hand in hand. Patients were admitted only if they had income and could afford to pay for the services. It was the physician who generated income, and good nurses were expected to help them continue to maintain power. Because the system rewarded people for being ill, there was little incentive to be healthy. Social values contributed to dependence on the health care system. From this milieu came the reformers (Bullough and Bullough, 1978; Davis, 1961; Kalisch and Kalisch, 1986; Stewart, 1950).

WHO WERE THE REFORMERS OF THE VICTORIAN ERA?

The Victorian era, although a time of repression for women, was also a time of reform. A list of important names in nursing reform would include M. Adelaide Nutting, Minnie Goodnow, Lavinia L. Dock, Annie W. Goodrich, Isabel Hampton Robb, Lilian D. Wald, Isabel M. Stewart, and Sophia Palmer, among others (Jamieson and Sewall, 1949; Kalisch and Kalisch, 1986). These women, who had in common a comfortable upper-middle–class background, intelligence, and education, also had in common a desire to reach beyond the constraints that society imposed on them. As society began to realize the important role that nurses played in treating the ill and injured, it also began to understand the need for training programs that would educate better nurses. Reformers focused on establishing standards for nursing education and practice. Among their accomplishments were the organization of the

American Nurses Association and the creation of its journal, the *American Journal of Nursing*, and the enactment of legislation to require the licensure of prepared nurses. This protected the public from inadequate care given by people who were not trained to nurse (Christy, 1971; Dock, 1900).

THE NURSE'S ROLE: THE STRUGGLE FOR DEFINITIONS

WHAT DO NURSES DO?

As a student, you study nursing texts that explain theories, skills, principles, and the care of patients. Every text has at least one introductory chapter that describes nursing and its significance. By examining many of these introductory chapters of nursing texts, you can generate a rather extensive list of roles (Anglin, 1991). From this list of roles, six major categories can be determined (Table 2-1). The most traditional role for nurses is that of **caregiver.** The nurse as **teacher** is often referred to when discussing patient care or nursing education. The role of **advocate** has been very controversial since 1900. Nurses were also expected to be **managers** ever since the first formal education or training program was instituted. Another interesting role for the nurse is that of **colleague.** The final role is that of **expert.**

WHAT IS THE TRADITIONAL ROLE OF A NURSE?

The role of the nurse as caregiver has engendered the least amount of controversy. This role has been thoroughly documented, not only in writing but through art, since

TABLE 2-1

What Nurses Do

Caregiver	Teacher	Advocate	Manager	Colleague	Expert
Care provider	Patient educator	Interpreter	Administrator	Collaborator	Academician
Comforter	Counselor	Learner	Coordinator	Communicator	Historian
Handmaiden	Patient teacher	Protector	Decision maker	Facilitator	Nursing
Healer		Risk-taker	Evaluator	Peer reviewer	instructor
Helper		Change	Initiator	Professional	Professional
Nurturer		agent	Leader	Specialist	educator
Practitioner			Planner		Researcher
Rehabilitator					Research
Support agent					consumer
					Teacher
					Theorist
					Practitioner
					Leader

early times. Nurses and nursing leaders agree that this is their primary role. As students, your caregiving skills will be measured constantly through skill laboratories, clinical evaluation proficiency, and eventually through licensure testing and staff evaluations. All of these mechanisms attempt to evaluate your ability to be a caregiver. When we think of the role of caregiver, we think of someone who is moved to take action so that suffering can be relieved. What is difficult to measure is the level of feeling related to caring. There is a great debate in nursing as to whether nurses can be taught to care. However, despite this controversy, the majority of nurses agree that they are caregivers. Because our current education is based on Nightingale's principles of caring, it is no surprise that all of you believe that you will provide care to those in need. You may choose to provide this care in various settings, but basically all of you desire to be caregivers and are expected to be so.

Caregiving is probably the only role on which there is agreement as to what it means and how we do it.

Imagine a nurse giving care. Generally, the picture that most often comes to mind is someone, usually female, in a white uniform caring for a patient who is ill. This picture is the romanticized version of caregiving continually portrayed in movies, television, and novels. We know that caregiving takes place in many settings: clinics, homes, hospitals, offices, businesses, and schools, among others. We can probably agree that caregiving is an important role for nurses and is probably why most of us chose nursing. Studies examining the role of caregiver continue, and our understanding of the role is expanding (Leininger, 1984; Watson, 1985; Benner, 1984). Without a doubt, this is an important role, one that is essential to nursing.

DID YOU KNOW YOU WOULD BE A TEACHER?

When you take care of patients, it soon becomes apparent that certain information must be shared with them so that they can participate in their care. Teaching patients about their therapy, condition, or choices is critical to the successful outcome of some prescribed treatments. For example, nurses have learned through research that knowledge can reduce anxiety before and after surgery. We teach patients about almost everything related to care. Knowledge can enhance compliance with medications and can encourage healthy lifestyles and behaviors. Teaching becomes especially important when patients have to make treatment choices and decisions about their care. With the volumes of information available regarding health care, it is even more important that nurses help patients understand what they need to know to make wise decisions. Without exception, standardized care plans have included as a nursing action *patient education*. Discharge plans also provide for patient education. Home care includes teaching as a reimbursable activity. Agency charting procedures all require documentation of patient education. All nursing textbooks include sections on what the nurse needs to emphasize regarding patient education. With all this evidence, there is little doubt that the teacher role is an important one for the nurse.

The role of the nurse as teacher of other nurses is rooted in the evolution of nursing education; however, as schools of nursing developed, nurses were taught by physicians. Gradually, nurses began supervising students of nursing and taught them on the job. Eventually, the influence of Nightingale resulted in qualified nurses teaching students about nursing. This model has prevailed for some time in nursing schools that have a great degree of credibility.

In America, the greatest impetus to nurses as teachers occurred in 1948 when recommendations from the Brown report included the separation of the nursing schools from hospital administrative budgets. This was a major step in nurses' gaining control over the budget and the educational processes of students (Brown, 1948). Numerous nursing curricula since 1900 have included sections on what the nurse needs to teach the patient about the illness. This continues to be a very important role for the nurse at a time when treatment choices and lifestyle choices are numerous.

Teaching is planned to strengthen a patient's knowledge of making decisions about treatment options and is an essential nursing intervention (Alfaro-LeFevre, 1998). In many ways the nurse as teacher is also an interpreter of information, and this leads us to the next role for discussion.

WHO WILL ADVOCATE?

A useful definition of the term *advocate* is "one who pleads a cause before another." The first advocacy issue, arising early in the 1900s, concerned nursing practice. Public health and visiting nurses were the majority (approximately 70%) and hospital nurses

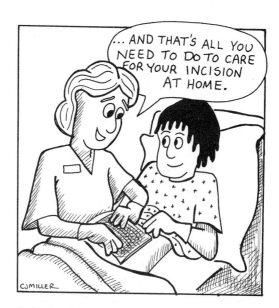

FIGURE 2-2
Did you know you would be a teacher?

were the minority (approximately 30%) of working nurses. Working as a private duty nurse or visiting nurse was a source of income for women who had no other means of support. Because there was no way to determine the credentials of the visiting nurse, many impostors worked in that capacity. Lavinia L. Dock, Sophia Palmer, and Annie W. Goodrich, three nursing leaders, deplored this situation and endeavored to protect the public from unscrupulous "nurses" (Dolan, 1969; Goodnow, 1936). Dock was an excellent nurse who believed in fairness to qualified nurses and to the public. She advocated that all practicing nurses be measured by a "fair-general-average standard," as determined by written examination, and rewarded with licensure upon attainment of the standard (Christy, 1971).

Palmer's proposed solutions were similar. Many hospitals were sending out inexperienced undergraduates to do private-duty nursing while keeping the income. She advocated a training school in which students of nursing would learn to give care under a qualified nurse and supported the implementation of a *registration* process for all qualified nurses to protect the public from incompetent, unqualified nurses.

Goodrich advocated compulsory legislation that would ensure that graduates or trained nurses would be the only ones who could work as nurses. She pleaded for the registration of qualified nurses, not only for the protection of the nurse, but for the protection of the community. Goodrich also fought against correspondence or home-study programs for nurses, which were a greater menace to the public's safety than people realized. Such legislation, she believed, would encourage talented young women who were intellectually prepared for scientific education to select nursing as a career. The role of the advocate as understood by these three early nursing leaders was to protect the public from unqualified nurses (Dock, 1900; Christy, 1969; Palmer, 1900).

From this beginning, the role of advocate grew. Public-health nurses served as advocates in factories and communities during the Industrial Revolution. Many municipal boards of health hired visiting nurses to work as inspectors in the factories to protect the workers from health hazards and to help prevent accidents. Communities were finding that the nurse as advocate for the factory worker had inestimable value. Visiting nurses were also proving very effective in preventing the spread of communicable diseases.

Hospital nurses also worked as advocates for the patients while giving care. Nurses were crucial in protecting patients from harm when they were too ill to protect themselves. Nurses were also responsible for providing measures to relieve pain, and they strove to make their patients happy and comfortable, even if it meant breaking the rules sometimes (Hill, 1900). During the 1970s and 1980s the responsibility of the nurse as advocate was expanded to include speaking for their clients when they could not speak for themselves (Sovie, 1978). Nurses returned to work in churches in the primary role of advocate under the Granger Westberg model for parish nursing. The members of the congregation where a parish nurse practiced found affirmation and support as they reached to improve their physical, emotional, and spiritual health (Striepe, 1987).

However, consumers, administrators, and courts do not share the perception of the nurse as advocate. The findings of a study done in 1983 indicated that consumers did not recognize the nurse as an initiator of health care (Miller, Mansen, and Lee,

1983). Consumers also believed that physicians would protect the rights of the patient. Miller, Mansen, and Lee (1983) concluded that although nurses were serving as mediators between patients and institutions, changes rarely occurred within the institutions as a result of this role. Patient advocacy was directly related to the power and authority allowed the nurse by the particular system. Nurses generally became advocates whenever the issue was care; however, they had little power to be truly effective as an advocate when the concerns involved the medical regimen or health care services (Miller, Mansen, and Lee, 1983). Examples of advocacy included questioning doctors' orders, promoting client comfort, and supporting patient decisions regarding health care choices.

Advocacy is a critical role for nurses today. Nurses are in a vital position to be effective in this role.

With the need for informed consent, advance directives, and treatment choices, patients more than ever need an advocate to interpret information, identify the risks and benefits of the various treatment options, and support the decision they make. Being an advocate does involve taking personal and professional risks. When the issue is care, nurses are willing advocates, but when the issue is the profession, nurses seem reluctant (Anglin, 1991).

WHY ARE NURSES MANAGERS?

Even Florence Nightingale recognized the need for nurses to be managers. She insisted that nurses needed to organize the care of the patient so that other nurses could carry on when they were not present. There were four major eras in the development of the nurse as manager. During the first period, lasting until about 1920, the nurse was known as the *charge nurse*. Charge nurses were responsible for teaching the nursing students what they needed to know and for directing the care that the students gave. The charge nurse was autocratic. This nurse had absolute authority over the student.

During the second era, lasting until 1949, the term *supervisor* was used to describe the role. The supervisor continued to be responsible for the students; however, the role had expanded to include enforcing agency policies, developing improvements in the care of the ill, and being responsible for the effective use of the ward's resources. The supervisor served on hospital committees but had no vote. Supervisors continued their autocratic management styles and established high standards of nursing practice. At the end of this period, management techniques were beginning to focus on a more humanistic approach, which was a more effective use of human resources. Nurses were more involved in the patient-care process. Hospital administrators were relying on nursing expertise to establish policies for patient care and hospital administration. This era ended with the publication of Esther Lucille Brown's report (1948) recommending that nursing education be separated from hospital administration.

During the third period, lasting until 1970, the nurse was referred to as a *coordinator*. The nurse coordinator no longer had responsibility for the nursing education of the students but was expected to motivate staff, be innovative, and solve problems. Coordinators were active in improving patient care and were expected to maintain harmony within the institution. Many nurse coordinators had few skills in and little knowledge of middle management and basically learned by trial and error how to be effective.

The last period, from 1970 to the present, is a series of waves. Nurses gained recognition as managers and were able to function in that role. Hospital nurses gained middle-management positions and proved their abilities. The period before diagnostic-related groups saw escalating hospital costs and growth in the numbers of employees and services. From this growth came significant efforts to control the costs of health care (Cohen, 1993). The term *manager* is used most often now in the nursing literature, but you may find it used to describe any of the four periods.

> No matter what time you might study, the expectation is that the nurse manager will coordinate patient care and supervise nurses in the delivery of quality care.

One cannot leave the discussion of this important role without some comments about the pressure of economics on the delivery of health care. Because nurse-managers are responsible for budgets and monitor reimbursement, the movement toward a case-management system is much like a tidal wave in nursing as a whole—unexpected and unprepared for. However, the reality is that nurses have always been case managers—not as contemporary critics might define it, but as the working nurse, especially in community health. Zander's classic interpretation of case management— i.e., a nurse manages nursing care while containing costs and maintaining quality (Zander, 1987; 1988)—has guided the practice of community-health nurses for as long as this area of practice has existed, even before the definition was developed. However, the model is relatively innovative in hospital settings (Cohen, 1993). The knowledge and skills required for the nurse as manager have become increasingly complex. Nurse-managers are expected to solve problems, evaluate care and personnel, develop budgets, delegate responsibility, negotiate, and be critical-thinkers in an effort to maintain harmony within the institution. Without a doubt, the role of the nurse as manager has evolved into a complex one that includes organizing patient care, directing personnel to achieve agency goals, and allocating resources (Anglin, 1991).

CAN NURSES BE COLLEAGUES?

The role of colleague is a vital one for any profession. The status of colleague within health care generates pictures of nurses, doctors, and pharmacists discussing, on an equal basis, problems and concerns related to health care. In nursing, however, a review of our history reveals that we have not quite achieved the status of colleague. Interdisciplinary collegial relationships currently are tenuous. More surprising is that, even among nurses, intradisciplinary collegial relationships are strained. Three periods in the evolution of this role can be identified.

The first period, that of the assistant role, ended in 1940. This early category of colleague was clearly defined by nursing leaders as one who was cooperative, loyal, and obedient to the physician and the hospital (Anglin, 1991). These characteristics were considered critical to being a competent nurse. In 1905, Jan Hodson actually set the standard by insisting that loyalty to the doctors was the most important factor for a faithful nurse to be successful. Hodson supported blind faith in carrying out doctors' orders, no matter how different or unusual. She also recommended a strong sense of responsibility when working with subordinates and superiors (Hodson, 1905; Anglin, 1991). However, she encouraged collegial exchange of information and emphasized asking for advice in serious or delicate matters (Hodson, 1905). Obviously, physicians encouraged and rewarded this type of subordinate role (Lawman, 1907; Aikens, 1935; Hamilton, 1949).

From 1941 to 1959, the role of colleague fell under the title of *coordinator*. A major effort to evaluate nursing service delivered during World War II revealed this more authoritarian principle of management (Brown, 1948). Nurses were caught between their hospital's administration, the physicians, and unfortunately, the highly authoritarian managers within their own profession. Few contributions from nurses were incorporated into the planning of the organizations. In public-health nursing, however, the role of colleague was fully realized (Brown, 1948). Public-health nurses served on boards of health and were major contributors in public-health planning and programs within local health departments. One important recommendation that came from the Brown report (1948) was that nurses should work to improve their actions and words based on their understanding of human behavior and learn to deal effectively with people. Brown continued by recommending an even more important goal for nurses. Once nurses learned to deal effectively with people, they could make major contributions to the total effort of health care delivery and other disciplines (Brown, 1948). Great emphasis was placed on developing collegial relationships for the good of the health care system. From these significant recommendations came team-nursing approaches to care and the coordination of activities for improved patient care. However, the theme of cooperation remained (Anglin, 1991).

Between 1960 and the present, the term *collaborator* has been adopted for this role. The root of this word means "to exchange information with the enemy." This may be the most fitting description of the role. Nurses were interested in developing collaborative relationships with doctors, pharmacists, and other health professionals. The literature is abundant with discussions of these relationships and consistently describes these relationships as collaborative (Hahm and Miller, 1961; Quint, 1967; Seward, 1969; Kelly, 1975; Wisener, 1978; Tourtillott, 1986).

WHERE DOES THIS LEAVE THE ROLE OF COLLEAGUE?

Nursing education has promoted the term *collaborator* over *colleague*. The dilemma is that employers neither recognize nor reward the role. Students in their educational experiences are seldom offered the opportunity to practice the role of colleague and therefore have only a vague understanding of the role. However, public-health nurses throughout American history have not only understood the role, but probably have attained a greater degree of collegiality than any other practice area of nursing. Public-health nurses are not the majority within the profession. Nevertheless, they continue to enjoy and maintain the essence of the role (Anglin, 1991). As a colleague, one recognizes nurses with expertise and relies on those nurses for their expertise in the interest of improving patient care and advancing the profession. The essence of the role is mutual respect and equality among professionals, both intradisciplinary and interdisciplinary (Anglin, 1991). Until nurses can respond to each other with respect, it will be difficult to move from collaborator to true colleague.

WHAT ABOUT EXPERTS?

There is one other role in which nurses are often found. For lack of a better name, this role is called *expert*. It is a conglomerate of advanced formal or informal education and acquired or recognized expertise. The role includes academicians, historians, nursing educators, clinicians, professional educators, researchers, research consumers, theorists, nurse technologists, and the leaders within the profession. The American Academy of Nursing recognizes some of these individuals and votes to bestow on them the honor of Fellow. There are many nurses who are experts in an area of practice, whether it be in clinics, at the bedside, in nursing homes, or in other settings. As nurses with special expertise, they are called on to provide testimony in courts and at government hearings or to share information and knowledge with other nurses, which is their obligation to the profession. This sharing can be done through mentoring, guest-speaking, performing in-services, offering continuing-education programs, contributing to publications, and writing technical articles. These experts are usually the nurses who create the momentum that moves the profession forward. This is a role that should be recognized, encouraged, and rewarded.

THE BEGINNING

What do nurses do? There is no simple answer. We agree that nurses care for patients—and hence are caregivers. We agree that nurses teach patients what they need to know to make informed choices—and thus are teachers. We also agree that the role of manager exists in some form, and so we manage our practice and patients' care. We can even define the role of advocate, although based on the history of the role, nurses are reluctant to take risks to fully carry the role into the future. The role of colleague is less clear. We are consistent in using the term *collaborator*; however, the term *colleague* is deemed more fitting for professionals, and that is the role to which we should aspire.

Finally, we have experts, who we may or may not recognize and upon whom the profession depends to provide the leadership for the whole. These roles merely provide a beginning for you to understand the profession you have chosen—nursing. May you become proficient in these roles and develop into an expert and then provide the leadership for nursing in the future.

The future is not the result of choices among
Alternative paths offered;
It is a place that is created,
Created first in the mind and will,
Created next in activity.
The future is not some place we are going to,
But one we are creating.
The paths to it are not found, but made.
And the activity of making them
Changes both the maker and the destiny.
—Anonymous (1987)

REFERENCES

Aikens CA: *Studies in nursing ethics*, Philadelphia, 1935, WB Saunders.

Alfaro-LeFevre R: *Applying nursing process: a step-by-step guide*, New York, 1998, Lippincott Williams & Wilkins.

Anglin LT: *The roles of nurses: a history, 1900 to 1988*, Ann Arbor, Mich, 1991, University of Michigan.

Benner P: *From novice to expert: excellence and power in clinical nursing practice*, Menlo Park, Calif, 1984, Addison-Wesley.

Bradford W: *History of Plymouth Plantation. Book II (1620)*, Plymouth, Mass, 1898, Wright & Potter.

Brown EL: *Nursing for the future*, New York, 1948, Russell Sage Foundation.

Bullough V, Bullough B: *The care of the sick: the emergence of modern nursing*, New York, 1978, Prodist.

Bullough V, Bullough B, Stanton MP: *Florence Nightingale and her era: a collection of new scholarship*, New York, 1990, Garland.

Christy TE: Portrait of a leader: Isabel Hampton Robb, *Nurs Outlook* 17(3):26-29, 1969.

Christy TE: First fifty years, *Am J Nurs* 71(9):1778-1784, 1971.

Cohen EL: *Nursing case management*, St Louis, 1993, Mosby.

Dalton R: Hospitals: their origins and history, *Dublin J Med Sci* 109(3), 17-19, 1900.

Dana CL: *The peaks of medical history*, New York, 1936, Paul B. Hoeber.

Davis MD: I was a student over 50 years ago, *Nurs Outlook* 61:62, 1961.

Dock L: What may we expect from the law? *Am J Nurs* 1:9, 1900.

Dodge BS: *The story of nursing*, ed 2, Boston, 1989, Little, Brown.

Dolan JA: *History of nursing*, Philadelphia, 1969, W. B. Saunders.

Donahue MP: *Nursing: the finest art*, St Louis, 1985, Mosby.

Goodnow M: *Outlines in the history of nursing*, Philadelphia, 1936, WB Saunders.

Hahm H, Miller D: Relationships between medical and nursing education, *J Nurs Educ* 39:849-851, 1961.

Hamilton JA: Success or failure in nursing administration, *Am J Nurs* 49:496, 1949.

Hill J: Private duty nursing from a nurse's point of view, *Am J Nurs* 1(2):129, 1900.

Hodson J: *How to become a trained nurse*, New York, 1905, William Abbott.

Jamieson EM, Sewall MF: *Trends in nursing history*. Philadelphia, 1949, WB Saunders.

Kalisch PA, Kalisch BJ: *The advance of American nursing*, Boston, 1986, Little, Brown.

Kelly LY: *Dimensions of professional nursing*, ed 3, New York, 1975, Macmillan.

Lawman JH: The evolution and development of the nurse, *Am J Nurs* 8:8, 1907.

Leininger M: *Care: the essence of nursing and health*, Thorofare, NJ, 1984, Charles B. Slack.

Miller BK, Mansen TJ, Lee H: Patient advocacy: do nurses have the power and authority to act as patient advocate? *Nurs Leadersh* 6(2):56-60, 1983.

Palmer S: The editor, *Am J Nurs* 1(4):166-169, 1900.

Quint GC: Role models and the professional nurse identity, *J Nurs Educ* 6:11, 1967.

Rybczynski W: *Home: a short history of an idea*, Middlesex, England, 1986, Penguin.

Seward JM: Role of the nurse: perceptions of nursing students and auxiliary nursing personnel, *Nurs Res* 18(2):164-169, 1969.

Sovie L: Nursing. In Chaska N, editor: The nursing profession, New York, 1978, GP Putnam's Sons.

Stewart IM: A half-century of nursing education. *Am J Nurs* 50:617, 1950.

Striepe J: *Nurses in churches: a manual for developing parish nurse services and networks*, Spencer, Iowa, 1987, Iowa Lake Area Agency on Aging.

Tourtillott EA: *Commitment—a lost characteristic*, New York, 1986, JB Lippincott.

Watson J: *Nursing: human science and human care—a theory of nursing*, East Norwalk, Conn, 1985, Appleton-Century-Crofts.

Wisener S: *The reality of primary nursing care: risks, roles and research. Role changes in primary nursing*, New York, 1978, National League of Nursing.

Zander K: Nursing case management: a classic, *Definition* 2(2):1-3, 1987.

Zander K: Managed care within acute care settings: design and implementation via nursing case management, *Health Care Supervisor* 6(2):24-43, 1988.

ADDITIONAL READINGS

Carr EH: *What is history?* New York, 1961, Vintage Books.

Christy TE: Nurses in American history: the fateful decade, 1890-1900, *Am J Nurs* 75(7):1163-1165, 1975.

Degler CN: *At odds*, New York, 1980, Oxford.

Leininger M: The leadership crisis in nursing: a cultural problem and challenge, *J Nurs Adm* 2(9):62, 1972.

Ryan MP: *Womanhood in America: from colonial times to the present*, New York, 1979, New Viewpoints.

Shattuck L: *Report of the Sanitary Commission of Massachusetts*, 1850, Cambridge, Mass, 1948, Harvard University Press.

Stille CJ: *History of the United States Sanitary Commission: being the general report of its work during the War of Rebellion*, Philadelphia, 1863, J. B. Lippincott.

Wormeley KP: *The United States Sanitary Commission: a sketch of its purposes and its work*, Boston, 1863, Little, Brown.

INTERNET RESOURCES

Nursing and Health Care

American Nurses Association
http://www.nursingworld.org

Nightingale
http://nightingale.con.utk.edu

Nursing and Health Care Resources on the Net

Nursing Net
http://www.nursingnet.org

University of Sheffield (England) School of Nursing and Midwifery
http://www.shef.ac.uk/uni/academic/N-Q/nm

Australian Science Archives Project
http://www.asap.unimelb.edu.au

History of Medicine Link

Karolinska Institute
http://www.mic.ki.se/History.html

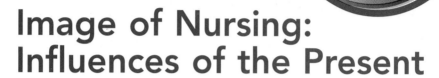
Image of Nursing: Influences of the Present

NELLIE NELSON, MSN, RN, CARN

Oh the power the gift He gives us, to see ourselves as others see us.
   —*Robert Burns, 1786*

We write our own destiny . . . We become what we do.
   —*Madame Chiang Kai-Shek*

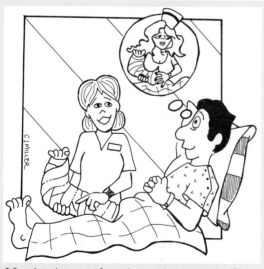

Nursing image—how is nursing perceived?

After completing this chapter, you should be able to:

- Identify selected historical educational studies and literature that have influenced the image of professional nursing.
- Describe different sociological models that characterize "professionalism."
- Apply Pavalko's characteristics as a framework to describe modern-day nursing practice.
- Identify the role that nursing organizations have in professional practice.
- Describe the role of credentialing and certification in professional practice.
- Examine two current nursing issues affecting nursing practice: advanced-practice nursing and community-based practice settings for nurses.

NURSING IMAGE—HOW IS IT PERCEIVED? What does it mean to be a professional nurse? How does the public view nursing? How does nursing define and view itself?

Within the profession of nursing there is no single definition of nursing on which all nurses agree. To describe the current image of the professional nurse would be analogous to the old Indian folk tale in which three blind men attempt to define an elephant by touching three separate parts of the animal.

Modern-day nursing has many exciting professional dimensions, one of which includes the debate surrounding its identification as a profession. A current movement in nursing is to change the public image of the nurse. This chapter discusses the development of nursing into a profession and explores the present and future dimensions of nursing's "image." Let's continue with nursing's historical journey by beginning with the question "What constitutes a profession?" Historical knowledge about our "rites of passage" gives us an appreciation of where nursing is today as a profession and what the future of nursing may hold for you, the recent graduate, in our complex and evolving health care world.

IMAGE OF NURSING

WHAT DO WE MEAN BY THE "IMAGE" OF NURSING?

Nursing has been identified as an "emerging profession" for at least 150 years. The image of professional nursing continues to evolve and is significantly affected by the media, women's issues and roles, and a high-technology health care environment. How nursing views itself in the evolution of the profession and how actively nurses are involved in the definition process will determine the image of nursing in the future.

Some say that the image of nursing is directly related to what the profession offers society and the value placed on that service (Schaffer, 1989). Nursing leaders have recognized that role behavior in professional nursing is related to the image of the nurse held by the consumer (i.e., the public). The most significant changes in the public's image of nursing have occurred within the past 50 years. Typically the public image of nursing does not accurately reflect the nurse's expertise and does not recognize the contributions nursing makes to health care.

Most nurses would like to be thought of as autonomous and competent decision-makers within their nursing practice areas. Throughout the 1990s, a nationwide advertising campaign supported by the National Commission on Nursing Implementation Project produced radio and television ads that said, "If caring were enough, anyone could be a nurse." Nurses of America, an advocate organization sponsored by the National League for Nursing (NLN), implemented a very successful program directed toward improving the image of nursing as depicted on television, on radio, in print, and on lecture circuits. Consultants were contracted to work with executives, politicians, and celebrities on presenting nursing in a positive manner. This approach reinforced the image of the modern-day professional nurse as having decision-making and problem-solving skills. Barbara Wallace, RNC, EdD, MPH, former executive director for Nurses of America and cohost of the ABC program "Health Beat," suggests that "if you tell a story about how nursing care made a difference, the conclusion will always be that it was the nurse who made the difference" (Wallace, 1999, p. 28).

In the early 1990s, *Media Watch*, a national newsletter, was published for three years by Nurses of America to address the image of nursing in the media. The newsletter was sponsored by the Tri-Council, comprising the American Nurses Association (ANA), the American Organization of Nurse Executives, and the NLN. The purpose of the newsletter was to inform the public about the role that the modern nurse has in health care delivery (Wallace, 1990). Nurses of America welcomed the reactions of professional nurses and nursing organizations to the way nursing was perceived by the media. The input from the professional community had a major impact on the nursing image in newspapers, in magazines, and on television. Remember the so-called television comedy "Nightingales"? Because of the outcry from professional nurses and the public against the negative way in which this program presented nurses, advertising support was withdrawn, and the program was canceled. However, because of media efforts during the past decade, the numbers of stories citing nurse experts and nursing research have increased tenfold (Wallace, 1999, p. 28). Dr. Eleanor Sullivan, RN, PhD, FAAN, president of Sigma Theta Tau International, acknowledges the key role of communication as the "stock in trade" of nurses and that the media can help promote the vital role of nurses in the health of the world (Sullivan, 1999).

Although the *Media Watch* newsletter is no longer published, many nursing organizations have taken charge in the promotion of nursing's image. Nursing associations are working together to promote a positive image and deal with nursing shortage issues. Nurses for a Healthier Tomorrow, an alliance of 37 nursing organizations, has launched a national media campaign that demonstrates, through print and broadcast media, the many opportunities for the career of nursing. One tangible example of this effort is the new Web site: http://www.nursesource.org.

Sigma Theta Tau International, the national honor society for nursing, is the coordinator of Nurses for a Healthier Tomorrow. Check out their Web site at http://www.nursingsociety.org. The ANA published a flyer titled, *Every Patient Deserves a Nurse*, along with other promotional materials. The promotional message of these materials reinforces the positive image of nurses as patient advocates and critical resources both to patients and families and emphasizes the right of people to a safe health care environment.

Sigma Theta Tau International also produced the television program *Nursing Approach*, from January 1993 to April 1994. This series aired weekly in 350 cities in the United States and Canada. In its 15 months of programming, *Nursing Approach* disseminated the latest nursing knowledge for patient care, presented by nurses in all areas of nursing research and clinical practice. This very positive television profile of nursing enhanced the professional image and the presence of men in nursing and used the media as an innovative tool to show the diverse role of nursing in caring for patients and families. The roles of nurses in 2001 movies, such as *Pearl Harbor*, show different roles of nursing through film media.

The image of nursing continues to evolve as media show the many roles of nurses in the restructuring of health care environments and in a variety of settings, such as emergency rooms and in war time (e.g., in Desert Storm). Studies continue to verify that competent nursing care affects mortality rates in critical-care patients and the future for many nursing jobs lies in the expanding role of nursing into community-based practice settings. The role and image of the nurse will continue to change as the many facets of health care delivery evolve into this century. How will nurses respond to these changes? The journey toward attaining a professional image has been and will continue to be challenging.

WHAT CONSTITUTES A PROFESSION?

There are many ways to describe a "professional." What meaning does the word have for you as a graduate professional nurse? Controversy over the definition of the term *professional* as it relates to nursing is not a new issue. Strauss (1966), a noted sociologist, found the word *professional* used in reference to nursing in a magazine article published in 1892 titled "Nursing, a New Profession for Women." The nurses of the twentieth and twenty-first centuries owe a lot to Isabel Adams Hampton (later Isabel Hampton Robb) for her visionary focus in the late 1800s. She was an outstanding advocate for the professionalization of nursing. In the textbook *Nursing Ethics* (1901), she wrote that

> The trained nurse, then, is no longer to be regarded as a better trained, more useful, higher class servant, but as one who has knowledge and is worthy of respect, consideration, and due recompense. . . . She is also essentially an instructor; part of her duties have to do with the prevention of disease and sickness, as well as the relief of suffering humanity. . . . These are some of the essentials in nursing by which it has become to be regarded as a profession, but there still remains much to be desired, much to work for, in order to add to its dignity and usefulness. As the standard of education and requirements become a higher character and the training more efficient, the trained nurse will draw nearer to science and its demands and take a greater share as a social factor in solving the world's needs.

Much analysis of the term has occurred in the literature since the early 1900s and continues through the current decade. How will the characteristics of professionalism affect the image of modern nursing?

Is social work a profession?, the classic work of Abraham Flexner, written in 1915, was used initially by the medical profession to begin to form its identity and redefine itself as a profession. As a sociologist, Flexner began examining his own profession. This was at a time when occupations such as medicine, social work, and nursing were moving away from their occupational focus and toward redefinition and professionalization. Flexner's criteria for defining a profession continue to provide a basis for the modern sociologist to use in addressing the question "What are the characteristics of a profession?" The main points include the following:

1. Professional activity is based on intellectual action, along with personal responsibility.
2. The practice of a profession is based on knowledge, not routine activities.

3. There is practical application rather than just theorizing.
4. There are techniques that can be taught.
5. A profession is organized internally.
6. A profession is motivated by altruism, with members working in some sense for the good of society.

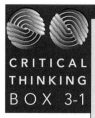

CRITICAL THINKING BOX 3-1

LEVENSTEIN'S CHARACTERISTICS OF A PROFESSION

What do you think about . . .

❑ The element of altruism
How do you define caring in your clinical practice?

❑ Code of ethics
Are you familiar with the ANA Code of Ethics?

❑ Collaboration with groups and individuals for the benefit of the patient

What other groups do you work with in your clinical setting that affect the health needs of the patient and family?

❑ Colleagueship demonstrated by:

An Organization for Licensing—

What is the role of the State Board of Nursing in your state?

A group that helps ensure quality—

Are you aware of the role of national nursing organizations that accredit nursing programs?

There are two national nursing organizations that accredit nursing programs; do you know what they are?

Peer evaluations of practitioners—

What is the role of job evaluations in terms of professional growth?

❑ Accountability for conduct and responsibility for practice decisions
Who monitors professional conduct issues from a legal and ethical point of view?
Does shared governance reflect more control of one's nursing practice?

❑ Strong research program
Are you aware that a national center for nursing research is now operating in Washington, DC?

In Caplow's classic work from the early 1950s, *The Sociology of Work*, several steps in the process of "becoming professional" were defined further, and the value of forming an association that defined a special membership was addressed. Caplow suggested that making a name change to clarify an area of work or practice would subsequently produce a new role. With the creation of this new role, the group would then establish a code of ethics and legal components for licensure to practice and educational control of the profession (Caplow, 1954). This process of becoming professional was taking place in nursing in 1897 with the establishment of the ANA. Other aspects of professionalization were also beginning to develop. For example, the *Code for Nurses* was suggested as early as 1926, although it wasn't written or published by the ANA until the early 1950s. Revisions were made in 1956, 1960, and 1976, with changes made in 1985 that included interpretative statements. In the summer of 2001 at the ANA convention, delegates again updated and changed the name to the *Code of Ethics for Nurses with Interpretive Statements* (http://www.ana.org/ethics/ecode.htm).

More than 50 years after Flexner's criteria and almost 20 years after Caplow's work, Pavalko (1971) described eight dimensions of a profession. Pavalko's dimensions of a profession and their specific application to nursing are examined in more detail in the next section. Nursing continues to apply these dimensions to support nursing's move away from the occupational focus on "professionalism." Is nursing a profession or semiprofession?

By responding to the questions in Critical Thinking Box 3-1, which presents a fourth model of professionalism, Levenstein's model, you will identify common themes in describing a profession. What are your thoughts about the nursing profession in light of these criteria?

Others have written about professions and their development, but these four sociological models present some logical characteristics for you to use to examine professionalism. According to Henshaw, a noted nursing leader and researcher, a profession includes "self-regulation and autonomy with ultimate loyalty and accountability to the professional group" (Talotta, 1990). Nursing is a dynamic profession and continues to strive to enhance a professional image—which leads us to the next question.

IS NURSING A PROFESSION?

Eunice Cole, past president of the ANA, described nursing as a dynamic profession that has established a code of ethics and standards of practice, education, service, and research components. The standards for both the professional and practical dimensions of nursing are continually reviewed and updated. Nurses, strong in numbers but splintered professionally in many ways, represent the largest group of health care providers in the United States. There are nearly 2.7 million registered nurses in the workforce with an average age of 45 years, and an estimated 71% of this population is working full time in nursing, with another 28% working part time (HRSA, 2000). By using Pavalko's eight dimensions to describe a profession, let's examine nursing and issues that challenge the collective whole.

1. A profession has relevance to social values.

Does nursing exist to serve self or others? Nursing historically had its roots in true altruism with lifelong service to others. Nursing defined itself in the ANA's Social Policy Statement (1988) as the "diagnosis and treatment of human responses to actual or potential health problems." As nurses, we focus not only on the treatment component of patient care, but also on wellness and health promotion issues, as a part of our nursing practice. The goal is to shift the focus of health care so that primary prevention becomes more valued. As this shift occurs, nurses will become increasingly important because of their ability to be teachers of health promotion activities and managers of wellness, activities that have an impact on social values.

2. A profession has a training or educational period.

According to Florence Nightingale, a nurse's education should involve not only a theory component, but also a practice component. An educational process for any professional is critical because it transmits the knowledge base of the profession and, through research and other scholarly endeavors, advances the practice of the profession. Luther Christman, noted nursing leader, has suggested that without a uniform educational base, it is difficult for nurses to communicate what they do as professionals, have clear standards of nursing care, stabilize colleagueship with other professionals, and ensure adequate funding of the profession (Deloughery, 1995). The diversity of educational programs for nurses has stimulated debate regarding the entry practice level for registered nurses. Some questions surrounding the issues include the following:

- Can 2-year programs continue to provide an adequate educational base for the profession?
- Is the nurse prepared for current and future nursing functions, if educated at the diploma level?
- How critical is it to complete a 4-year Bachelor of Science in Nursing (BSN) program to handle the challenges of the health care environment, complex patient-family needs, and the expanding community-based settings for clinical work?
- Will the Doctor of Nursing degree that was pioneered at Case Western University become the minimum background for entry into the profession?

These questions have been debated since the publication in 1965 of an ANA position paper that charged the profession with the goal of establishing nursing education at the baccalaureate level within 25 years. More than 30 years have passed since then, and the issue continues to challenge the profession. The inability of nursing organizations and educational systems at all levels to come to agreement on this issue has affected the solidarity of the profession. Only a few states have eliminated diploma programs, and only one state, North Dakota, has legally mandated the BSN as the degree for entry into practice. Other states (such as Maine and Idaho) in the mid 1990s had serious debate on regulatory issues concerning the BSN as the entry credential. Beyond this generic-degree controversy are the issues associated with specialization: What should the entry-level degree be to enter into specialty nursing practice: the Master of Science (MSN) degree or a doctorate (PhD)? This issue was not resolved in the twentieth-century. Will the twenty-first century bring a resolution to the issue?

3. Elements of self-motivation address the way in which the profession serves the patient or family and larger social system.

In 1990 the Tri-Council of Nursing, along with the American Association of Colleges of Nursing, designed a "Nursing Agenda for Health Care Reform" to collectively express the views of nurses concerning health care. Endorsed by 39 major specialty nursing organizations, along with the ANA and the NLN, this emphasized a restructured health care system that would provide universal access to health care, direct health care expenditures toward primary care, and reduce costs. Many of these features were included in health care reforms proposed by the Clinton administration.

Political activity is a way of translating social values into action. Nursing faces special challenges when, for example, nurses must "strike" for pay and benefits or demonstrate a united front to gain federal funding rather than continuing a passive role in such issues. The concept of nursing as truly altruistic stands in contrast to the prospect of a future generation of nurses who may view nursing as a job rather than a profession. As a graduate nurse, you are also a professional who will help effect many changes in the health care arena.

4. A profession has a code of ethics.

Nursing, like other professions, has ethical dimensions. As noted earlier in the chapter, the nursing *Code of Ethics* published by the ANA dates to the 1950s. Key points of the Code are given in Box 3-1. The Code of Ethics is discussed in more detail in Chapter 19.

5. A professional has a commitment to lifelong work.

By this statement, Pavalko means that a professional sees his or her career as more than just a steppingstone to another area of work or as an intermittent job. Nursing, however, is a female-dominated profession; role conflicts exist as the nurse is challenged with changing jobs and accepting part-time work to accommodate family or personal needs. Government data show that 81% of the nearly 2.7 million registered nurses work in health care (HRSA, 2000). Nursing is identified as one of the top five health occupations for the next decade for employability and new jobs (*Occupational Outlook Handbook*, 1998-1999). Thus, nursing as a career has great potential for financial rewards, involvement in a variety of professional endeavors, and commitment to lifelong work.

6. Members control their profession.

Nurses are not entirely autonomous. While nurses work under professional control, they are under legislative control as well. Among these controls are the 50 state boards of nursing, which control the scope of nursing practice within each state and professional practice standards that are supported both at local and national levels. In 1973 the ANA wrote the first *Standards of Nursing Practice* and since then has had a leadership role in the development of general and many specialty nursing practice standards.

Another publication by the ANA, the *Standards of Clinical Nursing Practice* (1991), discusses the use of nursing process and professional practice standards. The development of professional practice standards indicates to the larger social system that

BOX 3-1   Code of Ethics for Nurses

The ANA House of Delegates approved these nine provisions of the new *Code of Ethics for Nurses* at its June 30, 2001, meeting in Washington, DC. In July 2001 the Congress of Nursing Practice and Economics voted to accept the new language of the interpretive statements, resulting in a fully approved revised *Code of Ethics for Nurses with Interpretive Statements*, as follows.

1. The nurse, in all professional relationships, practices with compassion and respect for the inherent dignity, worth, and uniqueness of every individual, unrestricted by considerations of social or economic status, personal attributes, or the nature of health problems.

2. The nurse's primary commitment is to the patient, whether an individual, family, group, or community.

3. The nurse promotes, advocates for, and strives to protect the health, safety, and rights of the patient.

4. The nurse is responsible and accountable for individual nursing practice and determines the appropriate delegation of tasks consistent with the nurse's obligation to provide optimum patient care.

5. The nurse owes the same duties to self as to others, including the responsibility to preserve integrity and safety, to maintain competence, and to continue personal and professional growth.

6. The nurse participates in establishing, maintaining, and improving health care environments and conditions of employment conducive to the provision of quality health care and consistent with the values of the profession through individual and collective action.

7. The nurse participates in the advancement of the profession through contributions to practice, education, administration, and knowledge development.

8. The nurse collaborates with other health professionals and the public in promoting community, national, and international efforts to meet health needs.

9. The profession of nursing, as represented by associations and their members, is responsible for articulating nursing values, for maintaining the integrity of the profession and its practice, and for shaping social policy.

From American Nurses Association, http://www.ana.org/ethics/ecode.htm.

nursing can define and control its quality of practice. These national standards are incorporated into institutional standards to help guide nursing practice. Most recent publications by the ANA can be found on their Web site at http://www.nursingworld.org.

Nurses practice in varied settings, and the advanced-practice nurse may be in more of an autonomous professional practice role, such as the nurse midwife, psychiatric clinical specialist, or nurse practitioner.

In 1992 there were 100,000 advanced-practice nurses in the United States. In March 2000 the number of RNs with at least one advanced-practice credential was

196,000, with the largest percentage of that group working as nurse practitioners (HRSA, March 2000). These changes represent the largest-growing segment of specialty nursing practice. Advancing one's education level is often paired with increased autonomy.

The majority of nurses in this country work within a structured setting. Trends in those settings are slowly changing to give nurses a stronger voice. For example, nursing care delivery systems that have case management and shared governance reflect more progressive and autonomous environments (see Chapter 12). Nursing can control its scope of practice through professional organizations and publishing documents, along with an active voice in regulatory bodies such as state boards of nursing. Does nursing have more autonomy in the area of practice roles? Jean Steele, past president of the ANA Cabinet on Practice, stated that the hallmark of a profession is self-regulation. Nursing must continue to have a visible and vocal role in the evolution of clinical practice and professional standards as the art and science of nursing matures.

7. A profession has a theoretical framework on which professional practice is based.

Nursing continues to be based in the sciences and humanities, but nursing theory is evolving. It was not until the 1950s that nursing theory was "born." In 1952 Dr. Hildegard Peplau published a nursing model that described the importance of the "therapeutic relationship" in health and wellness. Since then, other nursing theorists such as Martha Rogers, Sister Callista Roy, Dorothea Orem, and Betty Neuman have contributed to our evolving theory-based nursing science.

8. Members of a profession have a common identity and a distinctive subculture.

The outward image of nursing has changed remarkably within the past 50 years. Nurses were once identified by how they looked rather than by what they did. The nursing cap and pin reflected the nurse's school and educational background. The modern-day trend emphasizes that it's not what is worn but what is done that reflects one's role in the nursing profession. The struggle to shift out of rigid dress codes was a major issue in the 1960s. Clothing and other symbols do identify a subculture, and changes in that identification process occur slowly. How many nurses do you know who wear their nursing cap in daily nursing practice? Does your school have a special nursing pin or cap? What kind of an image do you want to project as a professional nurse? (See Critical Thinking Box 3-2.)

Nursing colleagues reflect attitudes and values about the profession. Many schools of nursing have alumni associations, student nurse associations, and nursing honor societies or clubs on campus. These groups provide social interaction during the nursing education years and are great ways to build collegiality.

Belonging to a professional organization such as the ANA, the NLN, or a specialty organization helps professional nurses continue networking and maintain collegiality in our practice areas. In "The Future of Professionalism in Nursing," Sue Ellen Pinkerton, nurse executive, describes the nursing shortage and its impact on the key points of professionalism in today's work force and offers some perspectives on how the work environment can be a positive force (Pinkerton, 2001).

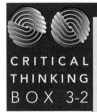

THINK ABOUT

What kind of image do you want to project as a "professional"?

❑ Look at several nursing journals, and note the dress code or uniform of the nurse. Does it portray a physical image of competence? Are the uniform, personal grooming, and style of interaction the kind of image you want to project as a recent graduate?

❑ What do professionals call each other in the clinical setting? Do you wear your name badge with proper credentials? Are you called by your first or last name?

❑ Do you wear your school pin? What other credentials and symbols indicate additional competence?

❑ Where do you see yourself in 5 years as a professional nurse? Does your career plan include formal education?

 "Nurses should choose optimism, making positive strides each day to celebrate who they are and the differences they make. Just a nurse—no, never."—Mellisa Fitzpatrick, 2001

Have the conflicts in educational preparation been resolved with the turn of the century? How will we use further refinement and application of nursing theories in our clinical practice? What can nurses do to have more control of nursing practice regardless of the clinical setting? Will there be an increase in the percentage of people who are choosing nursing as a career? What are the forces that will help nursing "come together" and become not only a true profession, but the largest and most powerful of all the health care professional groups (there is always strength in numbers)?

These are the kinds of problems that you, the graduate nurse, will be challenged with as you enter the real world of nursing. You can't afford to be uninvolved in your profession; you have a role and responsibility in charting your own destiny. Nursing is at one of the most exciting crossroads in its history. There are opportunities to refine the image of the professional nurse as the most powerful force in health care!

NURSING ORGANIZATIONS

WHAT SHOULD I KNOW ABOUT PROFESSIONAL ORGANIZATIONS?

Nursing organizations have significant roles in empowering nurses in their emerging professionalism. Yet many nurses do not belong to a national organization such as the ANA or the NLN or even to specialty-focused groups like the American Association of Critical Care Nurses (AACN) or the International Nurses Society on Addictions. Over the past few years, researchers have examined the issue of belonging to a professional organization, with no conclusive findings regarding why or how nurses choose nursing organizations. Some have suggested that organizations that represent nursing as a whole, such as the ANA and the NLN, do not meet the needs of the individual nurse practicing in today's changing health care environment.

In the early 1950s, belonging to a professional nursing group was popular. By the 1980s, membership in both the ANA and the NLN had declined by 10% to 15%, whereas the nursing population had increased by 150%. During this same period, specialty organizations such as the Association of Operating Room Nurses and the Oncology Nursing Society increased their membership. Does this shift in affiliation reflect a shift in practice settings from the generalist area to specialist areas and suggest that nurses are selecting a specialty organization that represents their current practice? Affiliation with a nursing organization to facilitate networking with colleagues is valuable and meaningful. As a recent graduate, you will need to examine your options for joining a professional group and then demonstrate your professional commitment by active involvement.

The question should be "Which ones should I join?" rather than "Should I even join an organization?" Some organizations give discount memberships to recent graduates the first 6 to 12 months after graduation and provide payment options (Figure 3-1). The next section reviews various organizations, with some historical notes to assist you in making the best choice as you begin your nursing career. A more complete directory of nursing organizations can be found in Appendix B.

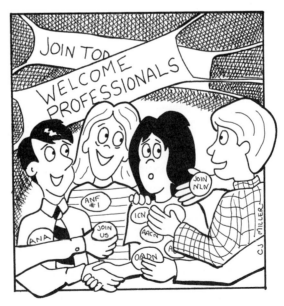

FIGURE 3-1
There is a nursing organization to fit your needs.

WHAT ORGANIZATIONS ARE AVAILABLE TO THE RECENT GRADUATE?

A few of these key professional organizations for individual and organizational membership are described in the next section in alphabetical order. Many of these organizations publish a newsletter or professional journal, and most have Web sites. Individual membership in one or more organizations is a great way to maintain current knowledge about changes in your career field.

American Nurses Association. The ANA is identified as the professional association for registered nurses. It was through the early efforts of Isabel Hampton Robb and others that the Nurses Associated Alumnae of the United States and Canada was formed. At the World's Fair in 1890 a group of 15 nursing leaders began discussions about forming a professional association. Six years later alumnae from the training schools organized the professional association now called the ANA. Canadian members split from the original group in 1911 and formed their own professional association. The ANA's organizational structure has undergone many changes over the years.

Currently when an individual joins the ANA, he or she joins the national organization along with the constituent associations at the state and local level. This method geographically groups smaller clusters of members together according to their practice interests. The ANA's current membership represents totals more than 180,000.

In 1974 an amendment to the Taft-Hartley Act allowed professional nursing organizations to be considered labor unions. After this significant event, some nursing administrators and managers withdrew their memberships in ANA because of the potential conflict of interest between professional affiliation and the workplace. However, this change generated another major nursing organization, the American Association of Nurse Executives (AONE).

The ANA has been at the forefront of policy issues and represents nursing in legislative activities. The ANA's cabinets and councils have provided standards of practice for both the generalist and the specialist. The 1988 *Social Policy Statement* document defines nursing practice at both the generalist and specialist levels. The ANA's certifying organization is the American Nurses Credentialing Center (ANCC), which has certified more than 150,000 RNs in different practice areas at both the generalist and the specialist level. The ANCC, a subsidiary of the ANA since 1991, identifies its mission as improving nursing practice and promoting quality health care service through several types of credentialing programs. The ANCC has created a modular approach to certification that enables the nurse to be recognized for multiple areas of expertise, not simply for competency in a core clinical specialty. There are 30 generalist care clinical specialties or advanced-practice care areas. In their "open door 2000" program, all qualified registered nurses, regardless of their educational preparation, can become certified as a generalist in any of the following specialty areas: gerontology, medical-surgical, pediatrics, perinatal, and psychiatric–mental health nursing.

In addition to certifying individual nurses, the organization also accredits educational providers (i.e., organizations that issue continuing-education credits for professional programs), recognizes excellence in Magnet nursing services, and educates the public about credentialing and professional nursing. This organization is electronically linked on the home page of the ANA (http://www.nursingworld.org).

American Nurses Foundation and the American Academy of Nursing. Two other organizations associated with the ANA are the American Nurses Foundation, founded in 1955, and the American Academy of Nursing (AAN), founded in 1973. Briefly described, these organizations serve special purposes in support of research and recognition of nursing colleagues. The American Nurses Foundation was established as a tax-exempt corporation to receive monies for nursing research. With the establishment of the National Nursing Research Institute, the focus has changed to one of support in the areas of policy-making and research or educational activities. The AAN has a membership of more than 1500 nursing leaders and was established as an honorary association for nurses who have made significant contributions to the nursing profession. When a nurse is elected to the AAN, the person is called a *Fellow*, and the credential following the individual's name is FAAN. The official publication of this organization is *Nursing Outlook*.

International Council of Nurses. The International Council of Nurses, established in 1899, is the international organization representing professional nurses. The focus of this nursing organization is on worldwide health care issues and nursing issues; it meets every 4 years and is headquartered in Geneva, Switzerland.

National League for Nursing. The NLN, established in 1952, can be traced to the 1893 organization of the American Society of Superintendents of Training Schools for Nurses of the United States and Canada. Between the late 1800s and the early 1900s seven nursing organizations formed and joined under the collective name and function of the NLN. One of the unique features of the NLN is that both individuals and agencies are members. The NLN adopted a strategic plan in 1995 to place community-based health care education and health care delivery at the center of its focus and activities (NLN, 1995). The NLN continues to foster improvement in nursing services and nursing education and offers annual educational summits for nursing faculty and leaders in all types of nursing-education programs to come together to discuss nursing education. A nonnurse can join the NLN to fulfill its purpose of promoting the consumer's voice in some nursing policies. Before 1997 the NLN functioned as an accrediting body in all levels of nursing education. In 1997 the NLN created an independent organization called the National League for Nursing Accrediting Commission, Inc. (NLNAC) to accredit educational and professional nursing programs. This organizational change was in response to the new standards established by the U.S. Department of Education. This step was taken to separate accrediting activities from membership activities and to respond to the Higher Education Act Amendment of 1992. Is your school an NLNAC-accredited institution? Visit their Web site at http://www.nlnac.org.

Some of the NLN's other activities include promoting educational workshops or institutes, maintaining a testing division, working with specialty organizations as their testing agency for certification, and providing consultation. The NLN has a biennial convention and publishes *N&HC: Perspectives on Community* (called *Nursing & Health Care* before 1995) bimonthly, *NLN Update*, and numerous other publications that can be obtained by calling (800) 669-1656 or by visiting their Web site at http://www.nln.org.

National Student Nurses' Association. The National Student Nurses' Association (NSNA) is a fully independent organization and publishes its own quarterly journal, *Imprint*. It was formed in 1952 for students enrolled in nursing programs. Becoming a member of the NSNA may be viewed as a way to begin the "professional" socialization process. Often, members of the NSNA serve on selected committees of the ANA and speak to the ANA House of Delegates regarding student-related issues. There are state and national chapters.

National Organization for Associate Degree Nursing. This group was organized in 1986 as an outgrowth of several state organizations. Texas was the first state to have a chapter, which was started in 1984. Membership is open to associate degree nursing graduates, educators, and students. Individuals, states, agencies, and other organizations may also join the organization. There are state and national chapters. The purposes of this organization are to represent associate nursing education and practice, to reinforce the value of an associate nursing education, to maintain endorsement of RN licensure from state to state, and to support the retention of the National Council Licensure Examination for Registered Nurses (NCLEX-RN) examination for associate nursing graduates. Visit their Web site at http://www.noadn.org.

American Association of Colleges of Nursing. This organization is the national voice for university and 4-year college educational programs in nursing and has a membership of more than 500 colleges. The mission of the organization is to "service the public interest by assisting deans and directors to improve and advance nursing education, research and practice" (American Association of Colleges of Nursing, 2000). This organization publishes a newsletter and a bimonthly nursing journal called the Journal of Professional Nursing. In the past few years it has formed a subsidiary for credentialing purposes. That organization is the Commission on Collegiate Nursing Education. This autonomous accreditation agency serves only baccalaureate and higher degree programs in the accreditation process. Additional information on either organization can be found on this Web site: http://www.aacn.nche.edu.

Specialty Practice Organizations. The past 15 years have demonstrated significant growth in specialty practice in nursing. Throughout the 1980s and 1990s, these organizations met annually as the National Federation of Specialty Nursing Certifying Organization to discuss issues in certification and nursing practice. This organization dissolved, and most of the specialty organizations joined the American Board of Nursing Specialties in 1991. The American Board of Nursing Specialties now represents the majority of specialty nursing organizations that promote specialty practice, in addition to the certification issues associated with specialty practice.

As a recent graduate, are you interested in a particular specialty nursing practice area? How do you anticipate obtaining a specialty credential, such as becoming certified as a generalist? How will you include membership in a professional organization in your 5-year career-educational plan?

Other Health-Related Organizations. The American Red Cross is part of approximately 120 Red Cross organizations around the world. Nurses of the American Red Cross pioneered public health nursing in the early 1900s. The American Red Cross is a voluntary agency that is supported by contributions and plays an important role in providing disaster relief and education in first aid and home health and in organizing volunteers to assist in hospitals and nursing homes.

In summary the roles that professional organizations have in enhancing the image of nursing are significant. Their impact is seen both in educational and practice issues for generalist and specialist nurse roles. Organizations provide a voice for nursing in policy issues and serve to unite nurses as a group of professionals. Ultimately it may be nursing organizations that will serve as the catalyst for change in the health care system, and their impact will be felt in the next century.

CREDENTIALING: LICENSURE AND CERTIFICATION

WHAT IS CREDENTIALING?

In the early days of nursing before the Nightingale era, anyone could say they were a nurse and practice their "trade" as they wished. It was only during the past century that nursing became a credentialed profession. A credential can be as simple as a written document of an individual's qualifications. A high school diploma is a credential that indicates a certain level of education has been attained. A credential can also signify a person's performance. The attainment of a title (e.g., FAAN) signifies excellence in performance; a postgraduate degree from an institution of higher learning (PhD or EdD) indicates success in terms of academic achievement and advanced nursing knowledge.

In nursing the educational credentials that an individual holds indicate not only academic achievement, but also that a minimum level of competency in nursing skills has been attained. Academic achievement is represented by an associate degree in nursing (ADN), a diploma in nursing, or a baccalaureate degree in nursing (BSN or BS). After academic preparation, you will have a legal credential—your nursing license—that permits you to practice as a RN. Additional nursing credentials may reflect areas of practice in special areas, such as Critical Care Registered Nurse (CCRN) and Certified Addictions Registered Nurse (CARN). Figure 3-2 summarizes how professional and legal regulations affect the individual, the institution, and the public.

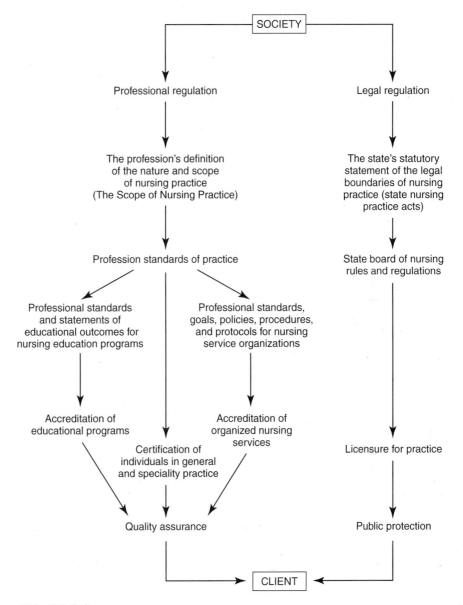

FIGURE 3-2
Flow chart on professional and legal regulation of practice. (From American Nurses Association: *The scope of nursing*, Kansas City, Mo, 1987, ANA.)

WHAT ARE REGISTRATION AND LICENSURE?

Licensure affords protection to the public by requiring the individual to demonstrate minimum competency by examination. By 1923 all 48 states had some form of nursing licensure in place. Nursing licensure is a process by which a governmental agency grants "legal" permission to an individual to practice nursing. This accountability is maintained through a governmental agency responsible for the licensing and registration process. The state boards of nursing are the governmental agencies responsible for this process. Boards of nursing vary in structure and design on the basis of the nurse practice act within each state. The state boards of nursing also exercise legal control over schools of nursing within their respective states. In 1978 all boards of nursing formed a national council, the National Council of State Boards of Nursing (NCSBN), to present a more collective front on nursing education and licensure.

All schools of nursing submit curricula for evaluation and approval by their state boards of nursing. The board of nursing within each state enforces the legal regulatory functions through the nurse practice act of that state. Without approval from the state board of nursing, the college would not be able to offer a nursing program. Each state's board of nursing has regulatory functions that are designed to delineate the scope of nursing practice and to protect the public. The NCSBN has adopted a Mutual Recognition Model of nurse licensure that will allow a nurse to have one license in their state of residence and practice in other states. Issues related to varied nurse practice acts and scope of practice will be challenging with this new approach to licensure without geographic boundaries. As of November 2001, 15 states have entered this type of nursing compact, and legislature is being presented in two additional states. For additional information about this project, view the NCSBN Web site at http://www.ncsbn.org (Kulig, 2001).

To practice nursing in United States, the graduate nurse must successfully complete the NCLEX-RN. After successful completion of the NCLEX-RN, the graduate nurse may use the title *registered nurse* and the initials RN after the surname. The NCSBN also controls the practice of vocational-practical nursing. It is the responsibility of graduate nurses to know the nurse practice act in the state in which they are working. States vary in the requirements to obtain and maintain the nursing license. Some states may require continuing-education credits to renew yearly licenses, whereas other states may consider continuing education as optional for professional growth. (Appendix A is a complete listing of the state boards of nursing and their addresses, or you can visit their Web sites for nursing education.)

Foreign nurse graduates who want to practice nursing in the United States must contact the board of nursing in the state in which they want to practice to obtain licensure because each state controls the requirements for licensure. The state's board of nursing will review the candidate's nursing education and make recommendations regarding requirements needed to obtain a license. Most states require that foreign nurses take the Committee on Graduates of Foreign Nursing Schools examination before the NCLEX-RN. This examination determines proficiency both in nursing and the English language, thus assisting in the prediction of success on the NCLEX-RN. All foreign graduates, regardless of licensure in their home countries, must successfully complete the NCLEX-RN.

HOW DO I OBTAIN A LICENSE?

Basically there are two different procedures for obtaining a license: licensure by examination (applying for an initial license) and licensure by endorsement (applying for a license in a state or jurisdiction when already licensed in another state). As a recent graduate, you will be applying for licensure by examination. What's involved in this process?

Licensure by Examination. First you must have graduated from an approved educational program and complete an application in the state in which you seek a license. There are several fees involved in the licensing process, and many states do not provide an interim work permit. The Computer Adaptive Testing process has decreased the time between the testing process and the receipt of the results by the NCLEX-CAT candidate. Chapter 24 discusses the NCLEX process in detail.

Be prepared during your last semester to save approximately $350 for both the NCLEX-RN and the license application fee.

If you plan on working in another state and want to take the examination in that state, be sure to contact that state early for application information. Many states require fingerprinting for both nurse assistant certificates and nursing licensure. Find out if your state has fingerprinting, and determine whether there are additional fees and legal issues associated with the process as you plan for graduation.

Licensure by Endorsement. *Endorsement* means that the license is granted without requiring that the examination be taken again. Is *endorsement* the same as *reciprocity*? No, *reciprocity* is the acceptance of a license by one state only if the other state does likewise. Each applicant is considered individually on the basis of the rules and regulations of the particular state board of nursing. Licensure by endorsement (not reciprocity) readily facilitates a nurse's transition when moving to another state. The NCSBN adopted Uniform Core Licensure Requirements for initial licensure of RNs and LPN/LVNs. These Uniform Core Licensure Requirements will promote consistency and a general understanding of the objective of nursing regulation while facilitating accessibility of care by easing nursing practice across state lines. These will not only assist in implementing compact nursing licensure, but also ensure mobility of licensed nurses while maintaining licensure standards critical to the public's health.

Currently there is one state, North Dakota, in which licensure by endorsement is available only to nurses with an educational credential of BSN. To be licensed as a registered nurse in North Dakota, you must have a baccalaureate degree; to practice as a practical nurse, you must have an associate's degree. At the time this regulation went into effect, the State Board of Nursing of North Dakota "grandfathered" all nurses then licensed in North Dakota, regardless of their educational preparation, but did not include nurses licensed in another state.

WHAT IS CERTIFICATION?

In the classic article on credentialing written by ANA in the late 1970s, *certification* is defined as a "voluntary process by which a nongovernmental agency or association certifies that an individual licensed to practice a profession has certain predetermined standards specified by that profession for specialty practice" (ANA, 1978-1979). Certification is a different credential than licensure and has a variety of interpretations—both for the nursing profession and the public. The nurse practice acts of some states require that the nurse become certified in some advanced-practice areas such as a nurse practitioner, nurse midwife, or clinical nurse specialist for advanced practice.

The movement toward certification in nursing practice areas has grown significantly within the past 40 years. It was in 1946 that credentialing was first required for entry into practice as a nurse anesthetist (i.e., Certified Registered Nurse Anesthetist, or CRNA). Twenty-five years later, nurse midwives followed suit by requiring certification through the American College of Nurse Midwives as an entry-level credential. In an article by Benner titled, "How to navigate specialty certification," she offers some helpful guidelines to select organizations and requirements for specialty certification. The nursing license is recognized as indicating minimum competency, whereas the certification credential indicates preparation beyond the minimum level. An August 2000 press release by the ANCC of the largest study ever conducted in the United States and Canada with credentialed nurses indicated that nurses who have professional certification made fewer health care errors (ANCC, 2000).

AT WHAT POINT IS CERTIFICATION OBTAINED—AT THE GENERALIST OR THE SPECIALIST LEVEL?

According to the ANA, a *generalist* is an RN who may practice in a general or special area of nursing. To be identified as a *specialist nurse*, the individual needs to have an advanced degree beyond the baccalaureate and to practice in a special area of nursing (ANA, 1990). Since the establishment of the first certification program by the ANA in 1973, certification is the credential that provides recognition of professional achievement in a defined functional or clinical area of nursing practice.

Specialty and generalist nursing organizations represent the largest number of nurses in the nation. More than 350,000 of the nearly 2.7 million RNs in this country hold certification in a specialty area of nursing (Miller, 2000). Research data from the ANCC indicate that there are 67 organizations that certify nurses, 95 different credentials, and more than 134 different specialty areas (Smolenski, 2001). Credentials, such as professional certification, are the stamps of quality and achievement to communicate professional competence. The process of becoming certified engages a full circle of accountability to patients and families, along with professional colleagues (Nardini, 2000).

WHAT IS ACCREDITATION?

The term *accreditation* is often confused with *certification*. The term is defined as a process by which a voluntary, nongovernmental agency or organization approves and grants status to institutions or programs (not individuals) that meet predetermined standards or outcomes. The accreditation of nursing programs by either the NLNAC or the Commission on Collegiate Nursing Education is an activity that you, the recent graduate, may have been involved with during your nursing education. The organizations that accredit programs were enumerated in an earlier part of this chapter.

Accreditation is a peer review and voluntary process. That use of standards and criteria are supported by member schools for the evaluation peer review process.

The process of accreditation is similar for both accrediting organizations—the Commission on Collegiate Nursing Education and the NLNAC. The NLNAC is the only organization that accredits all levels of nursing program education from the practical nurse to the graduate nurse. For the NLNAC, the peer evaluation process occurs after the college writes an extensive self-study of the nursing program by using a set of standards and criteria. A visit by a program evaluation team made up of peer educators occurs. Another level of review occurs after there is a site accreditation visit. A panel of objective national peer educators reviews the program's self-study report, the program evaluation visit team report, and all of the supporting documentation, noting strengths and concerns, and making a recommendation about the accreditation status. All recommendations from the four program review panels for each nursing education program (diploma, PN, ADN, and BSN or higher degree) are forwarded to the Commission of the NLNAC. The Commissioners are a cross section of professionals representing nursing education, nursing administration, and health care consumers; this is the decision-making body for NLNAC. A list of NLNAC schools is published yearly. Visit the Web site at http://www.nlnac.org.

WHAT NURSING JOURNALS OR LITERATURE ARE AVAILABLE?

Nursing journals were first published as a way of maintaining communication with other nurses. At the turn of the century, two nursing journals existed in the United States: *The Nightingale*, a monthly publication started by Sarah Post, and *The Trained Nurse* (later called *Nursing World*), started by Mary Francis. The *American Journal of Nursing* was first published in 1900 by the ANA and is still in publication today. *Nursing "Year"* and *RN* are two other widely read nursing journals, but they are not affiliated with any professional organization. Numerous nursing journals are published by specialty organizations, such as *Emergency Room Nursing*, *Oncology Nursing*, or *Addictions Nursing*.

Because of the changing health care environment and the proliferation of knowledge in health care and nursing, much of the knowledge acquired in your nursing education program may be out of date 5 years after you graduate. Naisbitt (1984) talks about this issue in *Megatrends* and concludes that we have moved from the Industrial Age to the Information Processing Age, with nursing in an information-provider role. Nursing journals continue to be a major link between nursing organizations and professionals in this age of information explosion. The proliferation of online journals and Web-based information resources will help you, as a recent graduate, obtain information on the "superhighway of information." Many nursing journals are available in an electronic format through subscription.

As a recent graduate, what type of journals do you subscribe to and read? It is critical for you to keep up with new information to maintain practice skills and a current knowledge base. You may consider subscribing to a professional journal, attending local nursing workshops, and using an online collection even before graduation to begin "lifelong learning" for your professional career.

CONTEMPORARY ISSUES

Florence Nightingale once described nursing as a "progressive art in which to stand still is to step backward." Her thoughts from more than 100 years ago still hold true today with regard to changes that are occurring in nursing professional practice areas. Major shifts in the health care setting mandate that modern-day nurses embrace flexibility and adaptability in their professional behaviors. The greater need for advanced-practice nurses represents a role shift that can move nursing forward to influence and effect a more powerful position as a profession. Flexibility in work behaviors, additional educational credentials, and certification can be viewed as positive responses to the changes taking place in health care. Opportunities have never been better for the recent graduate as your career launches you into the future. Let's look at two of the issues that will likely affect your professional practice.

WHAT IS GOING ON IN THE JOB MARKET?

All over this country the buzzwords of the business world—*reengineering*, *restructuring*, and *downsizing*—are becoming realities in health care settings. Lucille Joel remarks that, "burgeoning technology advances in medical science, shifts in demography and the economics of health care have dramatically changed hospital nursing practice" (Joel, 1994, p. 220). The acute-care setting that once was the major job placement area for recent graduates currently employs about 62% of the RN work force (HRSA, 2002).

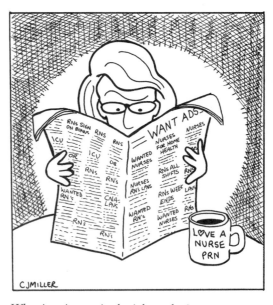

What is going on in the job market?

The reality of recent graduates who focus only on acute-care employment is that they may experience anxiety about future employment outside this setting as the health care market shifts. Data indicate that the greatest shift of nurses is in the increase in employment in the community-based setting, which represents nearly 20% of the current work force (HRSA, 2002). As the nation moves into managed care, which is influenced by insurance companies and other reimbursement mechanisms, some experts predict that one third to half of all hospitals will close their doors (Blancett and Flarey, 1995; Curtin, 1995). Hospitals have merged into a larger system, independent physicians have formed groups, and the downsizing of hospitals has occurred throughout the nation. Community-based care is favored over hospitalization, except for the very acutely ill patient populations. These kinds of major changes have a direct impact on the health professionals who represent the largest part of the work force of the inpatient environment—the nurses.

In the early 1990s a major downsizing of RN staff occurred through attrition and layoffs, with the increasing use of nonlicensed personnel adding to the nursing-care delivery system. There has been a remarkable shift in the downsizing of hospital beds, the shorter hospital stay, and transition and rehabilitation services and an expansion in community-based care. The demand for nurses is expected to increase because alternative settings for health care have created additional employment and professional opportunities.

As the employment trends reflect the decrease in jobs in traditional areas for RNs, they also reflect new employment opportunities. There is an ongoing shift to community-based care throughout the nation that includes rural and underserved areas, selected inner-city hospitals, and nursing home settings. Nursing education programs are preparing graduates for some of the new work areas through an increase in community-based clinical and senior preceptorships.

As the trend for traditional RN workplace setting is changing to a focus on community settings, the NCSBN research reveals that very few recent graduates are working in the community-based settings. The majority of recent graduates are working in hospitals providing direct patient care (NCSBN, 2000).

With today's job market changes, a major health care problem has developed in acute care. With the aging of RNs across the country, the increased level of patient acuity in the hospital, and the decreasing numbers of students in schools of nursing, a staffing crisis has again developed in acute-care hospitals. Nursing shortage is a cyclical phenomenon that has occurred throughout the history of nursing. There is major concern among nurse educators that the young adults who have previously come into nursing have too many other attractive opportunities available; thus there is a decline in the students enrolling in schools of nursing. With the graying of America, it is predicted that the staffing in acute-care hospitals by registered nurses is going to become an even more severe problem.

In today's market-driven reform of all health care jobs, the recent graduate must use a variety of strategies to maintain employability. A well-known consultant with expertise in corporate transitions and job markets has identified three characteristics that an individual needs for future job security in any area: *employability*, *vendor-mindedness*, and *resiliency* (Bridges, 1994).

Employability is the enhanced skills and knowledge that the nurse brings to the health care agency. The nurse's knowledge and abilities that enhance quality patient outcomes can translate into dollar savings for the institution. An ANCC study in 2000 demonstrated that nursing certification has a dramatic impact on practice outcomes (ANCC, 2000). *Vendor-mindedness* means that the nurse needs to ask, "What can I offer as a professional that would make the employer want my specific qualities and flexibility as an individual?" The movement toward contract work or pool work says to the employer that "I am flexible and able to meet the needs of the system, and I am your best asset as a valued worker . . . I can make a difference in the care of the patient."

Resiliency describes the professional's ability to blend into system needs in a chaotic time of health care change. The nurse who is shifted from the charge nurse position to staff level needs to keep a positive attitude within the job arena. Nurses need to promote job security within the system by adding new skills and abilities that help them maintain viability as professionals—perhaps cross-training to the home health department of the hospital or strengthening clinical skills through an added certification credential of management. The clinical role is demanding more delegation skills and fewer clinical skills with the influx of health care workers and the advent of working for several institutions rather than just one system (contract work).

A current knowledge base with critical-thinking qualities, a foundation in geriatrics or primary care, health teaching skills, and communication abilities are all qualities that enhance the value of the professional in any nursing role (Blancett and Flarey, 1995). In a classic article in the early 1990s, the ANA suggested that health care is moving toward a model founded on primary care, with the smallest portion of care being delivered at the most costly tertiary level. Five percent of the U.S. population consumes 58% of the health care dollars, whereas 75% of public and private health insurance dollars pay for hospitalization (ANA, 1993). The new model described in the literature would reverse the triangle (Fig. 3-3).

As Leah Curtin (1995) so succinctly stated, "Job security is not found in the job but rather in the person who holds the job. . . ." Nursing is a career, and nurses must take charge of their professional futures. The next section addresses one option that the recent nursing graduate may want to consider when making career plans.

WHAT ABOUT ADVANCED-PRACTICE NURSING?

A University of Colorado nursing professor, Dr. Loretta Ford, founded the first nurse practitioner (NP) program in 1965. As early as the mid-1960s, Dr. Ford believed that the NP would evolve from the graduate setting. Today there are more than 150 programs that educate NPs in a variety of clinical tracks, and more than 1000 publications address the role of the nurse practitioner (Watson, 1995). Advanced practice has since greatly diversified, with a variety of clinical roles, methods of educational preparation, and scopes of clinical practice, with more than 7.3% of today's registered nurses having advanced-practice credentials (HRSA, 2000). As master's degree programs proliferated in the 1970s with government funding, the clinical nurse specialist (CNS) emerged from university settings. The CNS had a focus area that was equated with graduate education. Ford, in 1965, had envisioned that the NP would evolve from graduate settings.

THE PROBLEM

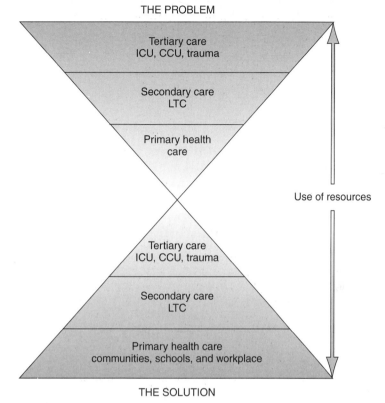

THE SOLUTION

FIGURE 3-3

Shifting the health care model. *(From American Nurses Association*: Primary health care: the nurse solution. Nursing facts, *Washington, DC, 1993, ANA.)*

Historically, NPs were able to enter the practice field in a variety of ways, as defined by the scope of their practice rather than their educational credentials. The scope of practice was defined by the board of nursing of the state in which the person was licensed as an RN. Thus, historically, a nurse could become an NP through a certificate program or other non–master's degree program. In 1987 the ANA, in its *Scope of Nursing* document, addressed the differences between the generalist and the specialist, making the distinction that the specialist has a graduate degree (ANA, 1987). Nurse practitioner programs have become integral parts of master's and even post-master's programs.

All types of advanced-practice nurse (APN) roles are responding to the changes in the health care arena. The need to redefine and clarify the terms and roles of professional nursing has never been more pressing, not only for the profession, but for the public. The movement toward a consensus on the definitions and the roles in advanced-practice nursing is occurring. Table 3-1 summarizes the terms and information regarding advanced-practice roles. As nursing struggles to develop this consensus, the issues of educational preparation and certification continue to challenge the profession. State boards of nursing reflect great variability in credentialing and advanced-practice roles in the legal language of scope of practice. For example, one of the oldest credentialed professional groups, nurse anesthetists, used certification—not education—to enter their professional specialty in 1952. Today, nurse anesthetists obtain certification at the graduate or the postgraduate level for entry into practice.

TABLE 3-1
Advanced-Practice Nursing

	Education	*What They Do*
Nurse Practitioner (NP)	Most of the approximately 150 NP education programs in the United States today confer a master's degree. At least 36 states require NPs to be nationally certified by the ANA or a specialty nursing organization. In March 2000, almost 45% of advanced-practice nurses were NPs.	Working in clinics, nursing homes, hospitals, or their own offices, NPs are qualified to handle a wide range of basic health problems. Most have a specialty— for example, adult, family, or pediatric health care. NPs conduct physical exams, take medical histories, diagnose and treat common acute minor illnesses or injuries, order and interpret lab tests and x-rays, and counsel and educate patients. In all states they may prescribe medication according to state law. Some work as independent practitioners and can be reimbursed by Medicare or Medicaid for services rendered. Others work for hospitals, HMOs, or private industry.
Certified Nurse-Midwife (CNM)	An average 1.5 years of specialized education beyond nursing school, either in an accredited certificate program or, like NPs, increasingly at the master's level.	CNMs provide well-woman gynecologic and low-risk obstetric care including prenatal, labor and delivery, and postpartum care. In 1998, the most current year data are available from the National Center for Health Statistics, there were 277,811 CNM-attended births in the United States. This accounted for 9% of all vaginal births that year. The number of CNM-attended births has increased every year since 1975. An ANA meta-analysis of CNM care found that nurse-midwives performed fewer fetal monitors, episiotomies, and forceps deliveries; administered fewer intravenous solutions; delivered fewer low birth-weight and premature infants; and had shorter patient hospital stays. CNMs have prescriptive authority in all 50 states.

(continued)

TABLE 3-1

Advanced-Practice Nursing *(Cont'd)*

	Education	*What They Do*
Clinical Nurse Specialist (CNS)	CNSs are the second-largest advanced-practice group. They are registered nurses with advanced nursing degrees—master's or doctoral—who are experts in a specialized area of clinical practice such as mental health, gerontology, cardiac or cancer care, or community or neonatal health. In 1998 it is estimated that there were 61,601 RNs prepared to practice as CNSs, including 7802 who were also licensed as NPs. Almost 91% of the 53,799 who were licensed solely as CNSs were employed in a nursing position; however, only 23% were practicing in a position with the title of CNS. Twenty-five percent were employed in nursing-education positions. Only 31% maintained national certification or state recognition, or both, as an advanced-practice nurse or CNS. In March 2000 almost 30% of advanced-practice nurses were CNSs.	CNSs work in hospitals, clinics, nursing homes, their own offices, and other community-based settings, such as industry, home care, and HMOs. Qualified to handle a wide range of physical and mental health problems, CNSs provide primary care and psychotherapy. They conduct health assessments, make diagnoses, deliver treatment, and develop quality-control methods. In addition to delivering direct patient care, CNSs work in consultation, research, education, and administration. Some work independently or in private practice and can be reimbursed by Medicare, Medicaid, Champus, and private insurers.
Certified Registered Nurse Anesthetist (CRNA)	CRNAs are registered nurses who complete a graduate program and meet national certification and recertification requirements.	In this oldest of the advanced nursing specialties, CRNAs administer approximately 65% of the 26 million anesthetics given to patients each year in the United States. As of October 2001, CRNAs were the sole anesthesia providers in nearly 50% of all hospitals and more than 65% of rural hospitals in the United States, enabling these health care facilities to provide obstetric, surgical, and trauma stabilization services. CRNAs provide anesthetics to patients in collaboration with surgeons, anesthesiologists, dentists, podiatrists, and other qualified health care professionals.

As more nurses in specialty practice organizations seek additional education credentials at the graduate level, certification will be offered both for the generalist and the specialist nurse.

Many barriers affect the growth of the role of advanced-practice nurse. Basic nursing education is slowly moving toward consensus. With improved articulation in educational programs, the terminology better defines the role and the scope of the advanced-practice nurse, and continued work with state licensing boards further supports the process. It has been suggested by the NCSBN that advanced-practice nurses have two levels of licensure rather than an RN license and certification in their field. Organizations such as the Pew Foundation challenge the system to reexamine these barriers, which often adversely affect the cost of the health care that advanced-practice nurses can deliver. The Pew publication "Reforming health care workforce regulation: policy considerations for the 21st century" (1994) explored how health care regulation protects the public health and proposed new approaches to health care work force regulation to better serve the public's needs. Pew also published a federal policy paper titled "Reforming Health Care Workforce for 2000" (1995) that identified nurse practitioners–advanced-practice nurses as part of the strategy to move the nation toward a more effective health care delivery system by 2005.

As a recent graduate you may want to explore the option of advanced-practice nursing as part of your long-term career goals. Both the NLN and the ANA have publications and videos about advanced-practice nursing. Check their Web sites for up-to-date information that may help you include specialty practice in the design of your 5-year career plan. In addition, reading about career roles for advanced practice and talking with APNs in your work sites can help you expand your career vision and plan for the future.

CONCLUSION

What are the ways in which nursing will be ready to meet the challenges of the changing health care environment? Does nursing clearly reflect professionalism? Is the image positive? Do we need to develop autonomy in practice? Who holds nursing accountable for practice in all areas? Is nursing ready to resolve educational splintering and work cooperatively at different levels of practice? Can nursing become more effective and active on the political front? How will research be used to advance practice both at the generalist and the specialist level? Is specialty practice and certification in that practice area the best method to affect clinical outcomes?

The questions go on and on. Answers to these questions will come from nurses in practice, education, and research in a collective fashion. Nurses in the United States have debated education issues for 120 years. These issues, which have a significant impact on nursing's professional image, must be resolved so nursing can move forward. As a recent graduate you will be a part of this exciting transition as nursing takes control and directs the course of its future.

As Winston Churchill said, "If we spend all our time debating the past, we shall lose the future."

REFERENCES

American Nurses Association: The study of credentialing in nursing: a new approach, vol 1-2 *Report of the committee*, Kansas City, Mo, 1978-1979, ANA.

American Nurses Association: *The scope of nursing*, Kansas City, Mo, 1987, ANA.

American Nurses Association: *Social policy statement*, Kansas City, Mo, 1988, ANA.

American Nurses Association: *The career credentials: professional certification. The 1990 certification catalog*, Kansas City, Mo, 1990, Center for Credentialing Services.

American Nurses Association: *Standards of clinical nursing practice*, Kansas City, Mo, 1991, ANA.

American Nurses Association: *American Nurse*, 24(10):16, 1992.

American Nurses Association: *Primary health care: the nurse solution, Nursing Facts*, Washington, DC, 1993, ANA.

American Nurses Credentialing Center: *1995 certification catalog*, Washington, DC, 1995: ANCC.

Benner J: How to navigate specialty certification, *Nursing* 30(8):52-53, 2000.

Blancett S, Flarey D: *Re-engineering in nursing and health care*, Baltimore, 1995, Aspen.

Bridges W: *Job shifts: how to prosper in a workplace without jobs*, New York, 1994, Addison-Wesley.

Caplow T: *The sociology of work*, Minneapolis, 1954, University of Minnesota.

Curtin L: Job security: is nothing sacred anymore? *Nurs Manage* 26(7):7-9, 1995.

Deloughery GL: *Issues and trends in nursing*, ed 2, St Louis, 1995, Mosby.

Flexner A: Is social work a profession? In *Proceedings of National Conference of Charities and Corrections*, Chicago, 1915, Hildeman.

Health Resources and Services Administration: *National sample survey of registered nurses*, Washington, DC, 2000, HRSA, Bureau of Health Professions, Division of Nursing.

Joel L: Viewpoints. In McCloskey J, Grace H, editors: *Current issues in nursing*, St Louis, 1994, Mosby.

Kulig N: Interstate licensure; nursing beyond your state's borders, *Nursing* 31(12):51, 2001.

Miller N: Leadership roundtable. *Nurs Econ*, 18(2), 2000.

Naisbitt J: *Megatrends*, New York, 1984, Warner.

Nardini J: Certification and credentialing—what does it mean to the patient? *Nephrol Nurs J*, 27(5), 2000.

National League for Nursing: *NLN updates*, New York, 1995, NLN.

Occupational outlook handbook, U.S. Department of Labor Government Bulletin 2500, 1998-1999.

Pavalko R: *Sociology of occupations and professions*, Itasca, Ill, 1971, Peacock.

Peplau H: *Interpersonal relationships in nursing*, New York, 1952, Putnam Press.

Pew Health Professions Commissions: *Reforming health care workforce for 2000—federal policy paper*, San Francisco, 1995, Center for the Health Professions.

Pinkerton SE: The future of professionalism in nursing, *Nurs Econ*, 2001.

Schaffer K: Research: future impact on image and retention, *Dimens Crit Care Nurs* 8(1), 1989.

Strauss A: *The structure and ideology of American nursing: an interpretation in the nursing profession*, New York, 1966, Wiley.

Sullivan E: *Reflections*, Sigma Theta Tau International, First Quarter, 4.

Talotta D: Role conceptions and professional role discrepancy among baccalaureate nursing students, *Image J Nurs Sch* 22(2):111-115, 1990.

Wallace B: Greetings from the executive director, *Media Watch* 1(1):1, 1990 (editorial).

Wallace B: *Reflections*, Sigma Theta Tau International, First Quarter, 28.

Watson J: Advanced nursing practice and what might be, *J Nurs Health Care*, 16(2):78-83, 1995.

ADDITIONAL READINGS

Aburdene P, Naisbitt J: *Megatrends for women,* New York, 1992, Villard.

Auttonberry D: The emerging role of the master's prepared nurse in marketing, *Nurs Manage* 19(9):40-42, 1988.

Gordon S: Prisoners of men's dreams, *Media Watch* 2(3), 1991.

Gordon S, Grady E: What's in a name? *Am J Nurs* 95(9):31-33, 1995.

Kaler SR, Levy DA, Schall M: Stereotypes of professional roles, *Image J Nurs Sch* 21(2):85-89, 1989.

Kalisch B, Kalisch P: Improving the image of nursing, *Am J Nurs* 83(1):48-52, 1983.

Levenstein A: The road to professional growth, *Nurs Manage* 15(7):60-61, 1984.

Naisbitt J. Aburdene P: *Megatrends 2000,* New York, 1990, William Morrow.

Pew Health Professions Commissions: *Reforming health care workforce regulation,* San Francisco, 1994, Center for the Health Professions.

INTERNET RESOURCES

National Student Nurses' Association
http://www.nsna.org
American Nurses Credentialing Center
http://www.nursingworld.org
National League for Nursing Accrediting Commission
http://www.nlnac.org

The following appendices list Web sites:

Appendix A: State Boards of Nursing

Appendix B: National Nursing Association

Appendix C: State Nursing Associations

Appendix E: Canadian Nursing Associations

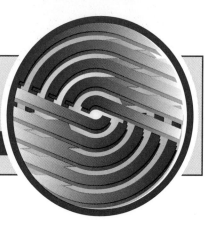

Nursing Education

GAYLE VARNELL, PhD, RN, CPNP

Education should not be a destination—but a path we travel all the days of our lives.

    —Anonymous

Education is the ability to listen to almost anything without losing your temper or your self-confidence.

    —Robert Frost

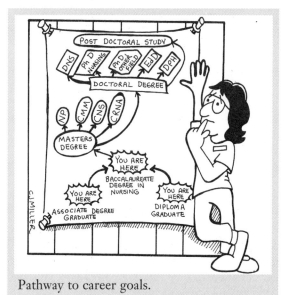

Pathway to career goals.

After completing this chapter, you should be able to:

■ Compare and contrast the types of educational preparation for nursing.

■ Describe the educational preparation for a graduate degree.

■ Compare and contrast the alternative options provided by career-ladder, external degree, Bachelor of Science in Nursing–completion, and university-without-walls programs.

■ Describe the purpose of nursing program accreditation.

■ Discuss the future of nursing education.

After struggling to complete your basic educational preparation for nursing, you are probably looking forward to that first paycheck as a registered nurse. The last thing on your mind is returning to school for more education! The purpose of this chapter is *not* to discuss the issue of entry into practice or to debate which educational program is best. Instead, the purpose of this chapter is to help you look at where you are educationally and to offer direction regarding educational opportunities to enhance your career goals. Before looking down the path at the variety of educational offerings available to help you meet those goals, let's look at the variety of pathways that lead to the basic educational preparation for an RN.

Which path did you travel? There are five paths that lead to one licensing examination: the National Council Licensure Examination for Registered Nurses (NCLEX-RN). The first three paths (diploma, associate's degree, and baccalaureate degree) are the most common and usually require a high school diploma or the equivalent for admission. The other, less common, paths are through master's and doctoral degree programs, both of which accept college graduates with liberal arts majors. Other paths that are becoming more popular are ladder programs (from practical nurse to associate degree nurse) and two-plus-two programs (from associate's degree to baccalaureate nurse).

PATH OF DIPLOMA EDUCATION

WHAT IS THE HISTORY OF DIPLOMA NURSING?

The oldest form of educational preparation leading to licensure as a RN in the United States is the diploma program. A large number of nurses practicing in the United States today received their basic educational preparation in a diploma program (Fig. 4-1). The first nurse training school was established at the New England Hospital for Women in 1872 (Kalisch and Kalisch, 1995). From that initial program, the number of diploma schools quickly increased from 15 in 1890 to 432 in 1900 (Bullough and Bullough, 1994). By the 1920s there were almost 2300 programs. However, during the Great Depression many of the hospital schools of nursing went bankrupt and had to close (Fitzpatrick, 1983).

In the beginning nursing education consisted of on-the-job training based mainly on the specific needs of the hospital in which the school of nursing was housed, not on the learning needs of the individual student. In other words, nursing students provided cheap or free labor.

These apprenticeship programs differed in quality and length. The size of the hospital influenced the experience of the nursing student. Larger hospitals offered more exposure to a variety of clinical experiences. Standardization of nursing programs was not considered until the publication of the National League for Nursing (NLN) (known earlier as the National League of Nursing Education) and the Winslow-Goldmark study of 1923. Standardization did not occur until the 1940s.

The theory classes taught in these early nursing schools were generally laid out in blocks of study that included medical nursing, surgical nursing, psychiatric nursing, obstetrics, pediatrics, operating room, and emergency department experience, in addition

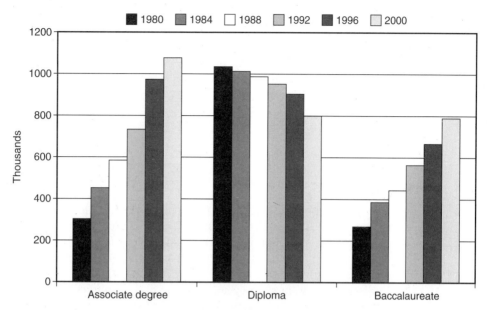

FIGURE 4-1

Basic Nursing Education of the Registered Nurse Population, 1980-2000
In March 2000 the distribution of the RN population according to the highest education
level, which incorporates any post-RN degree received, revealed that 22.3% (about 609,000)
reported having a diploma, 34.3% (about 925,000) reported having an associate degree, 32.7%
(about 881,000) reported having a baccalaureate degree, and 10.2% (about 275,000) reported
having a master's or doctoral degree. *(From Health Resources and Services Administration:* HRSA
Bureau of Health Professions Division of Nursing sample survey, *2000, HRSA.)*

to classes in anatomy, physiology, nutrition, pharmacology, the history of nursing, and
often a course called "professional adjustments." Nursing students would work on a
unit in the hospital, attend class for a few hours, and then return to work additional
hours on a unit. A typical day could be 12 or more hours in length. Nursing students
covered all three hospital shifts.

In the early diploma schools, a typical student was a single woman who lived in a
dormitory with other nursing students. There were strict codes of conduct that had
to be followed and rigid dress codes. Anyone who did not follow these rules was
subject to expulsion from the program. For example, married students were not
allowed in the program. If a student married, she hid her marriage or was subject to
expulsion from the program. In many of the diploma schools, these strict rules and
regulations were not relaxed until the 1960s.

Education in diploma schools emphasized the skills needed to care for the acutely
ill patient. Graduates received a diploma in nursing, not an academic degree. From
1872 until the mid-1960s, the hospital diploma program was the dominant nursing
program. In 1980, however, diploma schools accounted for only 8% of all nursing
education programs as compared with 80% during 1959 and 1960 (Rowland and
Rowland, 1984). The number of diploma schools has decreased to 86, or less than

10% (NLN, 2001). Perhaps one of the reasons for this decline was that the courses offered by hospitals frequently did not confer college credit. Students interested in furthering their nursing education would naturally be discouraged by the lack of transferability of the diploma education program. Although the majority of current diploma programs are associated with institutions of higher learning where the graduates receive some college credit, they still may not receive college credit for the nursing courses. Other diploma programs have evolved into what is called a *single-purpose institution*, having baccalaureate-degree–granting privileges for nursing only.

WHAT IS THE EDUCATIONAL PREPARATION OF THE DIPLOMA GRADUATE?

The current preparation of a diploma nurse varies in length from 1 to 3 years and takes place in a hospital school of nursing. This type of program may be under the direction of the hospital or incorporated independently. The diploma program may include general education subjects such as biology and physical and social sciences, in addition to nursing theory and practice. The diploma program serves qualified applicants who want an early and ongoing opportunity to be in contact with patients and other health care personnel (NLN, 1989a).

Graduates of diploma programs are prepared to function as beginning practitioners in acute, intermediate, long-term, and ambulatory health care facilities. Graduates of a diploma program are prepared for beginning supervisory or management positions in their hospital settings.

Standards and competencies for diploma programs are developed and maintained by the NLN Council of Diploma Programs. Graduates of diploma programs are eligible to take the NCLEX-RN state board examination for licensure.

The advantages of diploma programs include having nursing instructors who are actively involved in clinical practice. Graduates of diploma schools have the greatest amount of clinical experience in a hospital setting. Because there is a close relationship between the nursing school and the hospital, graduates are well prepared to function in that institution; on graduation, many graduates are employed by that hospital and therefore experience an easier role transition.

In diploma schools, theory and clinical practice are introduced concurrently. Diploma nursing students, according to Hocker (1984, p. 38), "are offered nursing theory equivalent to that offered in the other RN preparatory schools." Choinski et al (1978, p. 28) further state that nursing courses in baccalaureate programs usually are "limited to the last two academic years, or approximately 18 months, while diploma schools offer from 24 to 36 months of nursing theory and practice."

PATH OF ASSOCIATE DEGREE EDUCATION

WHAT IS THE HISTORY OF ASSOCIATE DEGREE NURSING?

The associate degree nursing program has the distinction of being the first and, to date, only educational program for nursing that was developed from planned research and controlled experimentation. Since its beginning in 1951, the associate degree nursing program has grown to more than 900 programs, producing more graduates annually than either diploma or baccalaureate programs. Graduates are employed in hospitals, outpatient departments, nursing homes, physicians' offices, and home care agencies.

In 1951 Mildred Montag published her doctoral dissertation, *The education of nursing technicians*, which proposed education for the RN in the community college. Dr. Montag suggested that the associate degree program be a terminal degree to prepare nurses for immediate employment. According to Dr. Montag, there was a need for a new type of nurse, the "nurse technician," whose role would be broader than that of a practical nurse but narrower than that of the professional nurse. The technical nurse was to function at the "bedside." The duties of the technical nurse, according to Dr. Montag, would include (1) giving general nursing care with supervision, (2) assisting in the planning of nursing care for clients, and (3) assisting in the evaluation of the nursing care given (Montag, 1951).

In 1952 an advisory committee was established by the American Association of Junior Colleges. Along with the NLN, this committee was to conduct cooperative research on nursing education in the community college. The goals of this Cooperative Research Project were threefold: (1) to describe the development of the associate degree nursing program, (2) to evaluate the associate degree graduates, and (3) to determine the future implications of the associate degree on nursing. The original project was directed by Dr. Montag at Teachers College of Columbia University and included seven junior colleges and one hospital from each of the six regions of the United States.

In the proposed technical nursing curriculum, there was to be a balance between general education and nursing courses. Unlike the diploma programs, the emphasis was to be on education, not service. At the end of 2 years, the student was to be awarded an associate's degree in nursing and was to be eligible to take the state board examinations for RN licensure. This degree was seen as terminal and not a step toward obtaining a baccalaureate degree (Montag, 1959).

WHAT IS THE EDUCATIONAL PREPARATION OF THE ASSOCIATE DEGREE GRADUATE?

The current preparation of an associate degree nurse usually begins within a community college, although some programs are based within a senior college or university. The program is 18 to 21 school calendar months in length. The NLN recommends that the program of learning be within 60 to 72 semester credits (90-108 quarter credits) and that there be a balanced distribution of no more than 60% of the total number of credits allocated to nursing courses (NLN, 2000). In some programs, the student must complete the general education and science course requirements before beginning the nursing courses. At the end of the program, the student receives an associate's degree in nursing.

Associate degree nursing education has helped to bring about a change in the type of student who enrolls in nursing programs. Traditionally, nursing students were usually single, white females younger than 19 years of age from middle-class families (Kaiser, 1975). Associate degree programs attract a more diverse student population of older individuals, minorities, men, and married women from a variety of educational backgrounds. Many of these individuals have baccalaureate and higher degrees in other fields of study and are seeking a second career. Along with their maturity, these students bring life experiences that are applicable to nursing. The students tend to be more goal-oriented and have a more realistic perspective of the work setting. The community college curriculum is conducive to students who want to attend school on a part-time basis.

Standards and competencies for associate degree programs are developed and maintained by the NLN Council of Associate Degree Programs. At the NLN 1998 Education Summit, the associate degree in nursing (ADN) competencies were revised to include multiculturalism, long-term care, systems management, and interdisciplinary collaboration. Graduates of associate degree programs are eligible to take the NCLEX-RN state board examination for licensure.

Dr. Montag's original proposal for the associate degree program to be a terminal degree is no longer applicable. In 1978, the American Nurses Association proposed a resolution regarding associate degree programs that stated that they be viewed as part of the career upward-mobility plan rather than as terminal programs. The associate degree program has provided students with the motivation to further their educations and the opportunity for career mobility. Although many nursing students end their education with an associate's degree, many enter the associate degree program with every intention of continuing their nursing education to the baccalaureate level and even further. There are 885 ADN programs in the United States (NLN, 2001).

PATH OF BACCALAUREATE EDUCATION

In this discussion, only the "generic" baccalaureate programs are addressed. A *generic student* is defined as a student who enters a baccalaureate nursing program with no training or education in nursing. A *generic program* is defined as a program that includes lower-division (freshman and sophomore) liberal arts and science courses with upper-division (junior and senior) nursing courses. RNs entering baccalaureate programs are discussed later in this chapter.

WHAT IS THE HISTORY OF BACCALAUREATE NURSING?

A few early training schools were affiliated with universities to provide some of the science courses. In 1889 Mercy Hospital in Chicago affiliated with Northwestern University. The science courses offered to nursing students were outside the academic curriculum and did not lead to a degree. Teacher's College of Columbia University also played a critical role in the establishment of baccalaureate nursing education by establishing a 1-year course in hospital economics in 1899. The course was extended to 2 years in 1905 (Anderson, 1981).

The early baccalaureate nursing programs were usually 5 years in length and consisted of the basic 3-year diploma program with an additional 2 years of liberal arts. In 1919 there were eight baccalaureate programs. At present there are 695 baccalaureate programs in the United States (NLN, 2001).

WHAT IS THE EDUCATIONAL PREPARATION OF THE BACCALAUREATE GRADUATE?

The current preparation of a baccalaureate nurse is 4 to 5 years in length (120-140 credits) and emphasizes courses in the liberal arts, sciences, and humanities. Approximately half to two thirds of the curriculum consists of nonnursing courses. To qualify for a baccalaureate program, the student must first meet all of the college's or the university's entrance requirements. Usual entrance requirements include college preparation courses in high school (e.g., foreign language, advanced science, and math courses) and a high cumulative grade-point average. Most colleges also require a college entrance examination such as the Scholastic Aptitude Test (SAT) or the American College Test (ACT).

During the first 2 years of college, the student is usually enrolled in liberal arts and science courses with other nonnursing students. It is not until late in the sophomore or early junior year that nursing courses are introduced. The emphasis in the baccalaureate nursing program is on developing critical decision-making skills, exercising independent nursing judgment, and acquiring research skills.

The graduate of a baccalaureate program must fulfill both the degree requirements of the nursing program and those of the college. On completion of the program, the usual degree awarded is a Bachelor of Science in Nursing (BSN).

The graduate of a baccalaureate program is prepared to provide health promotion and health restoration care for individuals, families, and groups in a variety of institutional and community settings. Graduates of baccalaureate nursing programs are eligible to take the NCLEX-RN state board examination for licensure.

NONTRADITIONAL PATHS FOR NURSING EDUCATION

WHAT ABOUT A MASTER'S DEGREE AS A PATH TO BECOMING AN RN?

Master's degree (MSN) programs are particularly attractive to the growing number of college graduates who later in their lives decide to enter nursing (Berlin and Bednash, 1995). There are a few colleges and universities that offer master's degree programs leading to the initial professional degree in nursing. Yale University, the University of Texas at Austin, and the University of Tennessee are among the institutions that have such programs. Generally the program is 2 years long. On graduation these students are expected to demonstrate the same entry-level competencies in nursing as baccalaureate graduates. MSN graduates are then eligible to take the NCLEX-RN.

WHAT ABOUT A DOCTORAL PATH TO BECOMING AN RN?

The last path, and the least common, leading to the RN licensure examination is the doctoral degree. This program was begun in 1979 at Case Western Reserve University. Rush University in Chicago initiated a similar program in 1988, and the

University of Colorado began one in 1990 (Forni, 1989). These programs provide basic nursing courses, along with advanced nursing courses. On completion the graduate is eligible to take the NCLEX-RN.

GRADUATE EDUCATION

WHAT ABOUT GRADUATE SCHOOL?

Whatever path you chose to become an RN, there is one thing for certain: It wasn't easy. After putting life, liberty, and the pursuit of happiness on hold while you worked toward becoming an RN, it may seem like pure insanity to subject yourself to more education!

Graduate nursing education, like other graduate programs, is responding to changes in social values, priorities in the public sector, and student demographics, in addition to technological advances, knowledge development, and maturity of the profession (McCloskey and Grace, 1997).

Graduate education programs are available on either a part-time or a full-time basis. Graduate programs require a good grade-point average at the undergraduate level. Prerequisites for most graduate programs are satisfactory scores on the Graduate Record Examination or the Miller Analogies Test, or both. It is strongly recommended that all students, whether they plan to pursue graduate studies or not, take the Graduate Record Examination after completing their undergraduate studies. Taking another test may be the last thing you want to do, but it is much easier to do it now, while the information is current in your mind, than later, when you decide that you want to continue your education.

WHAT IS THE HISTORY OF GRADUATE NURSING EDUCATION?

Graduate nursing programs in the United States originated during the late 1800s. As more nursing schools sought to strengthen their own programs, there was increased pressure on nursing instructors to obtain advanced preparation in education and clinical nursing specialties.

The Catholic University of America in Washington, DC, offered one of the early graduate programs for nurses. It began offering courses in nursing education in 1932 and conferring a master's degree in nursing education in 1935.

The NLN's Subcommittee on Graduate Education first published guidelines for organization, administration, curriculum, and testing in 1957. These guidelines have been revised throughout the years and reflect the focus in master's education on research and clinical specialization.

Until the 1960s the master's degree in nursing was viewed as a terminal degree. The goal of graduate education was to prepare nurses for teaching, administration, and supervisory positions. In the early 1970s the emphasis shifted to developing clinical skills and the roles of clinical specialists and nurse practitioners emerged. By the late 1970s the focus again shifted back to teaching, administration, and supervisory positions (McCloskey and Grace, 1997).

In response to health care reform, the number of master's programs has increased. The total number of master's programs is now 358 (NLN, 2001). A nurse may consider a master's or advanced degree in one of the following areas: administration, education, anesthesia, midwifery, practice, clinical nursing specialty, nursing informatics, or nursing research (Kelly, 2000).

WHY WOULD I WANT A MASTER'S DEGREE?

 You've got to be kidding! More school?

Sure, an advanced degree may not be in your career plans right now, but later on, after you have been practicing nursing, you may change your mind. Policy statements from the nursing profession reflect the need for more education in preparation for nursing's changing role, a result of health care reform. As care delivery moves increasingly from the acute-care center to the community setting, there will be an increased need for advanced clinical practice nurses. Nursing programs are already responding to this changing need. There has been an increase in the number of master's nurse practitioner programs, bringing the total to 199 programs in 1995 (NLN, 1997). Areas of specialty within the master's nurse practitioner programs include family, acute care, pediatric, psychiatric, geriatric, school health, and adult nursing practice. There are more family nurse practitioner programs than any other program.

According to the National Sample Survey of Registered Nurses March 2000 information on RNs prepared for advanced practice, there are 88,186 nurse practitioners, 54,374 clinical nurse specialists, 9,232 nurse-midwives, 29,844 nurse anesthetists, and 14,643 nurse practitioner/clinical nurse specialists (Fig. 4-2). To take advantage of these trends and better position yourself in the job market, you might find that the benefits of returning to school far outweigh the sacrifices.

Master's programs vary from institution to institution, as do the admission and course requirements and costs. The majority of programs are at least 1 full year in length, with many programs being expanded to 2 years. In the more traditional programs, the student takes the courses required for the degree and then, depending on institutional requirements, may also be required to take a written or oral comprehensive examination or write a thesis, or both. There are also nontraditional models that include outreach programs, summers-only programs, and RN-to-MSN tracks for RNs who do not have undergraduate degrees and RNs who have bachelor's degrees in other fields.

Advances in technology have also made it possible for graduate programs to become more creative in the way courses are being offered. It is now possible for students to obtain all or part of their course offerings by means of the Internet, distance-learning, computer-based programs, and teleconferencing. This flexibility is making it easier for students in rural communities and part-time students to obtain advanced degrees.

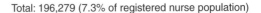

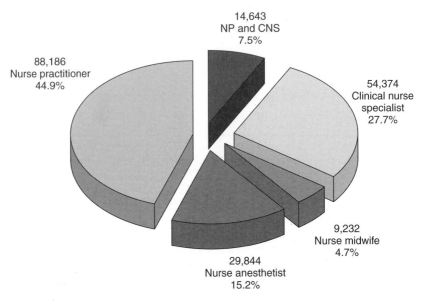

FIGURE 4-2
Registered Nurses Prepared for Advanced Practice, March 2000
Total: 196,279 (7.3% of Registered Nurse Population)
(From Health Resources and Services Administration: HRSA Bureau of Health Professions
Division of Nursing sample survey, *2000, the HRSA.)*
NP, Nurse practitioner; *CNS*, clinical nurse specialist.

In choosing a program for graduate studies, one of the best sources of information is the NLN's *Annual guide to graduate nursing education 1997*. In the future, we will see even more types of programs being designed to meet the needs of the returning graduate student.

HOW DO I KNOW WHICH MASTER'S DEGREE PROGRAM IS RIGHT FOR ME?

In choosing a program for graduate studies, one of the best sources of information is the NLN. The NLN also publishes a list of NLN-accredited programs in nursing education at the doctoral, master's, baccalaureate, associate's, and diploma levels, in addition to information on scholarships and loans for nursing education.

Your career goals and interests will help you to determine which choice is best for you. Keep in mind that one way to expand your nursing base is to attend a graduate school in a different area of the country than where you obtained your undergraduate education. A person's knowledge base is thought to be more marketable if they are not "inbred," which means that the person hasn't earned all of his or her degrees from one institution. If this is not a possibility for you, choose the next-best route to obtain your career goals. Consider all the options. After all, if you are going to expend the time, energy, and finances to obtain a graduate degree, you want to get the most from it.

WHY WOULD I WANT A DOCTORAL DEGREE?

Power, authority, and professional status are usually associated with a doctoral degree. Nurses with doctoral degrees provide leadership in the improvement of nursing practice and in the development of research and nursing education programs. It is no secret that the role of the nurse is changing and will continue to change as health care reform is being implemented. There is a growing need for administrators, policy analysts, clinical researchers, and clinical practitioners both within the community and governmental agencies. Nurses need to position themselves to take on these new leadership roles, and the way to do this is through advanced education, particularly at the doctoral level (Dennis, 1991).

There are two basic models of doctoral education in nursing: the academic degree, or Doctor of Philosophy (PhD), and the professional degree, or Doctor of Nursing Science (DNS, DSN, or DNSc). The total number of doctoral programs in nursing in the United States is now 75. The PhD continues to be the most highly esteemed degree in higher education. Nurses also have other doctoral degree options available to them, such as the Doctor of Education (EdD), the Doctor of Public Health (DPH), the Doctor of Philosophy in a discipline besides nursing, the nontraditional external-degree doctorate, and the Nurse Doctorate (ND).

The doctorate in nursing is basically a new concept. Before 1965 the most common doctoral degree earned by nurses was the EdD. It was not until the establishment of the federally supported Nurse Scientist Training Program in 1962 that a shift toward obtaining a PhD began. The DNS has been awarded since the early 1960s (Rowland and Rowland, 1984).

HOW DO I KNOW WHICH DOCTORAL PROGRAM IS RIGHT FOR ME?

As with the master's degree, it is important to look at your career goals before deciding which doctoral program is best for you. To help you with that task, look at the NLN publications specific to doctoral education. Ask yourself how much time you can devote to obtaining a doctorate degree. The average time needed to complete a doctoral program is 4.5 years (Rowland and Rowland, 1984). Can you be a full-time student, or must you continue to work? What do you plan to do with the degree once you get it?

"Today, a doctorate in nursing should be the first choice for nurses seeking doctoral education" (Allen, 1990). Is this a realistic goal? Is there an institution available to you that offers a doctorate in nursing or would you have to consider moving? What are your career and professional goals? Do you want to teach? The PhD is considered the research degree. It prepares an individual for a lifetime of intellectual inquiry and has an increased emphasis on postdoctoral study. In contrast, the DNS is viewed as the practical degree. The goal of this program is to prepare an advanced practitioner for the application of knowledge with an emphasis on research. The original intent of the DNS was to prepare nurses to do clinical research. Deans of nursing programs state that they prefer a PhD in nursing to a PhD in another discipline or a DNS (Allen, 1990).

OTHER TYPES OF NURSING EDUCATION

WHAT ARE THE OTHER AVAILABLE EDUCATIONAL OPTIONS?

In the 1960s baccalaureate programs made it very difficult for the RN to return to school to earn a baccalaureate in nursing. Most of the time these nurses found themselves receiving no credit for their past education or experience. A resolution passed in 1978 by the ANA that urged the creation of quality career-mobility programs with flexibility to assist individuals desiring academic degrees in nursing helped to change this philosophy. There are several basic patterns for achieving upward mobility in nursing, and within these basic patterns there are many variations. Career-ladder programs, BSN-completion programs, external-degree programs, and university-without-walls programs are the basic patterns that will be addressed in this section. In assessing the educational options that are available, one source of information is the *Directory of career mobility opportunities in nursing* published by the NLN. This directory, covering the United States and its jurisdictions, presents a current listing of nursing programs that give students mobility to advance their careers by offering varying degrees of credit for relevant education and experience. The potential student should also contact individual schools for information regarding their particular programs. Schools' addresses can be found in the NLN directory.

What Is a Career-Ladder Program? The career-ladder concept focuses on the articulation of educational programs to permit advanced placement without loss of credit or repetition. There are many variations on this type of program. Multiple-exit programs provide opportunities for students to exit and reenter the educational system at various designated times having gained specific education and skills. An example is a program that ranges from practical nurse to RN at the associate's, baccalaureate, master's, and doctoral levels. A student in such a program may decide to leave the educational system at the completion of a specific level and be eligible to take the licensure examination applicable to that educational level. On termination, the student may choose to work for a while and later return for more education at the next level without having to repeat courses on previously acquired knowledge or skills.

One such program is Project LINC (Ladders in Nursing Careers), which was developed in the city of New York for the purpose of providing educational advancement opportunities for individuals who are in entry- or midlevel jobs in nursing. It is a collaborative effort involving more than 40 hospitals and long-term care facilities in the New York metropolitan area and serves as a state and national model of educational mobility.

A growing number of basic nursing education programs within the community-college setting are beginning to offer career-ladder–type programs, affiliating themselves with upper-division colleges in the area. A student can enter the community college to spend 1 year studying to become a practical or vocational nurse. After a year, the student can decide to stop and take the practical nurse licensure examination or continue and complete the associate's degree in nursing. At the end of the second year, the student is eligible to take the RN licensure examination and may choose either to exit as an associate degree nurse or attend an affiliated upper-division college to obtain a baccalaureate degree.

What Is a BSN-Completion Program?

A BSN-completion program is a baccalaureate program designed for students who already possess either a diploma or an associate's degree in nursing and hold a current license to practice as an RN. Depending on the part of the country, these programs may also be known as *RN baccalaureate (RNB) programs*, *baccalaureate RN (BRN) programs*, *two-plus-two*, or *capstone programs*. In the majority of programs, nurses receive transfer credit in basic education courses taken at other institutions plus either some transfer credit for their previous nursing courses or the opportunity to receive nursing credit by passing a nursing challenge exam. The usual length of such programs is 2 years, depending on the number of course requirements completed at the time of admission to the program. In an effort to meet the needs of the returning student, many BSN-completion programs offer flexible class scheduling, which allows the student to continue working while going to school. Another innovation being implemented to address the needs of individuals seeking baccalaureate degrees in outlying geographic areas is telecommunication-assisted studies and Internet courses.

What Is an External-Degree Program?

The external-degree program gives credit for an individual's knowledge, regardless of how that knowledge was acquired. The external-degree program is a nontraditional program that allows a student to gain credit, meet external-degree requirements, and obtain a degree from a degree-granting institution without attending classes. Two examples of external-degree programs for RN education are the New York Board of Regents external degree programs (REX) for associate (ADN) and BSN education. Both of these programs are designed to allow individuals to obtain a degree in nursing without leaving their jobs or their communities. These programs are NLN-accredited. In these programs all students are required to pass specific college-level tests and performance examinations in two components: general education and nursing. Tests are administered in several cities throughout the United States. On completion of the external-degree program, students are eligible in most states to take the RN licensure exam. There are also external-degree programs in which a person can earn a doctoral degree.

What Is a University Without Walls?

The university-without-walls concept allows an RN to obtain a baccalaureate degree by taking courses at a local college or community college instead of on the university campus that will confer the degree. The student is usually assigned an on-campus adviser who helps plan the course of study to meet the college requirements. Past education and work experiences are taken into consideration. Instead of the traditional approach to grading and recording credit hours, a file is kept by the student and routinely reviewed with the on-campus adviser. When all the requirements are successfully met, a bachelor of arts degree is awarded.

Michigan State University School of Nursing and Skidmore College in Saratoga Springs, New York, offer university-without-walls programs. The advantages of this type of program include the following:

- Ability of an individual to remain employed while working on continuing education

- Flexibility of course design that gives credit for experience
- Elimination of travel costs
- Opportunity to apply newly acquired knowledge to the work setting
- Ability to accommodate older students, who may feel out of place in a regular college-campus setting.

In summary, there are many paths that all lead to the same destination: the opportunity to take the licensure examination to become an RN.

Internet Resources. Besides the traditional method of education, more and more colleges and universities are offering courses and even entire programs by means of the World Wide Web. One of the largest NLNAC (National League for Nursing Accrediting Commission)–approved programs for BSN completion and graduate education is the University of Phoenix, Online campus. Nursing education online is a rapidly expanding part of the Internet. At times it can be confusing and overwhelming trying to find these courses. There are several sites that are available to help locate the courses (and course descriptions) that are being taught on the Internet, in addition to the colleges and universities that are offering the courses. See the Internet resources listed at the end of this chapter.

ACCREDITATION

Why should you be concerned whether the nursing program you are attending, or thinking about attending, is accredited? Accreditation assures you, the student, and the public that educational standards over and above the legal requirements of the state have been achieved. It guarantees the student the opportunity to obtain a quality education. Accreditation is strictly a voluntary process. The U.S. Department of Education approves the professional association that is allowed to accredit nursing schools. Until 1997 the NLN was the only accrediting body for nursing programs. In 1997 the NLNAC was established, and responsibility for all accrediting activities was transferred to this new independent subsidiary. Around the same time, the American Association of Colleges of Nursing (AACN) sought recognition from the U.S. Department of Education to accredit baccalaureate and graduate degree nursing programs because membership in AACN is restricted to deans and directors of baccalaureate and graduate programs. The Task Force on Accreditation of Health Professions Education of the Pew Commission issued a report in June 1999. The accreditation report may be accessed on the UCSF Center for the Health Professions Web site at http://futurehealth.ucsf.edu.

Some graduate nursing programs require completion of an NLN-approved undergraduate program as a prerequisite for admission to their master's or doctoral program. The NLN publishes an official complete list of NLN-accredited programs annually. Accreditation becomes a major concern as more and more courses and programs are offered by means of distance-learning.

With two organizations offering accreditation to schools of nursing, it was difficult for schools of nursing to develop competency statements that were consistent. Rather than listing competency statements for three levels of nursing, the competency statement accepted by the 1996 annual meeting of the National Council of State Boards of Nursing (NCSBN) is presented. According to the NCSBN, "Competence is defined as the application of knowledge and the interpersonal, decision-making and psychomotor skills expected for the practice role, within the context of public health, safety and welfare" (NCSBN, 1996, p. 47).

It is the opinion of the NCSBN that a competency statement must be applicable to all nurses at every level of practice. This allows the state boards of nursing to hold the nurse accountable to their individual scopes of practice, which ensures the safety of the public. Standards for competency were established that specified expectations that were reasonable, enforceable, and essential to the safe and effective practice from the beginning nurse to the most experienced one (Fig. 4-3).

The promotion of competency requires a collaborative approach; it involves the individual nurse, employers of nurses, nursing educators, and the regulating board of nursing. The roles of each of these in competence accountability are described in Figure 4-3.

NURSING EDUCATION: FUTURE TRENDS

Education is a lifelong process and an empowering force that enables an individual to achieve higher goals. Student access to educational opportunities is paramount to nursing education. A chapter on nursing education would not be complete without taking a look at the future.

The Changing Student Profile. Future nursing programs will need to be flexible to meet the learning needs of a changing student population. It has previously been stated that there is a growing population of nontraditional students—individuals who are making midlife career changes in part because of job displacement or job dissatisfaction. The student population tends to be older, married, and with families. More poor, minority, and foreign students are looking toward nursing education for career opportunities. There is a growing number of students choosing to attend school part time.

These changes mean that nurse educators will have to further address the needs of the adult learner. More programs will be needed that permit part-time study and allow students to work while attending school. One option may be for more night or weekend course offerings. There will continue to be a need for emphasis on remedial education such as developmental courses in math, English, and English as a second language. The diversity in the student population means diversity in learning rates, which might be addressed with more self-paced learning modules.

Educational Mobility. Educational mobility will also need to be addressed further. A growing number of individuals in health care are seeking more education. The issue is not one of entry into practice, but rather of how to best facilitate the return of

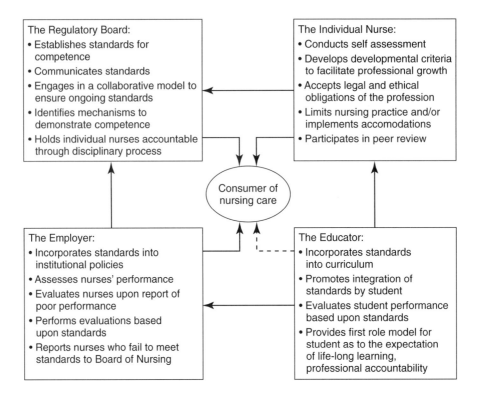

The Regulatory Board:
• Establishes standards for competence
• Communicates standards
• Engages in a collaborative model to ensure ongoing standards
• Identifies mechanisms to demonstrate competence
• Holds individual nurses accountable through disciplinary process

The Individual Nurse:
• Conducts self assessment
• Develops developmental criteria to facilitate professional growth
• Accepts legal and ethical obligations of the profession
• Limits nursing practice and/or implements accomodations
• Participates in peer review

Consumer of nursing care

The Employer:
• Incorporates standards into institutional policies
• Assesses nurses' performance
• Evaluates nurses upon report of poor performance
• Performs evaluations based upon standards
• Reports nurses who fail to meet standards to Board of Nursing

The Educator:
• Incorporates standards into curriculum
• Promotes integration of standards by student
• Evaluates student performance based upon standards
• Provides first role model for student as to the expectation of life-long learning, professional accountability

Actions of boards of nursing that assure competence to the public:
1. Establish competence requirements for safe and effective practice.
2. Communicate standards to the consumers, nurses, nursing educators, employers, and other regulators.
3. Hold individual nurses accountable for continued competence.
4. Engage in collaborative activities with nurses, educators, employers, and consumers to ensure nurses practice safely and effectively.
5. Identify a variety of techniques nurses may employ to demonstrate competence.
6. Discipline nurses who fail to meet standards for safe and effective practice.
7. Inform the public of disciplinary actions taken against nurses.
8. Establish nondisciplinary model to monitor and/or limit the practice of nurses who demonstrate inability to carry out essential nursing role functions.

FIGURE 4-3

Competence accountability
(From National Council of State Boards of Nursing: Definition of competence and standards for competence National Council of State Boards of Nursing, annual meeting: In Book of reports, Chicago, 1996, NCSBN, p. 51.)

these individuals to nursing school for educational advancement. Arkansas, California, Colorado, Florida, Hawaii, Maryland, Minnesota, Missouri, New Mexico, North Dakota, Texas, and Utah have already established statewide articulation programs to offer greater career mobility in nursing (McHugh, 1991). Additional states are currently studying articulation programs.

A Shortage of Qualified Nursing Faculty. Data on faculty reported by the AACN for 1999 and 2000 indicate that the average age of faculty has increased to a mean of 50.2 years for all faculty (AACN, 2000). Because of the decrease in the number of students entering the nursing profession and then choosing to teach, the number of qualified faculty will continue to decline. Predictions have one third of the nursing faculty retiring or resigning from 1992 through 2006 (Buerhaus, 2000).

Technology and Education. Educational learning will continue to change with technological advances in telecommunication and computer-assisted instruction. Nurses and nurse educators will need education to implement these advances into the curriculum and into nursing practice. As with cable television, which has extended the boundaries of the classroom, these new technologies will facilitate the offering of outreach programs.

Changing Health Care Settings. There has been a major shift from inpatient to outpatient nursing services as health care and nursing focuses on maintaining health rather then dealing with illness. However, with an increase in the age of the population there are more patients in the hospital with multiple chronic problems. Society is now developing a variety of new health care settings. Are nurses educated for these new roles? What will be the role of the advanced practitioner? Will there be enough nurses educationally prepared to meet these new challenges?

The Aging Population. There is a growing aging population. According to the Administration on Aging, by 2030 there will be approximately 70 million people over the age of 65 years, representing 20% of the population (2000). Naisbitt and Aburdene stated in their book *Megatrends 2000*, published in 1990, "If business and society can master the challenge of daycare, we will be one step closer to confronting the next great care giving task of the 1990s—eldercare." This is still a critical issue in the twenty-first century. Already the United States has well over 2000 adult daycare centers. Nursing educators need to address the provision of health care to the elderly and include it in the curricula.

What great opportunities in nursing!!

The future of nursing looks bright and exciting. With technological advances, changes in health care settings, increased demand for the services of the RN, and the shift back to the acute-care setting, nurses now have increased opportunities to chart their own destinies.

Nurses who have career plans and career goals will see the future trends in health care as a challenge and an opportunity for career growth in areas such as case manager, independent consultant, nurse practitioner, policy maker, or entrepreneur. In contrast, nurses without career goals may find themselves displaced or obsolete. There is not a more exciting time to be entering the profession of nursing than right now. Opportunities in nursing are wide open to those with the sensitivity and the creativity to embrace the future.

REFERENCES

Administration on Aging Web site http://www.aoa. gov/aoa/STATS/profile/default.htm#older. Accessed June 1, 2001.

American Association of Colleges of Nursing: *1999-2000 enrollments and graduations in baccalaureate and graduate programs in nursing*, Washington, DC, 2000, AACN.

Allen J: *Consumers guide to doctoral degree programs in nursing*, National League for Nursing Publication No. 15-2293, New York, 1990, NLN.

Anderson N.E: The historical development of American nursing education, *J Nurs Educ* 20(1):18-36, 1981.

Berlin L, Bednash G: *1994-1995 enrollments and graduations in baccalaureate and graduate programs in nursing*, AACN Publication No. 94-95-1, Washington, DC, 1995, AACN.

Buerhaus PI: A nursing shortage with a fundamental difference. *Syllabus Am Assoc Coll Nurs* 26(5):3-4, 7, 2000.

Bullough B, Bullough V: *Nursing issues for the nineties and beyond*, New York, 1994, Springer.

Choinski C, Hamer C, Hamm S, Macdonald M, et al: Sound off! Playing with the entry requirement: a game we can't afford, *RN* 41(12):27-32, 1978.

Definition of Competence and Standards for Competence National Council of State Boards of Nursing, Annual Meeting: *Book of reports*, NCSBN, 43-56, Chicago, 1996, the NCSBN.

Dennis KE: Components of the doctoral curriculum that build success in the clinical nurse researcher role, *J Prof Nurs* 7(3):160-165, 1991.

Fitzpatrick ML: *Prologue to professionalism: a history of nursing*, Bowie, Md, 1983, Robert J. Brady.

Forni PR: Models for doctoral programs: first professional degree or terminal degree? *Nurs Health Care* 10(8):429-434, 1989.

Health Resources and Services Administration (March 2000): HRSA Bureau of Health Professions Division of Nursing National Sample Survey, http://bhpr. hrsa.gov/dn/dn.html, accessed September 8, 2001.

Hocker BB: *Reflections of the characteristics of diploma programs and competencies of the graduates in the curriculum*, National League for Nursing Publication No. 16-1953, New York, 1984, the NLN.

Kaiser JE: *A comparison of students in practical nursing programs and in associate degree nursing programs*, National League for Nursing Publication No. 23-1592, New York, 1975, the NLN.

Kalisch PA, Kalisch BJ: *Advance of American nursing*, ed 3, Philadelphia, 1995, Lippincott Williams and Wilkins.

Kelly M: *NLN (National League for Nursing) official guide to graduate nursing schools*, Boston, 2000, Jones & Bartlett.

McCloskey J, Grace HK: *Current issues in nursing*, ed 5, St Louis, 1997, Mosby.

McHugh MK: Direct articulation of AD nursing students into an RN-to-BSN completion program: A research study, *J Nurs Educ* 30(7):293-296, 1991.

Montag ML: *The education of nursing technicians*, New York, 1951, GP Putnam's Sons.

Montag ML: *Community college education for nursing*, New York, 1959, McGraw-Hill.

Naisbitt J, Aburdene P: *Megatrends 2000: new directions for tomorrow*, New York, 1991, William Morrow.

National Council of State Boards of Nursing: Definition of competence and standards for competence, National Council of State Boards of Nursing annual meeting: In *Book of reports*, Chicago, 1996, NCSBN.

National Council of State Boards of Nursing: *MSR communiqué: Special edition*, June 1997, www.nscbn.org. Accessed June 8, 2001.

National League for Nursing: *Education for nursing: The diploma way 1989-1990*, Publication No. 16-1314, New York, 1989a, the NLN.

National League for Nursing: *Annual guide to undergraduate RN education*, ed 5, Publication No. 19-7378, New York, 1997, the NLN.

National League for Nursing: *Nursing data review 1997*, Publication No. 19-7327, New York, 1997, the NLN.

National League for Nursing: *Annual guide to graduate nursing education 1997*, Publication No. 19-7491, New York, 1997, the NLN.

National League for Nursing, Council of Associate Degree Nursing Competencies Task Force: *Educational competencies for graduates of associate degree nursing programs*, Bookcode 1404-6, New York, 2001, the NLN.

Rowland HS, Rowland B: *The nurse's almanac*, ed 2, Rockville, Md, 1984, Aspen.

ADDITIONAL READINGS

Heller BR, Oros MT, Durney-Crowley J: The future of nursing education. Ten trends to watch, *Nurs Health Care Perspect* 21(1):9-13, 2000.

Linderman C: The future of nursing education, *J Nurs Educ* 39(1):5-12, 2000.

Yeaworth RC, Benschoter RA, Meter R, Benson S: Telecommunications and nursing education, *J Prof Nurs* 11(4):227-232, 1995.

INTERNET RESOURCES

Here are some suggested search engines and related Web sites.

Included in this site are areas on distance education, continuing education, and virtual nursing education. Information on schools of nursing and doctoral programs throughout the world are also available.

Gradschools.com
http://www.gradschools.com/
This site contains a list of schools in the world that offer nursing and midwifery distance education graduate programs, including their university addresses, e-mail links, telephone numbers, and short descriptions of the available programs.

Petersons Guide Online
http://www.petersons.com/
This site offers a searchable database listing colleges and universities that offer bachelor degrees in nursing through a distance-education program. It also lists colleges and universities that offer master's degrees in nursing.

Virtual University
http://www.geteducated.com/vugaz.htm
This is a newsletter that has up-to-date information on courses online.

World Lecture Hall
http://www.utexas.edu/world/lecture/
This site contains links to pages created by faculty worldwide who are using the Web to deliver class materials.

UCSF Center for the Health Professions Web Site
http://futurehealth.ucsf.edu

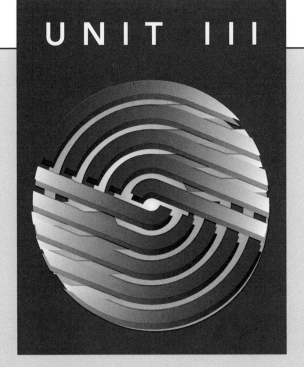

UNIT III

NURSING MANAGEMENT

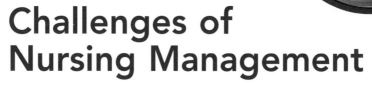

CHAPTER FIVE

Challenges of Nursing Management

CAROL SINGER, EDD, RN

When the best leader's work is done, the people say, "We did it ourselves!"
—*Lao-Tzu*

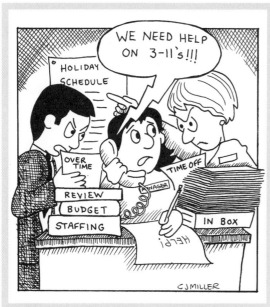

Nursing management can be challenging.

After completing this chapter, you should be able to:

- Differentiate between management and leadership.
- Describe various types of management.
- List characteristics of a good leader.
- Compare and contrast leadership styles.
- Distinguish between power and authority.
- Apply problem-solving strategies to clinical management situations.
- Use the decision-making process in clinical situations.
- Define the task and maintenance roles that group members assume to ensure effective group functioning.
- Identify the characteristics of effective work groups.
- Discuss the change process.

s you get closer to meeting your goal of being a "real" nurse, it is important to consider the role of the nurse as a leader and manager.

I don't want to be a manager, I'm a recent graduate!

I want to take care of patients, not be a paper pusher!

Not so!! Nursing in any role is a "people business," and dealing with people is what management is. When you accept your first position as a graduate nurse, you must realize that you are entering a work group where members spend at least one third of the day interacting with each other. Nurses must use interpersonal, leadership, and management skills to be effective in their roles.

Management requires different levels of functioning depending on the role of the individual nurse. For instance, as a recent graduate, you will have primary management responsibility for the patients for whom you are assigned to care. This may include planning and coordinating the care with other nursing personnel, such as nursing assistants. It may also require working with other members of the health team to meet patient needs. With more experience, you may become a team leader or charge nurse with responsibility for managing a group of staff members who provide care for a larger number of patients, perhaps even an entire unit.

MANAGEMENT VS. LEADERSHIP

WHAT IS THE DIFFERENCE BETWEEN MANAGEMENT AND LEADERSHIP?

Although the terms *management* and *leadership* are frequently interchanged, they do not have the same meaning. A leader selects and assumes the role; a manager is assigned or appointed to the role. Managers have responsibility for organizational goals and perform organizational tasks such as budget preparation and scheduling. Although it is desirable for managers to be good leaders and to be effective at influencing others, there are leaders who are not managers and, more frequently, managers who are not leaders! So, let's discuss in more detail what the actual differences are.

Management is a problem-oriented process with similarities to the nursing process. Management is needed whenever two or more individuals work together toward a common goal. The manager coordinates the activities of the group to maintain balance and direction. There are generally four functions that the manager performs: *planning* (what is to be done), *organizing* (how it is to be done), *directing* (who is to do it), and *controlling* (when and how it is done). All of these activities go on continually and simultaneously, with the percentage of time spent on each varying with the level of the manager and the characteristics of the group being managed. Managers must be attentive to both dimensions of their job: the mission and goals of the organization and the interpersonal relationships among the staff. The successful manager is one who respects the people of the organization as individuals and who cares how well the tasks are done.

Leadership, in contrast, is a way of behaving, an interpersonal ability to cause others to respond, not because they have to, but because they want to. Leadership is needed as much as management for effective group functioning, but each differs. The manager determines the agenda, sets time limits, and facilitates group functioning. The leader focuses a group's efforts on identifying goals and carrying out the activities needed to reach those goals.

> Florence Nightingale was an early nursing leader. What characteristics of a manager did she also demonstrate?

WHAT IS MEANT BY *MANAGEMENT STYLE?*

There are a variety of different management styles that you may come across in your nursing practice, but they basically are a continuum between *autocratic* and *laissez-faire* styles (Fig. 5-1).

The *autocratic manager* uses an authoritarian approach to direct the activities of others. This individual makes most of the decisions alone without input from other staff members. Under this style of management, the emphasis is on the tasks to be done, with little concern shown for the individual staff members who perform the tasks. The autocratic manager may be most effective in crisis situations, when structure and control are critical to success, as, for instance, during a cardiac arrest or code.

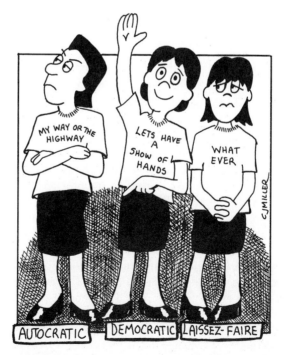

FIGURE 5-1
Management styles.

On the other end of the continuum is the *laissez-faire manager*, who maintains a permissive climate with little direction or control exerted. This manager allows staff members to make and implement decisions independently and relinquishes all power and responsibility to them. Although this style of management may function effectively in highly motivated groups, it is not usually effective in a bureaucratic health care setting that requires many different individuals and groups to interact.

In the middle of the continuum is the *democratic manager*. This individual is people-oriented and emphasizes effective group functioning. The goals of the group are identified, and the manager is perceived as a group member who is its organizer and who keeps it headed in the right direction. The environment is open, and communication flows both ways. The democratic manager encourages participation in decision making; he or she recognizes, however, that there are situations in which such participation may not be appropriate and is willing to assume responsibility for a decision when it is necessary.

As you can see, the continuum of management styles includes approaches ranging from almost total control to almost complete freedom for subordinates. Behaviors vary from telling others what to do to delegating authority for meeting objectives to the work group. In choosing a management style, the manager must decide between control and freedom and determine which trade-offs are acceptable in a particular situation.

 Look at managers on your clinical units—how do they fit into these categories?

WHAT ARE THE CHARACTERISTICS OF A GOOD LEADER?

The many attempts to define what makes a good leader have resulted in a variety of concepts and proposals. Researchers have tried to identify the characteristics or traits necessary to be a good leader. Several of these studies defined the concept of a "born leader," implying that the desired traits are inherited. Later research indicated that the effectiveness of the leader is influenced by the situation itself. It became clear that desired traits could be learned through education and experience. It also became clear that the most effective leadership style for one situation was not necessarily the most effective for another. Today it is recognized that leaders must have a variety of skills and possess the ability to select the most appropriate style for each situation. The concept of *contingency leadership* is sometimes used to refer to this flexible approach. The leader's style varies depending on the situation. Although this may sound complicated, it can be compared with your approach to patient care. You individualize a care plan on the basis of the needs of a particular patient, then you implement the care using available resources. The good leader brings the same flexible approach to each particular situation.

Leadership abilities can be further understood in relation to the two major components of management: *job-centered behavior* and *employee-centered behavior*. A leader's behavior may emphasize both areas, may be limited in both areas, or may be high in one area and low in the other. The leader who is high in both job-centered and employee-centered behaviors cares equally for the needs and feelings of the employee and the effective and efficient completion of the job. This individual uses democratic concepts in management and views the tasks to be accomplished from the standpoint of a team member. At the other extreme would be the leader who has little concern for either the employee or the task to be accomplished. This individual could be expected to approach management with a laissez-faire attitude.

Alternatively a leader who uses the autocratic style of management is probably high in job-centered behavior and low in employee-centered behavior. The leader who is high in employee-centered behavior and low in job-centered behavior would fall between the democratic and laissez-faire manager on the continuum. Let's look at the following few examples:

> Tom is a *high employee-centered* and *high job-centered* democratic leader. He is a person who cares equally about the employee as a person and getting the job done efficiently and effectively. Another type of leader is Jean, who is *high job-centered* and *low employee-centered*. She is a person who focuses on the job to be done with little concern for the needs or feelings of her employees. A great deal of work is accomplished with her autocratic style of management. Randy, in contrast, cares more for his employees and an individual's feelings and needs than getting the job done. He is a *high employee-centered* and *low job-centered* leader. Finally the laissez-faire leader, Laura, is the kind of person who just doesn't seem to care for either her employee's needs and feelings or the need to get the job done. She would be considered a *low employee-centered* and *low job-centered* leader.

Although most agree that every individual leans toward one of these four possible combinations, it has been found that fluctuations from one combination to another occur depending on the particular situation. In the health care setting, good leaders carefully balance job-centered and employee-centered behaviors to meet both staff and patient needs effectively.

Consider your educational and clinical experiences. What leadership qualities have you observed? What management characteristics have you observed? Are there specific personality traits that enhance a person's performance of these two roles?

A good leader works toward established goals and has a sense of purpose and direction (Critical Thinking Box 5-1). Rather than push staff members off in many directions, this leader uses personal attributes to organize the activities and pull the staff toward the goals. Remember, it is easier to pull than to push!

Let's take a moment now to summarize the main concepts of leadership that we have discussed.

- Leadership can be learned.
- Leaders are developers of people.

CRITICAL THINKING BOX 5-1

LEADERSHIP CHARACTERISTICS

Write a person's name in the left column and then list leadership characteristics of that individual in the spaces on the right. See if you can identify two people you know who have somewhat different characteristics, but are both good leaders!

Directions: To evaluate your views and determine your self-evaluation of your particular life situation, respond to the statements with the appropriate number.

❑ *Name*   ❑ *Leadership Characteristics*

1. _____   _____

   _____

   _____

   _____

   _____

   _____

2. _____   _____

   _____

   _____

   _____

Now, see if you can take those characteristics that you identified and fill in the blanks below!

A good leader has: e _ _ _ _ _ _ sm

se _ _ -c _ _ _ _ d _ _ ce

mat _ _ _ _ _

a concern for _ _ _ _ _ _

dec _ _ _ _ _ -m _ _ _ _ _ ab _ _ _ _ y

a s _ _ _ _ of _ _ _ or

A good leader also is: s _ _ _ ere

ta _ _ _ _ _

acc _ _ _ _ _ _ _ e

appr _ _ _ _ _ t _

- A person's style of leadership is dependent on that individual's basic personality and the particular situation in which he or she is functioning.
- The demands of the situation in which a leader is to function influence the qualities, characteristics, knowledge, and skills necessary for successful leadership.
- The degree to which the leader is knowledgeable and competent directly influences the subordinates' feelings of security and their ability to cooperate to meet goals.

POWER AND AUTHORITY IN NURSING MANAGEMENT

DO YOU KNOW THE DIFFERENCE BETWEEN POWER AND AUTHORITY?

Power is having the ability to effect change and influence others to meet identified goals. Authority relates to a specific position and the responsibility associated with it. The individual has the authority or the right to act in situations in which one is held responsible within the institutional hierarchy. Today there is much discussion in nursing about the importance of power and the concept of *empowerment*. To *empower* nurses is to provide them with more autonomy in their roles. The realization of greater power in the profession depends on the willingness of administrators to allocate it and nurses to accept it together with the accompanying responsibility.

 Remember, power and responsibility always go hand in hand!

WHAT ARE THE DIFFERENT TYPES OF POWER?

There are many different types of power, so let's discuss the most common.

Legitimate power is power connected to a position of authority. The individual has power as a result of the position. The head nurse has legitimate power and authority as a result of the position.

Referent power is power resulting from personal characteristics, often called *charisma*. Many successful leaders have referent power in that they are liked and admired by others primarily as individuals.

Reward power is closely linked with legitimate power in that it comes about because the individual has the power to provide or withhold rewards. If supervisors have the power to authorize salary increases or scheduling changes, then they have reward power.

Expert power is based on specialized knowledge, skills, or abilities that are recognized and respected by others. The individual is perceived as an expert in an area and has power in that area because of this expertise. For instance, the enterostomal therapist has expertise in the care of individuals who have had ostomies. Therefore staff nurses seek out the therapist as a resource and use the expert's knowledge to guide the care of these patients.

Information power is possessed by individuals who have knowledge that is needed by others to function effectively in their roles. This type of power is, perhaps, the most abused! An individual may, for example, withhold information from subordinates to maintain control. The leader who gives directions without providing needed information on rationale or constraints is abusing information power.

Coercive power is power derived from fear of consequences. It is easy to see how parents would have coercive power over children on the basis of the threat of punishment. This type of power can also be used against staff members when, for example, there is the threat of receiving unfavorable assignments.

Leaders and managers need to understand the concept of power and how it can be used and abused in working with others. Nurses, on the whole, need to identify ways to increase their power within the health team. Graduates need to be aware of and willing to implement methods and resources to increase their personal power. Staff nurses can develop expert power by increasing competency in their roles and in clinical skills. Refining interpersonal skills to enhance the ability to work with others can expand many types of power. These skills include communicating clearly and completely what people need to know and delegating tasks to those who know how to accomplish them. Demonstrating a willingness to give and receive feedback and being positive in communicating also are important. All of these are ways that can help individuals develop and enhance power in working with others. It is also important to recognize what detracts from power. Impressing others as disorganized, either in personal appearance or in work habits; engaging in petty criticism or gossip; and being unable to say "no" without qualification are some of the behaviors that can detract from power.

MANAGEMENT PROBLEM SOLVING

HOW ARE PROBLEM-SOLVING STRATEGIES USED IN MANAGEMENT?

Management is a problem-oriented process. The effective manager analyzes problems and makes decisions throughout all the planning, organizing, directing, and controlling functions of management. Problem solving can be readily compared with the nursing process (Table 5-1). The two are essentially the same, as can be seen by comparing the steps of one to the other.

As with the nursing process, problem solving does not always flow in an orderly manner from one step to the next. Throughout the process, feedback is sought, which may indicate a need for altering the plan to reach the desired objective. The most critical step in either process is identifying the problem (identified as the *nursing diagnosis* in the nursing process). Frequently what was originally identified as "the problem" may be too broad or unclear. Only the symptoms of the problem may be seen initially, or there may be several problems overlapping. If an approach is used to relieve only the symptoms, the problem will still exist. The good manager will guide the process of identifying the problem by asking questions such as "What is

☞TABLE 5-1

Nursing Process vs. Problem Solving

Nursing Process	*Problem Solving*
Assessment	Data gathering
Analysis/nursing diagnosis	Definition of problem
Development of plan	Identification of alternative solutions
Implementation of plan	Implementation of plan
Evaluation/reassessment	Evaluation of solution

happening?" "What is being done about it?" "Who is doing what?" and "Why?" It is important to differentiate among facts and opinions and to attempt to break down the information to its simplest terms. Think of it as being a detective looking for every clue!

Once the problem is clearly identified, the group should "brainstorm" all possible solutions. Often the first few alternatives are not the best or most practical. Identifying a number of viable alternatives usually provides more flexibility and creativity. All possible solutions must fall within existing constraints, such as staff abilities, available resources, and institutional policies. The more complex the problem, the more judgment is required. In some cases the problem may extend beyond the manager's scope of responsibility and authority and so it may be necessary to seek outside help.

Once all the alternatives are identified, each must be evaluated in relation to changes that would be required in existing policies, procedures, staffing, and so forth, and what effect these changes would have. Ask "What would happen if . . ." questions to clarify the short- and long-term implications of each alternative. Always keep in mind that the perfect solution is not possible in most situations.

Problem solving represents a choice made between possible alternatives that is thought to be the best solution for a particular situation. At its best, problem solving should involve ample discussion of the possible solutions by those who are affected by the situation and who possess the knowledge and power to support the possible solution. Once an alternative has been selected, it should be implemented unless new data or perspectives warrant a change. Feedback should be sought continuously to provide ongoing evaluation of the effectiveness of the solution. Remember that simply choosing the best alternative does not automatically ensure its acceptance by those who work with it!

Frequently, implementing the solution to a problem causes several other problems to arise. If that happens, don't let the new problems impede the implementation process; instead, pause and consider each individually, solve it, and then return to the original plan. After a period of trial, evaluate the progress made. A complete solution may not have been reached, but some progress should have been made. If not, a slight modification in the approach or a completely new alternative may be needed. The old adage "If at first you don't succeed, try, try again" is most appropriate when applying the problem-solving process! Remain positive, confident, and flexible! Eventually a possible solution will work! Let's apply the process to an actual problem.

> You are the head nurse on a busy medical-surgical unit with 32 patients. Staff members have complained to you that too much time is being spent during morning change-of-shift report. After asking questions and seeking out additional information, you determine that a more clear definition of the problem is that the night charge nurse does not give a clear, concise report. Involving the night charge nurse in the problem-solving process helps to define the problem, because the nurse does not have adequate knowledge of how to give a change-of-shift report.

Can you see how, once the problem has been clarified, it becomes more amenable to an acceptable, and perhaps even easy, solution?

HOW DO WE RELATE PROBLEM SOLVING AND DECISION MAKING?

By definition, problem solving and decision making are almost the same process, with one very notable difference. Decision making requires the definition of a clear objective to guide the process. A comparison of the steps of each illustrates this difference (Table 5-2). Although both problem solving and decision making are usually initiated in the presence of a problem, the objective in decision making may not be to solve the problem, but only to deal with its results. It also is important to distinguish between a good decision and a good outcome. A *good outcome* is the objective that is desired, and a *good decision* is one made systematically to reach this objective. A good decision may or may not result in a good outcome. Although it is desirable to have both good decisions and good outcomes, the good decision-maker is willing to act, even at the risk of a negative outcome.

> Susan is the evening charge nurse on a medical unit that has a total of 24 patients. One of the patients is terminally ill and seems to be having a particularly difficult evening. The patient requires basic comfort measures but little complex care. Susan has a choice of assigning the patient to another RN or to a nursing assistant. If she assigns the RN, the workload for the other staff will be heavier and she, herself, will have to administer medications. She decides to assign the RN to offer emotional and physical support to the patient. During the shift, the RN spends time sitting with the patient. Close to the end of the shift, the patient dies. Was this a good decision with a bad outcome or a good decision with a good outcome?

Decision making is values-based, and problem solving is a more scientific process. Nurses make decisions on the basis of personal values, life experiences, perceptions of the situation, knowledge of risks associated with possible decisions, and their individual ways of thinking. Because of these variables, it is possible, even probable, that two individuals given the same information and using the same decision-making process would arrive at different decisions.

In today's ever-changing health care environment, it is important for nurses and nurse managers to be effective in both problem solving and decision making. The good manager will evaluate the problem-solving or decision-making process on the basis of criteria that view the big picture. These criteria include the likely effects on the objective to be met, on the policies and resources of the organization, on the individuals

S TABLE 5-2

Problem Solving vs. Decision Making

Problem Solving	Decision Making
Define problem	Set objective
Identify alternative solutions	Identify and evaluate alternative decisions
Select solution and implement	Make decision and implement
Evaluate outcome	Evaluate outcome

involved, and on the product or service delivered. The quality of patient care is dependent on the ability of the nurse to effectively combine problem solving with decision making. To do so, nurses must be attuned to their individual value systems and understand their effect on thinking and perceiving. The values associated with a particular situation will limit the alternatives generated and the final decision. For this reason, the fact that nurses typically work in groups is beneficial to the decision-making process. Although the process is the same, groups generally offer the benefits of a broader knowledge base for defining objectives and more creativity in identifying alternatives. The effectiveness of the group decision-making process is dependent on the dynamics of the group. It is, therefore, important for nurses to understand the roles of individuals within the group and the dynamics involved in working in groups to take full advantage of the group process.

GROUP DYNAMICS

WHAT IS MEANT BY *GROUP DYNAMICS*?

Can you remember previous discussions in nursing school about group dynamics as they related to your peer group? How about in relation to therapeutic groups? The concepts are the same when talking about work groups!

Members of the nursing and health teams are interdependent in meeting patient needs. This interdependency involves continual interaction among members of different groups. If the staff forms a cohesive group, each member benefits from group participation by increasing his or her understanding and ability to give care. In addition, this cohesiveness will benefit groups that include patients and family members.

All groups go through phases, whether the group meets for a single time, once a year, or once a day. These phases are called the *initiation*, *working*, and *termination* phases. During the *initiation* phase, the goals and purposes of the group are defined, leadership evolves, and individual roles are determined. An important aspect of this phase is building rapport and trust among group members. The *working* phase begins once the initiation phase has been accomplished and the dynamics of the group are tentatively established. This phase deals with problem solving and the achievement of the goals of the group. Once the task is completed and problems have been resolved, the *termination* phase begins and the group attempts to bring closure to its activities. At this point, it is important to summarize the accomplishments of the group to make members feel good about themselves and the work that has been done.

WHAT TYPES OF ROLES ARE NEEDED TO PROMOTE GROUP FUNCTIONING?

There are two types of roles that group members perform. They are *task roles* and *maintenance roles*. *Task roles* are generally defined as follows:

- *Initiating* introductory activities: making suggestions and providing new ideas for group functioning.

- *Seeking information:* gathering facts and data, seeking advice and opinions, and asking questions.
- *Giving information:* offering information from other resources and sharing suggestions and ideas that support the group activity.
- *Clarifying:* rephrasing ideas, giving examples to explain suggestions, and tracking the progress made.
- *Coordinating:* reviewing group activities and demonstrating relationships between the group's activities and those of other groups.
- *Summarizing:* recording consensus of the group, summarizing the actions taken, and reviewing the group process.

Group maintenance roles are defined as follows:

- *Supporting:* showing concern for group members and being responsive to them.
- *Mediating:* trying to maintain harmony by seeking compromises and reducing differences among group members.
- *Gatekeeping:* encouraging participation from all group members.
- *Following:* compromising self when consensus of group supports another idea and promoting group harmony.
- *Reducing tension:* using humor or calling for breaks in activities to decrease tense and possibly disruptive situations.
- *Setting standards:* relating current group activity to standards already established by the group and guiding decision making to avoid conflict with the standards.

Both task and maintenance roles are necessary for the group process to be effective. Individual members generally assume one or more roles within the group on the basis of their personality and value system, as well as their position and status within the group. Each group will have a different dynamic as a result of these factors, even if the same members function in other groups as well.

WHAT EFFECT DOES THE LEADER HAVE ON THE GROUP?

The leader's philosophy, personality, self-concept, and interpersonal skills all influence the functioning of the group. A leader is most effective if members are respected as individuals who have unique contributions to make to the group process. Can you remember our earlier discussion of the characteristics of a good leader? The ability to influence and motivate others is particularly important in the group process.

Whenever the combination of people in a group is altered, the dynamics are changed. If the group is in the working phase, it will revert to the initiating phase when a new person or persons are added and will remain there until they have been assimilated into the group and a new dynamic has been formulated. The most effective groups are those that have had consistent membership and are highly developed. These groups demonstrate friendly and trusting relationships; the ability to work toward goals of varying difficulty; flexible, stable, and reliable participation of members; and productivity, with high-quality output. Leadership within these groups is democratic, and the members feel positive about their participation and the outcomes of the group process. Now let's apply these principles to a real situation!

When you graduate and accept a nursing position, you will become a new nurse in the work group, causing it to regress to the initiating phase. You must convince the members of the group that you are worthy of being included in the group. (If this is your first nursing position, you must also convince the group that you are worthy of entering the nursing profession!) To accomplish this task, you should anticipate the feelings of loneliness, isolation, and distance that accompany the initiating phase. Expect to feel that you are being excluded and understand that it is part of the process. Instead, put your energy into forming supportive professional relationships, including their social aspects. Seek and use feedback, and ask for help in areas that are not as familiar to you, such as priority setting. As you contribute your individual talents to the group, you will move from being a dependent new person to full group membership. It is important that you do not underestimate the length of time that may be needed to accomplish this task! Group processes proceed very slowly in most cases, and it may be 6 months or more before you are accepted as a full member of the work group. Don't be discouraged!

Remember that management skills come with experience in nursing, so don't be too hard on yourself during the transition phase. Identify nurse managers who have the skills you would like to incorporate into your management style. Look at the positive side of working for various nursing managers as a means to assist you in the development of your personal management style. Develop the ability to *think* like a nurse manager as you carry out your assignments—always look at the *big* picture.

THE CHALLENGE OF CHANGE

How many times have you heard staff nurses complain about how powerless they feel about the lack of control they have over their work environment? They state that they are frustrated that they cannot give the amount and quality of patient care that they desire and that staffing patterns are placing undue stress on them. Do they talk about quitting the acute-care environment and trying some other aspect of nursing (perhaps home health) as a less stressful option? Why don't they think about acting to change the situation rather than running away from it? Do they feel powerless to do so? Is it easier to withdraw and escape?

One thing we all know is that change is inevitable, particularly in today's health care delivery system. Economic factors have taken center stage and cutbacks in all aspects of health care services are occurring. But change can be like a truck with no driver at the wheel: It moves slowly and steadily toward you (Fig. 5-2). You have three options: You can move out of the situation and perhaps miss some opportunities; you can just stand there and withdraw, doing what you are told to just to avoid conflict; or you can start to run with it, jump on, and try to steer it in a positive direction.

So, how do you begin to direct the "change truck"? The first thing to know about the change process is that it, too, has similarities to problem solving and the nursing process. Let's lay them out and compare the three processes (Table 5-3).

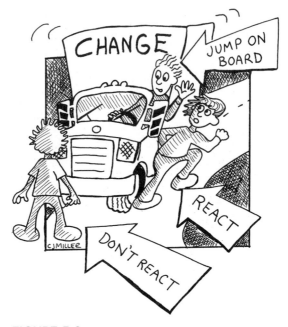

FIGURE 5-2
Change … React, don't react, or jump on board.

TABLE 5-3

Nursing Process vs. Problem Solving vs. Change Process

Nursing Process	Problem Solving	Change Process
Assessment	Data gathering	Recognition that a change is needed; collect data
Identification of possible nursing diagnoses	Definition of problem	Identification of problem to be solved
Selection of nursing diagnosis	Selection of one of possible alternatives	Selection of one of possible alternatives
Development of plan	Development of plan	Implementation of plan
Implementation of plan	Implementation of plan	Implementation of plan
Evaluation	Evaluation of solution	Evaluation of effects of change
Reassessment	Evaluation of solution	Stabilization of change in place

Look familiar? Maybe it's not that hard to take control and be a change agent! The first thing that you need to know about the change process is that resisting change is a natural response for most people. All of us are most comfortable in our state of "equilibrium," where we feel in control of what we are doing. To deal effectively with change, it is important to understand that every change involves adaptation. It requires a period of transition where the change can be understood, evaluated in light of its impact on the individual and, one hopes, eventually embraced.

There are various reasons why people resist change, and understanding them will help you to implement the change process more effectively. Following are the most common factors that cause resistance to change:

- A perceived threat to self in how the change will affect the individual personally
- A lack of understanding regarding the nature of the change
- A limited ability to emotionally cope with change
- A disagreement about the potential benefits of the change
- A fear of the impact of the change on self-confidence and self-esteem

Kurt Lewin sought to incorporate these concepts in his Change Theory. He identified three phases in an effective change process: *unfreezing, moving,* and *refreezing.* In the *unfreezing* phase, all of the factors that may cause resistance to change are considered. Others who may be affected by the change are sought out to determine whether they recognize that a change is needed and, secondly, their interest in participating in the process. You will need to determine whether the environment of the institution is receptive to change and then convince others to work with you. The *moving* phase occurs once a group of individuals has been recruited to take on responsibilities for implementing the change. The group begins to sort out what must be done and the sequence of actions that would be most effective. They identify individual(s) who have the *power* to assist in making the plan succeed. (*What types of power would be most effective?*) They also attempt to identify strategies to overcome the natural resistance to change—how to effect a cooperative approach to implement the change. Once developed, the plan is then put into place.

The *refreezing* phase occurs when the plan is in place and everyone involved knows what is happening and what to expect. Publicizing the ongoing assessment of the pros and cons of the plan is an important part of its ultimate success. Be certain someone is responsible for continuing to work on the plan so it doesn't lose momentum. Finally, make the changes stick—or *refreeze*—the change now becomes a part of everyday life and is no longer perceived as something new. Now let's apply this process to a real situation!

> Patti is working in a medical-surgical unit at a 200-bed acute-care hospital. She constantly hears her peers complaining about the lack of adequate nursing staff, and over the past 3 months, two full-time staff nurses have resigned. To cover the unit, part-time staff from temporary agencies and from the hospital staffing pool are being used to supplement the remaining regular staff. Because this staff has little orientation to the unit and frequently is placed where they are needed the most, the continuity of care and a potential for increased errors in patient care became a major concern.

Rather than continuing to complain about the situation or considering leaving it, Patti decided to act and try to steer the change truck. She approached a few of the nurses and initiated a discussion about the changes in staffing and how scheduling had become a nightmare for the charge nurse. She enlisted the support of several of the staff to begin problem solving possible solutions. They agreed that increased staffing was probably not a possible immediate solution and determined to work within the constraints that they had.

Several of the pool nurses were receptive to requesting their assignment be limited to this one unit and agreed to schedule their hours to complement each other. This, in essence, would add a shared full-time position, at no additional cost, and also would provide for consistency of patient care. When the proposal was presented to administration, they agreed to support the idea on the basis of its economic and patient-centered benefits.

React—move out of the way. Let the truck (change) pass you by. However, opportunities may be missed. Don't act—just stand there and let the truck run over you. It will leave you behind and more than likely in worse shape than when you started. Act—start running when you see it coming. Pace with it until you can decide when to jump on and steer it in the direction you want to move.

WHO INITIATES CHANGE AND WHY?

Another aspect to consider when evaluating change is who wants the change and why. Is it the system? Is it management? Is it you, the nurse? Or is it the patient? Change should be carefully planned and implemented for specific reasons. By identifying who is initiating the change, the implementation can be better understood.

System. The most common reason for change is that what you did before doesn't work anymore. For example, the handwritten medical record system is largely being replaced by the electronic medical record because the old system takes too much time, generates volumes of paper, and is not adequate to keep pace with the number of patients and the need to access key information quickly from various individuals outside the traditional hospital (home health nurse or hospice nurse at the patient's home).

Management. Change frequently occurs when new management enters the scene. This provides a new perspective and view regarding how the system operates. For example, a new vice president of nursing decides to implement critical pathways. The overall organization may benefit from the change; however, the employee may be wondering "How will the implementation of critical pathways change my job? Do I know how to implement a critical pathway?" (Critical Thinking Box 5-2.)

Patient. When "customers" are not happy, something within the system needs to change. What are the specific patient problems and how can they be resolved? For example, patients are complaining about lengthy admission procedures. Faxing physicians' orders or allowing "direct admit" to units may streamline the admission process.

Yourself. Sometimes we impose change on ourselves—we may or may not like it, but we see a need for it. Who ever wanted to go on a diet and enjoyed doing it? Stop to consider how you are going to implement the change. How will your work environment be affected? Can you delegate any part of it? If change involves other employees, make them a part of that change. They will own the results—that is, you will use the WIIFM principle (Wilson, 1996, p. 21).

CRITICAL THINKING BOX 5-2

What changes have you made in your life? _____

_____

How long did one new situation last before it changed again? _____

_____

You have just learned to deal successfully with the changes associated with being a student. Now you are facing the challenge of change again as you prepare for your role as a practicing registered nurse.

WIIFM Principle: What's In It For Me?

Again, change depends on your own perspective. You will be either actively involved in changes or choose to take a passive role. The choice is always yours. There are typical emotional phases encountered in the change process. It is important for nurse managers to recognize and plan interventions to effectively deal with these emotions. Table 5-4 summarizes the characteristics and helpful interventions associated with the change process. Only when you feel threatened by a change will you go through the steps (i.e., resistance, uncertainty, assimilation, transference, and

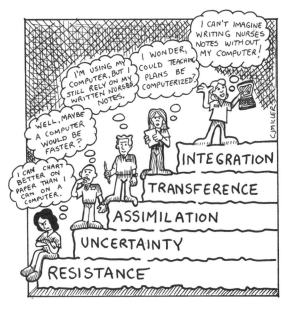

FIGURE 5-3
Five steps toward conquering change.

⑤TABLE 5-4

The Emotional Phases of the Change Process

Phase	Characteristics	Interventions
Equilibrium	High energy, feelings of balance and inner peace and harmony	Explain how changes will impact the status quo.
Denial	Denies reality that change will occur; experiences negative changes in physical health, emotional and cognitive behavior	Actively listen, be empathetic, and use reflective communication. Offer stress-management programs.
Anger	Blames others; may demonstrate envy, rage, or resentment	Be assertive and assist with problem solving. Encourage employee to determine the source of his or her anger.
Bargaining	Efforts made to try and eliminate the change; frequently talks in such terms as "If only ..."	Search for real needs and problems and explore ways of achieving outcomes through conflict management and win-win negotiation skills.
Chaos	Diffused energy; feelings of powerlessness and insecurity and a sense of disorientation	Encourage quiet time for reflection as inner search for identity and meaning occur. Listen.
Depression	No energy left; nothing seems to work; sorrow, self-pity; and feelings of emptiness	Encourage expression of sorrow and pain. Have lots of patience as employees learn to let go.
Resignation	Lack of enthusiasm as change is accepted passively	Allow employees to move at own pace.
Openness	Some renewal of energy and willingness to take on new roles or assignments resulting from change	Patiently explain again, in detail, the desired change.
Readiness	Willingly expends energy to explore new events that are occurring; reunification of emotions and cognition	Assume a directive management style; assign tasks, provide direction.
Reemergence	Feelings of empowerment as new projects and ideas are initiated	Mutually explore questions and develop an understanding of role and identity. Employees take actions based on own decisions.

(Adapted from Perlman D, Takacs GJ: The ten stages of change, Nurs Manage 21(4):34, 1990.)

integration) to conquer it (Wilson, 1996) (Fig. 5-3). All change will elicit some type of resistance. It is up to you to increase the impetus for change while decreasing resistance. The decision to be involved with change will help steer you in a direction that will be most beneficial.

REFERENCES

Wilson, P: *Change: coping with tomorrow today*, Shawnee Mission, Kan, 1996, National Press.

ADDITIONAL READINGS

Allen DW: How nurses become leaders. Perceptions and beliefs about leadership development, *J Nurs Adm* 28(9):15-20, 1998.

Badzek L, Cober S: 10 tips for success as a nurse manager, *Am J Nurs* 96(6):48-49, 1996.

Boston C, Vestal KW: Work transformation. Why the new health care imperative must focus both on people and processes, *Hosp Health Netw* 68(7):50-54, 1994.

Costelle-Nickitas DM: Get ready to take charge, *Am J Nurs* 97(5):16B-16J, 1997.

Curtin LL: Blessed are the flexible . . . , *Nurs Manage* 26(3):7-8, 1995.

Curtin LL: Management: Love it or leave it, *Nurs Manage* 26(6):7-8, 1995.

Kerfoot K: Management is taught, leadership is learned, *Nurs Econ* 16(3):144-145, 1998.

Medley F, Larochelle DR: Transformational leadership and job satisfaction, *Nurs Manage* 26(9):64JJ-64LL, 64NN, 1995.

Pedersen A, Easton LS: Teamwork: bringing order out of chaos, *Nurs Manage 26(6):34-35, 1995.*

Perra BM: The leader in you, *Nurs Manage* 30(1):35-39, 1999.

Peterson LW, Halsey J, Albrecht TL, McGough K: Communicating with staff nurses: support or hostility? *Nurs Manage* 26(6):36-38, 1995.

Strader MK, Decker PJ: *Role transition to patient care management*, Norwalk, Conn, 1994 Appleton & Lange.

Tappen RM, Weiss SA, Whitehead DK: *Essentials of nursing leadership and management*, Philadelphia, 1998, W.B. Saunders.

Yoder-Wise P: *Leading and managing in nursing*, ed 2, St Louis, 1999, Mosby.

INTERNET RESOURCES

Government

Achoo
http://www.achoo.com

Agency for Healthcare Research & Quality
http://www.ahcpr.gov

U.S. Centers for Disease Control
http://www.cdc.gov

U.S. Department of Health and Human Services
http://www.os.dhhs.gov

FedWorld
http://www.fedworld.gov

U.S. Food and Drug Administration
http://www.fda.gov

Centers for Medicare & Medicaid Services
http://cms.hhs.gov

Indian Health Service
http://www.ihs.gov

National Institutes of Health
http://www.nih.gov

U.S. Occupational Safety and Health Administration
http://www.osha.gov

U.S. Social Security Administration
http://www.ssa.gov

United Nations
http://www.un.org

U.S. Veterans Affairs
http://www.va.gov

World Health Organization
http://www.who.int

Hospitals

Health on the Net
http://www.hon.ch

Hospital Web
http://neuro-www.mgh.harvard.edu/hospitalweb.shtml

Occupational Health

Canadian Centre for Occupational Health & Safety (CCOHS)
http://www.ccohs.ca/resources

Safety Links Directory
http://www.pro-am.com/

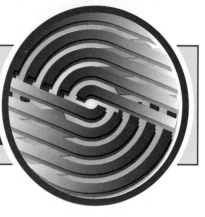

CHAPTER SIX

Group Process and Team Building

TOM GAGLIONE, RN, MN

A quality care team is made up of the interwoven skills, minds, and hearts of individuals who support each other as much as they support those in their care. The success of their outcomes lies in the common unity of their goal.

—*Tom Gaglione*

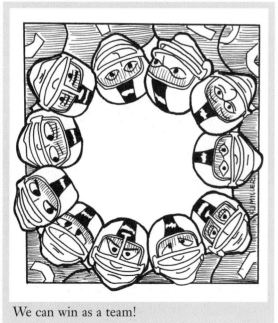

We can win as a team!

After completing this chapter, you should be able to:

- Identify different types of groups.
- Discuss group process.
- Analyze group member roles.
- Discuss team building.

GROUP PROCESS

WHAT IS A GROUP?

In choosing the world of nursing, you decided to leave an *informal group* of those who were trying to decide whether or not to become a nurse. Informal groups evolve spontaneously through social interaction and are not organized or structured. You entered a *formal group* as part of an aggregate, or cluster, of unique individuals who chose to join an organized, structured learning environment by applying and being accepted into nursing school. During your formal education, you were placed in clinical group rotations, which took the form of your first *real group*. This group was task-oriented and organized by its relationship to the criteria of your school's curriculum. Your *task group* may have been those of you who joined out of your class or clinical group to study for exams, which would have been made up of several classmates who would meet at certain times for a specific number of times to help each other gain the knowledge needed to pass the various written tests given during each rotation. On successful completion of the nursing program and the NCLEX exam, you gain access to your next group as a professional registered nurse. Your common bonds are the *RN* at the end of your signature, comparable nursing skills, and professional access to the area of your care-delivery sites. Two nurses can pass each other on the street and, unless they are in uniform or have their stethoscopes draped over the rearview mirror, are not able to recognize those in their common group. You may join nurse advocate groups, which, through their *committees* and *task forces*, work to address issues and support services in various areas of the nursing profession. Being a part of a group does not necessarily mean having personal or even professional relationships with others in your group. Groups can be obscure and minimally cohesive, such as in name or attributes only. Groups can also be highly organized and issues-oriented with a high degree of personal or professional interaction, such as the American Nursing Association.

WHAT IS GROUP PROCESS?

When we discuss the dynamics of groups, it's important to note that there are personality conflicts that tend to develop during the different cyclical phases of the group. In *forming* the group, think back to orientation day for nursing school. There you sit surrounded by some people you've never seen before and some you've known from your prenursing classes. A common bond is that you are all there for well-defined reasons, including finding out who is in your clinical group and who the instructors will be. Of course, the orientation is mandatory. You sit in the auditorium or classroom talking, listening, and watching those around you, playing your part in a form of controlled pandemonium. The pandemonium can actually be considered the *storming* phase. In the storming phase, you begin to act out the roles you normally portray in the presence of your peers, as you discussed your fears, fantasies, and hopes for a successful outcome to your nursing program (Tuckman, 1977).

Next you are divided into clinical groups. You now begin to reevaluate the personality composition of the new groups. As you begin to react to your new relationships, you begin to exhibit personality traits to establish the role you would like to be identified with in the group setting. Unfortunately, your unconscious defense mechanisms surface in the form of competitive conflict or one-upmanship within the group, with your hope that your response will secure the desired role in the group. It is at this time that *norming* begins to develop among members of the group, with the help of the clinical and lecture instructors. Norming occurs during the development of mutual goals and guidelines that help to redefine your behavioral roles in the group. This can allow for agreement in *performing* activities to help establish a purposeful clinical experience.

Groups can be multipurpose and multidynamic, as are the basic role choices of each participant in a group. When working in a group, the real fun and excitement start when group members begin responding to and dealing with the unconscious and semiconscious defense mechanisms of the individuals who act them out through the roles they play in the group. The responses of the defensive individual tend to be unproductive, time-consuming, and inappropriate to the harmony and overall function of a group effort. Of course they do give you something to talk and maybe laugh about later. In my years of nursing and group participation, the following tend to be my favorite dysfunctional group personalities.

The *self-servers* feel that the rules of the group don't apply to them. They show up late. They are usually unprepared to work. At times they will walk in and out of the group when it meets for superficial reasons, while appearing preoccupied with unrelated work or issues from outside of the group. When they do participate, their contributions are of little consequence. If they refuse to be functional members of the group, you may need to ask them to leave the group.

The first response of a *critical conservative* to a creative suggestion is, "No, it won't work" or "But it's always been done this way" and "How can you people succeed if you've never done this before?" They seem to have a criticism for any suggestion other than their own. If it isn't done their way, it just isn't right. They are obsessively negative and fearful of changes. It may be important to recognize the lessons of experiences and outcomes, but it is equally important to find new approaches to old problems.

The *motor mouths* talk just to hear themselves talk. They interrupt at any given moment to make statements or deliver a verbose response, possibly because they've been quiet for too long. Even when a person is talking, these people will talk over the speaker's words just to be the center of attention. At times the motor mouth begins to make a statement, only to ramble in and out of the group's issue, and ends up talking about unrelated issues that are usually about himself or herself. I suggest keeping a cloth gag nearby or redirecting their conversation to focusing on the issue and asking them for a short critical assessment of the issues in question.

The *mouse* is the silent observer fearful of voicing an opinion. Usually the mouse sits transfixed watching individuals take risks and responsibility for their input to the group. The mouse nods her head at appropriate times and answers questions in one or two words. The mouse may be a real addition to the group, especially if others in the group are able to find ways to engage and encourage the mouse to voice his opinions and feelings about the group issues. It's important to remember that they are some of the best observers and listeners; ask them for their input. You may find them to be a valuable asset to your team. Regardless of where you choose to work or the type of care-delivery system you are in, these group members are always there!

TEAM BUILDING

WHAT IS TEAM BUILDING?

Team building can be seen as a deliberate process of unifying a group of individuals into a functional working unit, accomplishing specific goals (Farley and Stoner, 1989). Another definition of a team is "a small number of people with complementary skills who are committed to a common purpose in performance of common goals, for which they hold themselves mutually accountable" (Katzenbach and Smith, 1993, p. 45). Katzenbach and Smith go on to say that there needs to be the right mix of attributes in three categories that help ensure a highly complementary and functional team. The three categories described are interpersonal skills, problem-solving and decision-making skills, and technical or functional expertise (Critical Thinking Box 6-1).

Teams are really just a formal way to actualize *collaboration*. Collaboration is at the heart of successful decision making. Collaboration among team members leverages skills, time, and resources for their own benefit and that of the organization. If you just examine the word *collaboration*, you will see that "co-labor" is the core of the word—meaning "working together toward some meaningful end."

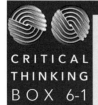

CRITICAL THINKING BOX 6-1

THINK ABOUT...

Try to assess and come to your own conclusion regarding the following hypothetical problem by picturing in your mind the who, what, and why before you read what the experts in the field would say.

You will be responsible for the care of your critically ill mother or father during his or her stay in the hospital over the next two months. I want you to assemble a team of your nursing peers to deliver care to your parent. The care will be based on the highest level of difficulty because of the serious nature of the diagnosis.

❏ Whom would you choose to help you?

❏ Why would you choose those specific nurses?

❏ What qualities would you want them to have when caring for your family member?

❏ What skill level would you want them to have to carry out the overall treatment plan?

❏ If some lacked skill levels to meet the treatment plan criteria, what would be an appropriate approach to this inadequacy?

When describing possible team performances along a functional curve, on the low side of the curve you might find the first three of the following descriptions as representative of our present health care delivery system.

A *basic team* is described as a group of nurses working as individual care deliverers with no incentives to work in conjunction with others to form a team. The *basic team* can be exemplified by a health care delivery site that is trying to cut costs by using agency staff or part-time nursing staff.

Pseudoteams have no common purposes or goals. They are designated as a team in name only for the benefit of the nursing administration or policy-makers. Members of pseudoteams generally are nurses, some of whom have been nursing most of their lives and may have lost their motivation, have a marginal level of professional skills, or have forgotten why they decided to become nurses. They usually know how to play the game and stay on the good side of the supervisors, and they usually work independently to hide their lack of skills while calling themselves team players. Others on a pseudoteam can be nurses—new to the field, overworked, underpaid, unappreciated, or easily intimidated. They just want to get through the shift.

The *potential team* is where nurses come together to form a team out of the need for mutual support and security, maybe because of their similarity in age or because of their newness to the field of nursing. Potential teams can consist of recent graduates and first- or second-year nurses. They have more in common with each other because they are able to identify with each other's newness and are willing to share their skills, working together for positive outcomes in care delivery.

A *real team* is made up of nurses with the highest level of skills to care for the acuity of those in their care. Each person on the team is goal-oriented and works as an interchangeable part of the team. They are supportive of each other and yet hold themselves mutually accountable for their outcomes. Examples of *real teams* are intensive care teams, emergency room teams, and flight nurses, who all have well-defined goals and work together toward a well-defined outcome. This type of *real team* effort is most obvious during codes, where the team members work together to render specific and complementary skills in a prescribed manner to save the patient. Ironically the general care units, where the goals are less well defined, can be rewarding and most challenging to the team approach. A good group leader and a motivated team who work to deliver quality care can help to make the difference in overall patient outcomes.

WHEN NURSES WORK AS A TRUE TEAM, EVERYONE INVOLVED BENEFITS!

In health care, the new imperative is quality care and service-oriented teams, as seen by Sovie (1992). It is also clear that teamwork is essential in care delivery outcomes and cost-control. Sovie also says that nurse managers and supervisors need to learn how to function in their capacity while being effective as team players. It might be argued that there is a difference between the previous concept of team nursing and the current concept of team nursing. The differences come in the form of an updated knowledge base and technological advances used in care delivery.

One of the most important ingredients in the team nursing approach is a positive psychological bond, which can bring the individuals of the team together. Without a positive cohesive bond, there will always be limits to the overall quality and function of the team. It should be possible to create a team approach to the overall health care delivery system. You as nurses are the unknown intervening variables that can either make or break the quality of the teamwork in team nursing. You and your colleagues, as a professional collective group, have the skills necessary to handle the multitude of problems associated with care delivery. The questions you may want to ask yourselves are as follows:

Are you as an individual mentally and emotionally prepared for real-world nursing?

Do you have a strong positive self-image?

Is your attitude about yourself and your peers conducive to team-directed nursing?

Are you willing to make difficult decisions in directing team care delivery?

Are you willing to relinquish control when necessary?

You may want to take the following into consideration:

> **Is management willing to support the nurses?**

> **Is the support constant, measurable, and appropriate to your needs?**

Research has shown that many staff nurses prefer to be dependent on their superiors for decision making and are less willing to assume responsibility for care coordination and team administration (Schmieding, 1990).

Nurses read the research to help formulate problem-solving models and innovative approaches in the development of care-delivery models. What is frequently left out is the extent of the role management is willing to play in helping to ensure the success of the new ideas. Is management willing to share control and leadership to help ensure a successful outcome in nurse-managed teams and care-delivery teams? I have been witness to many failed attempts at nurse leadership roles, the decentralization of authority, and shared governance. Some failures were caused by the last-minute intervention of management, usurping the authority from the nursing teams.

Following are some of the other factors responsible for various degrees of group or team failure:

- Nursing staff being unprepared or lacking the skills needed to work with other staff members in a unified team setting
- Nurses unwilling to move in and out of leadership roles to ensure the unity of the group and the best possible outcomes
- Management being pressured by upper management for faster adaptation to cost-cutting policies, which usually causes communication between management and nursing to consist of veiled threats, innuendoes, mixed messages, and other subtle negative forms that affect the morale of the nursing staff
- Nursing supervisors and administrative staff who appear to support shared governance but are unwilling to relinquish actual control of the nursing staff

Action always speaks louder than words. Work toward open and honest communication with administrators. Try to meet them halfway and find out what they are willing to do to support your teams or groups. How much interest do they have in the actual quality of health care delivery? Are they interested in learning the dynamics of your role as a nurse or the role of a nursing team? Let them know what type of support you need from them. Explain to them the importance of mutual respect and support in the overall quality of nursing care.

When forming teams or groups, realize that perfection is an illusion created in the mind of a critic. All of us have different skill levels. To function as a unified team, you will need to work with peers whose skills may need enhancing. You can help your peers by working side by side with them to build confidence while sharing in learning situations. Find ways of making the learning situations enjoyable, show a sense of humor, and give positive reinforcement whenever possible. Fear and guilt undermine confidence and destroy the cohesiveness of a team or group.

In the formation of any team or group, the mental and emotional stability of the individuals who make up the team or group will be reflected in their ability to establish a working rapport with the other team members. It is important for the stronger team members or group members to give their support and guidance. Their support can go a long way in building confidence in the other team members. The level of quality for any team is increased substantially by the comfort level among the individuals who make up the team.

The mix of complementary skill levels also gives comfort to the team or group as a whole. Taking inventory of technical or communication skills helps you identify other members' strengths when organizing the team members for emergency responses. The weaker team members should have support and guidance in the development of needed skills. Leadership roles in the team may be rotated to each member of the team. This allows the sharing of responsibilities related to the leadership role. Most people will gravitate to the role that they identify within the team. It will be important for the team members to communicate with each other, ensuring that each member's role remains positive and functional (Box 6-1). The tasks of the team or group will vary on the basis of the physician's treatment plan and the nursing plan of care, including the overall needs of the patient and family (Critical Thinking Box 6-2).

Like any other family member, we have periods when our personality renders us dysfunctional. At these times, our responses tend to have a negative impact on those who work with us. It may take our involvement in real life-and-death situations to snap us out of our dysfunctional responses.

A very important issue for nurses is self-recognition, along with positive forms of recognition from each other. In developing self-esteem and personal appreciation, we should think about what we do in our daily work. Who, besides you, your peers, and those in your care, recognizes your level of involvement? Who supports you after your efforts have saved someone's life? In reality we as nurses must be self-motivated, self-inspired, and self-supportive. The life and death responsibilities we assume may not be openly appreciated by those we work for or those outside of our profession. We as nurses, consciously or unconsciously, have chosen to place ourselves in harm's way. We are constantly aware of the possibility of carrying home a deadly disease to our family and friends. We care for the newborn and support the mother while preparing ourselves for the possibility of having to comfort the mother and father in the event that the baby dies. We care for adults and children with terminal diseases or physical abnormalities. We care for the elderly with respect and dignity while they

---

BOX 6-1 Basic Roles of Group Members

The following are some roles that individuals adopt when participating in a group. Each member may adopt more than one role.

❏ Opinion giver—states beliefs or values
❏ Opinion seeker—asks for clarification of beliefs or values
❏ Information giver—offers facts or personal experience
❏ Information seeker—asks for facts pertinent to what is being discussed
❏ Initiator—proposes new ideas on how the goal can be reached or how to view the problem
❏ Elaborator—expands on the idea of another; takes the idea and works out what would happen if it was adopted
❏ Coordinator—brings together ideas and suggestions
❏ Orientor—keeps the group focused on goals or questions the direction taken by the group
❏ Evaluator of critic—examines possible group solutions against group standards and goals
❏ Clarifier—checks out what someone said by restating or questioning
❏ Recorder—acts as the group's memory (e.g., takes notes)
❏ Summarizer—pulls together related ideas, restates suggestions, and offers decisions or conclusions

(From Sullivan EJ, Decker P: Effective leadership and management in nursing, ed 4, Menlo Park, Calif, 1997, Addison-Wesley, p. 144.)

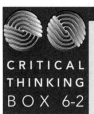

CRITICAL THINKING BOX 6-2

THINK ABOUT...

How is leading a group like the nursing process? The management process?
What motivates an individual to join a group? Stay in a group?
What group role do you adopt when participating in a group?

---

are healing, or we give support and comfort to them during the dying process. We may work in the area of hospice, where death is a daily expectation and nurses work to orchestrate a comfortable and dignified death. We work with our hands, hearts, and minds to relieve pain and suffering while helping those in our care to return to a normal healthy life.

Nurses experience the daily reality of life and death, working to restore life one minute while giving support and comfort to the dying in the next minute. Nurses are a major healing factor in a patient's response to the treatment plan. We help to instill a sense of well-being in those in our care when we work as a highly effective team and as individuals in our daily care delivery.

Nurses as a professional group can be a tremendous healing factor when we work together. As nurses we need to reach out in support of each other! As a formal group of professionals, we need to offer support and guidance to each other whenever possible. As a professional group of registered nurses, let us embrace each other as equals—with warmth, admiration, appreciation, and respect.

As graduating nurses, I truly admire you and your choice to dedicate your lives to the welfare of others. You have chosen to involve yourself in caring for those caught between life and death. It is critical for you as individual members of our nursing profession to grow in expertise, knowledge, wisdom, and self-awareness. You will be the guiding light for those who come after you. I hope that your experiences will be as wonderful for you as mine have been for me. I look forward to working side by side with you. Welcome to the team!

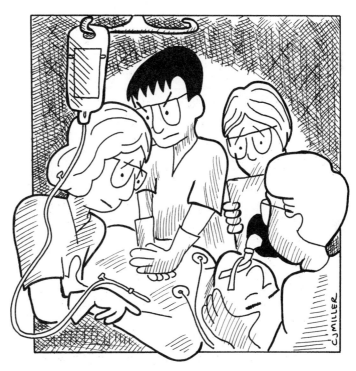

When nurses work as a team, everyone benefits.

REFERENCES

Farley MJ, Stoner MH: The nurse executive and interdisciplinary team building, *Nurs Adm Q* 13(2):24-30, 1989.

Katzenbach JR, Smith DK: *Wisdom of teams*, New York, 1993, Harper Business.

Schmieding NJ: A model for assessing nurse administrators' actions, *West J Nurs Resh* 12(3):293-306, 1990.

Sovie MD: Care and service teams: a new imperative, *Nurs Econ* 10(2):94-100, 125, 1992.

Sullivan EJ, Decker PJ: *Effective leadership and management in nursing*, ed 4, Menlo Park, Calif, 1997, Addison-Wesley.

Tuckman B, Jensen M: Stage of small group development revisited, *Group Organiz Stud* 2:419-427, 1977.

ADDITIONAL READINGS

Atwater D, Bass B: Transformational leadership in teams. In Bass BM, Avolio BJ, editors: *Improving organization effectiveness through transformational leadership*, Thousand Oaks, Calif, 1993, Sage.

Huber D: *Leadership and nursing care management*, Philadelphia, 1996, WB Saunders.

Orsburn JD, et al: *Self-directed work teams: the new American challenge*, New York, 1990, McGraw-Hill.

Rocchiccioli JT, Tilbury MS: *Clinical leadership in nursing: today's reality, tomorrow's vision*, Philadelphia, 1998, WB Saunders.

INTERNET RESOURCES

Center for the Study of Work Teams
http://www.workteams.unt.edu
Of interest are their archives of Work Teams Newsletters.
http://www.workteams.unt.edu/newsletter/Archive/archive-intro.htm

Team Building
http://www.mapnp.org/library/grp_skll/teams/teams.htm
Compilation of numerous sites and articles on team-building as a management strategy.

Team Building Super Site
http://www.teambuildinginc.com/ei_news.htm
Numerous online articles are available free of charge.

Experience-Based Learning
http://www.ebl.org
Provides information on active learning, teams, and group models for learning.

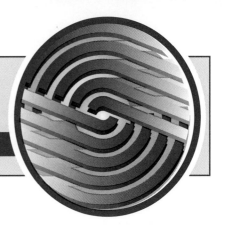

CHAPTER SEVEN

Effective Communication

LYNETTE W. JACK, PhD, RN, CARN

Nurse: "What seems to be the trouble?"

Patient: "I keep thinking no one can hear me."

Nurse: "What seems to be the trouble?"

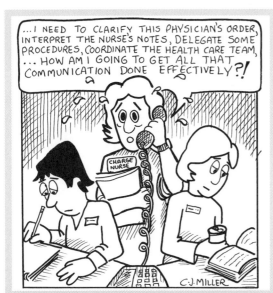

Communication should be clearly stated and directed to the appropriate responsible individual.

After completing this chapter, you should be able to:

- Describe the basic components of communication.
- Identify effective ways of communicating with other health care workers.
- Describe an assertive communication style.
- Apply effective communication skills in common nursing activities.

Y ou are probably wondering why there is a chapter in this book about communicating. After all, you've been talking with people for many years, and things seem to be going OK. Well, you're right—you do already have some communication skills. This chapter will help you apply what you do well to situations in the workplace that require effective communication skills. This chapter may also help you learn new ways of handling complex situations that commonly occur in nursing. So, if you're ready to proceed, let's briefly review some basic concepts about communication.

THE COMMUNICATION PROCESS

WHAT ARE THE PARTS OF THE COMMUNICATION PROCESS?

Communication begins with a person who creates a *message* on the basis of his or her own perception of a situation. This person is the *sender*, who transmits the message using words, actions, body language, tone of voice, and facial expression. The message goes to a *receiver*, who has to interpret and evaluate the message, including all the words and the signals. When the receiver sends a message back to the sender to let the sender know what he or she heard or saw, that is called *feedback*. So, communication is basically the giving and receiving of information that involves responding with meaning.

Much of the skill involved in effective communication involves how clear the message is. The actual words that are used are known as the message's *content*. Sometimes the words are very clear and the message is easily understood. But at other times, the words might mean different things to different people. The way in which the words are said may also change how they are interpreted. Check Critical Thinking Box 7-1 for an example of how many different ways information can be interpreted.

We all know that spoken words make up what we call *verbal communication*. When we include body movements, facial expressions, and tone of voice, we are adding the nonverbal communication components that make up nearly 90% of the message. An angry voice and crossed arms can change a friendly, supportive message to a hostile and critical one. The way we choose to communicate is known as *process*. The process may clarify the message or confuse the receiver. Consider the following one-act play as an example:

SCENE ONE

Susan has been working on a very busy surgical unit for 6 weeks since she graduated from nursing school. She is approached by the dietitian, who says to her, "I was so relieved when I got to the unit and saw that you had already requested a dietary modification for Mr. Smith following his surgery. Imagine that; I didn't even have to tell you to do it."

SCENE TWO

Susan: "Can you believe the arrogance of that dietitian? Just because she's been here forever and I'm new, does that give her the right to treat me like I'm a stupid third-grader?"

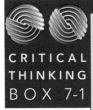

CRITICAL THINKING BOX 7-1

TRY THIS...

1. How many different ways can you communicate this sentence to change its meaning?
   "I don't care how you've done that procedure before; do it my way now."

   _____

   _____

   _____

   _____

2. When the instructor says to you:
   "Come to my office at 2:00. There's something I want to talk to you about."
   What are some possible interpretations of the message?

   _____

   _____

   _____

   _____

3. When a patient's spouse says to you:
   "I don't need your help when we go home."
   How many possible explanations can you come up with regarding the meaning of the communication?

   _____

   _____

   _____

   _____

Nancy (another recent graduate): "How do you know that's what she meant?"

Susan: "I could just tell by the frustration in her voice and how she moved away from me so quickly. It was as if she couldn't stand to talk to me anymore."

SCENE THREE (THE NEXT DAY ON THE UNIT)

Dietitian: "Susan, I wanted to thank you again for your initiative yesterday with Mr. Smith. I was having a particularly stressful day, and the thought of having to do one more task just seemed to overwhelm me. You really helped me out."

Susan: "I'm glad you said something about it. I wasn't sure what you meant then, and I feel much better."

Huber (2000) suggests several reasons why communication fails to be effective that can be applied to our one-act play. Nonverbal signals may mean different things to different people and can easily be misinterpreted. So can the words we use. In addition, if we are short of time, it is hard to hear clearly and remember pieces of important information. And finally, the personalities of the sender and the receiver may create a bias or distortion of the message.

WHAT ARE THE BASIC PRINCIPLES OF EFFECTIVE COMMUNICATION?

Here are some suggestions for improving our communication with others.

1. Communication is a process involving interaction between at least two people. Merely giving information is not communication unless the opportunity for a response is given.
2. The sender has a responsibility to make the message as clear as possible. You can verify what has been received by asking "Would you share with me how you interpreted what I just said?"
3. Whenever possible, use the simplest, most precise words you can. Your words must be understood by the listener.
4. Encourage the receiver of your message to provide feedback so you can verify that the message has been interpreted in the way it was intended. The receiver might say "So, what you're saying is . . . " or "Let me make sure I understand you. . . . "
5. Remember that nonverbal behavior communicates a message even when words are not used. Try to match your nonverbal behaviors to the feeling or tone of the message you want to send to others.
6. Your reputation and credibility will make it easier for you to communicate during difficult situations. When you are trustworthy, reliable, and competent, people will listen more carefully and be more likely to interpret your messages in a positive way.
7. Because communication is an interactive process, it is much more successful within the context of a sound relationship. To create and maintain that positive relationship with others, you need to acknowledge the needs, feelings, and contributions of others. This helps create a climate more open to communication.
8. Whenever possible, communicate directly with the person you want to receive your message. This allows for immediate feedback and verification and can reduce the chances of misunderstanding.
9. Concentrate on the communication happening in the present. Avoid the temptation to daydream or plan ahead what you might say or do next.
10. Be aware of your personal values and biases, and try to keep them from interfering with your ability to communicate.
11. When you are caring for a patient in his or her home, be especially respectful of the personal nature of the surroundings.

WHAT ARE FACILITATIVE MESSAGES?

Strayhorn (1977) divides messages into two types: facilitative and obstructive. Table 7-1 details some types of facilitative messages. These messages create a positive outcome in which the people communicating with each other feel good about their interaction. It may take some self-awareness and some practice to send facilitative messages, but it is worth it. Your relationships with other health care workers will be satisfying and, ultimately, the patients you care for will benefit.

⊜TABLE 7-1

Facilitative Messages

Type	Definition	Example	Effect
1. *I want* statement	Asks for a specific behavior	"I want you to let me practice this skill by myself and then check me in three days."	Simplest way to communicate what you want within a relationship
2. *I feel* statement	Shares your feeling in response to the other person's specific behavior	"I felt irritated just then when you told me to clean the nurses' station."	Allows you to get in touch with and share you feelings in a way undistorted by assumptions
3. *I like* and *I don't like* statements	Indicates your pleasure or displeasure with a specific behavior	"I liked it when you told me I did a good job with that patient."	Helps define what would make you happier; positive reinforcement most effective in changing another's behavior
4. Reflection	Tells the other person what you think you heard so he or she can verify or deny your interpretation	"Sounds like that really upset you."	Helps increase listening skills, reduces distorted messages, acknowledges feelings
5. Open-ended statement	Indicates general area of interest, but leaves specifics to other person	"Tell me your reactions to the new medication cart."	Offers attention and encourages communication to begin
6. Agreeing with part of a criticism or argument	Refuses to argue by agreeing or sympathizing with some part of the other's statement	The head nurse has just said to you, "You don't have any sense." You say, "It's true that I could be smarter than I am."	Avoids wasting time arguing; allows you to remember that you don't have to be perfect; focuses energy on negotiation of wants
7. Asking for more specific criticism	Allows you to ask what behaviors the critic didn't like, what behavior he or she would like in the future	The patient's family says, "You're doing that all wrong." You reply, "What would you like me to be doing instead?"	Turns an argument into an opportunity for productive negotiation; keeps anger at a minimum

(continued)

TABLE 7-1

Facilitative Messages *(Cont'd)*

Type	*Definition*	*Example*	*Effect*
8. Bargaining	Sender offers to sacrifice for the other if the other will sacrifice in return	"OK, I'm hearing that you don't want me to criticize you publicly. If I work on quitting doing that, will you work on asking me for help when you don't know how to do something?"	Offers positive incentives for meeting others' needs
9. Citing specific behaviors and observations	Names specific behaviors and events and describes them without drawing conclusions about meaning	"I noticed during the meeting that you weren't saying much, weren't smiling. I'm wondering what was going on."	Allows the other person to hear about his or her behavior and clarify what specific behaviors mean; reduces misperception
10. Asking for feedback	Asks the other person's reaction to what you have just said	"I'm interested in how you react to that idea."	Allows the sender to be sure the message was received as it was intended; allows further clarification
11. *You are good, you did something good, your something is good* statement	Conveys something was worthwhile	"You've really grown in your ability to handle complex situations." "That was good."	Draws attention to positive aspects of the other person and makes the other person feel good, appreciated
12. *I intend* statement	Conveys independent action the person plans to take	"I intend to be more careful about my charting."	Indicates the person accepts responsibility for his or her behavior
13. Communication postponement	Asks for postponement of a discussion until a more favorable time	"I'm feeling hurt and angry right now and would like some time to think before we talk more."	Allows you to be in emotional control

Modified from Strayhorn JM Jr: *Talking it out: a guide to effective communication and problem solving,* Champaign, Ill, 1977, Research Press, pp. 53-76.

Strayhorn (1977, p. 7) summarizes the benefits of learning to use facilitative messages: "If I can avoid antagonizing the other person, make my wishes known, find out the other person's wishes, explore various options, and make decisions accordingly, then I am much better equipped to bring happiness to others and to allow them to bring happiness to me."

WHAT ARE OBSTRUCTIVE MESSAGES?

Strayhorn (1977) says that obstructive messages generally make it much more difficult for people to communicate effectively within a positive relationship. Table 7-2 has some examples of obstructive messages. Noting the distinction between facilitative and obstructive messages will make you more attentive to the process of communication and more effective at getting your needs met. Try to identify facilitative and obstructive responses in Critical Thinking Box 7-2.

TABLE 7-2

Obstructive Messages

Type	Definition	Example	Effect
1. Communication cutoff	Statement or action that cuts off communication in order to avoid unpleasant feelings or to express hostility	"Just forget it—I won't ever bring it up again." "You don't care about me, just like everybody else."	Makes it impossible to negotiate a mutually acceptable solution to needs
2. Put-down question	Rhetorical question used to communicate a dissatisfied feeling in an indirect way	"What's the use in my doing anything for you when you always screw it up later anyway?"	Creates a need to attack or defend
3. *You are bad, you did something bad* statement	Conveys a negative value judgment about the other person	"You don't care about anybody but yourself."	Makes the other person feel threatened and less worthy; leads to further attack
4. *You should* statement	Statements that begin "you should have . . . ," "you shouldn't have . . . ," or "you ought to . . ."		

(continued)

⑤TABLE 7-2

Obstructive Messages *(Cont'd)*

Type	*Definition*	*Example*	*Effect*
5. Defending oneself	Response to criticism in which person tries to prove that what he or she did was right	"It wasn't my fault that patient started screaming; I was trying to be nice. That doctor sure was rough and uncaring, though."	Creates focus on placing blame, rather than looking for a solution
6. Sarcasm	Making a humorous statement, opposite of what is meant, to express hostility	"Oh sure, you're never late. We all really believe that."	Promotes attack and defense; allows the sender to avoid responsibility for expressing anger honestly and directly
7. Commanding	Directing another person to do something in an authoritarian voice that implies no choice	"You can't do that sort of thing around here."	Creates a power struggle and resentment
8. Expressing dissatisfaction through a third party	Communication not directed at the person to whom it is intended	Susan says to the head nurse, "You really ought to speak to Mary. She refuses to help any of the rest of us when we are really busy."	Allows attack and avoidance, may also lead to distorted messages
9. Assuming rather than checking it out	Assume your perception of an ambiguous or nonverbal message was correct without checking it out verbally	Susan sees the head nurse and a doctor in conversation at the door of one of her patient's rooms. The head nurse looks angry and is shaking her head. Susan concluded that they think she gave terrible care to that patient. In reality, they are talking about a hospital policy committee meeting.	Misunderstandings persist without being cleared up, and actions are based on mistaken assumptions

TABLE 7-2

Obstructive Messages *(Cont'd)*

Type	Definition	Example	Effect
10. Premature advice	Offer advice without first having encouraged the person to explore his or her feelings freely	Susan: "My head nurse really bothers me. She keeps giving me too much work." Mary: "If I were you, I'd tell her off. She has no right to treat you that way. Don't let her push you around."	Often the advice is not appropriate and closes off exploration of the real issue

Modified from Strayhorn JM Jr: *Talking it out: a guide to effective communication and problem solving*, Champaign, Ill, 1977, Research Press, pp. 53-76.

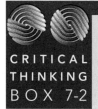

CRITICAL THINKING BOX 7-2

TRY THIS...

See if you can come up with some facilitative responses and some obstructive responses to these situations.

1. You are trying to finish your assignment, and your patient's family keeps asking you questions. This is interfering with your work.

_____

_____

_____

2. One of your co-workers repeatedly asks you for money and never pays you back.

_____

_____

_____

3. You need to be off this weekend to take care of a family emergency. Your head nurse tells you that her staffing needs must come first and you will have to work.

_____

_____

_____

COMMUNICATION IN THE WORKPLACE

COMMUNICATING WITH THE HEALTH CARE TEAM

Sharing information with the members of the health care team requires different approaches. This communication on a daily basis may involve delegation of a nursing procedure to an LVN (LPN) or aide, clarification of a physician's orders, reevaluation of a patient care assignment of another health care team member, or coordination of various hospital departments (radiology, dietary, pharmacy, and so on) to provide nursing care. Create role-playing situations with your peers by taking turns being in the supervisor and subordinate roles (Critical Thinking Box 7-3).

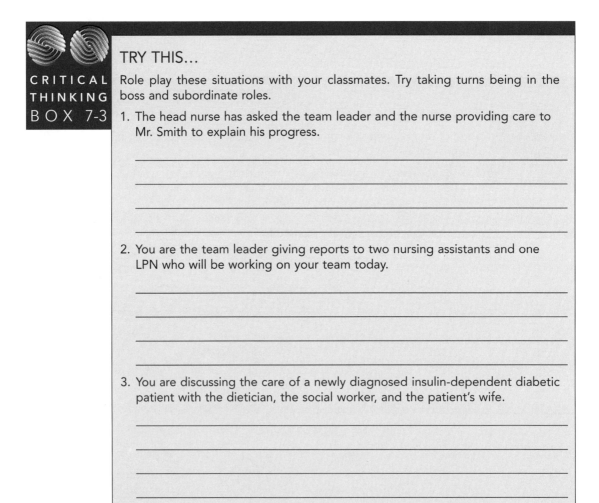

CRITICAL THINKING BOX 7-3

TRY THIS...

Role play these situations with your classmates. Try taking turns being in the boss and subordinate roles.

1. The head nurse has asked the team leader and the nurse providing care to Mr. Smith to explain his progress.

   _____

   _____

   _____

   _____

2. You are the team leader giving reports to two nursing assistants and one LPN who will be working on your team today.

   _____

   _____

   _____

   _____

3. You are discussing the care of a newly diagnosed insulin-dependent diabetic patient with the dietician, the social worker, and the patient's wife.

   _____

   _____

   _____

   _____

HOW CAN I COMMUNICATE EFFECTIVELY WITH MY SUPERVISOR?

Upward communication with supervisors takes on a formal nature. It is important to learn and then use the channels of communication. If you are a team member, this means you share information with your team leader. The team leader shares information with the supervisor, who shares information with the assistant vice president of nursing, who shares information with the vice president of nursing, and so on. You can see that there are many levels of nursing between the bedside nurse and the people with major decision-making responsibility.

Do you remember the game you played as a child in which someone whispers a secret to the next person, and each person repeats the secret down the line until the last person speaks the secret aloud? The secret may have started out as "Jenny was out picking berries today so she can bake a pie." By the end of the line, it may have become "Jenny is so allergic to cherries that she breaks out into hives." The point is that messages can get very distorted when they travel through many people in the upward flow of communication. Arredondo (2000) says it is important in communicating with superiors to state needs clearly, explain the rationales for requests, and suggest the benefits to the larger unit. It's also important to listen objectively to the response of the supervisor because there may be good reasons for granting or not granting the request.

Arredondo (2000) gives the following tips for talking to your supervisor:

1. Keep your supervisor informed.
2. If a problem is developing, make an appointment to talk it over. Have specific information available, especially written documentation of facts. Focus on problem solving, not just the problems.
3. Show that you have important information to share and a sense of responsibility.
4. Be careful which words you use. Avoid blaming others, exaggeration, and overly dramatic expressions.
5. Don't talk to your supervisor when angry, and don't respond with anger. Use "I" statements, and explain what you think.
6. If you want to present a new idea, give your supervisor a written proposal, then meet to discuss it after the supervisor has read it.
7. Accept feedback, and learn from it.
8. Never go above or around your supervisor. Always communicate directly with your supervisor first before going further up the chain of command.

HOW CAN I COMMUNICATE EFFECTIVELY WITH OTHER NURSING PERSONNEL?

When you speak with other professional nurses, you are communicating in a lateral, or horizontal, flow of information. This flow is based on a concept of equality, in which no person holds more power than the other. This type of communication is best done in a work climate that promotes a sense of trust and respect among colleagues. When nurses work well together, their cohesiveness makes success more likely. This takes work and the deliberate use of facilitative messages (Northouse, 2001).

Ideally, professional nurses should view themselves as equals in their interactions with members of other health care disciplines, and their approach to communication should be a lateral one, even with physicians. At the basis of this communication is the ability of the nurse to see himself or herself as competent and worthy of being an equal to physicians, social workers, dietitians, and others. To gain this self-confidence is a major goal of every recent graduate. The use of effective communication practices, as described in this chapter, will help you achieve that goal.

HOW CAN I COMMUNICATE EFFECTIVELY WITH PATIENT CARE ASSISTANTS?

Even a recent graduate will soon be providing direction to licensed nursing personnel and unlicensed assistive nursing personnel. (See Chapter 10 for further information on delegation.) It is important to remember that these people have needs for satisfaction and self-esteem, too. Directions do not need to be given in the form of authoritative commands unless an emergency demands immediate action in a prescribed way. Marquis and Huston (2000) suggest that when you provide direction, you need to think through exactly what you want to be done, by whom, and when. You need to get the full attention of the other person so that you know he or she is hearing you accurately. You should then give clear, simple instructions in step-by-step order, using a supportive tone of voice. Before the other person goes to do the task, ask for feedback to verify that he or she has accurately heard your instructions. Finally, follow-up is necessary to be sure your directions were carried out and to find out what happened, in case something more needs to be done. Involving these personnel who are at other levels of nursing care in the planning and evaluation of the care will increase their sense of responsibility for the outcomes and will help you to seem less authoritarian.

WHAT DOES MY IMAGE COMMUNICATE TO OTHERS?

 Remember that old saying "Don't judge a book by its cover"?

Unfortunately we know that most people don't follow that suggestion. People do get impressions about us from our image—the way we look, sound, talk, and act. Often we are less careful about the messages we send with our appearance and behavior than we are when we choose our words. But our image may speak louder than our words. Think about it. Would you feel comfortable accepting nutrition advice from a 300-pound nurse? How would you like it if your instructor criticized your professionalism while wearing dirty shoes, a wrinkled uniform, bright red nail polish, and four earrings in each earlobe? What would you think about a physician whose progress notes contain many misspelled words and poor grammar?

Communication is enhanced by your credibility. And people listen more to people they respect. Your image will help you communicate your professional credibility.

The place to start projecting a positive image is with the first impression your appearance creates (Vengel, 2000). Good personal hygiene is a must. Each day you have to pay attention to your grooming. This means a flattering, neat haircut; clean, well-fitting clothes; reasonable makeup and perfume; minimal jewelry; and clean, sensible shoes. Your image is improved greatly if your weight is appropriate for your height and bone structure. Your appearance at work should conform to the norms for professionals in your work setting; save your individuality for your personal time away from work.

Another aspect of your image is your depth and breadth of knowledge. You need to know your particular kind of nursing thoroughly if you want others' respect. But you also need to know something about a wide variety of subjects so you can have conversations with people beyond nursing. This means keeping up with current events, learning things about art or sports, and reading books. When people discover common interests, they are more willing to communicate with you.

Flexibility is necessary for effective communication with different kinds of people. This means that you are willing and able to adapt your behavior to relate more comfortably or effectively with others. Flexibility is part of a positive image because it says to people that you are willing to accept responsibility for changing your behavior to meet the professional needs or requirements of others.

People who achieve success in their professional careers are enthusiastic. They let others know they are happy to be at work. They work harder, longer, and more accurately. They are pleasant to be around. They are sincere in their efforts to create a professional image that can be trusted.

Take an inventory of your appearance, knowledge, and attitude. If you're not sure what kind of image you are communicating, ask several trusted friends.

WHAT DO I NEED TO KNOW ABOUT SEX DIFFERENCES IN COMMUNICATION STYLES?

Men and women view their work environments from different perspectives (Vengel, 2000; Mindell, 2001). Men often see the world from a logical, sequential, focused perspective. Women often tend to see the big picture and to seek solutions based on what makes people feel comfortable rather than on logic. Subtle communication differences can create barriers to open, healthy communication between men and women in the workplace. Men may ask fewer questions in a public situation, especially if they feel that their questions might suggest ignorance. Women seem to be more comfortable asking questions (Mindell, 2001). In fact there are times when a person can benefit from remaining silent and looking up information later in private so that others do not conclude that the asker lacks sufficient knowledge. At other times a person must be assertive and ask questions so that he or she does not threaten the health of patients.

Within the workplace, the dominant communication style is direct, confident, and assertive. This style may be more familiar to men because they are often raised hearing more aggressive, direct language from their parents, whereas many women may be more used to a soft, supportive tone of voice and choice of words. Cultural values learned in childhood also play a role in the communication style a person chooses. This style may have to be modified, however, to make interactions more successful. A woman who is communicating with a man may need to be more direct and assertive than usual, whereas a man may need to learn to be less aggressive in many situations.

Another sex difference in communication is related to childhood experiences with sports. Men often grow up with participation in team sports. They have worked toward a goal and have learned to strategize together for the good of the team, building a network of allies. Women have tended to be less involved with team sports than men. Women are more likely to have spent more time interacting with a few people they really like who share similar values and behaviors. Women are generally taught to be polite and to say nice things about and to others, whereas men are encouraged to do whatever it takes to help the team win. In the workplace, men and women need to understand their different points of view so that they can be team players and value cooperation and respectful relationships with each other.

To summarize, men and women have innately different communication styles, often developed from childhood experiences. To be successful in the workplace, we all have to learn as much as we can about communication differences, identify our own styles, and have the flexibility to use other communication techniques in situations that call for it.

WHAT SHOULD I KNOW ABOUT THE "GRAPEVINE?"

In addition to formal messages, informal communication flows upward, downward, and horizontally and is known as the *grapevine*. Whereas some people think of this kind of communication as gossip, others say it's the way things really get done. No matter how we describe the grapevine, we know it flourishes in all settings. People enjoy the satisfaction of the social interaction and recognition associated with the grapevine. It also provides information to employees that may not be easily obtained in any other way. It may, for example, be the quickest way to find out what the supervisor really values or what the new job openings are (Marquis and Huston, 2000).

Mindell (2001) provides the following tips for controlling the grapevine, which can provide much distorted information:

1. Provide factual information to answer questions before they are asked. Few employees get all the information they feel they need.
2. Communicate face-to-face whenever possible. Don't trust the accuracy of messages through a third party.
3. Whenever rumors are running through the grapevine, hold a meeting to provide information and answer questions.
4. Don't spread rumors. Make sure you have all the facts from their source.
5. Enlist the support of respected leaders to spread the truth.
6. Address significant issues as soon as possible with your manager so that negative feelings can be defused.
7. Make sure what is put in writing is clear and accurately understood.

HOW CAN I DEAL WITH CULTURAL DIVERSITY AT WORK?

Dochterman and Grace (2000) tell us that culture is a pattern of values and beliefs that is reflected in the behaviors we demonstrate. Whenever a group of people spend an extended period of time together, they develop a culture. Each of us comes from a cultural background, and we have beliefs, values, and behaviors that result from that background. In our workplaces we will encounter many different types of people coming from diverse cultural backgrounds. To communicate effectively, we need to understand our own culture as well as the other person's culture. In addition we must acknowledge and adhere to the cultural norms or rules that have developed in our workplace.

We must become aware of stereotypes that may interfere with our ability to see people as individuals. If we view people according to stereotypes, we might limit the way we perceive their communication. Even positive stereotypes make assumptions about people that may be inaccurate and thus may limit the nurse's ability to use all of his or her work skills effectively (Critical Thinking Box 7-4).

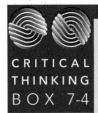

CRITICAL THINKING BOX 7-4

TRY THIS...

As you go about your work, take note of the various people you interact with and your reactions to them. Write them down so that you can reflect on them. What kinds of thoughts come to mind when you see a female executive, an African-American male, an Asian child, an older woman, or a handsome man dressed in a suit? How do your initial impressions impact on the way you communicate with each of these people?

Picture yourself in the homes of five of your clients. Choose people from different cultural backgrounds. How are their homes different? In what ways do their homes reflect their culture? What do you need to know about each culture so that you can provide care effectively while avoiding any stereotyped beliefs?

According to Arredondo (2000), communication goes through many filters when a person interacts with someone whom he or she perceives as different. Some of those filters are related to culture, sex, education level, age, and experience. When messages go through these filters, they may change because the actual communication symbols are interpreted according to a person's own cultural values and beliefs. This change may lead to misperceptions and misinterpretations. Communication is improved when we become more aware of the filters we use.

Within the work culture, people often communicate using jargon, inside jokes, or slang unique to the work setting. Acronyms are an example of jargon that health care workers understand but patients may not. It may seem to patients and their families that we are speaking in a code or foreign language. To interact effectively, we need to speak clearly, avoiding jargon or slang, and to keep our communication short and to-the-point. Long explanations can be confusing to people not familiar with the health care culture.

Differences in the cultural backgrounds of workers can be a real asset. Sometimes we may have to provide care to patients who speak languages other than English, and we may need the skills of co-workers to translate or interpret, especially when cultural values influence the interpretation of the patient's behavior. We need to understand and respect cultural differences in patients. We can learn how to do this by learning about the differences among our co-workers. Respect and empathy enhance communication with people from other cultures, whether those people are patients or co-workers (Dochterman and Grace, 2001).

COMPONENTS OF COMMUNICATION

HOW CAN I COMMUNICATE EFFECTIVELY IN WRITING?

Communication takes place not only when words are spoken, but also when they are written and then read by someone else. A big part of a nurse's overall effectiveness depends on the ability to write effectively. This includes written treatment plans, progress notes, job descriptions, consultation requests, referrals, and memos. Some of you may even write articles for nursing journals or chapters for textbooks!

Mindell provides some guidelines for writing (2001). Determine whether you need to write in a formal way. Most upward communication needs to be formal, which means you should use proper titles, format, grammar, spelling, and punctuation. Never allow something you have written to be sent without careful proofreading. Nothing creates a negative impression faster than sloppy work, misspelled words, or poor grammar. If you need to, ask someone else to do this proofreading; be sure it is done well. Take the time to make necessary revisions before sending your written work on.

Decide what your purpose is before you write (Marquis and Huston, 2000). This will help you to organize your thoughts so that everything you write helps you to meet your purpose. Learn to write exactly what you mean. Choose words that are clear and specific. Often this means simple, small words. Be careful to use technical words only when you are sure you are choosing the correct words and your reader will understand you. Keep your sentences short and simple, with only one idea in each sentence.

Try using the KISS principle. KISS Principle: Keep It Short and Simple.

When you learn to be clear and concise, you will write the essential information without a lot of flowery phrases. Your readers will be very grateful if they can follow your thoughts easily. Make your first sentence in each paragraph identify the key point for that paragraph. The reader shouldn't have to guess what you are trying to say. Use a format that guides the reader. This means that visually on each page, main points are easy to locate and concepts are identified by headings or titles. Remember, how well you write strongly influences how you are evaluated. What you put down on paper makes a lasting impression, and people will make judgments about your credibility and professionalism for a long time after you have actually written the words.

HOW CAN I LEARN TO SPEAK EFFECTIVELY?

From giving a report at the change-of-shift to explaining your plans for a new approach on the unit to the organization's administration, you will have lots of opportunities to make presentations.

 The first step in making effective presentations is to develop a positive attitude. ACCENTUATE the POSITIVE!

Many of us let our anxiety intimidate us. But public speaking can be a great chance to show off our skills, our ability to be creative, and our willingness to be a star entertainer. Think of your presentation as a wonderful opportunity to have the attention of others on just you, even if only for a few minutes (Arredondo, 2000).

 The second guiding principle in making good presentations is practice. PRACTICE makes PERFECT!

A well-planned rehearsal gives you a chance to see how long it will take you to say what you want and will help you feel more comfortable saying the words easily. Here are some tips on preparation from Kushner (1997).

1. Analyze your audience. What do they already know, and what do they need to know?
2. Have an objective or two for what you want your audience to get out of your presentation.
3. Do your homework. Know enough about your subject to make your talk clear and believable. Make sure you're able to answer at least a few questions.
4. Plan how you will make the presentation, including an outline of the content and the teaching strategies you might use. Visual aids or activities may be used to involve the audience in active participation.
5. If the speech or presentation is an important one and fairly formal, you may want to prepare a script. This means you write out exactly what you will say and have it typed double-spaced, with a wide margin on the left side. Here you can write notes to yourself about when to use your visual aids or when to pass out materials for the audience.
6. The more active your audience's participation, the longer they will pay attention. Choose at least one presentation strategy that involves them, such as question/answer, role playing, or small-group discussion. Key points you want your audience to remember should be highlighted visually on slides or overhead transparencies.
7. Use an attention grabber at the beginning to make sure your audience is listening. This may be a friendly greeting, a stimulating question, a startling statistic, a relevant story, or a quote by an expert.

8. Then tell your audience the purpose of the presentation and what it will cover in brief and concise words.

9. Visual aids should keep the presentation focused and organized. They help you hold your audience's attention.

10. In your closing, review what you've said, summarize the benefits or implications of what you've said, and reiterate any action you want taken.

11. Be sure to be familiar with the room and equipment you will be using. Make sure everything you need is there before you begin.

12. Make sure the spelling is correct on your visual aids and handouts.

13. Speak with confidence, energy, and enthusiasm.

14. Make as much eye contact as you can.

15. Use your hands and arms to make dramatic gestures. They add energy and interest.

WHAT LISTENING SKILLS DO I NEED TO DEVELOP?

Listening effectively is one of the most powerful communication tools you can have. It's more than just hearing the words of others. Listening involves concentrating all your energy on understanding and interpreting the message with the meaning the sender intended. Of the four verbal means of communication—writing, reading, speaking, and listening—listening requires most of our communication time. And yet we often pay the least attention to our listening skills (Mindell, 2001). It has been estimated that people actually remember only one third of the messages they have heard, although they spend 70% of their time listening (Marquis and Huston, 2000).

There are reasons why people are not good listeners (Arredondo, 2000). We simply don't pay enough attention; we hear what we want to hear and filter out the rest. Listening requires concentration, and that means doing nothing else at the same time. Some people think of listening as a passive behavior; they want to be in control by talking more. We think a lot faster than people speak, so we often think way ahead or think about other things or daydream. It may be that there are too many distractions that interfere with listening, such as background noises or movements.

One of the most problematic reasons for ineffective listening is that people allow their emotions to dictate what they hear or don't hear. We pay more attention to people we like or respect and less attention to people or messages that make us feel uncomfortable. If the message is making demands on us to do more, change what we do, or do better, we may stop listening to deal with our own feelings of anger, guilt, or anxiety. We may start planning our own defensive response while the other person is still talking.

> Think about situations you've been in where you've had difficulty listening, understanding, or remembering what was said. Consider these examples:
>
> ■ A psychiatric patient who has recently been admitted displays acutely psychotic thought processes by talking rapidly in pressured speech, using words and phrases so loosely connected that the whole conversation is disorganized and incomprehensible.
>
> ■ A head nurse spends 5 minutes screaming at her team leader, criticizing everything she has done that day, and then asks the team leader to carry out a very specific and detailed change in the physician's orders for a patient.

■ Another nurse asks you to hang an intravenous solution for the patient in room 1253 while you are writing some progress notes on a patient's chart. When you finish, you can't remember the room number where you agreed to hang the intravenous solution.

It becomes essential to develop effective listening skills (Arredondo, 2000). Following are some tips:

1. Make sure you can hear what is being said. Move closer, eliminate distracting noises, and, most of all, don't talk. You can't hear someone else when you're talking.
2. Focus your attention on what is being said. Actively concentrate by analyzing the key points as they are being said. Take notes. Don't do anything else while you are listening except concentrating on hearing and understanding what is being said.
3. Recognize and control your emotional response to what is being said. Focus on hearing and seeing accurately what is being communicated. You will have time to ask questions and explore feelings after the other person finishes.
4. Decide in the beginning that you will listen and accept the other person's needs and feelings, whatever they are. Improved understanding of the other person is gained through listening, and this understanding will help you to be more effective in solving problems and eliminating negative feelings.
5. Pay attention to nonverbal communication as you listen to the words. Much of the meaning comes through in the tone of voice, facial expressions, and body movements. You must listen with your eyes and your ears.
6. Fight off distractions. Don't let the speaker's style of communicating, his or her mannerisms, telephone calls, or other interruptions break your concentration.
7. If a lot of factual, important information is being given, take notes—but just jot down key words or numbers or the note-taking itself will become a distraction. You may also ask the speaker to put in writing what he or she has said.
8. Let the speaker tell the whole story. Make it a point not to interrupt. Try not to assume you know what is going to be said. Withhold formulating criticisms as you listen.
9. Make an effort to respond positively to the feelings being communicated. Empathy and acceptance will make it easier for the communication to continue.
10. React to the message, not the person. Ask yourself, "Are my feelings or biases interfering with my listening?"
11. Seek feedback of your understanding by verifying what you have heard.
12. Maintain a positive attitude about listening. Recognize that listening is necessary for success.
13. Allow yourself to hear all sides of an issue.

Identify the characteristics of your listening skills in Critical Thinking Box 7-5.

HOW CAN I USE NONVERBAL COMMUNICATION EFFECTIVELY?

Nonverbal communication uses movements, gestures, body position, and voice tone to transmit messages (Arredondo, 2000). To convey confidence and leadership ability, it is necessary to learn to use certain nonverbal signals effectively. Following are some tips:

CRITICAL THINKING BOX 7-5

TRY THIS...

Develop a listening action plan.

1. I listen most effectively when

_____

_____

_____

2. I have difficulty listening when

_____

_____

_____

3. My best listening skills are

_____

_____

_____

4. I need to improve on my skills at

_____

_____

_____

5. In order to improve my listening skills, I will

_____

_____

_____

1. Make eye contact with the person with whom you are talking. This helps the person interpret your message more favorably and says that you are giving your full attention to the conversation.
2. Stand up straight, with shoulders back. You may want to lean slightly forward toward the other individual to convey your interest.
3. Stand approximately 18 inches to 4 feet from the person you're talking to so that you don't invade personal space. Avoid personal contact unless you know the person well and it is a casual conversation.
4. Use a forceful voice without pauses to suggest confidence. Avoid a whining, nagging, or complaining tone. You may need to listen to your tape-recorded voice to get some insight into how you sound to others.

5. Stand with your toes pointed slightly outward and slightly apart. When you use your hands in gestures, keep your forearm up and the palm of your hand open. Avoid making a fist or shaking a pointing finger at the other person.

6. Avoid negative behaviors that detract from your verbal messages: nodding constantly, yawning, playing with your hair, scratching yourself, cracking your knuckles, or twiddling your thumbs.

WHAT SKILLS DO I NEED TO USE THE TELEPHONE EFFECTIVELY?

Many nurses spend time on the telephone talking with physicians, patients and their families, and other health care workers. Here are some tips for making telephone communication productive. It is always polite to ask the person you are calling if this is a convenient time to talk. You may encounter difficulties reaching people by telephone. If this "telephone tag" problem persists after two attempts, leave a message stating exactly when you will be available to talk (and then be there).

If you anticipate your conversation will involve complex information, make notes ahead of time so you can keep your conversation as focused and brief as possible. With detailed, critical information that is discussed over the telephone, it is wise to follow up with a written communication to that person. Important telephone calls should also be followed up in writing; this helps to clarify and confirm the information discussed. If your telephone conversation requires a follow-up action, you need to keep a written record.

It is difficult to focus on the telephone conversation if you are attempting to do something else. Your communication will be more effective if you do one thing at a time. (How many times have you been irritated by a driver who is also talking on a cellular telephone?) Once you have finished your discussion, get off the phone; don't chit-chat or gossip once the information has been communicated. Communicating with physicians on the telephone presents a challenge to recent graduates. Box 7-1 highlights some helpful tips.

 BOX 7-1   Tips for Communicating With Physicians on the Phone

1. Say who you are right away.
2. Don't apologize for phoning.
3. State your business briefly but completely.
4. Ask for specific orders when appropriate.
5. If you want the doctor to assess the patient, say so.
6. If the doctor is coming, ask when to expect him or her.
7. If you get cut off, call back.
8. Document attempts to reach a doctor.
9. If a doctor is rude or abusive, tell him or her so.
10. If you can't reach a doctor or get what you need, always tell your manager.

HOW CAN I COMMUNICATE EFFECTIVELY BY USING TECHNOLOGY?

Many of us are learning to use the technology that is changing our workplace and making communication easier. Although cellular telephones, fax machines, portable personal computers, modems, and voice mail may be conveniences, they must be used thoughtfully to make a positive contribution to your overall image as an effective communicator. Deep and Sussman (1995) give the following tips for the successful use of communications technology:

Don't misuse or overuse fax machines. Remember that the person on the other end must read every page faxed to him or her, so be brief. If you need to send a long document, use the mail. Send faxes only when you don't mind if the quality of the copy isn't first-rate because many people have fax machines that print less clearly than computers or even copying machines.

When you leave someone a voice-mail message, speak slowly and distinctly. This is especially important when you are leaving your telephone number so that the other person can return your call. It's frustrating to receive a message but not be able to understand the name or have to replay the message to get all of the digits in the phone number. Make your voice-mail message brief but complete, saying when you called, what you want the other person to do, and when you can be reached.

Don't leave callers on hold if you are using call waiting. Explain to the first caller that you must briefly answer another call, then take the number of the second caller, with the assurance that you will call back as soon as you finish your first call. This interruption should take no more than 10 seconds. Be sure to write down the telephone number of the second caller so that you don't forget it by the time you finish the first call.

When you call people, ask if they have time to talk and offer to call back at a more convenient time if necessary. People appreciate the courtesy and will be more likely to have a positive conversation with you if it is conveniently timed and is respectful of their busy schedules.

If you are conducting a conversation or a meeting with a speaker telephone or by means of a teleconference, make sure that each party to the call is introduced to the other people. Do not use the speaker telephone unless you are including a group in the conversation. Even with a conference call, there should be some structure to the discussion, including an agenda or a specified purpose and time for the call.

When you have business cards printed, include your e-mail address and your fax number. If you are sending messages by e-mail, be sure to read your words carefully before sending them. Because you are sending words without the benefit of clarifying nonverbal communication, the likelihood of being misinterpreted is greater. Make sure your messages are as clear as they can be. Include your name and subject in the e-mail note.

Do not send an emotional outburst in an e-mail. These messages can seem more hostile than you intended, and you can alienate or anger many people. If you cannot state your message in person, then don't send it by e-mail.

Learn to use basic computer software. Most people can effectively use fewer than half of the programs to which they have access. Know how to use word-processing software. This is especially helpful in making your communication easier and more credible.

When you need to send a personal message, especially a reminder or a thank-you, the most powerful way is to send a handwritten note. This conveys the importance you connect with the message and continues the interpersonal aspect of the communication. If you need to communicate something that you expect will have a real emotional impact, do it face-to-face. This communication style has more force, too, but it also allows you an opportunity to read the other person's nonverbal communication and offers a chance to negotiate a comfortable understanding following your message delivery.

GROUP COMMUNICATION

HOW CAN YOU IMPROVE COMMUNICATIONS IN A GROUP MEETING?

Nurses participate in many meetings, from patient care conferences to more formal committee meetings. Communication within a group of people can be an opportunity to influence the quality of care given to patients. When you participate as a member of a group, the following are positive behaviors that will help you to communicate effectively and will also help the group to accomplish its tasks more efficiently:

- Come prepared. Bring all the "stuff" you need.
- Listen. Be open to other viewpoints.
- Keep on track. Don't visit or chit-chat.
- Present your ideas or opinions. Ask other members for theirs.
- State disagreements. Be able to back them up.
- Clarify when needed. Don't assume.

All of us have been to and participated in meetings that were unorganized, confusing, and a waste of time. Critical Thinking Box 7-6 will help you to identify some unpleasant group meeting experiences and give you the opportunity to change future meetings.

WHAT ARE THE RESPONSIBILITES OF A GROUP LEADER?

If you are the leader of a group meeting, you have additional responsibilities. If you are organized and able to communicate effectively, the meeting is much more likely to run smoothly. This is especially important when you and your group members are busy. You can't afford to waste time sitting in an unproductive meeting. Nothing is as irritating as time spent arguing with others when you know your work is piling up on

CRITICAL
THINKING
BOX 7-6

TRY THIS...

Think of particularly unpleasant experiences you've had at meetings. You might think about meetings involving your clinical group or your class officers. Develop a list of ideas about what was wrong with those meetings.

_____

_____

_____

_____

_____

_____

_____

_____

_____

_____

your desk. If the irritation continues to build, you and the other group members will be less committed to the goals of the group and some will even stop coming. The key to effective meetings is the planning and organization that occurs before the meeting is actually held. Planning should allow the leader to think through what the meeting is for, who should be there, and how it should run (Huber, 2000). There should be a clear purpose for every meeting and every item on the agenda. Every item should require some action by the group. If the purpose could be achieved in another way, such as by making a telephone call or sending a memo, there should be no meeting.

It is the leader's responsibility to send out an agenda ahead of time and to indicate any preparations members need to make or materials they need to bring. The leader must also be concerned with the room where the meeting will be held. If you are making a formal presentation, some audio-visual equipment will be necessary and chairs will need to be arranged so that everyone can see the presenter and the audio-visuals. If the meeting is for discussion and decision making, a table at which everyone can sit face-to-face is more effective. Look at Figure 7-1. This type of note-taking clarifies who is responsible for what activities. Ask for a volunteer to keep track of the timeline information. At the conclusion of the meeting, summarize the decisions and identify the plan of action. Review the timeline information for clarity and understanding regarding group member responsibilities. At the end of the meeting, the time should be established for the next meeting. All members should receive a copy of the timeline information.

Inservice on Glucometer	Janet & Deb	5/24/03	
Revise Suction procedure	Sue & Bill	4/22/03	5/8/03
Review charting and report back to next Unit meeting	Tom & Amy	5/1/03	5/18/03

FIGURE 7-1
Action timeline for meetings.

ASSERTIVE COMMUNICATION

WHAT IS AN ASSERTIVE STYLE OF COMMUNICATION?

All of us have a style or way of communicating with others that is often based on our own personality and self-concept. In other words the kind of person we are and the way in which we see ourselves influence the process of communication. This style can be divided into three common types: passive or avoidant, aggressive, and assertive (Marquis and Huston, 2000). Following are some characteristics of each style:

Passive or avoidant behavior means that a person lets others push him around; doesn't stand up for himself; does what he's told, regardless of how he feels about it; is not able to share his feelings or needs with others; has difficulty asking for help; and feels hurt, anxious, or angry at others for taking advantage of him.

Aggressive behavior means that a person puts his or her own needs, rights, and feelings first and communicates that in an angry, dominating way; attempts to humiliate or "put down" other people; conveys a righteous, superior attitude; works at controlling or manipulating others; is seen by others as punishing, threatening, demanding, or hostile; and shows no concern for anyone else's feelings.

Assertive behavior means that a person stands up for herself in a way that doesn't violate the basic rights of another person; expresses her true feelings in an honest, direct manner; does not let others take advantage of her; shows respect for others' rights, needs, and feelings; sets goals and acts on those goals in a clear and consistent manner and takes responsibility for the consequences of those actions; is able to accept compliments and criticism; and acts in a way that enhances self-respect.

See if you can match the person with his or her style by using the descriptions you have just read.

■ JANE

Jane is a very shy, quiet senior nursing student who can't think straight when her instructor asks her questions in the clinical area. She wishes she could be more like her classmates, who seem to find it easy to talk about their experiences during clinical conference. During her evaluation, her instructor says she doesn't know enough theory and can't handle the pressures of the clinical unit. Jane says nothing and signs her evaluation. When she gets back to her room alone, she cries uncontrollably.

■ SUSAN

Susan is a senior nursing student who is highly verbal with her classmates. She is known to be opinionated and in every conference with her clinical group finds a chance to criticize someone. She blames the nursing staff on the clinical unit for making her look bad by giving her too much work to do and not enough time or help. When her instructor tells her she has not used enough theory in her written assignments, she says, "It's not my fault; you should have told me sooner."

■ MARK

Mark is a senior nursing student who is described by his clinical group as goal-oriented and confident. He wrote learning objectives for himself at the beginning of the last clinical experience and brought them with him, along with a self-evaluation, for his final evaluation conference. He listened to his instructor's suggestions, thanked her, and said, "I appreciate your concern for the quality of my nursing skills. I'm aware now of what I need to pay attention to in my first few months in my new job."

If you decided that Jane used a passive or avoidant style, Susan used an aggressive style, and Mark used an assertive style, you were right. Congratulations!

WHY AREN'T MORE NURSES ASSERTIVE?

It seems as though many nurses do not consistently act or communicate in an assertive way. Some have a hard time believing in their own rights, feelings, or needs. This difficulty may have gotten its start in childhood through exposure to many negative statements or experiences. It's important to recognize that communication style is learned and reinforced over time. While in nursing school and working in the nursing profession, additional experiences or comments may reinforce those negative messages about self-worth. It can be very difficult to change behavior, especially when risk-taking is necessary. The first step is to recognize what the barriers are. What is it that prevents you from being more assertive? Is it previously learned behavior, or are you afraid of the repercussions of assertive communication? Check the list in Box 7-2. If this list includes statements you feel are true, then you have identified some roadblocks to your ability to develop more assertive communication.

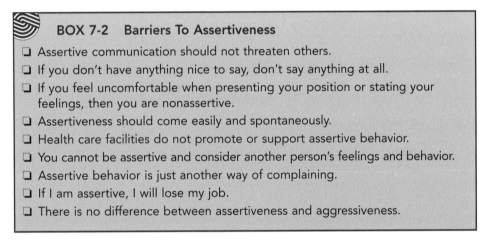

BOX 7-2   Barriers To Assertiveness
- ❏ Assertive communication should not threaten others.
- ❏ If you don't have anything nice to say, don't say anything at all.
- ❏ If you feel uncomfortable when presenting your position or stating your feelings, then you are nonassertive.
- ❏ Assertiveness should come easily and spontaneously.
- ❏ Health care facilities do not promote or support assertive behavior.
- ❏ You cannot be assertive and consider another person's feelings and behavior.
- ❏ Assertive behavior is just another way of complaining.
- ❏ If I am assertive, I will lose my job.
- ❏ There is no difference between assertiveness and aggressiveness.

Look over this list of barriers to assertive communication and think about yourself. Do any of these explain your feelings? Assertiveness takes self-awareness and practice. It will help you to identify and accept your position right now with regard to assertiveness so that you can make a plan to develop this skill.

WHAT ARE THE BENEFITS OF ASSERTIVENESS?

Assertive communication is the most effective way to let other people know what you feel, what you need, and what you are thinking. It helps you to feel good about yourself and allows you to treat others with respect. Being assertive helps you to avoid feeling guilty, angry, resentful, confused, or lonely. You have a greater chance to get your rights acknowledged and your needs met, which leads to a more satisfying life.

WHAT ARE MY BASIC RIGHTS AS A PERSON AND AS A NURSE?

As an adult human being, you have some legitimate rights. You may have to do some work to allow yourself to believe in your rights. You may have learned other values that make it difficult to accept the validity of these rights. But belief in your own value as a separate individual and confidence in the positive concepts associated with assertiveness as a communication style will help you to believe in your rights.

Consider the rights and responsibilities of the nurse. The issue of rights can become one-sided. When nurses consider rights, responsibilities must also be included. These rights are yours as a registered nurse; acquiring them and holding them are your responsibility (Chenevert, 1988).

HOW CAN I BEGIN TO PRACTICE ASSERTIVE COMMUNICATION?

There are a variety of ways to learn to be more assertive in your communication style, but they all involve self-awareness and practice. It may not feel totally comfortable at first, but as you work at it, assertive communication will come more naturally.

 Changing one's behavior requires a conscious decision.

You should practice being assertive in a situation where there is minimal risk to you, so that you can experience success. If sharing your feelings with your instructor or head nurse makes you extremely uncomfortable, set the situation aside. You can work on it after you are more confident. Share your feelings and practice being assertive with someone with whom you are comfortable. Personal risk should be at a minimum.

It is helpful to practice being assertive by yourself at first. Rehearse what you might say by talking to yourself while looking in a mirror. Once you feel more comfortable, ask a friend to help you practice. The two of you can role-play some assertive conversations. You may even want to videotape or audiotape your practice so you can get an idea of how you look and how you sound. When you are ready, try out your new assertive communication skills in a mildly uncomfortable situation you would like to change. Pay attention to how you feel. Ask for feedback from the other person. You'll then be able to evaluate your progress and decide what other information you want to practice.

WHAT ARE THE COMPONENTS OF ASSERTIVE COMMUNICATION?

When you communicate assertively, you are able to describe your own feelings and needs, listen to and acknowledge the other person's feelings and needs, define the problem clearly and nonjudgmentally, use body language confidently, and negotiate a workable compromise (Mindell, 2001).

Following are two ways to think about expressing your feelings and needs:

STRATEGY 1
I think . . .

I feel . . .

I want . . .

STRATEGY 2

I feel . . . about . . . because . . .

Let's look at an example for each of these.

> I think we've been working every evening for 2 weeks on that report for the nursing office.
>
> I feel tired and cranky because I'm not paying enough attention to my family's needs.
>
> I want to ask someone else to write a section of the report.
>
> I feel hurt and angry about Dr. Jones yelling at me in front of you because I need to feel competent and respected at work.

These statements can be successful when you maintain direct eye contact, stand up straight, and speak in a clear, audible, firm tone of voice. After expressing your own feelings and needs, it's helpful to seek clarification of the other person's feelings or needs. This can be done with the following questions:

"How do you feel about that?"

"What were you thinking and feeling at that time?"

"How would that affect you?"

With skillful listening and clear communication, the problem can be defined without placing blame or "putting down" the other person. Notice the use of "I" messages. That indicates willingness to accept responsibility for the process of defining the problem and negotiating a workable solution. To find a compromise, you have to be willing to meet the other person halfway. You may agree to try it your way one time and the other person's the next. Or you may both agree to change or give up something. You may do something for him or her if she does something else for you. Remember that in the work setting you cannot always have things exactly as you want them. You must be willing to change and compromise (Elgin, 2000).

WHAT ARE SOME EXAMPLES OF SITUATIONS IN WHICH ASSERTIVE COMMUNICATION WOULD BE HELPFUL?

Communicating Expectations

Supervisor: "You're being pulled to the orthopedic unit today because they're short-staffed."

Nurse: "I expect to be oriented into the unit and the equipment before I give nursing care because I haven't worked on that unit in more than a year."

Saying No

Physician: "Come with me right now. I need some help doing a procedure on Mr. Smith."

Nurse: "No, I can't come with you right now. I'm doing a nursing assessment on Mrs. Anderson. I'll be finished in 20 minutes and will help you then."

Accepting Criticism

Head Nurse: "It seems to me that you aren't very good at doing care plans, and they're never done on time."

Nurse: "I have been falling behind on my care plans. I would like to look at some examples of good care plans. Do you think you could help me with that? I'd be willing to spend some time at home reviewing them."

Accepting Compliments

Home care patient's spouse: "You give really thorough care. It's obvious you know what you're doing."

Nurse: "Thank you. Your feedback is important to me."

Giving Criticism

Nurse: "I want to talk with you about your care of Mrs. Samuelson. I found her sitting in a wheelchair alone in the hallway. It is your responsibility to make sure that she is not left alone, so that nothing happens to her."

Aide: "I don't think that's my job."

Nurse: "We talked about your responsibilities this morning when you got your assignment. I expect you to complete your assignment as directed or ask for help."

Providing Feedback

Head Nurse: "I wanted to tell you that I have noticed an improvement in your relationship with Dr. Turner. He has not complained about his patients' care for 2 weeks, and yesterday he told me that he had a satisfying discussion with you about home health care options for Mrs. Atkins."

Nurse: "Thank you. I have been working very hard at not responding angrily to his sarcastic comments and criticisms."

Asking for Help

Nurse: "It is hard for me to do this because I expect myself to care for all patients without difficulty. But I am having a hard time with Mr. Jones. He seems to have a way of pushing my buttons so I get angry."

Community Health Nurse Supervisor: "Are you asking me for something?"

Nurse: "Yes. I need help in understanding why I get so angry at him, and I want to know how to handle him in a more positive way."

Remember that you need to evaluate how your assertive communication feels to you and you need to seek feedback from other people about how you are being interpreted. You need to know whether people perceive you as aggressive rather than assertive. It may mean modifying your communication to make sure you are standing up for yourself without violating the rights of others.

It should also be noted that some situations will not get resolved just because you communicated assertively. Finding a workable solution is a process involving other people who must take responsibility for their own feelings and needs. When others are unable to acknowledge their feelings, to listen, or to negotiate a compromise, your assertive communication may make you feel better about yourself but may not produce an immediate solution. But keep trying. Persistence pays off.

Remember, too, that there are some situations in which you must simply follow orders. You can't always meet your own needs; you must do what a physician or your head nurse tells you to do. Sometimes you must put aside your own needs to meet the needs of the patients you are caring for. However, your judgment will increase as you gain experience, and you will recognize ways to communicate your needs and feelings, with the goal of improving the processes and procedures used in your work setting.

Now that you have learned a lot about communicating effectively, try doing the student exercise in Critical Thinking Box 7-7. And happy communicating!

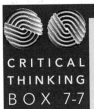

CRITICAL THINKING BOX 7-7

COMMUNICATIONS EXERCISE

Directions: Use the following situations to reflect on key points covered in this chapter. Think of a way to communicate effectively in each situation. You may want to consider your own individual solutions and then role play or discuss your ideas with a group of your classmates.

1. Develop a list of 10 patients who are hospitalized on your unit. Give for each patient some personal information, a diagnosis, and some data about his or her progress during the last 24 hours. Use the information you have listed to give a change of shift report to the four staff members who will be caring for these patients during the next 8 hours.

2. You have asked to speak to Dr. Sanders about your concerns in caring for one of her patients who has required much physical care since she has gone home from the hospital. Dr. Sanders has a reputation for being cold, aloof, and sarcastic. You have never spoken directly to her alone before.

3. You are a member of the home health care agency's procedures committee. After attending the last meeting, you have been given the responsibility for drafting a revision to the procedure used when administering controlled substances. You know that you need more information before you can begin your work. Send a memo to at least three different members of the agency staff identifying what information you would like them to provide for you. Do a follow-up phone call to make sure you get all the information you need.

REFERENCES

Arredondo L: *Communicating effectively*, New York, 2000, McGraw-Hill.

Chenevert M: *Pro-nurse handbook*, ed 3, St Louis, 1988, Mosby.

Deep S, Sussman L: *Smart moves for people in charge*, Reading, Mass, 1995, Addison-Wesley.

Dochterman J, Grace H: *Current issues in nursing*, ed 6, St Louis, 2000, Mosby.

Elgin S: *The gentle art of verbal self-defense at work*, Paramus, NJ, 2000, Prentice Hall.

Huber D: *Leadership and nursing care management*, Philadelphia, 2000, WB Saunders.

Kushner M: *Successful presentations for dummies*, Foster City, Calif, 1997, IDG.

Marquis B, Huston C: *Leadership roles and management functions in nursing: theory and application*, ed 3, Philadelphia, 2000, JB Lippincott.

Mindell P: *How to say it for women: communicating with confidence and power using the language of success*, Paramus, NJ, 2001, Prentice Hall.

Northouse P: *Leadership theory and practice*, ed 2, Thousand Oaks, Calif, 2001, Sage.

Strayhorn JM Jr: *Talking it out: a guide to effective communication and problem solving*, Champaign, Ill, 1977, Research.

Vengel A: *The influence edge: how to persuade others to help you achieve your goals*, San Francisco, 2000, Berrett-Koehler Communications.

ADDITIONAL SOURCES

Albert B: *Fat free meetings: how to make them fast, focused, and fun*, Princeton, NJ, 1996, Peterson's.

Buresh B, Gordon S:. Subtle self-sabotage, *Am J Nurs* 96(4):22-24, 1996.

Chenevert M: STAT: *Special techniques in assertiveness training for women in the health professions*, ed 2, St Louis, 1983, Mosby.

Davis M, Eshelman E, McKay M: *The relaxation and stress reduction workshop*, ed 5, Oakland, Calif, 2000, New Harbinger.

Pratt J: Giving effective feedback, *Home Health Care Manage Prac* 10(2):76-78, 1998.

INTERNET RESOURCES

10 Tips for Effective Communication
http://nsweb.nursingspectrum.com/cfforms/tipsforeffectivecommunication.cfm
Article from Nursing Spectrum outlining tips for better communication.

Communication Styles
http://www.nsba.org/sbot/toolkit/CommStyl.html
http://www.siu.edu/offices/counsel/talk.htm
Offers an assertiveness quiz.

CommunicATER
http://www.communicater.com/services.html
Consultation services about health care coaching.

About Communications
http://www.cyberparent.com/talk/

Tips on Gender Communication
http://www.bbraham.com/html/gender.html

Interpersonal Communication
http://www.pertinent.com/pertinfo/business/communication
Compilation of hyperlinks to various articles.

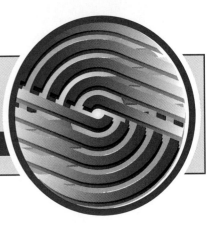

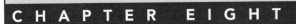

Conflict Management

JOANN ZERWEKH, EdD, RN, FNP, CS

Everything that irritates us about others can lead us to an understanding of ourselves.

—*Carl Jung*

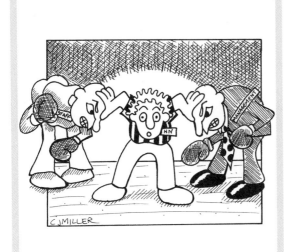

There is a better approach to conflict resolution than fighting it out.

After completing this chapter, you should be able to do the following:

- Identify common factors that lead to conflict.
- Discuss five methods to resolve conflict.
- Discuss techniques to use in dealing with difficult people.
- Discuss solutions and alternatives in dealing with anger.
- Identify situations of sexual harassment in the workplace and discuss possible solutions.

Can you imagine a world without conflict? Why, it would be a world without change! Conflict is inevitable wherever there are people with differing backgrounds, needs, values, and priorities. The presence of conflict in a situation is not necessarily negative but may, in fact, have some positive results. As a process, conflict is neutral. Following are some possible outcomes of conflict:

- Disturbing issues are brought out into the open, which may avert a more serious conflict.
- Group cohesiveness may increase as individuals resolve issues.
- New leadership may develop as a consequence of resolution.
- The results of conflict can be constructive, which occurs when productive outcomes are achieved; or destructive, leading to poor communication and creating dissatisfaction.

CONFLICT

WHAT CAUSES CONFLICT?

Let's look at some common factors of conflict as they relate to nursing.

Role conflict. When two people have the same or related responsibilities with ambiguous boundaries, the potential for conflict exists. For example, a nurse on the 11 PM to 7 AM shift may be uncertain whether he or the nurse on the 7 AM to 3 PM shift is responsible for administering enemas until clear on a patient scheduled for a barium enema.

Communication conflict. Failing to discuss differences with one another can lead to problems with communication. Communication is a two-way process; when one person is unclear in a communication, the process falls apart. A recent graduate may find that with a busy schedule, numerous patient demands, and a shortage of time, it is easy to forget to notify a patient's family of a change in visiting hours—a great annoyance to the family members who cannot visit when they arrive.

Goal conflict. We all have unique goals and objectives for what we hope to achieve in our places of employment. When one nurse places his or her personal achievement and advancement above everyone else's, conflict can occur.

Personality conflict. Wouldn't it be great if we got along with everyone? Of course we all know that there are just some people with whom we have a difficult time. The situation is all too familiar, and many times we may find ourselves with such thoughts as "I'll try and overlook her negative, lousy behavior; after all she doesn't have much of a family life." Trying to change another person's personality is like guaranteeing an unhappy ending to a story.

Ethical or values conflict. During a cardiac arrest, a young graduate nurse has difficulty with the physician's order of "No Code," on a young adolescent patient.

She has difficulty taking care of the adolescent because he reminds her of her younger brother who died tragically in an automobile accident.

Conflicts in nursing may fit into one or more of the aforementioned categories. Consider some common areas of conflict among nursing staff, including scheduling days off, determining vacation leave, assigning committees, patient care assignments, and performance appraisal, to name just a few.

WHAT ARE COMMON AREAS OF CONFLICT BETWEEN NURSES AND PATIENTS—AND BETWEEN NURSES AND PATIENTS' FAMILIES?

Guttenberg (1983) identifies five common areas of conflict among nurses and their patients and families.

1. Quality of Care

This is by far the most common area of conflict and the easiest to remedy. Families typically are concerned with how well their loved one is being attended to, how friendly the nurses are, how well the hospital or home health services are provided and coordinated, and how flexible the hospital is with visiting hours and meeting their special needs.

2. Treatment Decisions

This area of conflict often arises between the family of an elderly adult and the nurse. A physician may order a treatment with which the family does not agree. In this situation it is very important that the nurse not defend the physician's orders or attempt to persuade or establish with the family that the physician or nurse knows what's best for the patient. In these situations the issue is rarely the treatment itself but rather the family's desire to decide what's right for their loved one. Be sure to clarify the orders and explain to the family that you are supposed to carry them out unless the family negotiates directly with the physician to change them.

3. Family Involvement

The situation of a young adult diagnosed with cancer illustrates numerous issues that may arise concerning the presence of family members during procedures and the extent of their involvement in the overall care. Such issues are based on the family's real need to feel significant and adequate in meeting the young adult's needs.

4. Quality of Parental Care

This can become an issue when nurses are unhappy with how the parents are participating in their child's care. It is helpful to offer parenting classes, to encourage parents to meet other parents, and to model positive parenting techniques.

5. Staff Inconsistency

This is another easily preventable issue. Make sure that each shift is consistent in enforcing hospital policies and that they notify other shifts of any attempts at manipulation by family members or patients.

CONFLICT RESOLUTION

WHAT ARE WAYS TO RESOLVE CONFLICT?

Unresolved conflicts waste time and energy and reduce productivity and cooperation among the people with whom you work. In contrast, when conflicts are resolved, they strengthen relationships and improve the performance of everyone involved. The key to successfully managing conflict is tailoring your response to fit each conflict situation instead of just relying on one particular technique. Each technique represents a different way to achieve the outcome you want and to help the other person achieve at least part of the outcome that he or she wants. How do you know which technique to use? That depends on the following:

- How much power do you have in this situation as compared with the other person?
- How much do you value your relationship with the person with whom you are in conflict?
- How much time is available to resolve the conflict?

An example of a model for conflict resolution can be found in Figure 8-1. This model incorporates several views on conflict resolution. Filley (1975) described three basic strategies for dealing with conflict according to outcome: win-win, lose-lose, and win-lose. Various others have identified five responses to resolve conflict. They are as follows: competition, accommodation, avoidance, compromise, and cooperation. Let's look at an example and apply the model.

> Suppose the head nurse on your unit has posted the vacations for the month of December. You, as a recent graduate, have requested to be off during Christmas so that you can be with your family. You notice on the schedule that none of the recent graduates has received the Christmas holidays off. You feel that this is unfair because you have not had an opportunity to be with your family during the Christmas holidays. How can you resolve this conflict?

Competition. This is an example of the *win-lose* situation. In this situation, force— or the use of power—occurs. It sets up a type of competition between you and your head nurse. Typically competition is used to resolve conflict when one person has more power in a situation than the other. *In the given situation, the head nurse refuses your request for Christmas vacation, explaining that the staff members with more seniority have priority for vacation at Christmastime.*

Avoidance. Avoidance is unassertive and uncooperative, and leads to a *lose-lose* situation. In some situations, avoidance is not considered a true form of conflict resolution because the conflict is not resolved and neither party is satisfied. *In the given situation, you would not have approached the head nurse with the Christmas schedule issue.* Usually both persons involved feel frustrated and angry. There are some situations in which avoiding the issue might be appropriate, such as when tempers are

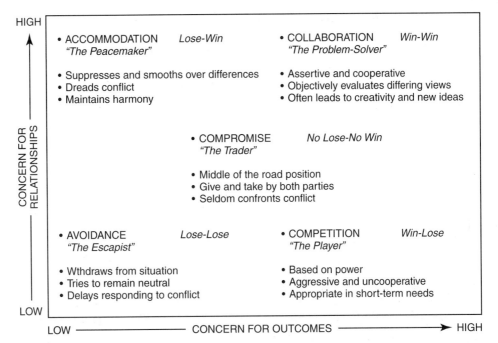

HIGH

• ACCOMMODATION   *Lose-Win*
"The Peacemaker"

• Suppresses and smooths over differences
• Dreads conflict
• Maintains harmony

• COLLABORATION   *Win-Win*
"The Problem-Solver"

• Assertive and cooperative
• Objectively evaluates differing views
• Often leads to creativity and new ideas

• COMPROMISE   *No Lose-No Win*
"The Trader"

• Middle of the road position
• Give and take by both parties
• Seldom confronts conflict

• AVOIDANCE   *Lose-Lose*
"The Escapist"

• Wthdraws from situation
• Tries to remain neutral
• Delays responding to conflict

• COMPETITION   *Win-Lose*
"The Player"

• Based on power
• Aggressive and uncooperative
• Appropriate in short-term needs

CONCERN FOR RELATIONSHIPS

LOW

LOW —————— CONCERN FOR OUTCOMES ——————→ HIGH

FIGURE 8-1

Model for conflict resolution.
(Modified from Douglas E, Bushardt W: Interpersonal conflict: strategies and guidelines for resolution, J AMRA 56(18), 1988; and Sullivan E, Decker P: Effective management in nursing, *Menlo Park, Calif, 1988, Addison-Wesley.)*

flaring or when strong anger is present. However, this is only a short-term strategy; it is important to get back to the problem after emotions have cooled.

Accommodation. *In the given situation, the head nurse would basically put her own concern aside and let you have your way, possibly even working in the scheduled slot for you.* Accommodation is the *lose-win* situation, in which you accommodate the other person at your own expense but often end up feeling resentful and angry. The head nurse loses and the graduate nurse wins in this situation, which may set up conflict among staff and other recent graduates. When is accommodation the best response? Is it when conflict would create serious disruption, such as arguing, or when the person you are in conflict with has the power to resolve the conflict unilaterally? Basically, in this response to conflict, differences are suppressed or played down while agreement is emphasized.

Compromise. Compromise or bargaining is the strategy that recognizes the importance of both the resolution of the problem and the relationship between the two people. Compromise is a moderately assertive and cooperative step in the right direction in which one creates a *modified win-lose* outcome. *In the given situation, the head nurse compromises with you by allowing you to have Christmas Eve off with your family, but* *not the entire week. The problem lies in the reduced staffing that will occur for a short period of time. The compromise may not be totally satisfactory for either party, but it may be offered as a temporary solution until more options become available.*

Collaboration. Collaboration is the strategy that involves a high level of concern for the problem, the outcome, and the relationship. It deals with confrontation and problem solving. The needs, feelings, and desires of both parties are taken into consideration and reexamined while searching for proper ways to agree on goals. Collaboration is a *win-win* solution, a commitment to resolve the issues at the base of the conflict. It is fully assertive and cooperative. *In the given situation you and the head nurse discuss the week of Christmas vacation and the staffing needs and agree that you will work the first three days of that week and the head nurse will work the second half of that week. You also agree to be there the first part of the week to complete the audit on the charts from the previous week for the head nurse. In this situation both persons are satisfied and there is no compromising what is most important to each person. That is, the head nurse gets her audit completed and the recent graduate gets to spend half of the Christmas week with her family.* What is your particular style for resolving conflict (Critical Thinking Box 8-1)?

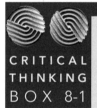

CRITICAL THINKING BOX 8-1

CONFLICT QUESTIONNAIRE

Directions: Consider situations in which you find your wishes differing from those of another person. For each of the following statements, think how likely you are to respond in that way to such a situation. Check the rating that best corresponds to your response.

	Very Unlikely	Unlikely	Likely	Very Likely
1. I am usually firm in pursuing my goals.	_____	_____	_____	_____
2. I try to win my position.	_____	_____	_____	_____
3. I give up some points in exchange for others.	_____	_____	_____	_____
4. I feel that differences are not always worth worrying about.	_____	_____	_____	_____
5. I try to find a position that is between others and mine.	_____	_____	_____	_____
6. In approaching a negotiation, I try to consider the other person's wishes.	_____	_____	_____	_____
7. I try to show the logic and benefits of my position.	_____	_____	_____	_____
8. I always lean toward a direct discussion of the problem.	_____	_____	_____	_____

CRITICAL THINKING BOX 8-1

CONFLICT QUESTIONNAIRE *(Cont'd)*

	Very Unlikely	Unlikely	Likely	Very Likely
9. I try to find a fair combination of gains and losses for both of us.	_____	_____	_____	_____
10. I attempt to work through our differences immediately.	_____	_____	_____	_____
11. I try to avoid creating unpleasantness for myself.	_____	_____	_____	_____
12. I might try to soothe other's feelings and preserve our relationship.	_____	_____	_____	_____
13. I attempt to get all concerns and issues immediately out.	_____	_____	_____	_____
14. I sometimes avoid taking positions that create controversy.	_____	_____	_____	_____
15. I try not to hurt the other's feelings.	_____	_____	_____	_____

SCORING: Very Unlikely = 1; Unlikely = 2; Likely = 3; Very Likely = 4.

	Item:	Item:	Item:	
COMPETING:	1 _____	2 _____	7 _____	TOTAL _____
COLLABORATING:	8 _____	10 _____	13 _____	TOTAL _____
COMPROMISING:	3 _____	5 _____	9 _____	TOTAL _____
AVOIDING:	4 _____	11 _____	14 _____	TOTAL _____
ACCOMMODATING:	6 _____	12 _____	15 _____	TOTAL _____

From Thomas KW: Toward multi dimensional values in teaching: the example of conflict behaviors, *Academy of Management Rev* 2:487.

WHAT ARE SOME BASIC GUIDELINES FOR WHICH TECHNIQUE TO USE?

In some situations, certain techniques and responses work best. You may have to use accommodation or avoidance when you lack the power to change the situation. When you have conflict in a relationship that you value, it might be more helpful to use accommodation, compromise, or collaboration. When there is no immediate, pressing sense of time to solve an issue, then any of the five techniques can be used. However, when you're facing an emergency situation or a rapidly approaching deadline, your best bet is to use competition or accommodation. Just remember the following key behaviors in managing conflict:

- Deal with issues, not personalities.
- Take responsibility for yourself and your participation.
- Communicate openly.
- Listen actively.
- Sort out the issues.
- Identify key themes in the discussion.
- Weigh the consequences.

Suppose that you follow all of these suggestions and you still are confronted with that difficult situation or that difficult person. Read on. . . .

DEALING WITH DIFFICULT PEOPLE

WHAT ARE SOME TECHNIQUES FOR HANDLING DIFFICULT PEOPLE?

Now that we've discussed types of conflict management techniques, we are ready to look at techniques for handling difficult people. How do you deal with an abusive physician or supervisor? How do you react when someone constantly complains and gripes about something? How do you deal with the know-it-all who won't even listen to your thoughts on an issue?

I'm sure if you haven't by now, you will, in the near future, run into a *Sherman tank* (Fig. 8-2). According to Bramson (1981), Sherman tanks are the attackers. They come out charging and are often abusive, abrupt, and intimidating. But more importantly, they tend to be downright overwhelming.

> Remember Dr. Smith, who flew into a tirade because you forgot to have a suture removal set at his patient's bedside at 8 AM sharp? Remember how you felt . . . My heart was beating so loud I could hear it and was sure everyone else around could hear it, too. I was so furious at him for the comments he made.

In understanding Sherman tanks, it is important to realize that they have a strong need to prove to themselves and to others that their view of the situation is what's right. They have a very strong sense of what others ought to do but often lack the caring and the trust that would be helpful in getting something done. They usually achieve what they want, but to do so costs them a lot of disagreements and lost friendships and uncomfortable relationships with their co-workers. Sherman tanks are often very confident and tend to devalue those who they feel are not confident. Unfortunately, they demean others in a way that makes them look very self-important and superior. How do you cope with a Sherman tank? The most important thing is to keep your fear and anger under control and avoid an outright confrontation about who's right and who's wrong. Following are some specific things you should do:

- Don't get run over, step aside.
- Stand up for yourself. Defend yourself, but without fighting.
- Give them a little time to run down and express what they might be ranting about.

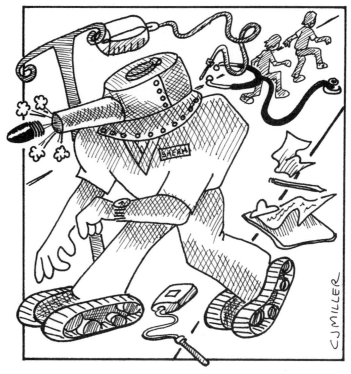

FIGURE 8-2
Sherman tank.

- Sometimes, it is necessary to be rude; get your word in any which way you can.
- If possible, try to get them to sit down. Be sure to maintain eye contact with them while you are stating your opinions and perceptions very forcefully.
- Don't argue with them or try to cut them down.
- When they finally hear you, be ready to be friendly.

Next to the Sherman tanks are the *snipers* (Fig. 8-3) . The snipers are the pot-shot artists. They are not as openly aggressive as the Sherman tanks. Their weapons are their innuendoes, their digs, and their nonplayful teasing, which is definitely aimed to hurt you. Snipers tend to choose a hidden rather than a frontal attack. They prefer to undercut you and make you look ridiculous. So, when you're dealing with a sniper, remember to expose the attack, that is, "smoke them out." Ask them very calmly:

> "That sounded like a put-down. Did you really mean it that way?" Or you might say,
>
> "Do I understand that you don't like what I'm saying? It sounds as if you are making fun of me. Are you?"

When a sniper is giving you criticism, be sure to get group confirmation or denial. Ask questions or make statements such as, "Does anyone else see the issue this way?" "It seems as though we have a difference of opinion," or "Exactly what is the issue

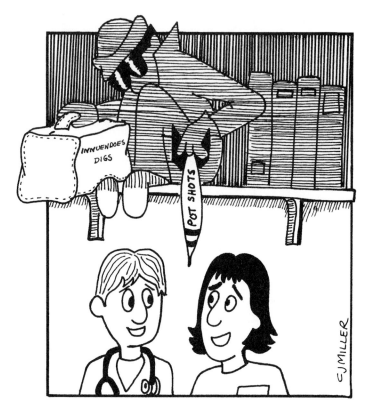

FIGURE 8-3
The sniper.

here? What is it that you don't like about what occurred?" One way to prevent sniping is by setting up regular problem-solving meetings with that person.

Another difficult person to cope with is the *constant complainer*. They often feel as though they are powerless and get attention—but seldom action—on their problem. A complainer points out real problems but does it from a very nonconstructive stance. Coping with a complainer can be a challenge. First it's important to listen to the complaints, then acknowledge them and make sure you understand what the person said by paraphrasing it or checking out your perception of how the person feels. Don't necessarily agree with them; with a complainer it's important to move into a problem-solving mode by asking very specific, informative questions and encouraging them to submit complaints in writing. For example, try communicating with the constant complainer in the following manner:

"Did I understand you to say that you are having difficulty with your patient assignment?"

"Would it be helpful if I went to the pharmacy for you, so that you could complete your chart on your preoperative patient?"

Next are the maddening ones: the *clams* (Fig. 8-4). The clams have an entirely different tactic from the previous three. They just refuse to respond when you need

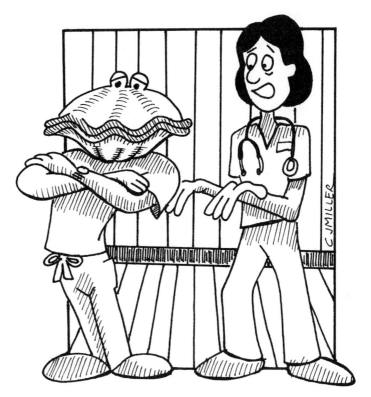

FIGURE 8-4
The clam.

an answer or want conversation. It might be helpful to try to read a clam's nonverbal communication. Watch out for wrinkled brows, a frown, or a sigh. How to deal with a clam? Try to get them to open up by using open-ended questions and waiting very quietly for a response. Don't fill in their silence with your conversation. Give yourself enough time to wait with composure. Sometimes a little "clamming" on your own part might be helpful by using the technique called the "friendly, silent stare," or FSS. The way to set up the FSS is to have a very inquisitive, expectant expression on your face with raised eyebrows, wide eyes, and maybe a slight smile—all nonverbal cues to the clam that you're waiting for a response. When clams finally open up, be very attentive. Watch your own impulses—don't bubble over with happiness that they've finally given you two moments of their time. Avoid the polite ending; in other words, get up and say, "This was important to me. I'm not going to let this issue drop. I'll be back to talk to you tomorrow at 2 o'clock." Don't be the nice guy and say, "Thanks for coming in. Have a nice weekend. I'll see you tomorrow." Be very direct, and inform the clam what you're going to do, especially if the desired discussion did not occur.

WHAT IS ANGER?

Anger is something that we feel. Usually when we get angry we assume it's because we're upset about what someone has done to us. Often we want to pay them back or take out our rage on them. Usually when anger occurs, it's hard to see beyond the moment because most people are consumed with thoughts of revenge or the wrongdoing that has occurred to them. Weiss and Cain (1991) state that "Anger is often a cover-up emotion . . . that disguises what is really going on inside you." Yet anger is a signal, and according to Lerner (1985), it's "one worth listening to." She goes on further to say that

> Our anger may be a message that we are being hurt, that our rights are being violated, that our needs or wants are not being adequately met, or simply that something is not right. Our anger may tell us that we are not addressing an important emotional issue in our lives, or that too much of ourselves—our beliefs, values, desires, or ambitions—are being compromised in a relationship. Our anger may be a signal that we are doing more and giving more than we can comfortably do or give. Or our anger may warn us that others are doing too much for us, at the expense of our own competence and growth. Just as physical pain tells us to take our hand off the hot stove, the pain of our anger preserves the very integrity of our self. Our anger can motivate us to say "no" to the ways in which we are defined by others and "yes" to the dictates of our inner self.

No matter what, when feelings of frustration, disappointment, or powerlessness take over, there is no doubt anger is in the making. Anger seems to begin in situations fraught with threats and anxiety.

Anger has two faces. One is *guilt*, which is anger aimed inward at what we did or did not do, and the other is *resentment*, which is anger directed toward others at what they did or did not do. The following is true about both guilt and resentment: They both accumulate over time and lead to a cycle of negative energy that poisons our relationships and stifles our personal growth.

However, there is another side of the coin. If feeling angry signifies a problem, then ventilating anger does not necessarily solve it. Actually, ventilating anger may serve to maintain it if change and successful resolution do not occur. Tavris (1984) suggests that we teach two things about dealing with anger: first, how to think about anger and second, how to reduce the tension. More about this later in the chapter.

Lerner (1985) gives some helpful advice on how to determine your characteristic style of managing anger. Box 8-1 has a summary of five different anger styles. Just think about anger from a cardiovascular point of view. Most authorities consider anger one of the most damaging and dangerous emotions because your pulse and blood pressure become elevated, sometimes to dangerous heights.

WHAT IS THE SOLUTION FOR DEALING WITH ANGER?

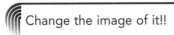 Change the image of it!!

BOX 8-1 Characteristic Styles of Managing Anger

Pursuers

❑ React to anxiety by seeking greater togetherness in a relationship.

❑ Place a high value on talking things out and expressing feelings.

❑ Feel rejected and take it personally when someone close to them wants more time and space alone or away from the relationship.

❑ Tend to pursue harder and then coldly withdraw when an important person seeks distance.

❑ May negatively label themselves as "too dependent" or "too demanding" in a relationship.

❑ Tend to criticize their partner as someone who can't handle feelings or tolerate closeness.

Distancers

❑ Seek emotional distance or physical space when stress is high.

❑ Consider themselves to be self-reliant and private persons—more "do-it-yourselfers" than help-seekers.

❑ Have difficulty showing their needy, vulnerable, and dependent sides.

❑ Receive such labels as "emotionally unavailable," "withholding," and "unable to deal with feeling" from significant others.

❑ Manage anxiety in personal relationships by intensifying work-related projects.

❑ May cut off a relationship entirely when things get intense.

❑ Open up most freely when they are not pushed or pursued.

Underfunctioners

❑ Tend to have several areas where they just can't get organized.

❑ Become less competent under stress, thus inviting others to take over.

❑ Tend to develop physical or emotional symptoms when stress is high in either the family or the work situation.

❑ May become the focus of family gossip.

❑ Earn such labels as the "patient," the "fragile one," "the sick one," the "problem," or the "irresponsible one."

❑ Have difficulty showing their strong, competent side to intimate others.

Overfunctioners

❑ Know what's best not only for themselves but for others as well.

❑ Move in quickly to advise, rescue, and take over when stress hits.

❑ Have difficulty staying out and allowing others to struggle with their own problems.

❑ Avoid worrying about their own personal goals and problems by focusing on others.

❑ Have difficulty sharing their own vulnerable, underfunctioning side, especially with those people who are viewed as having problems.

❑ May be labeled the person who is "always reliable" or "always together."

Blamers

❑ Respond to anxiety with emotional intensity and fighting.

(continued)

> ### BOX 8-1 Characteristic Styles of Managing Anger *(Cont'd)*
> ❑ Have a short fuse.
> ❑ Expend high levels of energy trying to change someone who does not want to change.
> ❑ Engage in repetitive cycles of fighting that relieve tension but perpetuate the old pattern.
> ❑ Hold another person responsible for one's own feelings and actions.
> ❑ See others as the sole obstacle to making changes.
>
> (Modified from Lerner H: *The dance of anger: a woman's guide to changing the patterns of intimate relationships*, New York, 1985, HarperCollins.)

Stop. Appraise the situation. Don't do a thing. You're at a pivot point. You have two ways to go: One is to get angry, the other is to reappraise the situation. Try to look at a way to reinterpret the annoying comment. Consider the following example:

> "Who does that head nurse think he is to treat me like I'm a dummy!" or "How could someone be so thoughtless as to not remember my birthday!" You can reinterpret these and say to yourself, "Maybe if they weren't so unhappy, they wouldn't have considered doing such a thing" or "Maybe that person's having a rough day." The important thing here is to empathize with the person and to try to find justifications for the behavior that was so annoying to you.

Look. What image (*shoulds*, *musts*, or *need to's*) about yourself or another is about to be or has been breached? In other words what has just occurred that has led you to feel angry at yourself or another?

> After receiving the end-of-shift report and making rounds to her patients, a recent graduate goes into a patient's room to take vital signs. Within moments the patient has a cardiac arrest. Two hours later while completing her chart, the recent graduate states guiltily, "I should have taken those vital signs earlier. It just needs to be the first thing I do when I get on the unit. I should have been on top of this. I must do better." Notice the self-criticism in the recent graduate's comments. Guilt, like resentment, can be a habit. It demonstrates—too clearly—how we respond to a situation in a negative manner. To help you get in touch with these feelings, try eliminating the words *must* and *should* from your vocabulary for just an hour. It's quite surprising to find out how frequently we use these terms.

Change. How do you change the image? One of the ways is to use humor. Humor makes the anger (guilt and resentment) tolerable. Remember that it's difficult to laugh and frown at the same time. (It only takes 15 facial muscles to laugh, but twice that many to frown.) If reappraising the situation and humor fail as ways to deal with your anger, some suggest venting the anger—for example, by getting mad, yelling, shouting, telling someone off, or breaking things. Although this might make us feel better momentarily, in the long run such outbursts make us feel worse.

Why does this method of venting anger, that is, letting it all hang out, make us feel worse? First off think of all the physiologic changes that are occurring in your body: blood pressure, pulse, and respirations increase; the muscles contract; and adrenalin is released. Sound familiar? It's the "fight or flight" adrenal response. Can it be healthy to maintain a constant state of stress and readiness to respond? Another disadvantage of an uninhibited outburst of anger is that it may lead the other person to retaliate.

It might be important to recognize the difference between venting and acknowledging our anger. A typical expression of anger might be something such as the following:

> "Hey, you turkey, what do you think you're doing? Don't you know how to put that catheter in? Are you stupid or something? Either you figure it out, or you get out of here. You hear me?"

This approach is insulting, demeaning, and accusatory. It's also likely to lead to some type of provoking comment. In contrast when we acknowledge our feelings, we make statements such as *"I feel angry about . . . ,"* *"I feel hurt about . . . ,"* and *"I feel guilty about . . . ."* The use of "I" statements is our first step toward taking responsibility for ourselves by owning up to our own feelings instead of blaming others.

Venting anger simply doesn't work unless you want to intimidate those around you, coerce them into submission with a hot temper, or, better yet, look childish while ranting, raving, and beating the floor or each other with foam bats. So, what does work?

- First, acknowledge the anger (*face it*): Ask "What am I feeling? Anger? Guilt? Rage? Resentment?"
- Second, identify the provoking or triggering situation (*embrace it*): Ask "What caused this feeling? Whose problem is it?"
- Third, determine what changes need to occur (*erase it*): Ask "What can I change? Can I accept what I cannot change?" Then take action and let go of the rest. Other ways to deal with anger and get out of the vicious cycle of guilt and resentment include the following:

 Move.

Get active. Try exercise or anything involving physical activity such as walking, aerobics, and running. Clean out the garage or a kitchen drawer. If you are sitting, get up. If you are in bed, move your arms around. Just get up and do something!

 Focus.

Refocus on something positive. Think of your cup as half full, not half empty. Look at the provoking situation: "My head nurse won't give me Christmas off.

However, I am not scheduled to work either Christmas Eve or New Year's Eve. So, by working Christmas Day, I'm assured the other days off."

 Breathe.

Pay attention to your breathing. Slow it down. Take deep, slow breaths, feeling the air move through your nose and down into your lungs. Check out your body for areas of tenseness. Often anger can be felt as tightness in the chest and abdomen.

Conflict is an inevitable part of our day-to-day experience. How we negotiate and handle conflict and anger may not always be easy. You might be thinking right now "This looks good on paper, but in real life, it's not that easy to put into practice." If you are feeling this way, take a risk at changing your approach and viewpoint.

 The important thing is learning about yourself.

How do you deal with conflict? How do you handle difficult people? How do you respond when angry?

SEXUAL HARASSMENT IN THE WORKPLACE

Today sexual harassment as a source of conflict has been taken seriously, as evidenced by the widespread visibility and increased recognition of the issue. The potential impact of harassment on nursing students both in the classroom and in the practice area is significant. According to Dowell (1992), nursing administrators and educators must be proactive in writing and implementing policies regarding sexual harassment. In a study by Libbus and Bowman (1994), 70% of female staff nurses surveyed reported sexual harassment by male patients and co-workers, with the most common complaint being sexual remarks and inappropriate touching. In addition, in a survey of nursing administrators, 68.8% of those who responded reported sexist attitudes among employees in their organizations and 47.7% reported observing instances of sexual harassment (Blancett and Sullivan, 1993). These studies reflect the prevalence of sexual harassment in health care settings.

The issue of sexual harassment came to the forefront during the 1991 confirmation hearings of Supreme Court Justice Clarence Thomas (Allen, 1992). Now a once-feared and secretive problem is openly discussed in newspapers and by the media. As awareness about sexual harassment increased, we all realized how little we knew about it and what we could do about it. The majority of cases involve women who report being harassed by men. In nursing the stereotypical situation of sexual harassment involves a nurse (i.e., a woman) and a doctor (i.e., a man) because of the large number of nurses who are women. However, with the increase in the number of men entering the nursing profession, there is the potential for men to experience sexual harassment by women in the workplace.

WHAT IS SEXUAL HARASSMENT?

According to Friedman (1992, p. 9), "*sexual harassment* refers to conduct, typically experienced as offensive in nature, in which unwanted sexual advances are made in the context of a relationship of unequal power or authority." He goes on to explain that victims of sexual harassment are subjected to sexually oriented verbal comments, unwanted touching, and requests for sexual favors. The typical problem, known as *quid pro quo harassment*, arises when unwelcome sexual advances have been made and an employee is required to submit to those demands as a condition either of employment or of promotions. "Hostile work environment" has been used as a legal claim to show that "the atmosphere in the work (or other) environment is so uncomfortable or offensive by virtue of sexual advances, sexual requests, or sexual innuendoes that it amounts to a hostile environment" (Friedman, 1992, p. 16). Let's look at hypothetical examples of how sexual harassment can affect nursing.

> Tracey, a recent graduate working in the surgical area of the hospital, had been receiving compliments from the chief of surgery. Eventually he asked her out and told her that if she would have an affair with him, he would make certain she was promoted to shift supervisor as soon as the position became vacant.

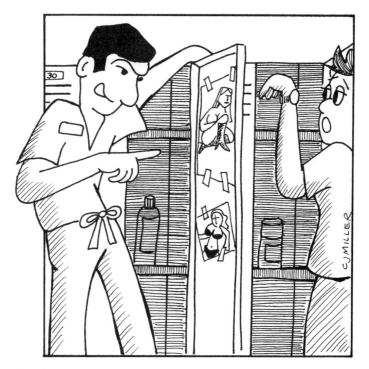

Sexual harassment

Lisa, the evening charge nurse, was quite excited that Tom, a recent graduate, was going to work on her unit. Lisa pursued Tom by repeatedly asking him for assistance with patient care and when she called him into her office, she would touch him.

WHAT CAN I DO ABOUT IT?

There are two ways to deal with this type of workplace conflict: informally and formally through a grievance procedure. Start with the most direct measure. Ask the person to STOP! Tell the harasser in clear terms that the behavior makes you uncomfortable and that you want it to stop immediately. Also, you might want to put your statement in writing to the person, keeping a copy for yourself. Tell other people, such as family, friends, personal physician, or minister, what is happening and how you are dealing with it. Friedman (1992) suggests keeping a written journal of harassing events, along with all attempts the victim has used to try and stop the harassment. The need to exercise power and control, rather than sexual desire, is frequently the motive of the sexual harasser (perpetrator). If sexual harassment is occurring as a result of miscommunication and misinterpretation of actions and is primarily sexually driven, not power-driven, then telling the perpetrator to stop will often clear up any misconceptions. However, if the perpetrator is power-driven, the harassment will continue as long as he or she views the victim as passive, powerless, and frightened. What may be most difficult for the recent graduate is facing the fear that surrounds threats of job insecurity or public embarrassment (Friedman, 1992).

If a direct request to the perpetrator to stop does not work, then an informal complaint may be effective, especially if both parties realize a problem exists and want it to be solved. The goal of the informal method is to stop the harassment but not punish the perpetrator. This method assists the person filing the complaint in maintaining some type of harmonious relationship with the perpetrator. "A formal grievance usually requires filing a written complaint with an official group such as a hearing" (Friedman, 1992, p. 65). This is a legal procedure that is guided and regulated by federal and state laws specific to this type of grievance. Before a 1991 amendment to the Civil Rights Act (Title VII), the means of correcting this bad situation—making it right or compensating the victim for difficulty encountered— were quite restricted. What has occurred as a result of this act is that victims of intentional discrimination may now seek compensatory and punitive damages. Each state has an Equal Employment Opportunity Commission, which has as its specific charge the enforcement of Title VII.

Sexual harassment may be one form of conflict you are faced with in the workplace. Learning to deal with your feelings and being aware of actions to take should this unpleasant situation occur are important. When this type of situation is resolved in a constructive, positive manner, it allows you an opportunity to feel better about your ability to deal with conflict.

REFERENCES

Allen A: Equal opportunity in the workplace, *J Post Anesth Nurs* 7(2):132-134, 1992.

Blancett SS, Sullivan PA: Ethics survey results, *J Nurs Adm* 23(3):9-13, 1993.

Bramson R: *Coping with difficult people*, New York, 1981, National Press Publications.

Dowell M: Sexual harassment in academia: legal and administrative challenges, *J Nurs Educ* 31(1):5-9, 1992.

Filley AC: *Interpersonal conflict resolution*, Glenview, Ill, 1975, Scott Foresman & Co.

Friedman J: *Sexual harassment: what it is, what it isn't, what it does to you, and what you can do about it*, Deerfield Beach, Fla, 1992, Health Communications.

Guttenberg RM: How to stay cool in a conflict and turn it into cooperation, *Nurs Life* 3(3):25-29, 1983.

Lerner H: *The dance of anger: a woman's guide to changing the patterns of intimate relationships*, New York, 1985, Harper & Row.

Libbus MK, Bowman KG: Sexual harassment of female registered nurses in hospitals, *J Nurs Adm* 24(6):26-31, 1994.

Tavris C: Feeling angry? Letting off steam may not help, *Nurs Life* 4(5):59-61, 1984.

Weiss L, Cain L: *Power lines: what to say in problem situations*, Dallas, Texas, 1991, Taylor.

ADDITIONAL SOURCES

Davidhizar R, Giger J: When subordinates go over your head. The manipulative employee, *J Nurs Adm* 20(9):29-34, 1990.

Eubanks P: Preventive measures key to sexual harassment policies, *Hospitals* 65(22):35-36, 1991.

James J: Learning the art of verbal self-defense, *Nursing* 22(1):108-109, 1992.

Jones MA, Bushardt SC, Cadenhead G: A paradigm for effective resolution of interpersonal conflict, *Nurs Manage* 21(2):64B, 64F, 64J, 64L, 1990.

Neuhs HP: Sexual harassment: a concern for nursing administrators, *J Nurs Adm* 24(5):47-52, 1994.

McWilliams JR, McWilliams P: *Life 101: everything we wish we had learned about life in school—but didn't*, Philadelphia, 1991, Bantam.

McWilliams JR, McWilliams P: *You can't afford the luxury of negative thought*, Philadelphia, 1991, Bantam.

Scafa W: Unacceptable advances, *Nurs Times* 88(26):66-67, 1992.

Valente S: Handling criticism, *Nursing* 22(3):93-94, 96, 1992.

INTERNET RESOURCES

Negotiation
http://pertinent.com/pertinfo/business/negotiation/index.html
Compilation of negotiation article hyperlinks at this Web site.

Negotiation & Resolving Conflicts: an Overview
http://web.cba.neu.edu/~ewertheim/interper/negot3.htm

10 Negotiation Tips
http://www.bbraham.com/html/negotiation.html

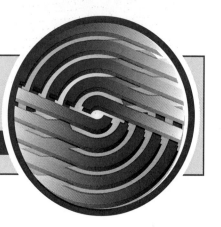

Time Management

SHARON DECKER, RN, CS, MSN, CCRN

Gain control of your time, and you will gain control of your life.
   —*Anonymous*

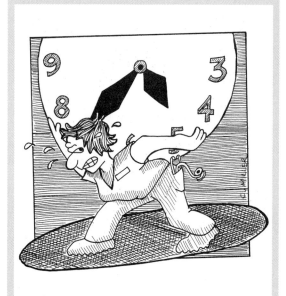

Is time managing you, or are you managing time?

After completing this chapter, you should be able to:

- Identify and describe your individual time styles.
- Discuss strategies that increase organizational skills.
- Describe time-management strategies.
- Discuss principles of priority-setting.

There are so many activities that individuals need to accomplish at any one time that deciding "how to get it all done" and "what to do when" is a daily challenge that is sometimes overwhelming. Nursing school complicates the daily routine. This relentless competition for our attention is described by the term *timelock* (Keyes, 1991).

MANAGING TIME

Regrettably, there is no way to alter the minutes in an hour and the hours in a day. Although we cannot create more actual time, we can alter the choices we make of how to use time. When employers of recent graduates were asked to identify behaviors seen as being deficit in the graduate, lack of organizational and time-management skills were noted as concerns. The methods and strategies identified by time-management experts can help you cope with timelock.

This section introduces you to the principles of effective time management. You will learn how to gain control of your time, increase your organizational skills, and reduce time waste. You will learn strategies for using the newly acquired hours to achieve your personal and professional goals.

BALANCE IS THE KEY

Making time to meet your individual, family, and professional needs and goals is vital to your overall success. If you neglect your health maintenance needs, completing school may be jeopardized. Putting off assignments until the last minute can lead to extreme anxiety and, thus, stressful behavior, which negatively affects personal health and interpersonal relationships. Integrating the principles of time management into your daily life can help you achieve both your personal and professional goals.

WHAT ARE YOUR BIOLOGIC RHYTHMS, AND HOW DO YOU USE THEM?

Individuals have different biorhythms that affect their energy levels during the day and even in different seasons. Rest and sleep are essential for optimal health and emotional and physical responsiveness. Some individuals function best when they go to bed by mid-evening and awake at the "crack of dawn," ready to tackle difficult tasks. Others are more energetic in the midafternoon, early evening, or even in the middle of the night.

 Whenever possible, schedule difficult activities at your high-energy times.

When possible, get 8 solid hours of sleep. Maintaining a regular sleep–wake rhythm with adequate hours of sleep has both physiologic and psychologic restorative effects. Disruption of this rhythm causes chronic fatigue and decreases one's coping abilities and performance. Factors affecting rest and sleep include anxiety, work schedules, diet, and the use of alcohol and nicotine.

Engage in a relaxing activity 1 hour before going to bed; for example, take a warm bath, read an interesting novel, or learn to initiate progressive relaxation techniques.

Motivate yourself in the morning by reading an inspiring quote, listening to upbeat music, or doing stretching exercises. Take time for a balanced breakfast and visualize your day. Take periodic breaks or switch activities throughout your day to maintain a high energy level. Tension can be released by simple stretching exercises and even laughter.

Alternate mental and physical tasks. This strategy includes taking periodic breaks from studying to engage in a short game of basketball or a short run with the vacuum cleaner.

WHAT IS MEANT BY RIGHT- AND LEFT-BRAIN DOMINANCE, AND WHERE IS *MY* BRAIN?

People use time in relation to their characteristic brain dominance; left, right, or both (Fig. 9-1).

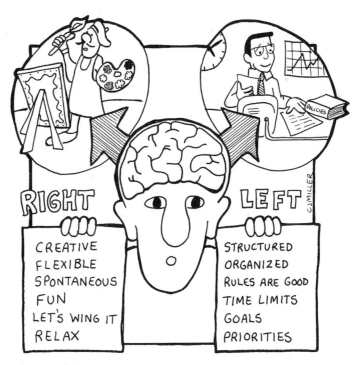

FIGURE 9-1
Are you right- or left-brain dominant?

Left-brain–dominant people approach time with logic and orderliness. Their thinking structures time by minutes and hours. They tend to schedule activities in time segments and carry them out in the sequence ordered. Left-brain–dominant people like to know the rules and play by them. They are usually able to meet their goals, but if this behavior is carried to an extreme, the individual is in danger of overwork at the expense of creative and relaxing activities.

Right-brain–dominant people resist rules and schedules. They prefer looking at a project as a whole and completing it in their own way and time. These are creative, flexible thinkers. However, if their behaviors are taken to an extreme, they can fail to meet needed completion times, which can induce guilt.

Some people are neither left-brain–dominant nor right-brain–dominant and, thus, are more mixed in their behaviors. Everyone uses both sides of the brain to some extent and thus has the benefits of their full capacities. The use of lists and calendars engages the left brain, whereas techniques such as the use of colored folders and whimsical office supplies help individuals to use right-brain holistic thinking to solve problems.

Which are you?

I am left-brain–dominant.

I am right-brain–dominant.

I am left-brain–dominant and right-brain–dominant.

In addition to assessing your own dominant time style, it is helpful to be aware of the time styles of the people with whom you live and work. Heaping rigid rules on a right-brain–dominant person will lead to increased resistance and frustration for everyone. Better to assign them clean-up of the kitchen or utility room to be completed by a specific time; if necessary, inform them of the consequences of it not being done. It would be appropriate to have some right-brain–dominant persons on the recruitment and retention committee and some left-brain–dominant persons on the policy and procedures committee.

Knowing your time style can help you maximize your strengths and modify your weaknesses. Individual time styles can be modified, but it is wasted energy to fight or work against natural inclination. Once you are aware of your time style, you can begin to create more time for what you want and need to do by increasing your organizational skills.

HOW CAN I MANAGE MY PHYSICAL ENVIRONMENT?

 A place for everything and everything in its place.

Organizing and maintaining your physical environment at home, school, and work can dramatically reduce hours of time and the emotional frustration associated with "looking for stuff."

At home, set up a specific work area for such things as school supplies, papers, and books. A separate area, corner, closet, drawer, or cupboard should be set up where you can pay bills, send letters, order take-out food, and take care of other household chores. At school and at work, a locker with extra supplies is also helpful. If none is available, use a compartmentalized carrier of some sort for essential items. At the beginning of your orientation to a new unit, take time for a "scavenger hunt." Tour the area and locate frequently used items.

- *Compartmentalize* your areas, carrying bags, even purses. Again, it may not be the time spent locating items that is so wasteful but the accompanying anxiety, fear, or frustration of not finding something or of not having what you need. Men usually carry their keys in a specific pocket; women should keep their keys in a specific pocket of a purse or tote bag. Put papers associated with a class or project in a folder, box, or other designated container.

   When practicing nursing, have a pen, pencil, notepaper, scissors, penlight, keys, change, or any other necessary items in a holder that can fit in a uniform pocket and be transferred to another uniform the next day. Such inexpensive, serviceable holders can be ordered from nursing journals. Organize supplies by the type of procedure for quick access. An intravenous start tray and cart with all the needed equipment for insertion of a central line are examples of such time-savers.

- *Color-code* files, keys, socks, and whatever you can. Office supply stores are good sources of color-coded items. Color-coding keys with a plastic cover enables you to immediately pick out your car key, house key, or locker key. Drug syringes are color-coded for accurate and rapid identification in a resuscitation situation. One clinical research team copies their material on purple paper so that all nurses gathering the data can easily identify the correct forms.

- *Convenience*. Move and keep frequently used items nearest to where they are used. Keep extra nurse's notes in the area where nurses on the unit do charting. Store infrequently used items farther away. A work team needs to agree on where essential items are to be stored in consistently designated places. At home, holiday decorations or out-of-season clothes can be put away in hard-to-reach cabinets or closets.

- *Declutter the clutter*. Anything you have not used in a year or more can likely be thrown out or put up for resale. The rare items you might later wish you had not thrown out can probably be replaced and do not justify the storage space and handling that would be required by the other unused ones. At work, designate one person to regularly clear work areas of clutter.

When in doubt, throw it out.

- *Maintenance*. Keep supplies in stock at home and work. Interrupting activities to make a trip for a needed piece of equipment is a definite time-waster. If hours are lost looking for or waiting for a wheelchair, more wheelchairs should be purchased. Set up a system with the biomedical department for equipment maintenance.

Ensure that when equipment is being serviced, a replacement is available immediately. It is also vital to have environmental problems attended to as soon as possible. Poor lighting, extreme temperatures, or any other environmental condition in need of repair drains everyone's energy and can be another source of physical and mental frustration. If no one calls maintenance to fix the thermostat in a patient's room, the patient's physical and mental health may be impaired. Likewise, the staff will be interrupted frequently over a 24-hour or several-day period while everyone lets the next shift handle it.

WHAT ABOUT ALL THE PAPERWORK—HOW CAN I MANAGE IT?

Handling each piece of paper only one time is a great time-saver. Whenever possible, spend 30 seconds filing an important paper in the appropriate folder. This technique can save you 30 minutes of searching time when you need to use the information again. Following are five ways to deal with paper:

- File it.
- Forward it.
- Respond to it—on the same sheet if possible.
- Delegate it.
- Discard it.

Use the A-B-C system when items cannot be handled at once because of your time commitments. Sort mail and messages by relative importance. The A pile will require action as soon as possible. The B pile will wait until you can get to it (i.e., B items may become A items later, especially if they have time-dates). The C items can wait until you can "get around to doing them." Because of their relative unimportance, most of the C-pile items can usually be discarded at some point.

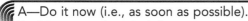

A—Do it now (i.e., as soon as possible).
B—Necessary, but do it later.
C—When I get to it.

In a nursing setting, pace your paperwork by charting throughout the day instead of at the end of the shift. Waiting until the last hour of the shift, when you are likely to be fatigued, reduces accuracy and completeness. Standardized, preprinted change-of-shift reports and other kinds of flow charts also help to document objective data effectively and efficiently. There is now "light at the end of the tunnel": Bedside and other computers are likely to become the major method of communication in your professional lifetime.

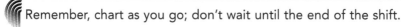

Remember, chart as you go; don't wait until the end of the shift.

WHAT ABOUT MANAGING THE TELEPHONE?

Polite comments at the beginning and end of a telephone conversation are necessary to maintain positive interpersonal communications. However, when time limits are necessary, focus the conversation on the business at hand. Some possible phrases include "How can I help you?" or "I called to . . . ." To end the conversation, summarize the actions to be followed through: "I understand, I am to find out about . . . and get back to you by the end of the week. Thanks for calling." Professional courtesy demands you turn off your cellular phone while in the classroom, during clinical, and while attending a workshop.

Having conversations to maintain friendships, to touch base with a relative, to relax yourself, to vent your emotions, or to serve similar social purposes can be combined with routine housekeeping duties. Who hasn't swept the floor, put away dishes, sorted mail, or cleaned out a drawer while chatting with a friend?

 One time-management principle is "don't agonize, organize!"

WHAT ABOUT ALL THAT E-MAIL?

Set aside time daily to read and answer your e-mail. This could be one of your first tasks in the morning while you are enjoying your coffee. Don't let e-mail pile up in your inbox. Read it, answer it, and, if important, transfer it to a designated folder or delete it. When you are communicating with your instructor by means of e-mail, be sure that you include in your subject line what class you are in (e.g., Nursing 202). Many instructors manage their e-mail by sorting it with respect to class, so a standardized subject line helps with their time management. Your e-mail program may have parameters that you can set up so that any message with a certain address goes directly into a special file, such as into a file for newsletters you receive. This helps move information out of the inbox and keeps you organized. Spend some time in your e-mail program. Look at all of the functions and what they do. Use your e-mail program to your best advantage—it can become your best friend in terms of helping you organize your e-mails in folders.

 Use your delete key aggressively, and eliminate junk e-mail without reading it.

HOW CAN I DEAL WITH ALL THE INTERRUPTIONS?

Interruptions are one of the major threats to effective time management. Not only is time taken away from goal-directed activities, but additional time is needed to get refreshed and back on track. Of course some interruptions are inevitable, but they can be minimized. Begin by recognizing when you are interrupting yourself. Do you start one task and then begin another rather than concentrating on completing the first? Do you respond to added distractions (television, ringing telephones, chatty friends) at times when task completion is required? In these instances, you are cooperating with the interruption and allowing yourself to be interrupted. When possible, in nonemergency situations, use your time-management strategies and communication skills to remain focused on the task at hand. People will accept that you may need to get back to them when you have finished what you are doing. Write down when and where you can reach them and then follow through. Turn off your telephone's ringer and let the message service or answering machine pick up the calls, but check it every hour or so. This way you can return the calls you want to respond to and at your convenience.

Responding to interruptions can also mean you are doing your job. For example, when you are interrupted to answer a patient's call light or answer a physician's telephone call, you are doing your job. These activities are part of your nursing responsibilities. They may not be of an urgent nature and can be delayed a short time, or they may be urgent and necessitate immediate response; either way, you will need to deal with them eventually. Rather than feeling that you have been interrupted, remind yourself that what you are doing is accomplishing part of your job. There are many aspects of your job that you cannot control, but you can always choose how you respond.

Everyone needs some totally uninterrupted time in which to relax, refocus, and reenergize. During clinical experience, at work, or at home, spend a few minutes in a quiet place by yourself (e.g., the nurses' lounge, the chapel, an empty patient room, a bedroom at home) to evaluate what is happening or what needs to happen next. Take several deep, slow breaths, read, meditate, space-out, relax, or get in touch with yourself. (Parents with small children can take turns watching their children so each adult can have some uninterrupted private time.) Again, taking a break from fast-paced activity and relaxing will reenergize you and result in more productive use of time. (If now is a good time to take a break from this chapter, we'll proceed when you get back!)

HOW CAN I MANAGE MY CALENDAR?

Calendars are available to schedule to-do activities by the month, week, and day. You gain control of your life by completing a schedule (Tables 9-1 and 9-2). Scheduling provides you with a method to allocate time for specific tasks and is a constant reminder of your tasks, due dates, and deadlines. Schedule only what can realistically be accomplished and leave extra time before and after every major activity. Tasks, meetings, and travel can take longer than anticipated, so give yourself some time to transition from one project to another. Schedule personal time in your calendar. If someone wants to meet with you during this time, just say, "I'm sorry, I've got an important appointment. When would be another convenient time?"

Leave white space (nothing) in your schedule so you will have time for yourself and family, or schedule uninterruptible time for both.

TABLE 9-1

Weekly Personal Calendar

Monday	*Tuesday*	*Wednesday*	*Thursday*	*Friday*
Cleaners 9 AM workout	Pick up health insurance forms 3:30 PM carpool	4 PM workout	4-7 PM professional organization meeting	9 AM workout

TABLE 9-2

Daily Nursing To-Do List

(A) Immediate activities			
A-1	Check IV tube		Mr. D, Room 20
A-2	Assess chest tube		Mrs. B, Room 15
A-3	Suction ET tube		Ms. F, Room 12
(A) Scheduled items			
A-4	9:00 AM	Dressing change	Ms. P, Room 10
A-5	10:00 AM	Medications	Ms. B, Ms P, Ms J
A-6	12:00 PM	CT scan	Ms. W, Room 25
A-7	2:00 PM	Medications	Mr. D, Ms P
A-8	3:00 PM	Change-of-shift report	
(B) To be done when time allows			
B-1	Diabetic teaching		Mr. X, Room 17
B-2	Social service consultation		Mr. X, Room 17
(C) If time available			
C	See new videos in tape library		
C	Reorganize reference materials on unit		

IV, Intravenous; *ET*, endotracheal; *CT*, computed tomography

At the beginning of each week, review the activities scheduled for the week to avoid unexpected "surprises." Overscheduling of more tasks than any human being can do in 1 day inevitably leads to frustration. Build in some flexibility. It will not always be possible to follow your exact schedule. However, when you do get "derailed," having a plan will help you get back on track with a minimum of time and effort.

Strategy: Leave some extra time before and after every major event to allow for transition.

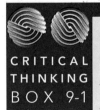

Develop your time calendar—will it be a week-at-a-glance or a month-at-a-glance? Think about what works the best for you.

_____

_____

_____

MANAGING TASKS

HOW DO I DEAL WITH PROCRASTINATION?

Everyone procrastinates, especially when a task is unpleasant, overwhelming, or can't be done perfectly. Often the amount of time spent worrying about or anticipating doing something takes more time than actually doing it! The anticipation itself can also be worse than the actuality, draining your energy and accomplishment. Here are some tips for getting started.

Consider the Consequences. Ask yourself what will happen if you do something and what will happen if you don't do it. If there are no negative outcomes of not doing something, there is no point in spending time doing it. You can eliminate that activity!

 If something will happen because you don't do it, then, of course, you need to get started.

The Earlier, the Better. Most projects take longer than planned, and glitches happen; for example, coffee spills all over your study notes the night before the test, your computer crashes, or your dog eats your notes. To compensate for the inevitable delays and avoid crises, start in advance and plan for your project to take three times longer than you think. Be realistic and use your common sense in scheduling this time frame.

 Schedule times to work on your project, and track your progress on a calendar.

"By the Inch, It's a Cinch." Break projects into small, manageable pieces; gather all the resources required to finish the project; and plan to do only the first step initially. For example, to study for a test, first collect all the related notes and books in one place. Next, review the subject areas likely to be tested. If you are having difficulty getting started, plan to work on these steps for only 5 to 10 minutes. (Anybody can do just about anything for 5 to 10 minutes, eh?) Frequently, this will create enough momentum to get you going. When you have to stop, leave yourself a note regarding what the next steps should be. Here are some hints for effective studying.

- Study difficult subjects or concepts first.
- Study in short "chunks" of 20 minutes' time.
- Take a brief break after every 20 minutes of studying.
- Schedule study time when you are at your best.
- Use waiting times. (Compile and carry 3 by 5 notecards wherever you go. This should contain information you need to review and can be pulled out anywhere—even when you are standing in that long line at the checkout counter.)
- Keep a calendar for the semester that includes all of your assignments, tests, and papers. Use a different color for entering deadlines for each course.
- Make a weekly to-do list. Prioritize this list and cross off each task as you complete it.

Before beginning a project, know what you are doing. Determine the goals, benefits, costs, and timetable for the endeavor. If you are working in a group, at the beginning of the project, make sure everyone understands their responsibilities; you should also designate who is in charge of organizing group meetings. Leave time during the project for unexpected delays and to revisit and modify your goals. Be flexible.

Reward Yourself. Bribing yourself with a reward can help you get started and keep you going. "If I concentrate well for 1 hour on reading the assigned chapter, then I can watch my favorite television show guilt-free." Often, the stress reduction that comes from working on the project that has been put off is a reward in itself!

 Schedule a time for celebration and self-reward with all of your projects.

Avoid the Myth of Perfection. Many of us were brought up with the well-intentioned philosophy that "Anything worth doing is worth doing well." This

CRITICAL THINKING BOX 9-2

What do you do to reward yourself for a job done well?

_____

_____

_____

_____

usually meant "worth doing perfectly." The fear of not doing something well enough or perfectly also feeds the tendency to procrastinate.

Certainly, everyone needs to make the best effort they can, but not everything needs to be done perfectly. Consider what the standard needed is—not the standard of perfection possible—and how you can meet it with a minimum amount of time and effort. Effective procrastination (i.e., procrastination that is used appropriately) is recognizing when a task should be purposefully postponed. This technique is a conscious decision and is used when time is needed to accomplish a task with a higher priority. Here are some hints for managing procrastination.

- Set priorities.
- Break a task into separate small steps.
- Establish multiple, specific, and realistic short-term goals.
- Get started by taking one step at a time.
- Reward yourself as you accomplish each short-term goal.
- Delegate tasks when possible.
- Be realistic.

MANAGING OTHERS

Communicating and getting along with other people are always a challenge. Most people are easy to be with and are straightforward and supportive. They add to your energy and ability to function effectively and contribute to your goal attainment. However, some people drain energy from others and from organizational accomplishment through their whining, overcriticizing, negative thinking, chronic lateness, poor crisis management, overdependency, aggression, and similar unproductive behaviors. Occasional exhibitions of such behavior in relation to personal crises that happens to everyone can be dealt with easily. It is the people who use these behaviors as their everyday *modus operandi* (method of operating) who interfere with attainment of individual and organizational goals. Even in the best of human relationships, conflict and extreme emotions are inevitable. To protect your time and achieve your goals, it may be necessary to limit your time with such individuals. Avoidance is one strategy. Learning to say "no" and assertive communication can help as well. The content and skills mentioned in Chapter 7, Effective Communication, and Chapter 8, Conflict Management, provide assistance in learning these skills.

Minimize the time spent with individuals who constantly complain and criticize. Use assertive communication and communicate directly with the person with whom you are having a problem.

WHAT ABOUT DELEGATION AND TIME MANAGEMENT?

You do not have to handle everything personally. Use your delegation skills at home to identify tasks and activities that can be completed by others, leaving you more time to study and concentrate on important projects.

Delegate the laundry and save yourself 1 to 2 hours per week. With this strategy you could gain 4 free hours in a month.

MANAGING YOUR GOALS

Goals are the incremental steps required to achieve long-term success. Personal and professional goals are critical to lifestyle management. Keeping your goals in mind enables you to plan and carry out activities that contribute to your goals and eliminate or reduce those that do not. Be realistic when setting your goals: Allow enough time to complete them appropriately. Activities that contribute to goals are your high-payoff, high-priority activities and those that don't are low-payoff, low-priority activities. Your goals should be demanding enough that completion provides a feeling of satisfaction.

Many goal-directed activities need to be scheduled with completion times. This is sometimes called *deadlining* the to-do list; the use of the term *completion times* may seem less stress-producing than the use of *deadlines*. All kinds of calendars are available to schedule to-do activities by the month, week, and day. There are organizer notebooks and computerized organizers. It is also easy to make your own forms. Knowing your goals and priorities promotes flexible rescheduling, resulting in more effective time management and successful accomplishment.

BEGIN BY LISTING

It will be helpful to list all your goal-related activities on a master to-do list. Another approach, which is also a useful learning exercise, is to record all your activities in a time log as they occur (e.g., record them every day for several days or a week). This will give you an overview of how you are using your time and provide a baseline for a to-do list. Either way, decide the order in which to do the activities in your list. You will have to decide the order in which your activities need to be completed—in other words, you will have to prioritize.

Cross out items on your to-do list, cards, and schedule as you do them. This will give you immediate, positive feedback—an instant reward for your efforts and progress. When the inevitable interruptions occur, scan the to-do list and reevaluate your priorities in relation to your remaining time.

 Reward yourself as you cross out items on your to-do list.

PRIORITIZE WITH THE ABC SYSTEM

Scan your list and decide which are A, B, or C items. The activities that are most closely related to your goals are the high-payoff ones; these are A priorities. Effective use of your time-management skills demands that you focus most of your energy on A-priority items. List these according to the urgency of the time limits. Train yourself to do the hardest task first. Attending to the hardest activity first reduces the nagging anxiety that you "should be . . ." and helps you make progress early to identify, gain control of, and possibly prevent additional problems. This is an example of the classic time-management principle, Pareto's 80/20 Rule.

According to Pareto, an early 1900s economist, 20% of the effort produces 80% of the results. For, example, spending 20% of your time studying the hardest course can produce 80% success. In your home, 80% of what needs cleaning is in the kitchen and bathroom; spend 20% of your cleaning time on these two rooms and 80% of the cleaning will be done. Eighty percent of your nursing care will be with 20% of your patients. This illustrates that there are proportionally greater results in concentrating at least 20% of your efforts on higher-payoff priorities. You will need to balance your priorities because it is impossible to achieve our best at all times.

The B items also contribute to goal achievement and, so, are high-payoff, but they are generally less urgent and can be delayed for awhile. Eventually many B items become A items, especially as completion times approach. It is also possible to do some B items in short periods of time, reading an article as you wait in a long line or "waste" time waiting for someone.

Items that do not substantially contribute to goals or are time-limited are C items. These activities really can wait until you get around to them. Keep a list of things to be done when time permits. Some C items may never be accomplished. If you have trouble throwing out mail, announcements of coming events, and so forth, put them in a C drawer. About once a month, go through the C drawer; many of these items will now be outdated and can be thrown out. Of course, some C items become B or A priorities. However, many C items will fit the "nothing will happen if you don't do something" category.

Develop daily (or time) benchmarks, which allows you to assess your daily progress in relation to the time spent on a specific project.

KEEP IT GOING

Continuously review your lists, schedules, and outcomes, and reward yourself for achieving your goals. As you evaluate and revise accordingly, ask yourself: "Did I have a plan with priorities in writing?" "Was I doing high-payoff activities that pertain to my goals?" "Was I doing the right job at the right time?"

No one is perfect. Omissions and errors will occur and are good learning experiences. Don't waste time regretting failure or feeling guilty about what you didn't do; consider these learning experiences of "what not to do" and opportunities for learning "what to do." Remind yourself that there is always time for important things and that if it's important enough, you will do it.

MANAGING TIME IN THE CLINICAL SETTING

One of the main sources of job dissatisfaction reported by nurses is too little time. This "limited time" to provide patient care has been accelerated by the nursing shortage and the increase in numbers of patients and the acuity of these patients. In response to this issue, nurses must develop competent skills in time management and priority-setting. Nurses can use several techniques to maximize the time spent providing patient care. Remember the 80/20 Rule discussed earlier in this chapter? Here is another example—20% of your patients will require 80% of your time! Those 20% should be the sickest patients; when their care and needs are met first, then the rest of the assignment is much easier. It will be important to determine which patients require the most time (the 80%): do they require time that can be delegated to someone else, or do they require the time because they are the most unstable and ill patients (Fig. 9-2)?

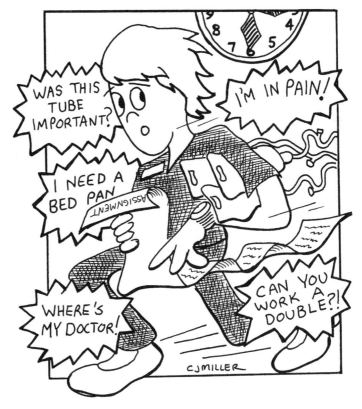

FIGURE 9-2
Time management and work organization can be challenging.

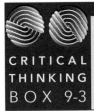

CRITICAL THINKING BOX 9-3

Develop a flow sheet to organize your time and patient care for your clinical schedule. Obtain an assignment for an RN on one of the units to which you are assigned for clinical. Can your prioritize and delegate this RN's assignment appropriately?

GET ORGANIZED BEFORE THE SHIFT REPORT

Develop your personal flow sheet, or use one provided by the agency to write down information you need to begin coordinating care for a group of patients. Modify this form as you discover areas needing improvement. Make several copies so you will always have one handy. Avoid gossiping and other distractions as you receive a report and begin to fill out your time-management (or work organization) form. Get the information needed to plan the care for your patients, and begin to organize your shift activities (Fig. 9-3).

Name: Susan

Time	Activities	Room 416	Room 417	Room 418
7-8	✓ MAR Shift report ✓ Vitals	✓ Bld Sugar 7:30 insulin	I.V. @ 125/hr. turn ✓ pulses	7:45 pre-op NPO ✓ consent form
8-9	assessments meal trays	meds x3-9 up for meals	meds x2-9 if leg dsg. assist c̄ meal	To OR
9-10		Shower Chg bed ✓ pain meds	Complete bath ✓ pulses turn	
10-11	Chart			Chg bed
11-12	meal trays lunch	up for meals ✓ Bld sugar insulin?	turn ✓ pulses assist c̄ meal	
12-1	Chart assessment	meds x2 -12	IVPB-12	Return fm. OR? N.G. suction I.V.
1-2		diabetic teaching	turn ✓ pulses if. leg dressing change	
2-3	IVPB IV's report info			

FIGURE 9-3
Work organization sheet.

PRIORITIZE YOUR CARE

Setting priorities has become difficult in relation to the dichotomy between the expected outcomes of efficiency and effectiveness and the perceived limitation of resources, including "time." Priority-setting is not only based on patient needs, but it is influenced by the needs of the organization and the accountability of the nurse. Priorities are established and reprioritized throughout the day according to patients' assessed needs and unscheduled interruptions, both minor and emergent. Plan your day around the patient you perceive to be the sickest. This is the patient who is at the greatest risk of harm if you do not address his needs first. Do the initial status and environmental assessment on that patient first. Go to the patient's room immediately after report and make sure that he/she is safe at this time. You will also see what needs to be done or brought to the room the next time you are there; make a note of it on your work organization form. Then, proceed to your next sickest patient. Those at the end of your list are probably more capable of self-care and are stable.

Prioritize patients by using the ABC system or Maslow's Hierarchy of Needs. Of highest priority are the patients with problems or potential problems related to the airway, next are those having any difficulty with breathing, and then circulation. When using Maslow's Hierarchy of Needs to assist with prioritization, you need to meet physiologic needs first: that is, resolve any difficulty with oxygenation first.

For example, a characteristic assignment for the day could be:

A patient who is 1 day postoperative and wants something for pain.

A geriatric patient who is vomiting.

A patient with diabetes who is angry about the care from the last shift.

A geriatric patient who has soiled the bed with urine.

Which of these patients needs your immediate attention? Most likely the one who is vomiting because he is at increased risk for aspiration, then probably the patient who is in pain, then the angry patient, and so on. With each patient, you may spend less than 5 minutes in the room before you move on to the next patient. But you will have a good idea of what each patient's immediate needs are.

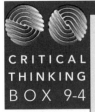

CRITICAL THINKING BOX 9-4

How do the nurses on your clinical unit prioritize their time and their patients?

_____

_____

Identify the busiest times on the unit—don't schedule a dressing change when medications need to be given. Plan on preparing medications at least 30 to 45 minutes before the hour they are due. This will provide you some time to research any medications with which you are unfamiliar. Don't procrastinate; start your medication administration 30 minutes early, leaving more time to get nursing care done later. If you have dressing changes for several patients, start with the cleanest and progress to the more contaminated wounds. If you have diabetic teaching for three patients, maybe you can get them together and do it at one time.

PLAN TIME FOR CHARTING

Do not put charting off until the end of the shift. On a busy unit, you will forget half of what you have done for all your patients by the end of the day. How many times have you seen staff nurses staying late so they can complete their charting? Make notes for charting on your work organization form and cross through it when it is charted. As you are providing patient care, make notes on your forms for charting. Plan on stopping about three to four times a shift to make charting entries. Don't obliterate anything on your form because you will need the information for an accurate shift report.

Watch those nurses who always seem to get everything done, done well, and still enjoy nursing. Ask them about their "secrets" of time management, and try out some of their tips.

CRITICAL THINKING BOX 9-5

When would you schedule charting time in your current daily clinical schedule?

_____

_____

_____

REQUEST CONSISTENT PATIENT ASSIGNMENTS WHENEVER POSSIBLE

This allows you to develop relationships with your patients and their families and promotes time management as you become familiar with the special needs of these patients.

ORGANIZE YOUR WORK BY PATIENT

By using this technique the nurse maximizes the number of tasks that can be accomplished with each visit to the patient. The nurse thinks strategically about "How can

I multitask or accomplish several objectives in one visit to the patient?" By using this technique the nurse would combine the assessment, administration of medications, and teaching during one patient visit (Fig. 9-3).

DEVELOP AND USE ASSERTIVE COMMUNICATION

Assertive communication is a technique used to get one's needs met without purposely hurting others. It incorporates the principles of therapeutic communication, active listening skills, and a willingness to compromise. When you use these skills, you will be able to express yourself more effectively during challenging situations and handle confrontation in a professional manner. When you are confronted by a situation that provokes anger, take a deep breath, pull yourself away, get your emotions under control, and then approach the individual privately in a nonthreatening manner. Following are some hints for using assertive communication:

- Use *I* statements: "I am really upset . . . ."
- Describe the behavior that has upset you and focus on the present: "You have been having excessive personal telephone calls over the past 2 days . . . ."
- Discuss the consequences of the behavior: "This behavior is contrary to the agency policy and could result in . . . ."
- State how the behavior needs to be modified and the time for this change: "You must immediately stop this interruption to your work and request that only emergency phone calls be . . . ."

WHAT ABOUT DELEGATING AND TIME MANAGEMENT?

Multiple studies have demonstrated that about 50% of nursing time is spent on nonnursing activities. These include cleaning, running errands, clerical duties, and stocking supplies. Appropriate delegation of nonnursing tasks can provide the nurse with additional time to dedicate to patient care. Some patient care tasks can be delegated once the training and competence of unlicensed personnel have been verified. These requirements vary in different states and institutions.

Delegation includes more than asking someone to do something. Delegation has been defined by the American Nurses Association as "the transfer of responsibility for the performance of an activity from one individual to another, with the former retaining accountability for the outcome" (ANA, 1995). This definition emphasizes that delegation increases the responsibility and accountability of the registered nurse (RN). Be sure you know the delegation rules and regulations of your state's nursing practice act. You will also need to know the delegation policies and job descriptions of nursing team members in your employing agency. (*See* Chapter 10 for more information on delegation.)

In general, women have more difficulty delegating than men do because of their socialization. Women are socialized to please others and to anticipate and meet the needs of others. Because the majority of the nursing profession remains female, you can understand the magnitude of the problem. In today's society, women, men, and nurses have so many responsibilities that sharing and delegating some of them are essential.

To increase delegation skills, it is sometimes necessary to overcome the myth of perfection. In teaching or training someone else to do a delegated task, initially they may or may not be able to perform the activity as well as you can; however, it is not important that they do this perfectly, in the way you do it, or even as well as you do. What is important is that they meet the standards required to complete the task adequately. As long as safety is not compromised, it is more effective time management to delegate to others. With experience, most people will improve (and may even surpass you).

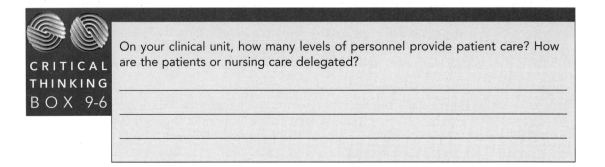

CRITICAL THINKING BOX 9-6

On your clinical unit, how many levels of personnel provide patient care? How are the patients or nursing care delegated?

_____

_____

_____

HOW DO I KNOW WHAT AND WHEN I CAN DELEGATE?

As previously stated, knowing the nurse practice act of your state, in addition to the policies for each institution, is critical in delegating appropriately and safely. Once that has been established, then consider some general guidelines regarding what and when to delegate.

You should not delegate to anyone other than another RN the task of assessment to determine changes in a patient's condition. Licensed practical nurses or vocational nurses perform patient assessment (gathering data), but it is the RN who must confirm and interpret these findings. Assessment should not be delegated when a decision needs to be made regarding patient care, the patient's condition is changing, or there is a new patient the RN has not previously assessed.

According to the nursing process, after assessment and analyzing comes planning. This is another role of the RN. Data can be gathered from a number of sources, including input from a vocational nurse or unlicensed assistive personnel (i.e., a patient care attendant or nursing assistant). Ultimately it is the responsibility of the RN to determine the immediate plan of care and the comprehensive plan of care for the patient.

Another area of the nursing process that is reserved for the RN is the area of evaluations. It is the RN's responsibility to determine the patient's response to procedures, medications, nursing care, and so forth. Nursing judgment based on the assessment and evaluation of the patient must also remain the responsibility of the RN. It all comes down to the RN's responsibility in implementing the nursing process. Time management with delegation can help the RN more effectively implement the nursing process.

Determine which patients are the most stable and whose positive progress can be anticipated. The stable patients with predictable progress should be the first to be delegated. The unstable, unpredictable patient should only be delegated to an RN. An RN should be assigned to any patient who is undergoing a procedure or treatment that may cause them to become unstable.

When you are dealing with unlicensed assistive personnel, you can delegate to them those activities that are standard with specific guidelines that are unchanging. For example, feeding, dressing, bathing, obtaining equipment for the nursing staff, picking up meal trays, refilling water containers, straightening up cluttered rooms— all of these activities should have guidelines according to the institution policies, fit within the job description, and be followed by the unlicensed assistive personnel.

Patient teaching and discharge planning are also the responsibility of the RN. It is the RN's responsibility to determine the patient's learning needs and to establish a teaching plan. It is also the RN's responsibility to coordinate and implement the discharge planning. The RN should request input from all nursing personnel who have assisted to provide care for this patient or who are involved (e.g., dietary, physical therapy) in the care of the patient. It is important that once the RN implements the teaching plan, the other RNs, licensed practical nurses, vocational nurses, and unlicensed assistive personnel are aware of what the patient has been taught so they may follow-up and report any pertinent observations to the RN.

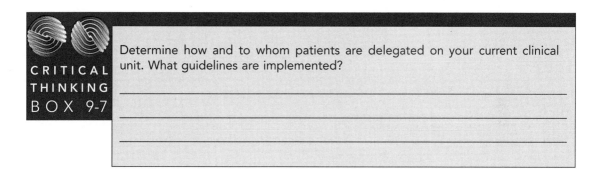

CRITICAL THINKING BOX 9-7

Determine how and to whom patients are delegated on your current clinical unit. What guidelines are implemented?

_____

_____

_____

Nursing care makes a difference in patient outcomes. This care is more than providing tasks. It incorporates assessment, care planning, initiation of interventions, interdisciplinary collaboration, and outcome evaluations. It includes patient and family teaching, therapeutic communication, counseling, discharge planning, and teaching. To maximize the impact nursing care can have on patient outcomes, nurses must develop and integrate multiple strategies to promote effective time management.

You will find that once you get organized with your clinical schedule, you will become a more effective nurse and begin to have the time to perform the type of nursing care that you were taught. Often you will hear nurses complain about not having enough time in clinical to provide the type of bath or teaching they would like to do because of the lack of time. Check them out—most often they are the most guilty of wasting time (e.g., taking time to gossip after report, wasting time complaining that they do not have enough time, not delegating effectively, allowing unnecessary interruptions, not organizing their patient care, or not delegating when appropriate). Wow, all the things that this chapter is all about!

REFERENCES

American Nurses Association: *The ANA basic guide to safe delegation*, Washington, DC, 1995, ANA.

Keyes R: *Timelock: how life got so hectic and what you can do about it*, New York, 1991, HarperCollins.

ADDITIONAL RESOURCES

Antai-Otong D: Creative stress-management techiques for self-renewal, *Dermatol Nurs* 13(1):31-32, 35-39, 2001.

Bowers BJ, Lauring C, Jacobson N: How nurses manage time and work in long-term care, *J Adv Nurs* 33(4):484-491, 2001.

Covey S: *The seven habits of highly effective people, ed 1*, New York, 1990, Simon & Schuster.

Davidson SB, Scott R, Minarik P: Thinking critically about delegation, *Am J Nurs* 99(6):61-62, 1999.

Laborde SA, Lee JA: Skills needed for promotion in the nursing profession, *J Nurs Adm* 30(9):432-439, 2000.

Nyberg DB: Successful delegation skills enhance patient care, *AORN J* 69(4):851-856, 1999.

Hansten R, Washburn M: Why don't nurses delegate? *J Nurs Adm* 26(12):24-28, 1996.

Tillman HJ, Salyer J, Corley MC, Mark BA: Environmental turbulence: staff nurse perspectives, *J Nurs Adm* 27(11):15-22, 1997.

INTERNET RESOURCES

Here are some Web sites on time management.

Mind Tools
http://www.mindtools.com
Good listing of time-management tools; also provides information on creativity, dealing with stress, and methods to improve memory.

Time Management Tips
http://www.gmu.edu/gmu/personal/time.html

Personal Time Management for Busy Managers
http://www.ee.ed.ac.uk/~gerard/Management/art2.html

Bigtimes Top Tips
http://www.bigtimes.co.uk/Top_Tips/top_tips.html

Time Management Guide
http://members.aol.com/rslts/tmmap.html

Time Management Principles
http://www.d.umn.edu/student/loon/acad/strat/time_man_princ.htm

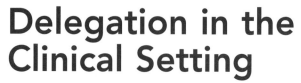

CHAPTER TEN

Delegation in the Clinical Setting

RUTH HANSTEN, PhD, MBA, BSN, FACHE

MARILYNN JACKSON, PhD, MA, BSN

Let whoever is in charge keep this simple question in her head (NOT how can I always do the right thing myself but) how can I provide for this right thing always to be done?

—Florence Nightingale

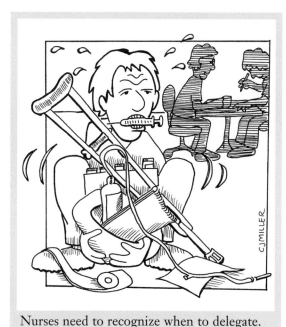

Nurses need to recognize when to delegate.

After completing this chapter, you should be able to:

- Define the operational terms *delegation*, *supervision*, and *accountability*.
- Delegate tasks successfully on the basis of outcomes.
- Select the right person for the right task.
- Apply the "four Cs" of initial direction for a clear understanding of your expectations.
- Provide reciprocal feedback for the effective evaluation of the delegate's performance.

Unless you are practicing on a deserted island with only one patient and you as the health care provider, chances are great that you will be working with other members of the health care team. How do you make effective use of the resources they have to offer? What is your role as the registered nurse (RN) on the team in terms of making these decisions? Your ability to effectively delegate tasks that need to be done, on the basis of desired outcomes, will go a long way in determining the success of the efforts of your work.

WHAT DOES *DELEGATION* MEAN?

We begin where we always must, with an understanding of the terms under discussion. Fortunately, there have been many people hard at work for the past several years, creating operational definitions of the term *delegation* to assist us in standardizing our approach. It helps if everyone is talking about the same thing when in the heat of controversy! Clinical delegation has been with us since the dawn of team nursing, but in the past several years it has taken on new meaning as we have seen the addition of many types of assistive personnel in our care-delivery models. Many RNs are uncomfortable with the idea of someone "practicing on their license," or at the very least, taking away the tasks they like to do best. Let's take a look at delegation and accountability to clarify the issue that many RNs perceive as someone practicing on their license. It helps to clear the air by beginning with the vocabulary and achieving an understanding of the basic concepts we are talking about.

Delegation: "Transferring to a competent individual the authority to perform a selected nursing task in a selected situation. The nurse retains the accountability for the delegation" (NCSBN position paper, 1995).

As you can see, this is a very generic definition, used as a standard across the country; most states have incorporated similar definitions into their nurse practice acts. (Have you reviewed your state nurse practice act lately?) A good deal of decision making is left to you as the RN. *You* will be selecting what task and in what situation to delegate. You will make a decision to delegate on the basis of your assessment of the desired outcome and the competency of the individual delegate. This is certainly more involved than a simple process for time management! In the pages ahead, we discuss steps that use the "four rights" that will assist you in this practice, making it easier for you to maximize the work of your team in a safe manner.

Supervision: "The provision of guidance or direction, evaluation and follow-up by the licensed nurse for accomplishment of a nursing task delegated to unlicensed assistive personnel" (NCSBN position paper, 1995).

It is often confusing to nurses regarding whether they are supervising another individual. This responsibility does not belong to only the one with the title of manager or house supervisor; rather, the expectation by law is that any time you delegate a task to someone else, you will be held accountable for the initial direction you give and the timely follow-up (periodic inspection) to evaluate the performance of the task. Delegation and supervision are integrated processes: Once you delegate, you must supervise.

WHO IS ACCOUNTABLE HERE?

One of the biggest questions concerning teamwork and delegation is the issue of personal accountability. The definition of delegation already notes that the nurse is accountable for the total nursing care of the individuals. What does this really mean?

 Accountability: "Being answerable for what one has done, and standing behind that decision and/or action" (Hansten and Washburn, 1998).

Accountability has gotten a lot of "bad press" lately, and many nurses feel that being accountable means "I am the one to blame." With that kind of attitude, no wonder there is reluctance to delegate! What is the point if someone else is going to make a mistake and you are going to be taking the blame? (Notice how we focus on the negative and forget that accountability also means taking the credit for the positive results we achieve through the actions and decisions we make.) Here is an important reminder about accountability before you take the weight of the world on your shoulders:

 "The delegate is accountable for accepting the delegation and for his/her own actions in carrying out the task" (NCSBN, 1995, p. 3).

It's important to focus on what you are accountable for in this process and to let the delegate also assume his or her own level of accountability. Remember, you are accountable for the following:

- Making the decision to delegate in the first place.
- Assessing the patient's needs.
- Planning the desired outcome.
- Assessing the competency of the delegate.
- Giving clear directions and obtaining acceptance from the delegate.
- Following up on the completion of the task, providing feedback to the delegate.

What if the delegate makes a mistake doing the task? What are you accountable for? Let's consider the following example:

It's 7 AM on your busy medical-surgical unit. You scan your assignment quickly, reviewing the high points with your nursing assistant before going into report. With trays coming at 7:30, you remind your assistant that your patient in room 210 will be going to surgery this morning and is to have nothing to eat or drink. Coming out of report, you make brief rounds, only to find that (you guessed it!) your patient in room 210 is happily drinking her morning coffee.

What are you accountable for?

Did you delegate correctly?

What do you do now?

In your review of the previous guidelines, you identified that you did indeed delegate appropriately. Your communication may or may not have been as complete as it needed to be (more about that later). You are accountable for correcting the clinical effects of this error: Did the patient drink too much coffee, requiring that surgery be canceled or delayed? You will call the operating room and make the appropriate adjustments in this patient's care on the basis of the decision regarding her surgery time. What about the nursing assistant? You are also accountable for following up with her regarding her performance, giving the appropriate feedback so that she understands her level of personal accountability as well. For more on the "how-to's," read on as we discuss the four rights of clinical delegation.

THE FOUR RIGHTS OF CLINICAL DELEGATION*
Right task
Right person
Right communication
Right feedback

THE RIGHT TASK

The first part of any decision regarding delegation is the determination of what needs to be done and then identifying if this is a task that can be delegated to someone else. Many nurses, unfortunately, suffer from "supernurse syndrome" and believe that no task should be delegated because no one can do it better, faster, or easier than they can (Fig. 10-1). In comparison, other nurses may be all too eager to delegate the least desirable tasks to someone else. A word of caution is necessary here: If we focus only on making task lists for people to do, we eliminate the very core of our purpose.

*Note: The National Council of State Boards of Nursing describes the "Five Rights of Delegation," discussing the "right circumstance" as an additional consideration for the nurse. "Right Circumstances—appropriate client setting, available resources, and consideration of other relevant factors," suggests that the staffing mix, community needs, teaching obligations, and the type of patients being cared for should also be considered (NCSBN, 1995).

Remember, your role as the RN on the team involves the coordination and planning of care, with your primary focus on identifying with the patient and the physician the desired outcomes for your patients. Once determined, interventions will be readily apparent, and the decision regarding possible delegation of these tasks must be made.

WHAT CAN I DELEGATE?

Fortunately, there are several references to assist you in making this determination. The first place we recommend looking is in the nurse practice act for your state. At this point, the majority of state boards have addressed the issue of delegation and have developed rules that may offer specific guidelines regarding who can do what. The scope of practice for each level of care provider usually includes a description of the tasks that may be performed at that level.

The next place to look is in your organization, getting a copy of the job description and the skills checklist for each care provider. This will give you a very specific list of tasks to work from, but remember, there are other considerations. Simply because the skills checklist includes ambulation of patients, it may not be advisable to delegate the first ambulation of a postoperative total hip replacement patient to the new patient care assistant (*see* Critical Thinking Box 10-1).

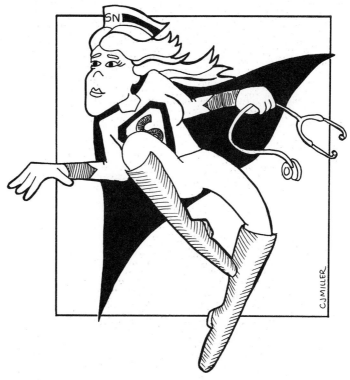

FIGURE 10-1
Many nurses suffer from "supernurse syndrome."

IN YOUR ORGANIZATION, CAN YOU DELEGATE THE FOLLOWING TASKS?

YES   NO

_____   _____   Foley insertion

_____   _____   Taking vital signs

_____   _____   Feeding a patient

_____   _____   Hygienic care

_____   _____   Medication administration

_____   _____   Discontinuing an IV line

_____   _____   Teaching insulin administration

IV, Intravenous.

IS THERE ANYTHING I CAN'T DELEGATE?

Again, your first resource is the law. Many states are very specific in their description of what cannot be delegated and therefore belongs only to the RN's scope of practice. The National Council of State Boards of Nursing (NCSBN) reminds us that

> Nursing is a knowledge-based process discipline and cannot be reduced solely to a list of tasks. The licensed nurse's specialized education, professional judgment and discretion are essential for quality nursing care. . . . While nursing tasks may be delegated, the licensed nurse's generalist knowledge of patient care indicates that the practice-pervasive functions of assessment, evaluation and nursing judgment must not be delegated. (NCSBN, 1995)

According to nurse-attorney Joanne P. Sheehan, nurses can't delegate the following:

- Assessments that identify needs and problems and diagnose human responses.
- Any aspect of planning, including the development of comprehensive approaches to the total care plan.
- Any provision of health counseling, teaching, or referrals to other health care providers.
- Therapeutic nursing techniques and comprehensive care planning. (Sheehan, 2001, p. 22)

If you have questions and need clarification for your state, call the board of nursing for assistance. You can get their information on the National Council of State Boards of Nursing (NCSBN) Web site at http://www.ncsbn.org. Be aware that your state may have introduced or passed a bill that may affect your practice with residents of neighboring states. As of July 2001, 18 states had passed or are in the process of approving interstate compact licensure regulation legislation designed to allow nurses to practice across state lines because of Internet consultation, telenursing, or other technology that would broadcast nursing practice across state borders (NCSBN, 2001). If you have questions and need clarification in your state, call the board of nursing for assistance (see Critical Thinking Box 10-2).

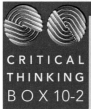

CRITICAL THINKING BOX 10-2

WHERE TO LOOK FOR DETERMINATION OF THE RIGHT TASK

Nurse practice act
Employee job description
Skills checklist
Demonstrated competency

Beyond the law, your employer will have job descriptions and skills checklists that should clearly define the role of the caregiver. If you have not seen these items, be sure to review them soon. This is the baseline for determining "who does what" and selecting the right task to delegate. As many organizations develop creative assistant roles to leverage the professional judgment of scarce registered nursing personnel, the scope of practice of each role is defined first by law. If the organization extends the role of a patient care technician to include preoperative teaching, you want to be aware that this is clearly an RN function and not allowed by law to be delegated to the technician. A job description and a policy would not override the legal limits of the scope of practice.

With the right task selected according to the scope of practice, the policies in your agency, and your assessment of the situation, there is still work to be done. Who will do this task? (*See* Fig. 10-2.)

THE RIGHT PERSON

Matching a task that can be delegated to the right person involves that definition of delegation once again. Nurses must *select* the right task for a *competent* person in a *selected* situation. We've already discussed how you would determine the correct task. But how do we select the right person in the right situation?

HOW CAN I USE OUTCOMES IN DELEGATING?

In planning for the right person to do a task, focusing on outcomes is essential (*see* Critical Thinking Box 10-3). For example, two patients can be admitted to a hospital. Each of these individuals will need a bath today (task), but who will do the bath is related to the outcome you are trying to achieve. For Mr. Peterson, who has been homeless and is in dire need of hygienic care so that you can perform a complete and accurate skin assessment, the *priority outcome you and your patient desire* is that

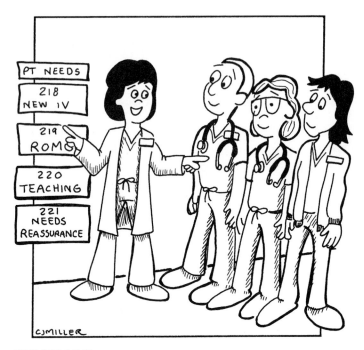

FIGURE 10-2
It can be difficult to know who is the best person to handle a given situation.

Mr. Peterson will be clean. With Ms. Ibutu, who is a paraplegic, today is the day that *her caregivers and she will demonstrate how they'll assess the skin for areas of breakdown and how to perform range of motion to her lower extremities.* The RN's decision about who will do the task is dependent on the plan of care and the goals that the team has established in the discussion with the patient or family (see Table 10-1).

This same logic applies when you've heard in report that a patient is unstable. In your current care-delivery system on your unit, the licensed practical nurse (LPN) (or licensed vocational nurse [LVN]) may carry out the initial vital sign data-gathering in your postoperative intensive care unit (ICU). Suppose, for example, that the report you received stated that there had been increasing cherry red drainage in the chest tube and that the patient's cardiac monitor showed supraventricular tachycardia, with increasing respiratory rate. On the basis of the outcome for the shift, Mr. Handelsky will maintain cardiorespiratory homeostasis and continue on critical path for first day postthoracotomy. Using your insight that his condition may be deteriorating, you may make a different decision regarding who will be there for initial patient contact. If the assistant working with you today is an experienced team member, you may choose to send him in to see the patient immediately while you check on another critical patient. Or if the assistant is a float from an agency, known to you only by initial questioning, you may immediately make a visit to see Mr. Handelsky, beginning to set up the plan for the data-gathering and schedule for

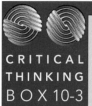

TALKING ABOUT OUTCOMES: WHAT'S IN IT FOR ME?

- ❏ Provides a method to decide appropriate assignments: who should be doing what task
- ❏ Gives you a sense of purpose for the shift (short term) and long term
- ❏ Enhances your ability to motivate co-workers along a track to achieving the outcomes
- ❏ Clarifies your role as leader of the team
- ❏ Verifies and clarifies patient/family expectations when outcomes are discussed and planned with them
- ❏ Promotes job satisfaction for the whole team

TABLE 10-1

Using Outcomes in Delegating

Patient	Outcome	Task/Process	Who will perform it?
Mr. Peterson	Patient will be clean	Bath	Nursing assistant or other care associate
Ms. Ibutu	Patient and caregivers will know how to perform skin assessment and range of motion	Bath with education regarding home care	*RN:* teaching plan; OT, PT, or rehabilitation aide may also assist
Mr. Handelsky	1. Patient will maintain cardiorespiratory homeostasis and continue on care path day 1 2. Patient will be free of pain and comfortable for this shift. Long-term outcome, pain-free death	Initial baseline vital signs and assessment, close monitoring Pain assessment and treatment, comfort measures (repositioning skin care)	*RN:* assessment and interpretation of data *LPN:* data-gathering and reporting *RN:* initial plan for comfort measures and pain assessment *Assistant:* comfort measures, report of progress

RN, Registered nurse; *OT*, occupational therapist; *PT*, physical therapist; *LPN*, licensed practical nurse.

reporting you'll expect from your assistant. This would be a very different process if the outcome you'd want to achieve with this patient would be pain relief and comfort with an impending death.

Take a moment to consider the outcomes for a particularly difficult patient you've been dealing with lately. Were you clear on outcomes? If so, have you shared them with colleagues?

Focusing on outcomes takes time. But, as many have often said, "If you fail to plan, you plan to fail." Why should an RN focus on outcomes? Discussion of goals not only establishes *who* should be doing what task, but also allows RNs to motivate others. How many of us jump on a train if we don't know where it's going? A purpose and a destination allow all of the team members to function more effectively. When assistive personnel are given the same assignment daily, without variation, without any understanding of *why* they are doing what they are doing, it's similar to being an assembly line worker putting widgets in a machine. Satisfaction and motivation of co-workers generally come from the feeling that they are making a difference in the lives of their patients.

In a similar manner, you as the leader of the team would feel much better at the end of your shift or assignment if you could feel comfortable with the outcomes you have assisted the patient in achieving. You could actually verify the outcomes and plan with the patients, much as you were always told to do by the teachers in your nursing program! Much time is saved by streamlining the care to the patient's expectations.

Again, the RN is accountable for the patient, for determining the situation in which delegation will be used, and for the selection of the right person to do the right task, in addition to the periodic inspection and follow-up of those they supervise.

THE RIGHT CIRCUMSTANCES

The NCSBN describes "Five Rights of Delegation," discussing the "right circumstance" as an additional consideration for the nurse. "Right Circumstances—appropriate client setting, available resources, and consideration of other relevant factors;" suggests that the staffing mix, community needs, and teaching obligations, in addition to the type of patients being cared for, should also be considered (NCSBN, 1995). Different rules for delegation may apply regarding what and how an RN must delegate in home care, long-term care, or in community homes for the developmentally disabled or group boarding homes for assisted living (Hansten, Washburn, and Kenyon, 1999, p. 316).

HOW CAN I DETERMINE THE STRENGTHS AND WEAKNESSES OF TEAM MEMBERS?

Often motivated by the fear that a delegate may make a mistake in an assigned task, nurses focus on the potential weaknesses of their team members. As nurses, we are educated to anticipate the worst so we can prevent accidents, adverse drug reactions, and negative sequelae to disease processes and treatments alike. Prudent as this approach may be for the safety of all concerned, it's worthwhile to discuss the need to be clear on the strengths of the team members as well.

Recall the last time you were given specific, positive feedback about your performance as an RN. (We hope this occurs often!) How did you feel? Most of us are energized and restored by the reinforcement that our hard work has been recognized. When working with assistive personnel or any other colleague, the recognition of strengths will begin to get us on the right track in our relationship.

Assigning tasks on the basis of the strengths of the person will allow the individual and the patient to experience the very best care. Now, as a supervising RN, you're in a new position with respect to the long-term performance of delegates. If assistive personnel are assigned only those tasks they are good at, they may not grow in their abilities and skills. This mistake is exemplified by a hospital that had created a new multiskilled Patient Care Assistant (PCA) role with Certified Nursing Assistants (CNAs). These CNAs had been trained to do phlebotomies as well, as authorized by the state board. Phlebotomists had been eliminated but were given the option of training for the new PCA role. When all of the PCAs worked together, the lab tests were drawn by those who had been phlebotomists because they were more comfortable with that skill. You can certainly imagine the chagrin of the supervising nurses when all the PCAs who were former phlebotomists were off on vacation and maternity leave. None of the PCAs who were formerly CNAs had become proficient at this skill! Recognize strengths, and encourage the best patient care possible by using them, but challenge delegates to grow too.

The dreaded weaknesses in performance of team members can often be prevented by asking the right questions before delegation. Nurses can be reticent about asking personnel such as float or agency replacement staff about whether they feel comfortable in completing the assignment they've received. Float and temporary personnel tell us that they'd *prefer* being asked about their competency at the beginning of a shift or assignment, with the offer of help and clarification, rather than having to locate an RN to request information. The American Nurses Association Code of Ethics states, "The nurse is responsible and accountable for individual nursing practice and determines the appropriate delegation of tasks consistent with the nurse's obligation to provide optimum patient care" (ANA, 2001, http://www.ana.org/ethics/chcode.htm). Be assured that although it is the responsibility of the RN to assess the competency of those they supervise, the delegate must be "accountable for accepting the delegation and for his/her own actions in carrying out the task" (NCSBN, 1995). The RN who is familiar with the situation, however, must ask the correct questions to determine whether the person is competent.

> For example, if an RN were planning to ask a nursing assistant to feed a baby with respiratory difficulties, based on the outcome that the baby would be able to ingest 12 ounces of formula this shift, what questions might the RN ask to determine the potential strengths and weaknesses? If the individual has not had experience in this procedure, how could the nurse ensure future competency? In this situation, an RN would certainly ask questions about past experiences with feeding babies with difficulty swallowing. If the delegate assures the RN that she is competent, the RN may go further in asking what the CNA would do if coughing or choking occurred. Depending on the situation, the RN would probably want to demonstrate feeding techniques and observe the skills to ensure the competency of the delegate.

WHAT ARE THE CAUSES OF PERFORMANCE WEAKNESSES?

Let's take a look at an example of a performance weakness and try to determine what the potential causes may be.

> In this scenario, you are an RN working a night shift on a hematology-oncology unit, and an agency nursing assistant, Pam, comes to work with you this shift. Pam is excited about the possibilities of interviewing for a regular night shift position and would love to work extra on holidays and weekends. As you begin to discuss her assignment for the night, she states, "Oh, I forgot to tell you, I don't ever take patients who are HIV (human immunodeficiency virus)–positive! Ever!"

There are some potential costs and benefits to your response to this statement. As the charge nurse, you could ignore this statement and continue with your work. You may decide this person has problems, and you may elect to deny her request for an interview. Or you may determine there is something behind her refusal. How you respond may cost you a potentially valuable staff member and could upset the other members of your staff and the patients. Avoiding the problem or accommodating her refusal could become a terrible headache for making assignments and would be contrary to the mission of your organization.

Experience has shown that there are several potential causes of performance inadequacies (*see* Critical Thinking Box 10-4). One of the most common causes is that the employee is not aware of what is expected of him or her. Does Pam know that at this facility, it is part of your policy that everyone takes care of all patients, whether or not they are known to be HIV-positive? Perhaps being aware of this expectation would assist Pam in making her decision about whether to apply for work on this unit.

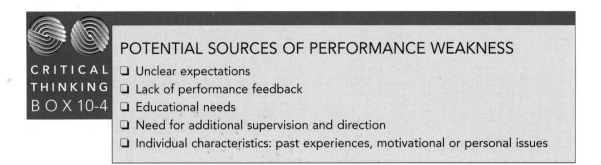

CRITICAL THINKING BOX 10-4

POTENTIAL SOURCES OF PERFORMANCE WEAKNESS

❏ Unclear expectations
❏ Lack of performance feedback
❏ Educational needs
❏ Need for additional supervision and direction
❏ Individual characteristics: past experiences, motivational or personal issues

Often, being clear about expectations is not enough. Each of us has some blind spots in his or her own performance. Perhaps we think we are doing just fine, meeting performance competencies and beyond, but colleagues have noted that we aren't performing procedures according to policy. If these observations are not shared, we will blithely believe we're doing great. Another common cause of performance difficulties is that no one has shared their perceptions of our performance with us. Pam may have adopted this attitude regarding other patients in other work settings, and because of the desperation for her help, no one had shared the fact that this behavior falls short of competencies in her job description.

Another common origin of performance weakness is an educational need. Does Pam need more education about how HIV infection is transmitted and how it is prevented? Surely she had to complete some content regarding this in her CNA certification course, but it seems she didn't internalize this content. Or is there a personal problem? She may have just witnessed the death of a loved one from acquired immune deficiency syndrome (AIDS) and feel unable to cope with seeing others with this disease for the short term.

The amount of supervision needed can be another source of performance problems. As an RN, you must determine the degree of "periodic inspection" needed by the delegate. Some people require additional direction but are still able to do the job competently. In the absence of that direction, they will be unable to create positive patient outcomes. Nurses tell us they wish that the assistive personnel on their staff would be "self-directed and take initiative without being told." We question whether an RN's hope that all will do their jobs without interaction or supervision on his or her part fits with the definition of supervision! Again, as leader, the RN must determine how much supervision is needed for the individual delegate, just as we determine the degree of observation needed for each patient on the basis of our assessment of their needs. In Pam's case, her reluctance to work with patients with HIV may have nothing to do with supervision but may reflect a need for guidance, education, or a frank discussion of expectations.

As the RN who is supervising Pam, what steps would you take to determine the cause of Pam's performance weakness, the assertion she refused to care for patients with HIV? What questions would you ask? How would you respond so that you could continue to use Pam's services this shift, maintain the integrity of your mission, and preserve the potential for hiring a new employee?

Matching the right person with the right task is the second step in the circular process of delegation. This process includes planning and articulating priority patient outcomes, assessing the competency of the delegate to perform the task, determining the potential strengths and weaknesses of the assistive personnel, and planning how much supervision is needed. To ensure that the right task will be done by the right person, additional clarification of expectations, performance feedback, and planning for education needs may be necessary; these steps will promote the long-term success of the team. The *right communication* will begin that clarification process, bringing us to the next step in the four rights of delegation.

THE RIGHT COMMUNICATION

HOW CAN I GET THE DELEGATE TO UNDERSTAND WHAT I WANT?

No matter what, it always comes back to communication. How clear you make your initial direction will be the cornerstone in determining the success of your delegated task and, ultimately, the performance of your team. The bottom line, whether the patient outcome was achieved, hinges on your ability to give initial direction that clearly defines your expectations of the delegate in performing the assigned task. It is not surprising that this is a step that is often done poorly or left out entirely because the assumption is made that the individual "knows what the job is and should just do it."

The first component of supervision, according to its definition, is the provision of initial direction. Achieving a balance in which we provide enough information for the person to understand the request without overstating the case and risking confusion or condescension requires that we tread a fine line. The use of the "four Cs" of initial direction will help you to plan your communication (*see* Critical Thinking Box 10-5).

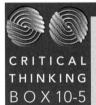

CRITICAL THINKING BOX 10-5

THE FOUR Cs OF INITIAL DIRECTION

CLEAR: Does the team member understand what I am saying?

CONCISE: Have I confused the direction by giving too much unnecessary information?

CORRECT: Is the direction according to policy, procedure, job desciption, and the law?

COMPLETE: Does the delegate have all the information necessary to complete the task?

Let's assume that you are working in a home health agency and you are planning the care for a patient with congestive heart failure. You have made your initial visit, assessing the patient and planning the outcomes you and the team will work toward in the next 3 weeks. Your patient is taking diuretics and antihypertensives, in addition to potassium supplements and being on a restricted diet. She is frequently short of breath and requires an assistant three times per week for hygienic care. In addition to providing hygienic care, you would like that assistant to monitor the blood pressure on the days you are not making a visit and to notify you if the blood pressure is outside of the range 120 to 170 systolic and 50 to 90 diastolic. Using the four Cs listed, you can evaluate your communication.

"Mrs. Jones has a heart condition and high blood pressure that requires medication and constant monitoring. One of our goals is to help Mrs. Jones have a stable blood pressure, in a range that is normal for her. On the days that you are visiting and giving the patient her bath, I would also like you to take her blood pressure. If it is outside the range of 120 to 170 systolic and 50 to 90 diastolic, I would like you to let me know. We may need to adjust her medication, change her diet, or call her physician for different orders."

Clear: Does the home health aide understand what is being asked of her? This direction is fairly straightforward: an easily understood instruction of taking the blood pressure.

Concise: Have you confused the assistant by giving too much information? Or is it enough for her to complete the task? Only the assistant can help you with this determination. You will need to ask directly, "Am I confusing you, or do you have enough information to do the job?" Every individual has different needs. However, you will want to make certain to check this out; some people will not be honest or accurate in their assessments of their understanding or abilities, leading to trouble later. Many of us are reluctant to ask questions, being afraid to admit our need for additional information. (We don't want to look like we don't know what we're doing!) This reluctance can ultimately result in harm to the patient because assumptions are made that the direction was understood when, in fact, it was not.

Correct: Can a home health aide monitor blood pressures? Where would you look for additional information if you weren't sure?

Complete: Does the assistant have enough information to fulfill your expectations? Once again, you will need to ask the delegate for clarification of his or her understanding of what you are asking. If you expect this assistant to also note the respirations and alert you to increased effort of breathing, have you shared that in your initial direction? Or did you assume she would naturally observe all vital signs because you alerted her to the patient's condition (and besides, she's a good assistant)? In our attempts not to appear condescending (I don't want to insult this assistant by reminding her to note the respirations— she'd think I didn't trust her to think!), we may often choose not to be as complete as we should be in giving initial direction.

Another common pitfall is the rationale that comes from working with someone over a period of time. A working relationship develops, and a routine or pattern of performance is established. When this happens, we start talking less and less to the other individual, believing that "she knows what I expect her to do." Consider the following situation:

You are working on a surgical unit in a partnership with Sam, an LPN you have been working with for the past year. Your easygoing style has led to a comfortable reliance on each other and the feeling that each knows what the other expects. On this particular evening shift, you are traveling down the hall, intent on medicating one of your patients. You also see a postanesthesia care unit (PACU) nurse bring one of your patients back from surgery. Seeing Sam coming your way, you state, "Sam, the postop is back in room 103." Evaluate your initial direction.

Did you believe that Sam just *knew* you wanted him to check on the patient, get the first set of vital signs, position the patient, check the dressing and the drains, and note the status of the intravenous tube?

Thirty minutes later, you are standing at the nurses' station, noting an order. Sam is charting. You ask him, "Sam, how's the patient in room 103 doing?" Expecting a brief report, you are surprised when Sam says, "I don't know. I thought you were going to take him." What went wrong?

No matter how long you have been working with someone, the right communication is essential to ensure the success of teamwork. Sam didn't *accept* the delegated task (remember what the delegate is accountable for?) because he did not understand what you meant. Be sure that you check the delegate's understanding of what you are saying. Failing to do this may result in unmet expectations, which lead to anger and frustration. More importantly, the patient will not receive the optimal care that both of you want to provide.

You've carefully assessed the patient, determined your plan on the basis of outcomes, and selected the right task to delegate to the right person. You have even given clear initial direction as part of the right communication. Now what? The final right of delegation is also a part of supervision: the periodic inspection of the actual act. Read on as we continue with a discussion of the right feedback.

THE RIGHT FEEDBACK

HOW CAN I EFFECTIVELY GIVE AND RECEIVE FEEDBACK?

Many nurses have shared their discomfort with giving and receiving feedback from co-workers. Few of us enjoy telling co-workers how they are doing or hearing about how we may have missed the mark! (*See* Fig. 10-3.) When supervising others, it's absolutely necessary to give feedback during your "periodic inspection." By following a formula for giving and receiving feedback and practicing it daily, RNs are assisted in the difficult job of correcting the performance of others. The reciprocal feedback process also permits you, as supervising RN, to hear how your own supervisory performance and communication affected the outcomes of the team (*see* Critical Thinking Box 10-6).

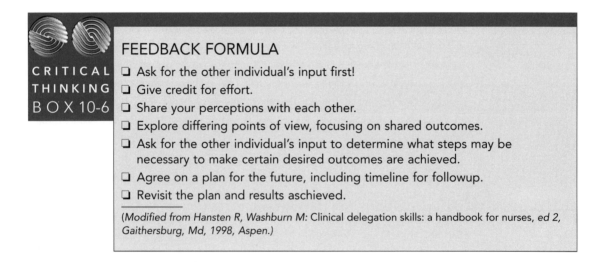

CRITICAL THINKING BOX 10-6

FEEDBACK FORMULA
❏ Ask for the other individual's input first!
❏ Give credit for effort.
❏ Share your perceptions with each other.
❏ Explore differing points of view, focusing on shared outcomes.
❏ Ask for the other individual's input to determine what steps may be necessary to make certain desired outcomes are achieved.
❏ Agree on a plan for the future, including timeline for followup.
❏ Revisit the plan and results aschieved.

(*Modified from Hansten R, Washburn M:* Clinical delegation skills: a handbook for nurses, *ed 2, Gaithersburg, Md, 1998, Aspen.*)

Let's look at how this process can be used in a situation in which positive feedback is intended.

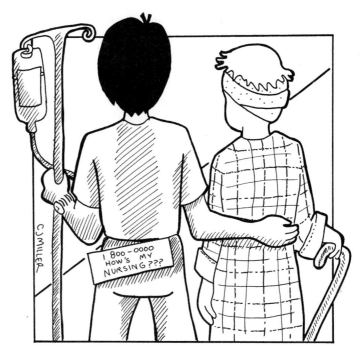

FIGURE 10-3
Providing feedback to the people you supervise doesn't have to be intimidating.

An RN (Pat) is working with a float RN (Julia) for the first time. Julia is new in the pool but is an experienced nurse. Pat is so pleased with Julia's experience and performance that she's gone off to have a nice long break and lunch with an old friend from the third floor. She's also taken time to meet with a colleague from the evening shift regarding a unit problem. Unfortunately, she hasn't been present on the unit much today. When Pat is having lunch with her friend, she exclaims, "That new float Julia is just excellent! If it weren't for her, I couldn't be here having lunch with you. I hope that she knows how organized and valuable she is!" Her friend, Alex, states, "Well, you know you should tell **her**, not just me, about this." When Pat returns to the floor, flushed with good intentions of making Julia's day with effusive praise, she tells Julia about how lucky she has been to work with her today.

Because all of us crave positive feedback and Julia is new to your organization, will Julia tell Pat that she's been trying to find her for hours? Probably not. But she *may* tell others that "Pat is one of those 'dump and run' nurses. I don't want to work on that floor again!" What if Pat asked *first*, "How have things been going for you today, Julia? I know this is your first day on the unit." Julia may have determined it was possible (and expected) to give reciprocal feedback: "I've been trying to find you! I have completed everything, but it hasn't been easy. Where have you been?" The best intentions can be destroyed by not asking the other individual for input first.

If you plan to give some negative feedback to an individual, you'll also need to ask their input first. For example:

> You've just noted that the night shift CNA didn't chart the intakes and outputs (I and O's) on three patients on your telemetry unit. You've called him and are thinking about how to discuss this with him in a positive manner, yet you know that he isn't going to want to chat because it is about time for him to get some rest.

If you said, "Why didn't you put the I and O's on the charts!?" the CNA would react defensively. If you state, "How was your night? I noted the I and O's are not on the charts," you've allowed the person to respond with what happened. If this CNA went home early with the flu or the unit experienced three codes, it would not be an effective or popular action to pounce on the team member for missing data.

This brings us to the next step in the process—giving credit for what has been accomplished. Let's return to Pat and Julia. At this point, Julia's input has been received. Pat can state, "Well, I can see I didn't help you as much as I should have and I forgot to give you my beeper number. But I do want you to know that I've checked on all of our patients, and they are very happy with their care today." After hearing input and giving credit where it is due, exploration of the gaps in the relationship and their communication and initial direction at the beginning of the shift can now be undertaken with open and frank discussion.

The discussion of differences will progress most smoothly if each party recognizes that they share common objectives: safe, effective care of the patients on their unit, as reflected in the fulfillment of shared, planned outcomes or goals determined by collaborative discussion among patients and care team members. When difficulties or conflicts occur, remember the reason you are both there: *the patients.*

Julia and Pat may clarify what happened and what actions each may take to ensure that the missed communication doesn't happen again in the future. Don't try to "fix" the situation for the other individual or prescribe what you'll do for them. The other individual will know what he or she needs to do to achieve your shared outcomes. For example, Pat may have decided that what would fix it for Julia would be to convene an hour before shift tomorrow and go through the unit manuals and read procedures. However, the most Julia may need is a beeper number and some more discussion and planning about assignments at the beginning of the shift.

Why wait for the other individual to come up with ideas when we can solve it for them? RNs who lead teams throughout the nation tell us that their work lives would be much better if everyone were behaving in an *accountable* manner. When we ask others for their step-by-step plan to prevent the problem in the future, it helps them determine that they are accountable for their own performance. In our scene with the missing I and O data, the RN will ask, "How can you make sure those I and O's are charted before you leave in the future? What will work for you?" This type of statement confers the necessary respect for the delegate's ability to determine how to adapt his work performance.

Don't miss the final steps in the formula. The individuals must agree on how they'll proceed in the future and when they'll revisit the problem or issue again. Julia may determine that she'll remind Pat in the future when she gets to the unit that she'll need her beeper number and a plan for the day. Then when the next shift is completed, they'll want to compare notes about how the shift has proceeded and whether patient outcomes have been achieved. The CNA may decide to ask the RN next week whether she's noted any missing I and O's. The pair will be able to evaluate whether the CNA's charting plan has been effective and can proceed to celebrate the success of the plan or to try other interventions.

Practice using the feedback formula. Remember the following three most important points:

- Ask for the other person's input first.
- Give credit for accomplishments and efforts.
- Ask the other individual to come up with steps for resolving the issue.

How would you use this formula to tell a supervisor that you are concerned about how long it's been since you've heard about your intershift transfer and you're getting worried about whether it will take place? How would you give positive feedback to an individual on your team who has been improving his ability to get out on time? What about a delegate who is "missing in action," the person you can't seem to locate when you need her?

HOW CAN I PRACTICE DELEGATION SKILLS?

We often hope for an exact prescription for what to delegate, when, and how. Because nursing assessment and professional judgment are necessary for clinical delegation, each situation will be different. Whether you work in an intensive care unit in a large tertiary hospital or a rural long-term care facility, the template of the delegation process—*matching the right task with the right delegate, communicating effectively, and offering and receiving feedback*—will be similar. To judge your comfort and assess your ability to integrate this process in your daily work life, complete the exercise in Critical Thinking Box 10-7. Good luck!

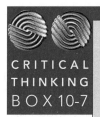

CRITICAL THINKING BOX 10-7

ASSESSING YOUR DELEGATION SKILLS

Assemble these documents:

❑ Your state nurse practice act
❑ Your job description and those of co-workers and delegates
❑ Skills checklists
❑ The patient list or assignment form from your unit
❑ A list of the usual staffing complement for your shift

1. Using the above, determine the short-term outcomes for an average patient assignment based on the information you've been given in a report. What tasks could be delegated to the individuals you have on staff? When will you complete further assessment of the patient situations?

(continued)

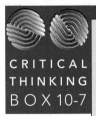

CRITICAL THINKING BOX 10-7

ASSESSING YOUR DELEGATION SKILLS *(Cont'd)*

2. Based on the outcomes and job descriptions, how will you determine the competency of individuals to complete the tasks you have determined could be delegated?

3. How will you communicate the team's plan using outcomes in your discussion?

4. How often will you communicate with the delegates, based on their need for supervision and patient complexity and dynamics? Have you used the four Cs?

5. How will you evaluate the effectiveness of your plan? How will you give positive feedback to the team?

6. A mistake was made by a delegate. You determined the person was competent, but the procedure was done improperly. For what are you accoutable? How will you give feedback to the individual, encouraging his or her growth and accountability?

7. Have you implemented the Four Rights of Delegation?

REFERENCES

American Nurses Association: *Code of ethics for nurses*, 2001, accessed January 10, 2002. http://www.ana.org/ethics/chcode.htm

California State Board of Nursing (BRN): *Advisory statement on unlicensed assistive personnel*, Sacramento, Calif, 1994, State Board.

Hansten R, Washburn M: *Clinical delegation skills: a handbook for professional practice*, ed 2, Gaithersburg, Md, 1998, Aspen.

Hansten R, Washburn M, Kenyon V: *Home care nursing delegation skills: a handbook for practice*, Gaithersburg, Md, 1999, Aspen.

National Council of State Boards of Nursing: *Concept paper on delegation*, Chicago, 1990, NCSBN.

National Council of State Boards of Nursing: *Delegation: concepts and decision making process*, Chicago, 1995, NCSBN.

National Council of State Boards of Nursing: *Nursing regulation: mutual recognition*, Chicago, 2001, NCSBN.

Sheehan JP: UAP delegation: a step-by-step process, *Nurs Manage* 32(4):22-24, 2001.

ADDITIONAL RESOURCES

Anthony MK, et al: Congruence between registered nurses and unlicensed assistive personnel perception of nursing practice, *Nurs Econ* 18(6):285-293, 2000.

Boucher MA: Delegation alert! *Am J Nurs* 98(2):26-33, 1998

Canavan K: Combating dangerous delegation, *Am J Nurs* 97(5):57-58, 1997.

Coburn JM, Sturdevant NJ: The acquisition of delegation skills: collaboration between education and service, *Nurse Educ* 17(6):32-34, 1992.

Hansten RI: Delegation: learning when and how to let go, *Nursing* 21(4):126, 128, 131, 1991.

Hansten R, Washburn M: *I light the lamp*, Vancouver, Wash, 1990, Applied Therapeutics.

Hansten R, Washburn M: Working with people, *Am J Nurs* 92(8):56-59, 1992.

Hansten R, Washburn M, O'Neill L: Clinical delegation skills: patient care management skills for the nineties. . . . and beyond [workshop], Seattle, 1990, Washington Organization of Nurse Executives.

Herrick K, Hansten R, Washburn M, O'Neill L, et al: My license is not on the line: the art of delegation, *Nurs Manage* 25(2):48-50, 1994.

Johnson SH: Teaching nursing delegation: analyzing nurse practice acts, *J Contin Educ Nurs* 27(2):52-58, 1996.

McClung TM: Assessing the reported financial benefits of unlicensed assistive personnel in nursing, *J Nurs Adm* 30(11):530-534, 2000.

Thomas S, Hume G: Delegation competencies: beginning practitioners' reflections, *Nurse Educ* 23(1):38-41, 1998.

Washburn M: Delegation: the art of getting things done through others, *Ariz Nurse Times*, 1991.

Westfall P: Nurse attorney organizations makes UAP recommendations—the American Association of Nurse Attorneys, *Insight* 7(2):1-3, 1998.

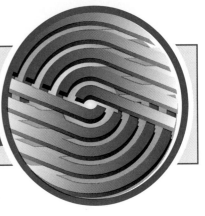

CHAPTER ELEVEN

Using Nursing Research in Practice

ELA-JOY LEHRMAN, MS, MAEd, PhD, RN, CNM

Knowledge can be used deliberately for the guidance of practice decisions and the development of theoretical explanations, as well as researchable questions.

—*Ada Sue Hinshaw*

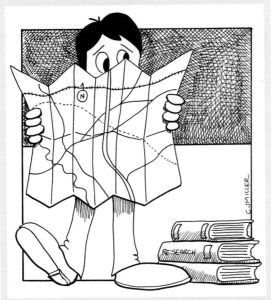

Nursing research is the road map to professional practice.

After completing this chapter, you should be able to:

- Identify the steps in the process of research use.
- Discuss the difference between conducting research and research use.
- Identify the characteristics of your practice context.
- Describe the function of the National Institute of Nursing Research.

RESEARCH USE

With the increasing competition in health care delivery, nurses can no longer rely on their traditional knowledge as the basis for providing nursing care. At a time when improved patient outcomes must be documented, the age-old wisdom that "nurses provide the best care" is no longer adequate. Nursing practice must have a sound scientific base like that obtained through nursing research and must be able to demonstrate cost-effective, predictable, measurable practice outcomes. Although more research is needed to expand nursing's scientific base, an even larger need is to apply existing nursing research findings; that is, there needs to be more research use.

WHAT IS RESEARCH USE?

Research use is the process of systematically integrating the findings of completed nursing research studies into clinical nursing practice (Horsley et al, 1983). In research use, the emphasis is on the reliance on already existing data (findings) from previous nursing research studies to modify a current nursing practice. A major component of the process of research use is reviewing completed nursing research studies that have been published in the literature. In contrast, conducting new research involves the collection of new data to answer a specific clinical practice question. The use of nursing research in practice is a step-by-step process incorporating critical thinking and decision making to ensure that a change in practice has a sound basis in nursing science.

WHAT STEPS ARE INCLUDED IN THE USE OF NURSING RESEARCH IN PRACTICE?

Step 1: Preusing. The first step in the use of nursing research in nursing practice is the recognition that some aspect of nursing practice could be done in a more efficient, a more beneficial, or simply a different way. This begins an exploratory phase in which nursing colleagues in the practice setting are consulted regarding their opinions about the need to find a new approach for some aspect of nursing practice. An early question should be, "Is the current practice research-based?" When current practice is research-based, the next question should be "Is the research on which the practice is based outdated?" (e.g., the specific details of taking temperatures with mercury thermometers became outdated when digital thermometers were used exclusively in practice).

Consensus building constitutes a second phase of step 1 that is used to identify the specific practice to be changed. The incorporation of the principles of change theory will increase the possibility of success. (See Chapter 5 for information about the change theory.) In any practice setting in which there are several nurses, a change will be more acceptable if those affected by the change are included in the decisions related to the change. This consensus is crucial for successful research use.

The third and final phase of step 1 delineates the aspect of nursing practice that will be changed into a concise statement of the *practice problem*. This statement will answer the question "In our current nursing practice, what do we want to change, improve, or make more efficient?" The narrower and more specific the statement of the practice problem, the easier your task will be in step 2.

Step 2: Assessing. The second step in research use is the identification plus critical evaluation of published research that is related to the practice problem you have identified (Fig. 11-1). Nursing literature is searched to identify those studies that deal with your practice problem. Although some studies may have explored the exact practice problem that you are examining, it is likely that most research will have approached the problem from a different point of view. Your task will be to analyze the research reports critically to determine which findings are adaptable to your practice problem and context. Organizing and summarizing the adaptable findings into an outline format will provide you with your primary working document for the remainder of the use plan (Box 11-1). Box 11-2 contains suggestions on reading a nursing research article.

The advent of the Internet and online searches has made a thorough search of the current literature easier. However, the volume of materials now available also increases the complexity of a review of literature. For example, the keywords used in a search can either return no articles or hundreds of articles. One technique is to

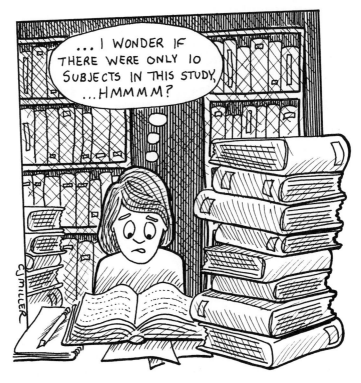

FIGURE 11-1
Nine out of ten nurses recommend...

BOX 11-1 Questions To Ask When Analyzing a Research Article for Potential Use of Findings in Nursing Practice

1a. The **Purpose** of the study is:

1b. The importance of this study to nursing practice is:

2. The **Research Question/Hypothesis** is:
   (If the question/hypothesis is *not* stated, it could be):

3a. The **Independent Variable** (s) is/are:

3b. The **Dependent Variable(s)** is/are:
   (If there are no independent and dependent variables, the **Research Variable(s)** is/are):

3c. **Definition(s)** of the variable(s) of interest to me is/are:

4. The **Conceptual Model/Theoretical Framework** linked with this study is:

5a. The content areas in the **Review of Related Literature** are:

5b. The review does/does not evaluate both supporting and nonsupporting studies:

6a. The **Research Design** used for the study is:

6b. The design is/is not appropriate for the research question:

6c. The control(s) used in this study is/are:

6d. The **Study Setting** is:

7a. The **Target Population** is:

7b. The **Sampling Method** is:

7c. The **Sampling Method** is/is not appropriate for the design:

7d. The criteria for participants are:

7e. The sample included _____ participants

7f. The sample is/is not representative of the population:

8a. The **Study Instrument(s)** is/are:

8b. Instrument validity and reliability information is presented and are of adequate levels for confidence in using the results:

9a. The **Data Collection Method(s)** is/are:

9b. The data collection method(s) is/are—is not/are not appropriate for this study:

10. Steps were taken to protect the **Rights of Human Subjects**:

11a. The **Data Analysis Procedure(s)** is/are:

11b. The data analysis method(s) is/are appropriate for the level of data collected and the research question/hypothesis:

11c. The research question/hypothesis is/is not supported:

12. The author(s) major **Conclusions and/or Implications for Nursing Practice** are:

begin searching the most recent year and then move back one year at a time until an adequate research base is identified. Keep in mind, however, that the classical research studies may not be available online, so you may need to make a trip to the stacks in the library. Box 11-3 contains hints on conducting a search in the library.

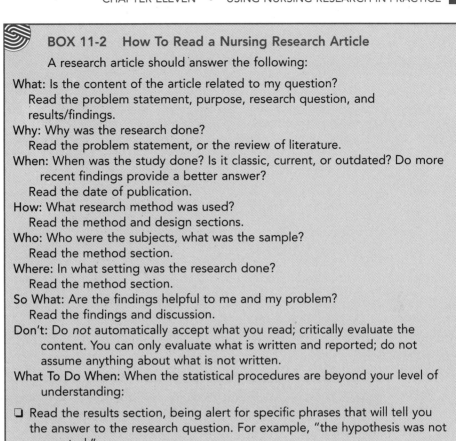

BOX 11-2   How To Read a Nursing Research Article

A research article should answer the following:

What: Is the content of the article related to my question?
Read the problem statement, purpose, research question, and results/findings.

Why: Why was the research done?
Read the problem statement, or the review of literature.

When: When was the study done? Is it classic, current, or outdated? Do more recent findings provide a better answer?
Read the date of publication.

How: What research method was used?
Read the method and design sections.

Who: Who were the subjects, what was the sample?
Read the method section.

Where: In what setting was the research done?
Read the method section.

So What: Are the findings helpful to me and my problem?
Read the findings and discussion.

Don't: Do *not* automatically accept what you read; critically evaluate the content. You can only evaluate what is written and reported; do not assume anything about what is not written.

What To Do When: When the statistical procedures are beyond your level of understanding:

❑ Read the results section, being alert for specific phrases that will tell you the answer to the research question. For example, "the hypothesis was not supported."
❑ Look at the tables; tables should be understandable without the narrative.
❑ Assume that the appropriate statistical analysis was done correctly and that the researcher has interpreted the results correctly.
❑ Have someone who understands the statistics read the article and get his or her opinion or get a consultant.

Step 3: Planning. Planning of research use is accomplished in three phases. The first phase involves determining the new approach, or *innovation*, that will be used on the basis of the findings from the review of the literature. Prior research findings will be used to design the innovation in the context of your practice setting (e.g., intensive care unit, ambulatory care, home care). The expected *practice outcomes* should also be determined on the basis of the literature and may need to be adjusted according to the characteristics of your particular practice.

Phase two of planning is the establishment of a systematic method for implementing the new approach. A *specific plan* should be established and followed so that the new approach is applied appropriately. Policies and procedures for implementation may need to be written. This phase may include staff training for the new approach.

> **BOX 11-3   Hints for Conducting a Literature Search in the Library**
>
> 1. Do some narrowing before you go to the library. Think about some key terms or alternate terms for your problem. Be prepared to narrow or expand your search, depending on what you find.
> 2. Plan to spend time in the library, but do not waste valuable time. Ask the library personnel to help you get started.
> 3. Begin by identifying the major professional nursing journals that publish nursing research, and start your literature review with those. If your problem is in a specialty area, review specialty journals.
> 4. Use the card catalogue if you come up with nothing when using a computer search.
> 5. If you find one article related to your problem, look at that author's reference list for other articles and journals.
> 6. Look at the table of contents in the journal where you found one related article.
> 7. Look at the section of books or journals in the library stacks that are about your problem.
> 8. Know the limitations of the library where you do your search; use interlibrary loan as needed.

The third phase of planning involves establishing a *method for evaluating* the practice outcomes, or effects, of the new approach. The outcomes are usually some specific improvements in patient care. Ideally your evaluation will indicate both the quality and the quantity of the change in the outcome.

Step 4: Implementing. Step 4 involves the implementation or application of the new approach, along with the collection of the evaluation data. By following the specific plan that you established in step 3, the new approach will be introduced into practice. It is important that you begin collecting your evaluation data at the same time so that you can clearly determine the effect of the new approach.

Step 5: Evaluating. Step 5 involves the evaluation of the implementation to determine whether the new approach improved practice outcomes. Whether you will continue using the new approach in the practice setting may also be determined on the basis of new technology, economic considerations, or changes in staffing. If there is no change in outcomes, you may want to return to the previous practice. The evaluation phase may lead to another research use project; for example, if the practice problem is significant and the practice outcomes were not improved, another new approach may be tried.

RESEARCH USE: WHAT IS IT NOT?

Research use does *not* entail simply taking the findings of a single research study and using those findings in nursing practice. Research studies are replicated to rule out chance findings and to validate the original study. Similar studies with different populations are conducted to determine the applicability of findings to different groups of people. For these reasons, research use encompasses the findings of many studies to develop the new approach that will be put into practice.

Data are collected in the process of research use. However, research use is not the collection of data to answer a research question, as is the case when conducting research. The data collected in research use are needed for evaluation to determine whether there is some advantage to the new approach in the practice setting.

Research use should not be confused with review use. Review use involves a quality-control/risk-management process to evaluate the appropriate use of resources related to a specific treatment. Review use does not entail the use of nursing research findings during the process of evaluation.

When you review the nursing research literature for research use, as mentioned previously, there is no assurance that you will find studies that are directly applicable to your practice situation. Your specific question may not have been answered. You may have to either adapt the findings from the literature or conduct your own research.

DEFINING YOUR PRACTICE CONTEXT

Your practice context will determine to what degree you can use the findings from nursing research. A *practice context* entails a blending of all those factors and systems that contribute to the delivery of nursing care. This blend includes the health, social, and ethnic characteristics of the patient population served; the type of practice setting; the economic constraints of the setting; the type of health care–delivery system; the existing policies and procedures; the staffing pattern; and the administrative structure. Each factor or system can be either enabling or inhibiting, but it is the practice context as a whole that is evaluated to determine the use of nursing research.

WHAT ARE THE HEALTH, SOCIAL, AND ETHNIC CHARACTERISTICS OF THE PATIENT POPULATION BEING SERVED?

To begin defining your practice context, you will need to identify any characteristics that are specific to the group of people who will be receiving nursing care. Is there some particular health characteristic that should be considered? For example, if you teach prenatal classes, the health characteristic will be pregnancy. Are there some particular social and ethnic characteristics that need consideration? If your prenatal classes are for pregnant teenagers who are single, this social characteristic needs special consideration. Be as thorough and as specific as possible in identifying these characteristics.

WHAT ARE THE HEALTH-CARE DELIVERY CHARACTERISTICS OF YOUR SETTING?

As you continue to define your practice context, specify the type of practice setting, the economic constraints of the setting, the type of health-care delivery system, the existing policies and procedures, the staffing patterns, and the administrative structures.

In other words, include all the characteristics of the care setting that will either contribute to or inhibit the process of research use. If your practice setting is a hospital where there is a limit to the length of stay for a particular surgery, then a new approach that would increase that length of stay would not be an appropriate one for implementation. Furthermore, when implementing a new approach in practice, care must be taken to preserve or improve the current health-care delivery standards.

WHAT ARE THE MOTIVATORS AND BARRIERS FOR INCORPORATING NURSING RESEARCH INTO YOUR PRACTICE?

Identify your bridges (motivators) and roadblocks (barriers) in the practice setting (Critical Thinking Box 11-1). The more individuals in the practice setting from whom you can attain consensus on the new approach to practice, the easier it will be to implement. Those who understand the need for making a change in practice will be more likely to support the change. (See Chapter 5 for information on change theory.) Those who feel that they had a part in the decision making surrounding the new approach are also more likely to promote it. In both instances, these colleagues become motivators for the implementation of innovation and change.

CRITICAL THINKING BOX 11-1

THINK ABOUT...

What are the barriers that might inhibit your use of research findings?

_____

_____

_____

How would you go about minimizing the barriers?

_____

_____

_____

As with any change process that involves a group of people, it is very likely that a small number of individuals in the practice setting will be very resistant to the new approach. Those who are resistant may present barriers that prevent the full implementation of the new process. They may complain about lack of time to learn the new approach, for example, in an effort to avoid being a part of what they do not support. These colleagues and budgetary and personnel constraints are examples of barriers.

In addition, the research literature may present barriers to implementing a new approach. For example, if there are only a few research studies reported in the nursing literature that are related to your practice problem, then the lack of replication of the findings may prevent you from developing a research-based approach for your particular practice problem. Another barrier is the time lag from the completion of a research project until the project report is published. This time lag, which may be a few years, may make the research findings obsolete. For example, research related to glass oral thermometers would be obsolete if your practice setting uses electronic ear thermometers.

A COMPARISON OF PROCESS: RESEARCH UTILIZATION COMPARED WITH NURSING RESEARCH AND THE CONDUCT OF RESEARCH

HOW IS THE USE OF RESEARCH IN PRACTICE DIFFERENT FROM CONDUCTING RESEARCH?

As illustrated in Table 11-1, the major steps involved in both conducting and utilizing research are the same. Both are problem-solving processes involving critical thinking. For example, a clinical practice problem may provide the impetus to conduct and use research. However, there are differences. Conducting research taps into the "ways of knowing," whereas using research taps into the "ways of doing."

When we conduct research, whether in the clinical setting or the laboratory, the primary activity undertaken is the systematic collection of new data. Following specific steps called the protocol, we gather information that will answer a specific research question. For many nursing studies, the *research question* arises from a situation in nursing practice that needs an answer.

The *utilization of research* involves the systematic process of integrating the findings of completed nursing research studies into clinical nursing practice. Research utilization also entails reviewing research that has already been completed to develop a new approach to nursing practice. All three processes, research utilization, nursing research, and the nursing process, have the same five major steps. However, the specific tasks for each process are different.

WHAT IS THE RELATIONSHIP BETWEEN NURSING THEORY AND RESEARCH UTILIZATION?

Nursing theory used as the theoretical framework of a research study is essential for the continued development of nursing theories; research findings will support or suggest the modification of theory. In contrast, when a specific nursing theory is used as the framework for nursing practice, the focus is on the intervention. The intervention that is designed in the planning phase of research utilization must be consistent with the theory. For example, if Orem's theory of self-care requisites is used for nursing practice, a successful intervention would be one that emphasizes self-care rather than care received from others.

TABLE 11-1

Comparison of Processes: An Overview of the Nursing Process, Conducting Research, and Research Utilization

Nursing Process	Conducting Research	Research Utilization
Preprocess Establish a nurse-patient relationship	Preplanning Identify the need for a research study Determine feasibility Scan the literature	Preuse Identify a practice problem that needs a new approach Obtain consensus
Assessing Gather data	Assessing Identify the problem State research purpose Begin to formulate the research question Review the literature	Assessing Identify and critically evaluate published research related to your practice problem Identify the findings that are adaptable to your problem and your context
Planning Diagnose Set goals Prioritize Determine nursing interventions Formulate care plan	Planning Identify and define the variables Select a conceptual or theoretical model Select research design Finalize research question Plan data analysis Write research proposal Negotiate a site for data collection Complete human subjects review	Planning Determine the new approach and the desired outcomes Establish a systematic method for implementing the new approach Establish a method for evaluating the outcomes of the new approach
Implementing Initiate the plan	Implementing Prepare questionnaires Train data collectors Obtain subject sample Collect the data Prepare data for analysis	Implementing Begin using the new approach Collect data about the outcomes of the new approach
Evaluating Determine the patient response	Evaluating Analyze the data Organize the data Answer the research question Interpret the results Report the findings Plan next project	Evaluation of the implementation Determine whether the practice change improved patient outcomes Decide whether to continue using the new approach

THE NATIONAL INSTITUTE OF NURSING RESEARCH

WHAT IS ITS FUNCTION?

The National Institute of Nursing Research (NINR) is a branch of the National Institutes of Health, which is under the jurisdiction of the U.S. Department of Health and Human Services. Each institute within the National Institutes of Health focuses on a specific area of health care research; the NINR is a major source of federal funding for nursing research. The NINR also supports education in research methods, research career development, and excellence in nursing science.

Another function of the NINR is establishing a National Nursing Research Agenda. The agenda is composed of priority topics for nursing research. These topics may be related to a national health need, or they may be in an area that requires research for the development of nursing science. Nurses incorporate topics from the agenda in research grant proposals that will be submitted to the NINR. For more information online, visit the NINR Web site at http://www.nih.gov/ninr.

THE AGENCY FOR HEALTH CARE POLICY AND RESEARCH

WHAT IS ITS FUNCTION?

As part of the Omnibus Budget Reconciliation Act of 1989, the Agency for Health Care Policy and Research was established to enhance the quality and effectiveness of health care services. The Agency for Health Care Policy and Research conducts and supports general health services research; develops clinical practice guidelines; and disseminates research findings and guidelines to health care providers, policymakers, and the public. The Agency for Health Care Policy and Research has several components that can be useful to the nurse wanting to incorporate research findings into clinical practice: The Center for Medical Effectiveness Research, the Center for General Health Services Extramural Research, the Center for General Health Services Intramural Research, the Center for Research Dissemination and Liaison, the Office of Health Technology Assessment, and the Office of Science and Data Development. Several versions of the clinical practice guidelines are produced to meet different needs (e.g., *Clinical Practice Guideline*, *Quick Reference Guide for Clinicians*, and the *Consumer Version*). Following are some examples included in the clinical practice guidelines: management of cancer pain, acute low-back problems in adults, and treatment of pressure ulcers.

REFERENCES

Horsley JA, et al: *Using research to improve nursing practice: a guide*, New York, 1983, Grune & Stratton.

ADDITIONAL RESOURCES

Bandsman EL, Bandsman B: *Critical thinking in nursing*, Norwalk, Conn, 1988, Appleton & Lange.

Burns N, Grove SK: *Understanding nursing research*, Philadelphia, 1995, WB Saunders.

Burns N, Grove SK: *The practice of nursing research: conduct, critique, and utilization*, ed 3, Philadelphia, 1997, WB Saunders.

Fawcett J: *Analysis and evaluation of conceptual models of nursing*, ed 3, Philadelphia, 1995, FA Davis.

Fitzpatrick J, Whall A: *Conceptual models of nursing*, Norwalk, Conn, 1989, Appleton & Lange.

Hinshaw AS: Response to "Structuring the nursing knowledge system: a typology of four domains," *Sch Inq Nurs Pract* 1(2):111-114, 1987.

Phillips L: *A clinician's guide to the critique and utilization of nursing research*, Norwalk, Conn, 1986, Appleton-Century-Crofts.

Polit D, Hungler B: *Nursing research: methods, appraisal, and utilization*, Philadelphia, 1993, JB Lippincott.

Polit D, Hungler B: *Nursing research: principles and methods*, Philadelphia, 1995, JB Lippincott.

Woods N, Catanzaro M: *Nursing research: theory and practice*, St Louis, 1988, Mosby.

Yura H, Walsh M: *The nursing process*, Norwalk, Conn, 1983, Appleton-Century-Crofts.

INTERNET RESOURCES

Here is a sample of Internet sites that can be used to locate nursing research studies.

George Mason University
http://apollo.gmu.edu/index.html

Grant and Research Resources, GrantsNet
http://www.grantsnet.org

National Institute of Nursing Research
http://www.nih.gov.ninr

U.S. National Library of Medicine
http://www.nlm.nih.gov

Sigma Theta Tau International Nursing Honor Society
http://www.nursingsociety.org/

Here is a sample of databases that contain research articles.

Alt-HealthWatch
http://www.uwp.edu/information.services/library/artand/althlth.htm

Cinahl
http://www.cinahl.com

ERIC (Educational Resources Information Center)
http://www.askeric.org

Medline
http://www.ncbi.nlm.nih.gov

Medscape
http://www.medscape.com

ProQuest
http://www.umi.com

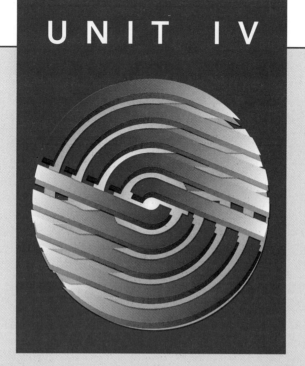

HEALTH CARE DELIVERY SYSTEM

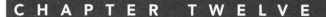

The Health Care Organization and Patterns of Nursing Care Delivery

SUSAN SPORTSMAN, RN, PhD

Every patient deserves a nurse.

—*American Nurses Association*

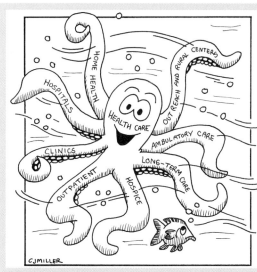

Health care organizations should all be within reach.

After completing this chapter, you should be able to:

- Describe changes occurring in the health care delivery system.
- Identify trends affecting the health care delivery system.
- Identify components of a hospital's organizational structure.
- Differentiate between a centralized and a decentralized organizational structure.
- Discuss various models of hospital organization.
- Discuss patterns of nursing care delivery systems.
- Describe strategies to coordinate care and reduce costs.
- Describe factors that influence staffing and scheduling in nursing care delivery.

HEALTH CARE DELIVERY SYSTEM

The United States health care delivery system has been rapidly and constantly changing for the last 25 years. This change is likely to escalate in the future. Nurses practicing in any health care environment must embrace change and be willing to contribute to solving problems that arise because of the change and complexity of the system.

WHAT IS CAUSING THESE DRAMATIC CHANGES?

There is general consensus by society that health care in the United States costs too much. These costs do not seem to be coming down. For example, the cost to care for Medicare patients in 2001 is expected to be 10% more than it was in 2000 (*The Atlanta Journal-Constitution*, August 15, 2001). There are various factors that influence the continuing rise in cost, including expanding technology, emphasis on acute care rather than prevention, and insurance reimbursement that rewards increased spending. Various approaches have been introduced into the health care scene in an effort to control costs. These include the following:

- Managed-care strategies by insurance companies and all types of provider groups to make sure that care is appropriate, provided in the least-restrictive setting possible, and cost-effective (i.e., the cost doesn't outweigh the benefits the patient receives)
- Changes in reimbursement methods to hospitals, physicians, and other providers to encourage them to provide health promotion/risk-reduction screening activities for their patients
- Restructuring of hospitals and other health care organizations ("downsizing" or "right-sizing") to reduce costs
- Mergers of various types of entities in an effort to provide a continuum of services in large organizations rather than in many small ones

These factors, along with the continued recognition that many in our country have limited (or no) access to health care, as well as the growing shortage of health care professionals, has encouraged numerous changes in the way health care is delivered.

The radical reshaping of health care is influenced by the two following contradictory forces: (1) the recognition that access to care must be improved through government intervention and (2) the increasing notion of competitive free-market forces in health care. At various points in history since 1922, the United States has considered a national health plan approach, in which minimal health coverage would be available to everyone in the country. Such a plan would eliminate the problem of millions of people who have no health coverage. In 1994 President Bill Clinton introduced a health reform package aimed at improving access. This plan did not pass into law; however, there continues to be discussion regarding how the government (either state or federal) can increase health care benefits available to everyone in a way that is affordable for the government.

Many people have begun to question the value of extremely costly technological interventions that may prolong life only briefly, or prolong life but not improve the quality of life for the patient. Recognition has grown that money spent on preventive health care and wellness teaching might lower costs for later acute care. People, through their elected officials, have said that they are unwilling to pay the high price for the health care that they are receiving. Many changes are being introduced at a fast pace to address this mandate from society.

The health care reform program presented to Congress by President Clinton in 1994 represents the belief that government must be actively involved in the planning and regulation of services. In a nutshell, this program would have provided minimal health coverage to everyone in the United States, thereby eliminating the problem of millions of people who have no health care coverage at all. The proposal would have set up a governmental structure through which tax dollars could be channeled and disbursed to payers and providers to provide patient care. However, the Clinton plan did not make it through Congress for a variety of reasons. Although some states, such as Hawaii, are providing a form of universal coverage (health coverage for everyone), we are, in general, left with essentially the same governmental structure for health care programs that we have had in place for the last 50 years.

The second and equally strong belief in the United States is that government should not be involved in health care and free-market forces should reign. A competitive free-market system in health care currently seems to be the major influence in this country. Proponents of this approach believe that if appropriate competitive forces are allowed to operate in the health care industry, market forces will bring down the cost of health care. Deregulating health care and eliminating the role of the government will enable competition to bring about necessary savings.

Free-market forces are currently a major influence in the way health care is being delivered. Fierce competition has developed among insurance companies to offer such programs as health maintenance plans. Providers—physicians, nurse practitioners, and hospitals—are under increasing pressure to lower their costs dramatically to obtain the right to have insurance companies send patients to them. The competition among insurance companies is fueled by the fact that employers are shopping among the companies to get the lowest prices for their employees' health coverage. Employee health care represents a major cost of doing business in this country and one that cuts deeply into employers' profits. Reducing these costs can enable a company to offer to their potential customers a more price-competitive product. These dramatic changes are influencing major trends that affect the practice of nursing.

TRENDS

WHAT IS MEANT BY THE CORPORATIZATION OF HEALTH CARE?

Small, stand-alone physicians' offices, hospitals, and other kinds of facilities will probably not make it in this new world of health care. To achieve large economies of scale with lower costs, the *corporatization* of health care is taking place. Small operating facilities such as hospitals or physicians' offices are merging into large-scale organizations so that duplicate processes and redundant facilities, equipment, and procedures can be eliminated and costs reduced. Just as the small, stand-alone corner grocery store has been merged into large chains, the small, stand-alone physicians' offices and hospitals are being merged into large regional and national conglomerate groups. Health care is adopting the business practices of corporate America at a rapid rate.

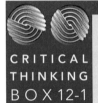

CRITICAL THINKING BOX 12-1

How will the move of small clinics to larger regional physician groups affect the public's access to health care?

The emphasis in health care has been and continues to be on a shift from nonprofit to for-profit status. National for-profit chains are now purchasing many nonprofit hospitals. Nonprofit organizations do not pay taxes and return their earnings to the community. For-profit organizations pay taxes and return their earnings to stockholders. A few years ago almost all hospitals were nonprofit. Now we see a fast-moving trend that, if it continues, will result in a large number of hospitals being owned by for-profit organizations. Therefore nurses must move from being not only patient care–centered to also being experts in the business side of health care. Whether the organization is for-profit or nonprofit, the environment in which the nurse will most likely work is a large corporate system that emphasizes the business side and the patient care side of health care.

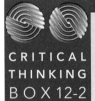

CRITICAL THINKING BOX 12-2

Should a hospital be allowed to operate as a for-profit organization? Are for-profit hospitals managed more efficiently?

WHAT IS MEANT BY INTEGRATED HEALTH CARE DELIVERY SYSTEMS?

Individual health care organizations that merge into systems to provide all needed services under one corporate umbrella are known as *integrated health care delivery systems*. These systems may offer prevention services such as wellness programs, acute- and long-term care facilities and home health and hospice services. The system may own the individual entities or may contract with them to provide specialty services. With integrated health care systems, employers and insurance companies have the ability to contract with one system to meet all the health care needs of the employees or members rather than negotiating multiple contracts with many organizations. Nurses will increasingly work within systems that offer a high degree of continuity of care among the various health care organizations. Patients should also enjoy a sense of seamlessness in the delivery system, as they move from the hospital to the nursing home, the hospice, or the rehabilitation center.

How Are We Building Integrated Delivery Networks? Small physician practices are merging into large ones. Small, standalone hospitals are merging into systems that include several hospitals. Health care facilities that have had a long history of competing are now merging to become one entity. Consequently the staff has to learn to work together as a family rather than as competitors. Mergers force organizations with very different cultures to amalgamate into a new entity that is a hybrid of the old ones. There is often much despair and fear with respect to job security when mergers are announced. The challenge to do work in a different way in order to save costs is also a threat to many people.

HOW ARE REIMBURSEMENT SYSTEMS CHANGING?

Health care reimbursement continues to move rapidly toward such mechanisms as Health Maintenance Organizations (HMOs) and away from fee-for-service arrangements. In the past providers such as hospitals and physicians were paid for procedures rendered to patients. Under this fee-for-service model, there were dollars available for repair work (acute care) but not for maintenance. Medicare introduced the prospective payment system in the early 1980s, marking the beginning of a movement to control costs. Under this system, a fixed fee was paid to the hospital according to a reimbursement rate that was preset for the diagnosis given at discharge. A hospital that could treat a particular diagnosis with a shorter length of stay and reduced consumption of resources, such as unnecessary intensive care stay, would show a smaller loss for caring for this kind of patient. This practice began the trend to pay for health care at a prearranged rate rather than as billed.

Historically in the automobile industry, cars were serviced in repair shops when they broke down and we paid whatever price was charged for the parts and labor involved in the repair. Health care in the past was built around such a "repair-shop" model. Automobile manufacturers then developed preventive maintenance contracts in which they guaranteed the buyer they would take care of any repair work necessary within a given number of miles driven. As time went on, the miles allowed became much greater as the quality of automobiles improved. Service contracts are now common when one buys a variety of appliances.

Health care is also moving in the direction of "preventative maintenance." Under *capitation*, employers pay a set fee each month to an insurance organization for their employees to receive health care. That amount does not vary even if an employee gets sick, is hospitalized, or never needs health care. Under this kind of contract, there is an incentive for the insurance company to work aggressively to keep employees healthy. If they are hospitalized, a great expense must be paid out of the proceeds from the monthly fee. These new reimbursement methodologies place much more emphasis on wellness, disease prevention, and patient self-management of health and illness. The health care providers actually lose money if patients do not stay healthy and consequently overuse hospitalization.

HMOs are a form of health insurance that has become very popular in the last decade. An annual payment is made by or for beneficiaries to a group of providers that delivers all of the health care services covered under the plan, including physician and hospital services. There are four kinds of HMOs.

- In the *staff model*, physicians are employed by a health plan and work on salary.
- In the *group model*, a single group of physicians contracts with a health plan to deliver services.
- In the *network model*, a health plan contracts with multiple physician groups to provide services to enrollees.
- In the *independent practice association (IPA)*, the plan contracts with a variety of physicians who work in independent practice or multispecialty groups to provide services to enrollees. Physicians working in network and IPA models usually provide services to HMO enrollees and patients with other kinds of insurance. HMOs sometimes own their own hospitals, but they most commonly pay hospitals for needed services through a discounted payment mechanism or a per-case reimbursement mechanism.

HMOs have grown in the past few years because they provide a strong incentive to avoid hospitalization, which consequently reduces health care costs. HMO members often like the ease of utilizing health care with an HMO because there are fewer uncovered services and forms to fill out. There are now HMO options available for Medicare and Medicaid beneficiaries.

Preferred provider organizations (PPOs) are another form of health plan. In general, beneficiaries use physicians who have agreed to provide services at a lower price to the insurer. The beneficiary is given an incentive to use particular physicians because there is usually a lower insurance premium or reduction of co-payments.

TYPES OF ORGANIZATIONS

All organizations design themselves in response to the trends with which they are dealing. The structure determines what the organization will be like. There are many different kinds of organizational design in health care, depending on the services provided and the philosophy of the institutions. Box 12-1 outlines various types of organizations in health care and the services typically provided. Regardless of the type of organization, the structure can range from highly centralized to highly decentralized. To determine whether an organization is centralized or decentralized, one must know where the majority of the decisions are made and how much flexibility and autonomy people in various parts of the organization are given. The organizational structure in hospitals tends to be more formal (and often more centralized) than the organization of other health care entities such as clinics or home health care. Regardless of where you work, the organizational structure will affect the decision-making process.

BOX 12-1   Types of health care organizations

ACUTE CARE HOSPITALS
Care provided to individuals who require close observation and equipment that cannot be provided in the home
- ❏ General hospitals
- ❏ Children's hospitals
- ❏ Emergency care centers
- ❏ Women's hospitals
- ❏ Oncology hospitals

PSYCHIATRIC HOSPITALS
Care provided to individuals experiencing acute and chronic emotional and behavior problems

COMMUNITY MENTAL HEALTH CENTERS
Care provided to psyhiatric patients to assist them in controlling emotions and behavior without hospital admission

LONG-TERM CARE FACILITIES
Care provided to chronically ill patients to maintain their physical, social, and psychological well-being
- ❏ Skilled care facilities
- ❏ Intermediate care facilities

DAY CARE CENTERS AND HOMES FOR ELDERLY
Care provided for clients who cannot be left alone during the day but can be cared for in a home setting with assistance

AMBULATORY CARE
Care provided to clients who come to the health care facility, receive care, and return home or are admitted to an acute care hositpal
- ❏ Nurse managed clinics
- ❏ Outpatient clinics
- ❏ Emergency clinics
- ❏ Health centers
- ❏ Physician offices
- ❏ Renal dialysis center
- ❏ Rehabilitation centers

HOME HEALTH CARE
Care provided within the patient's home
- ❏ Hospice
- ❏ Follow up care from an acute care hospital
- ❏ Follow up care from ambulatory centers
- ❏ Well-baby visits

WHAT IS THE DIFFERENCE BETWEEN A DECENTRALIZED AND A CENTRALIZED ORGANIZATION?

In centralized organizations, the control of financial management and changes regarding nursing care delivery come from a central authority. In the most centralized structure, this activity comes from the chief nursing officer. Centralized structures are common in small organizations. As organizations become more decentralized, activities are transferred from the chief nursing officer to the nurse manager or supervisor and perhaps even to the bedside nurse. Nursing structures have evolved from organizations that historically were very centralized. Because nursing was traditionally perceived as a practice that needed much managing, we have many legacies of this centralized management style.

In a decentralized organization, subordinates are given a wide range of authority that involves decision-making and even policy formulation. The trend in the last few years has been toward decentralized structures. Much research has shown that when people are given responsibility and accountability, their involvement in the work, motivation, and job satisfaction increase. As nursing has become a more autonomous profession, the move toward decentralized structures has been a natural outgrowth. However, not everyone is ready for decentralized structures. Some nurses are not interested in taking on additional accountability and authority. They prefer to work in a setting where there is less personal responsibility and accountability and where nurse managers or other supervisors in the setting can positively direct them. Not all organizations are moving in this direction either, so there are options available in choosing the kind of organization that fits you best.

HOW DO OTHER MODELS OF ORGANIZATION WORK?

New models have been adapted that reflect principles of business applied to health care. For example, many hospitals are organized around product lines or service lines—in effect, a hospital within a hospital. Small, unique, autonomous units are developed that can concentrate their interests on a specific kind of patient and care. For example, a women's health center, a children's hospital, a sports medicine center, and an oncology center are all examples of organizing around a certain kind of patient and care. A women's center can be organized within a hospital to bring together all the services women potentially use under one administrator. Obstetrics and gynecology services and psychiatric/psychosocial services, plastic surgery, osteoporosis care, exercise groups, and educational classes might all be coordinated under the accountability of one administrator. A definite marketing plan to attract potential patients to this unit will be in place. In this kind of structure, nurses either can work for the administrator (product/service line manager), who may or may not be a nurse, or can report to the nursing division. Or the nursing staff can be responsible both to the product line manager and to someone in the nursing division. When people have more than one boss, this concept is described as *matrix management*. In a situation in which nursing staff are accountable both to the product line/service line manager and the chief nursing officer, these two people must have clear roles and set the individual expectations for the performance of the nursing staff.

As organizations design themselves, they determine their priorities and how people work within the organizations. The role of the nurse in a centralized structure is much different than in a decentralized or matrix structure. There is no right answer to the kind of organization design that is best. All organizations work well in specific situations. However, not all people work well in all types of organizations. Some people do not like the abstract matrix model, whereas others find great freedom in this model. Some nurses are flexible enough to work in any model. Box 12-1 identifies types of health care organizations. Depending on your beliefs and your needs, you will find an organizational structure that fits you best and meets your long-range goals.

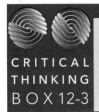

CRITICAL THINKING BOX 12-3

Consider the facilities in your community that provide health care: Do they have a centralized or decentralized type of organization?

WHAT PURPOSE IS SERVED BY ORGANIZATIONAL CHARTS?

Organizational charts are maps that determine who reports to whom. Some organizational charts will show many managers between the chief nursing officer and the staff nurse. These charts will be pyramidal in design. Other organizational charts will be more flattened" and will show fewer people between the chief nursing officer and the nurse at the bedside (Figs. 12-1 and 12-2). The shape of the chart is dependent, in part, on the size of the organization, but it is also dependent on the style of governance. An organizational chart will describe your relationship to the chief nursing officer and chief executive officer and will also identify patterns of formal communication.

HOW DO ORGANIZATIONS FUNCTION, AND WHAT ARE THEIR COMMUNICATION PATTERNS?

Organizational charts also reflect the formal communication patterns expected in the entity. There are five types of communication networks which often appear in organizational communication. These are illustrated in Figure 12-3 and include the *circle, all-channel, Y, wheel, and chain.* As you can see by the structure, the Y organization shows a situation in which two employees report directly to a supervisor within a continuing chain of command. If you are assigned to complex tasks, they are more easily done in less centralized, formal communication networks, such as the all channel. Simple tasks are handled most efficiently in centralized networks such as the wheel. It also would stand to reason that it might be very difficult to accomplish a complex task in an organization that is like the chain (Sullivan, Decker, and Jamerson, 2000).

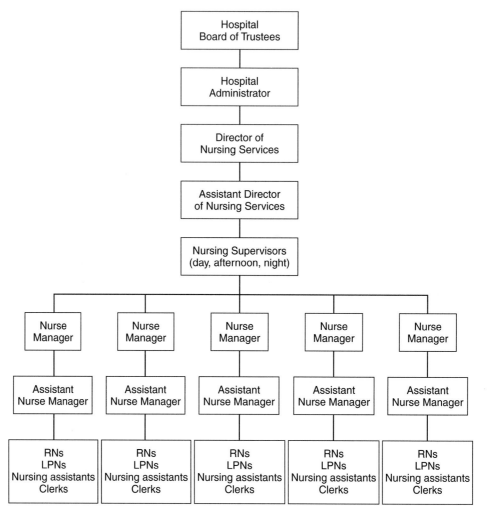

FIGURE 12-1
Cenralized organizational structure
LPN, Licensed practical nurse; *RN*, registered nurse.

Committees also provide a clue to the running of the organization. In some organizations, the committee structure is very important and powerful. Some committees, such as task forces or councils, actually make decisions autonomously. In other organizations, they are merely advisory, and in some organizations they do not exist. If you have an interest in working within the organization in addition to providing direct patient care, knowledge of the organizational chart would be important to you.

Another way organizations get work done is through participation. *Participative management* is a term for allowing the staff nurse to participate in and provide advice about issues, but not to make actual decisions about the management of the unit or facility. *Shared governance*, which is a step beyond participative management, came into

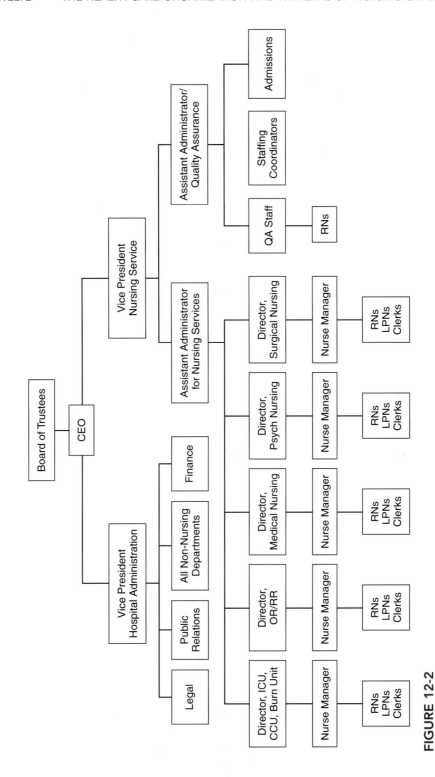

FIGURE 12-2

Decentralized organizational structure

CCU, Coronary care unit; *CEO*, chief executive officer; *ICU*, intensive care unit; *OR*, operating room; *QA*, quality assurance; *RR*, recovery

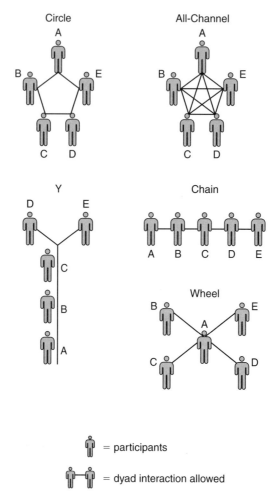

= participants

= dyad interaction allowed

FIGURE 12-3
Types of communication networks.

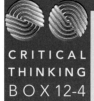

CRITICAL THINKING BOX 12-4

How do nursing faculty serve on the committees of the college and of the nursing department? Is it important for nursing faculty to represent education in hospital-based committees dealing with the delivery of nursing care?

being as a way to share certain aspects of the management of the unit or department of nursing with the staff nurses. Over time, staff nurses take on more responsibility and accountability for self-scheduling, quality-improvement programs, recruitment/ retention programs, and other aspects of managing the unit or department.

An advanced form of the shared governance model is the *self-governed model*, in which staff nurses take on virtually full accountability for running a unit. A chairperson is usually elected for a defined term to lead the group. This person coordinates the work of the unit as others take on accountability over time for different aspects such as financial management and quality. Self-governed units are not very common as yet, but shared governance and participatory management are becoming much more so. Depending on the amount of autonomy and decision making you want in your work life, you will prefer one of these organizational structures to another.

Another way the nursing staff communicates to the organization is through a union. In a union structure, the staff chooses to have a union speak for them instead of speaking directly for themselves. The union designates a representative who speaks for the group of nurses who have delegated that responsibility. In this kind of structure, the nurse speaks to management through the union representative. For more information, *see* Chapter 18.

Nursing departments and facilities choose to reward people in a variety of ways. For example, some units have a clinical ladder that rewards clinical expertise or professional accomplishments. Other organizations do not reward individual differences with merit pay but instead provide monetary rewards on the basis of the union contract or across-the-board "cost-of-living" raises. A trend that is gaining popularity is to reward team performance rather than individual performance. Organizations also reward informally by various recognition programs and celebrations. Depending on your needs, you will fit with one reward structure better than another. Consider the "perks" and benefits that motivate you; are these available in the organization that you are considering? (*See* Critical Thinking Boxes 12-5 and 12-6.)

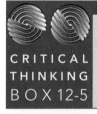

CRITICAL THINKING BOX 12-5

What are the values that drive your behavior? Do these values correlate with the values that drive an organization?

CRITICAL THINKING BOX 12-6

THINK ABOUT...

My mission statement: At the end of my life when I look back and say I have been happy and successful in my career, I will have accomplished the following mission:

_____

_____

_____

PATTERNS OF NURSING CARE DELIVERY

HOW IS THE DELIVERY OF NURSING CARE ORGANIZED IN AN INSTITUTION?

Over the years, the delivery of nursing care has been done in many ways (Fig. 12-4). While you were in school, you probably studied one or more methods of care delivery. You may have learned that various nursing care delivery systems are distinct from one another. In the real world, you seldom find pure forms of these systems. Consequently, you must be prepared to work in systems that may be a combination of those you learned about in school. One system is not better or worse than another. Various systems are tailor-made to meet the individual needs of the people in the organization and the types of patients served.

Originally nursing was organized around the private duty model. Registered nurses (RNs) were hired by the patient and provided nursing to one person. Student nurses staffed the hospital. RNs worked as special duty nurses or in the community doing home care.

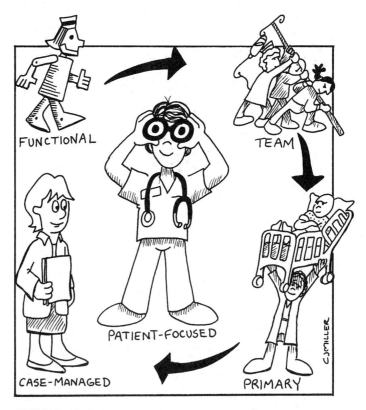

FIGURE 12-4
Evolving patterns of nursing care delivery.

The movement to use RNs as employees of hospitals came with the outbreak of World War II. Because nurses were required to work in hospitals, the terrific shortage of nurses during the war effort forced organizations to develop alternative models of nursing. The positions of aides and vocational nurses/licensed practical nurses came into being, and in some states they were allowed to perform functions such as administration of medication and treatments. This functional kind of nursing, which broke nursing care into a series of tasks performed by many people, resulted in a fragmented, impersonal kind of care (Fig. 12-5).

In the 1950s team nursing evolved. In this type of nursing, groups of patients are assigned to a team headed by a team leader, usually an RN, who coordinates the care for a designated group of patients (Fig. 12-6). The team leader determines work assignments for the team on the basis of the acuity level of the group of patients and the ability of individual team members. A team may be composed of the following:

- An RN who is team leader
- Two licensed vocational nurses/licensed practical nurses assigned to patient care
- Two nursing assistants or patient care aides

Good communication is essential between the team members and the team leader. The team conference is a vital part of this approach. The purpose of the conference is to assess the needs of the group of patients and to develop or revise their individual plans of care. It is imperative that the team leader continuously evaluates and

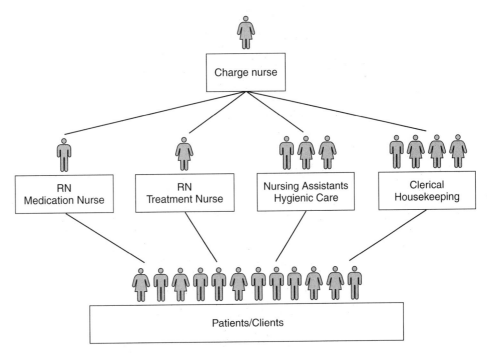

FIGURE 12-5
Lines of authority: functional nursing.

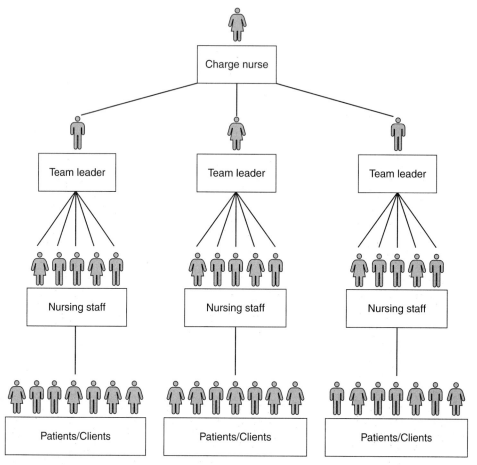

FIGURE 12-6
Lines of authority: team nursing.

communicates changes in a patient's plan of care to team members. This role often requires the RN to be available throughout the shift, thus limiting his or her delivery of bedside care. Even though team nursing evolved in the 1950s, there are components of it that remain in delivery systems today.

In the 1960s and 1970s primary nursing evolved. In this system, a nurse plans and directs the care of a patient over a 24-hour period. The fragmentation between shifts and nurses is eliminated because one nurse is accountable for planning the care of the patient around the clock. Progress reports, referrals, and discharge planning are usually the responsibility of the primary nurse. When the primary nurse is off duty, an associate nurse continues the plan of care. An RN may be the primary nurse to some of the assigned patients and an associate nurse to others. Some forms of primary nursing evolved into an all-RN staff (Fig. 12-7). Currently we find primary nursing being mixed and modified with nurse extenders such as paired partners, or partners in care, who are trained care assistants, working in a synergistic manner with the RN. Although team nursing took the RN away from bedside care, primary and modified primary care have put the nurse back in close contact with the patient.

WHAT IS PATIENT-FOCUSED CARE?

Patient-focused care is another delivery system that has evolved over the last decade. In the past traditional nursing services, such as phlebotomy and diet instruction, have been given to members of departments that do not report to nursing. These ancillary workers spend a great deal of time in transit from one unit to another. Time would also be lost when there was no work for this single-function member to do. The trend now is to centralize these functions on the unit under the direction of the RN and to cross-train ancillary workers to perform more than one function, thus increasing their levels of productivity. The patient comes into contact with fewer people under this organizational framework. Those who work directly with the patient are unit-based, and they are cross-trained in more than one function. They know the patient very well because they spend more time in direct care than in transit. An RN who is familiar with the plan of care supervises them. This model also moves the RN to a higher level of function because the RN is now accountable for a fuller range of services to the patient. Tasks that do not require an RN are delegated to the ancillary worker under the supervision of the RN.

WHAT IS CASE MANAGMENT?

In today's health care environment, case management is one of the strategies suggested to ensure the coordination of care while reducing costs. Although case

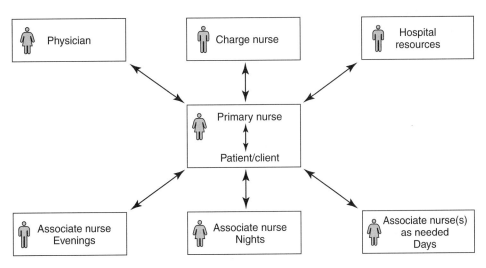

FIGURE 12-7
Lines of authority: primary-care nursing.

management in acute-care hospitals is relatively new, it has been used for many years in long-term or community-based care as a way to make sure that health care services were coordinated (Fig. 12-8).

According to the Case Management Society of America, case management is a collaborative process that assesses, plans, implements, coordinates, monitors, and evaluates options and services to meet a person's health needs. The case manager uses communication and available resources to promote quality, cost-effective care (http://www.cmsa.org). Case management, like the nursing process, is based on steps, which are circular. Table 12-1 outlines the components of the case-management process.

Case managers work in all types of health care organizations (acute-care, subacute-care, rehabilitation, psychiatric/substance abuse, and a variety of community service agencies). In addition, they may work for insurance or utilization management companies or in employee health in large businesses. Registered nurses, social workers, and therapists may all be case managers; although how they perform their role depends on the scope of practice of their discipline. All case managers must be skilled at communication, critical thinking, negotiation, and collaboration. They must be knowledgeable about resources available to patients. The case manager not only deals with the individual patient, but also with the family and other support systems of the patient (Sportsman and Hawley, 1998).

Case management is effective in providing care, but all patients do not need this intensity of interaction. To provide such care to all patients would be wastefully expensive. Patients should only be assigned a case manager if they:

- Have complicated health care needs.
- Are receiving care that is very expensive as well as complicated.
- Pose discharge-planning problems.

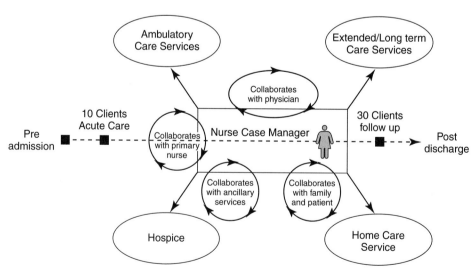

FIGURE 12-8
Case-management structure.

⊛ TABLE 12-1

Components of the Case-Management Process

Steps in the Process	*Definition*	*Activities to be Accomplished by Case Manager*
Assessment	Process of collecting pertinent information about a person's situation to identify needs and develop a plan.	■ Identify factors likely to affect treatment or recovery (e.g., age; identified chief complaint; other medical conditions; mental, social, psychosocial, or emotional problems; use of medications; financial status; lifestyle; occupational issues; support systems). ■ Determine what social and community resources are available to patient. ■ Determine patient's financial resources, including available insurance benefits. ■ Identify patient's/significant other's expectation and understanding of the problem.
Reassessment occurs periodically as new information becomes available or as changes occur.		■ Identify abnormal coping patterns, unusual family dynamics, or potential barriers to recovery. ■ Gather information regarding abnormalities from multiple sources (e.g., patient record, other providers, patient, significant other). ■ Organize and classify data collected, identifying patterns to determine what is pertinent.
Planning	Process of setting goals and objectives and determining actions necessary to meet them. The plan must be time-specific, and steps to the plan should include the sequence, duration, and frequency of the actions. Care maps, critical paths, and/or disease-management protocols may be used to develop the plan.	■ Develop goals, objectives, and actions in collaboration with other caregivers, the patient, significant other, insurance companies, or employers and other interested parties. ■ Determine the costs and benefits of available resources. If patients need treatment for which they have no coverage, look for alternative sources of care.
Implement	Process through which the agreed-on plan is enacted.	■ Refer patient/significant other to services. ■ Help patient to self-refer. ■ Educate patient regarding options.

(continued)

≋TABLE 12-1

Components of the Case-Management Process *(Cont'd)*

Steps in the Process	Definition	Activities to be Accomplished by Case Manager
Coordinate and monitor	Process by which the resources are secured and integrated to accomplish the goals/objectives of the plan. Case manager is responsible for smooth implementation of care. Care maps, critical pathways, and disease-management protocols and checklists may be used to document this process.	▪ Communicate the results of referrals and treatment to other caregivers. ▪ Monitor issues that affect the patient's recovery or integration back into the community (home support, physical and environmental barriers, occupation, educational level, and so forth). ▪ Maintain communication with insurance plans or others paying for services. ▪ Follow-up with patient and others periodically throughout episode of care. ▪ Evaluate possible barriers to care or patient compliance (lack of understanding, lack of transportation, family support, scheduling conflicts, and so forth).
Evaluation	Process of measuring quality and outcomes of products and services to determine whether the activities have produced the desired effect. Evaluation data may also be used to modify existing programs, plan new ones, or develop clinical benchmarks.	▪ Evaluate the frequency and the duration of treatment for appropriateness. ▪ Compare actual outcomes with expected ones. If goals/objectives have not been reached, determine why not. ▪ Revise the plan on the basis of feedback gathered from the evaluation.

(Modified from Ling C: Why and what you should know about case management, *Health Week*, February 2, 1998)

   ▪ Receive care from multiple providers.
   ▪ Are likely to have significant physical or psychosocial problems (Sportsman and Hawley, 1998).

WHAT TOOLS ARE USED TO SUPPORT CASE MANAGEMENT?

Clinical pathways and disease-management protocols are similar strategies that support the work of the case manager and help to reduce expensive variations in care. Clinical pathways, which are also known as *care maps or collaborative plans of care*, are interdisciplinary plans of care that outline the optimal sequencing and timing of interventions for patients with a particular diagnosis, procedure, or symptom (Ignatavicius and Hausman, 1995, p. 10). The terminology usually associated with clinical pathways includes the following:

- *Patient outcomes*—a list of outcomes expected by the time of the discharge from the health care setting
- *Timelines*—the specific timing for the sequence of health care interventions
- *Collaboration*—joint effort by multiple health care professionals
- *Comprehensive aspect of care*—a component that tracks the primary health care intervention, such as diagnostics, treatments, or medications (Ignatavicius and Hausman, 1995, p. 10)

Table 12-2 is a scheme of a clinical pathway that takes into account the number of days allocated by the patient's diagnosis, in addition to information for teaching and discharge.

Disease management, also called *population-based care* or *continuous health care improvement*, is an integrated system of interventions, measurements, and refinements of health care delivery designed to optimize clinical and economic outcomes within a specific population (Gurnee and Da Silva, 1997). Managed-care organizations often enroll members who have a specific disease in a program tailored for the needs of patients with that condition. The programs focus on prevention and educational activities when members are NOT in the acute stage of the disease so that they will be prepared to understand and manage symptoms throughout their lives. Nurses, often employed by health plans, are frequently involved in this component of disease management. Disease-management protocols also outline standard interventions to be implemented during the acute stage of the illness, although physicians or other providers may make modifications to provide individualized care. Disease-management programs are primarily for patients with chronic diseases that occur frequently, those that vary widely in treatment options, and those that are very expensive to treat. The disease must also respond well to preventive or self-care interventions (Finkelman, 2000, pp. 171-173).

Both critical pathways and disease-management protocols are generally based on clinical guidelines, which incorporate nationally acceptable ways to care for a specific disease. These guidelines are typically developed by government agencies, such as the Agency for Healthcare Research and Quality, professional organizations such as the American Medical Association, or an organization devoted to a specific disease, such as the American Heart Association.

HOW ARE NURSING WORK ASSIGNMENTS DETERMINED?

How your work assignment is determined will vary with individual institutions. A real problem for a health care institution is the fact that patient acuity fluctuates dramatically from day to day and from season to season. For example, over the Christmas holidays there is often a significant decrease in the number of elective surgeries. In response, some hospitals may close units. By contrast, in the middle of the influenza season, the hospital might be full and understaffed. The amount of staff assigned must reflect the needs of patients. When there are more and sicker patients, more staff is needed. When patients are not as acutely ill or there are fewer of them, or both, less staff is required.

Nursing has tried a variety of approaches to anticipate the number and qualifications of nurses that will be needed for a specific period of time for a specific

TABLE 12-2

Clinical Pathway Major Chest Procedures—4-Day Recovery

Time Frame Location / Date/Unit	1 TCI → OR → CVICU → RNF		2 POD #1		3 POD #2		4 POD #3		Discharge POD #4	
	Date	Unit	Date	Unit	Date	Unit	Date	Unit	Date	Unit
Patient Satisfaction	What can we do to enhance your stay with us?		What can we do to enhance your stay with us?		What can we do to enhance your stay with us?		What can we do to enhance your stay with us?		What can we do to enhance your stay with us?	
Discharge Planning	Patient verbalizes expected LOS and postop activity. PERS initiated. Patient's primary support person identified.		Verbalizes understanding of progress. Patient's needs indentified and notify as needed for D/C.		Verbalizes understanding of progress. Patient's needs identified and notify as needed for D/C.		Verify all medications, supplies, services are arranged for discharge.		Discharge instructions given to patient.	
Patient Education	Instruct family to go to surgical waiting room. Orient patient during emergence from anesthesia.		Reinforce IS, C & DB exercises, pain management, and ambulation. Provide patient/family with info R/T discharge needs.		Provide patient/family with information R/T discharge needs/procedures and progress.		Provide patient/family with information R/T discharge needs/procedures and progress.		Discharge instructions R/T medications, activity, diet, treatments, and incisional care.	
Tests/Procedures/Consults	CXR, CBC, KP6; ABGs, BPH/Ventolin q6°; respiratory therapy; pain management; CHIRP.		CXR, oximetry. Radiation oncology prn. Hemo/oncology prn. Home health care prn.		CXR, oximetry. Respiratory therapy.		Oximetry. Pulmonary rehab prn.			
Allied Health Interventions			Respiratory Tx per respiratory consult algorithm.		Respiratory Tx per respiratory consult algorithm.					
Nursing/Medical	Monitor rhythm; VS routine; I & O; wt		Telemetry; I & O; wt qd; VS routine; IS		D/C telemetry; D/C I & O; wt qd; VS		Wt qd; VS routine; IS 10×/hr		VS routine; IS 10×/hr w.a.	

(continued)

TABLE 12-2

Clinical Pathway Major Chest Procedures—4-Day Recovery (Cont'd)

Time Frame Location	1 TCI → OR → CVICU → RNF		2 POD #1		3 POD #2		4 POD #3		Discharge POD #4	
Date/Unit	Date	Unit	Date	Unit	Date	Unit	Date	Unit	Date	Unit
Interventions		qd; O₂ N/C; Chest tubes to suction; Foley; wean from vent.		10×/hr w.a.; C & DB; D/C 1 CT; epidural pain control, D/C Foley.		routine, IS 10×/hr; C & DB; epidural pain control (to be D/C when last CT out); D/C CT; wean O₂ to room air; remove incisional dressings and begin wound care.		pain control with PO.		
Mobility		BR; turn q2°, HOB↑ 30°; up in chair after extub.		OOB with assistance and chair 1 qs.		Chair qs and ambulate hall TID.		UAL.		UAL.
Nutrition		NPO; ice chips; clear liquids D5 1/2NS + 20 KCl.		Clear liquids → full liquid diet; IV to HL if tolerating liquids.		Advance diet as tolerated.		Preop diet.		Preop diet.
Outcomes Criteria		Admission assessment completed. Anesthesia consult documented. Patient assessment completed and WNL. Patient premedicated. Patient/family satisfaction addressed.		Patient with adequate oxygenation per pulse oximentry; hemodynamocally stable; alert and oriented ×3. Adequate pain control. Patient/family satisfaction addressed.		Tolerate diet. Has BM normal for patient. Comfort level maintained. Ambulate W/O SOB. Patient/family satisfaction addressed.		Tolerate diet. Has BM normal for patient. Comfort level maintained. Ambulate W/O SOB. Breath sounds and secretions clear. Patient/family satisfaction addressed.		Breath sounds and secretions clear. Ambulates independently W/O SOB. Infection free. Patient/family satisfaction addressed.

From Phipps, Sands, Marek (1999), Med-Sung, Nursing, Mosby.

4/1/97 (1:\cct\thoracic\75a-fdr) Thoracic FDR—4 Day Recovery, Courtesy The Cleveland Clinic Foundation, 1997. This is a general guideline to *assist* in the management of patients. This guideline is not designated to replace clinical judgement or individual patient needs.

CXR, Chest x-ray; *HOB*, head of bed; *IS*, incentive spirometry; *qs*, quantity sufficient; *CHIRP*, rehab program; *OOB*, out of bed; *D/C* discharge; *CT*, chest tube; *C & DB*, cough and deep breathe; *R/T*, routine; *UAL*, up ad lib; *W/O*, without, *SOB*, short of breath; *WA*, when awake; *HL*, heparin lock.

group of patients. In fact, regulatory agencies such as the Joint Commission for the Accreditation of Healthcare Organizations require that staffing be based on some sort of organized system. A *patient classification* or *acuity system* is used in many acute-care hospitals to estimate the intensity of nursing care required to meet patient needs. In addition, staffing in organizations may be based on budgeted *hours per patient per day*. Hours per patient per day are calculated by the number of patient care staff working during a 24-hour period and divided by the number of patients served in a day. However, the most accurate way of determining optimal staffing is through the judgment of a good experienced nurse who is knowledgeable about quality and fiscal management.

In 1998 the American Nurses Association identified principles of staffing to help nurses ensure adequate staffing in all situations. These nine principles are divided into three categories: (1) patient care–related, (2) staff-related, and (3) institution/organization–related. In the area of patient care–related, appropriate staffing levels must reflect both individual patient needs and the needs of the group receiving care. The American Nurses Association notes that the concept of hours per patient per day should be questioned because one formula will not fit all situations. Instead they suggest that the number of patients, the intensity of their need, the expertise of the caregivers, and the environment in which care is given must all be considered when determining staffing patterns (http://www.nursingworld.org/readroom/stffprnc.htm).

WHAT ABOUT SCHEDULING PATTERNS?

Nursing has also always been concerned about staff scheduling practices and options. That's why there are numerous scheduling patterns other than the typical 8-hour shift 5 days a week. From working 10-hour days 4 days a week to the weekend alternative (known as the *Baylor plan*) of two 12-hour weekend shifts for 36 hours of pay, nurses have tried numerous patterns and combinations of shifts. Despite the best scheduling patterns and innovative approaches, staffing crises *always* occur—family emergencies, sick calls, and so on. Regardless of the staffing pattern, if you are in charge, someone has to cover the shift. *See* Critical Thinking Box 12-7 for suggestions on dealing with the problem.

Another aspect of scheduling is the impact it has on how nurses are paid. Some nurses have gone so far in their quest for professional stature that they work under a salary model rather than an hourly model. It is difficult to be classified as a professional and work under the hourly wage system. In some organizations, the entire nursing department or separate units have converted to an all-salary model. The advantage of this model is that the nurse receives a given salary regardless of the number of patients and amount of care given. When there are more patients, they work harder but do not receive overtime pay. When there are fewer patients, they work less but do not experience a loss of income because they are not sent home without pay or forced to take vacation time. In a salary model, which is really a professional model, the nurse works until the job gets done. Some days this might take 4 hours, some days it might take 12 hours. Over a period of months, the nurses track their overtime and develop a fair, equitable system of sharing the overtime and also the time off when there are too few patients. In reality, many other positions in

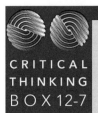

CRITICAL THINKING BOX 12-7

THINK ABOUT ...

How Do You Handle a Staffing Crisis?

❏ Assess unit census, acuity, and patient classification systems—can you safely do without the absent nurse?

❏ Does your organization have a float pool within the staff, or are agency or outside staff available?

❏ Check on your part-time staff to work an extra shift.

❏ Will another staff member cover the extra shift for a day off later in the schedule?

❏ Can you do with partial shift coverage during the "peak" shift hours? *Example: Have a night shift nurse stay over for the first 4 hours of the day shift.*

❏ Ask a staff member to work a double shift—either stay late, or come in early.

❏ Work it yourself. (It may initially solve the problem but leave the rest of your job undone.)

Can you think of some other alternatives?

the hospital are paid this way. Traditionally, billing clerks and admitting clerks are paid a set salary and are not sent home when the census fluctuates. Other professionals such as social workers and pharmacists are paid on a salary model.

In these models, the nursing staff members work among themselves to determine the work schedule. Obviously, to go to a salary model, working relationships on a unit must be very good.

WHAT ABOUT QUALITY PATIENT CARE?

Over time, the way we have looked at quality in nursing has changed. Much of what has been done to control quality has been directed by the accreditation bodies, such as the Joint Commission on the Accreditation of Healthcare Organizations, and by professional practice standards. When we examined the quality of care, it was done retrospectively to first examine the care provided and then to determine whether we did, or did not, do a good job. The problem with that approach is that many mistakes happen along the way that are not caught until well after the fact. We have also tried to improve quality by looking at problems and identifying the area that would benefit most from change.

Now the watchword in health care is *continuous quality improvement*. This approach emphasizes continually looking for opportunities to improve. Even if we think we are doing a good job, we are relentless in our pursuit to do even better. We look not only at what the nurse does in the pursuit of quality, but also at how the systems of the unit in the hospital can be improved to provide better care at lower cost.

The responsibility for the delivery of quality care was previously vested in the quality assurance department of a hospital. Now it rests with the individual nurse providing direct patient care. As nursing has become more of an autonomous profession, the accountability for quality care has been shifted to the individual practitioner. Therefore a big part of your practice will be to do a better job than you did yesterday. The organization of quality monitoring may also now be at the unit level. People who work in various units are responsible for validating quality care, with each unit determining how to measure the quality of care in its own way.

Quality is also measured against the standards of those who receive the care. It does us no good to provide our own idea of excellent nursing care if it does not meet the expectations of our patients, their families, and the people who pay for the care. Therefore the perception of quality as measured by patients, physicians, other departments, and other professionals is becoming much more important. Patients expect certain things from their visit. If we do not know what their expectations are and do not meet their standards, they perceive that we deliver poor-quality care. In addition to providing excellence in terms of professional nursing care, you will also be charged with the responsibility of delivering care that meets the expectations of all the patients.

Currently there are systemwide concerns about the quality of health care in the United States. In response to concerns about strategies that reduce cost without considering the impact on the quality of care, there has recently been an increased national emphasis on quality of care and patient safety. The Institute of Medicine recently released two reports critical of the quality of care in the United States. The first, "To err is human," was released in 1999, and the second, "Crossing the quality chasm," was released in 2000. In 2001 the Agency for Healthcare Quality and Research released an analysis of whether specific patient safety practices are effective. Other governmental agencies and watchdog groups have also done similar projects. In addition, the U.S. Congress and various state legislatures have passed or are currently considering patient safety regulations. The issue of patient safety and quality at the national level will ultimately affect the way you practice in any clinical setting.

HOW CAN NURSES DECREASE THE COST OF HEALTH CARE?

Of course we cannot talk about delivering nursing care without also considering how much it costs. Today nurses are being challenged to provide excellent care with fewer dollars than in the past. To do so, we must take on increased responsibility for the cost of health care. There is no single entity to blame for the rising cost of health care. We cannot blame the cost on hospitals, insurance companies, or physicians alone. However, health care professionals can make choices that dictate how much or how little society will pay for their services. Nurses can help to reduce these costs by becoming more knowledgeable about the cost of the equipment (intravenous tubing, syringes, incontinence pads, and so forth) that they use. Our choice of supplies can have an effect on whether the cost of care will be exorbitant or minimal. Nurses can also help reduce costs by developing and carrying out programs in preventive health care. Educating health care consumers, whether at their bedsides or in community settings, is another way to reduce costs.

Such interventions will lead to less medication consumption preoperatively and postoperatively and fewer hospital admissions for patients who understand and manage their illnesses. Controlling the cost of nursing care will be a big part of your practice and will be grounds for much discussion.

CONCLUSION

New models of health care delivery are being developed in which we look at the desired outcome and manage backwards to achieve it with the shortest length of stay and the lowest level of expenses. Many payers, through HMOs and other models, are developing new ways of paying for health care. It is common for payers to pay a certain amount (e.g., Medicare) regardless of the course of the patient's illness. Prospective payments provide us with the same number of dollars no matter how quickly the patients leave the hospital or how much longer they have to stay because of complications. This is certainly a trend that will continue. We will be challenged to develop more innovative and creative ways of attaining excellence in patient care with limited dollars. We can do that. Nurses have always been very cost-conscious. We are now being provided with more opportunities to meet that challenge.

REFERENCES

Finkelman AW: *Managed care: a nursing perspective*, ed 1, Upper Saddle River, NJ, 2000, Prentice Hall.

Gurnee MC, Da Silva RV: Constructing disease management programs, *Manag Care* 6(6):67-70, 75-76, 1997.

Ignatavicius DD, Hausman KA: *Clinical pathways for collaborative practice*, Philadelphia, 1995, WB Saunders.

Ling C: Why and what you should know about case management, *Health Week* February 2, 1998.

Agency for Healthcare Research and Quality: *Making health care safer: a critical analysis of patient safety practices* [summary], Publication No. 01-E057, Rockville, Md, AHRQ.

Sportsman S, Hawley L: *Case management in a managed care environment* [Web-based course offered by University On-Line/Health Exec Inc.], January 1998.

Sullivan EJ, Decker PJ, Jamerson P: *Effective leadership and management in nursing*, ed 5, Philadelphia, 2000, Prentice Hall.

ADDITIONAL READINGS

Bennett R: Is managed care in your future? *Nurs Homes Long Term Care Manage* 48(8):28-31. 1999.

Broadwell M: *The new supervisor: how to thrive in your first year as a manager*, ed 5, New York, 1998, Perseus.

O'Brien LJ: *Bad medicine: how the American medical establishment is ruining our healthcare system*, New York, 1999, Prometheus.

INTERNET RESOURCES

Agency for Healthcare Research and Quality
http://www.ahrq.gov

American Nurses Association
http://www.nursingworld.org

Case Management Society of America
http://www.cmsa.org

Citizens' Council on Health Care
http://www.cchc-mn.org
A resource for designing the future of health care.

Duke University Center for Health Policy, Law and Management

Duke Health Policy Cyberexchange Home Page
http://www.hpolicy.duke.edu/cyberexchange

Healthcare Internet Services
http://www.healthcareinternet.com
Provides consulting services to health care organizations in the areas of Web site development, design, and marketing. Sites are user-friendly with point-and-click update capabilities. This site also provides links to more than 500 health care–related sites.

Health Reform Online Home
http://www.worldbank.org/healthreform
The World Bank's comprehensive online resource center on health sector reform efforts around the world.

Healthy People 2010
http://www.health.gov/healthypeople

Institute of Medicine Reports

To err is human: building a safer health system (1999)
http://www.nap.edu/books/0309068371/html/

Crossing the quality chasm: a new health system for the 21st century (2001)
http://www.nap.edu/books/0309072808/html/

Online home of *Managed Care* magazine
http://managedcaremag.com

National Academy for State Health Policy (NASHP)
http://www.nashp.org
Nonprofit. Nonpartisan. Public policy think tank addressing pressing health care policy issues of concern to state governments.

Sigma Theta Tau International Honor Society for Nurses
http://www.nursingsociety.org

Joint Commission on Accreditation of Healthcare Organizations
http://www.jcaho.org

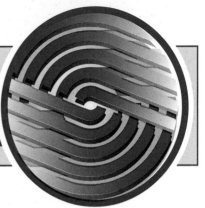

CHAPTER THIRTEEN

Health in Community: Nursing's Role

ISELA LUNA, PhD, RN, CLNC

Today it is fashionable to talk about the poor. Unfortunately, it is not fashionable to talk with them.

—Mother Teresa

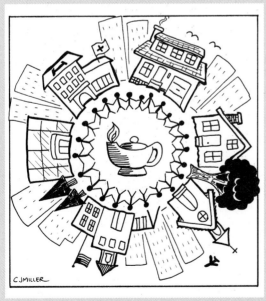

Nursing is a vital part of community health.

After completing this chapter, you should be able to:

■ Identify essential players in community health and nursing.

■ Differentiate between community-based and community development practices.

■ Identify concepts in community that are related to improving health care access.

■ Identify concepts in developing community partnerships.

■ Identify strategies in community health that are useful in influencing policy.

A ccess to health care in America is a right, not a privilege. As our world becomes increasingly complex with different information inputs, we seem to lose sight of our most fundamental values. Many believe that improving access to health care can be one of many answers to closing the gap on the health disparities of the present American population. Many people, both laypersons and health professionals, also agree that the only way to cut health care costs and reform the U.S. health care system is to improve the overall health of the community. There is a belief that if the social health of the population improves, people will live healthier lives, access emergency care less often, and need less acute care, which is very expensive. However, not many organizations are willing to invest the time and money into creating a healthier community.

Those who invest in the health of communities wonder if it is really fair for some of us to pay for the not-so-healthy choices that others make. Whatever the case may be, improving the health of the community is an idea that is reaching the agendas of health care organizations, for-profit and nonprofit organizations, schools, government agencies, and industry because of the associated expenses of illness.

Increasing access, however, is a little more complicated than giving handouts to the poor and disenfranchised. Increasing access to health care cannot be the work of a single organization or government entity. It will be the result of a wide, organized, and planned community effort, that values, above all else, human rights and human relationships. This work may well be done within the framework of community health nursing. The twenty-first century is an exciting time to be a nurse. It provides the opportunity to bridge the gap between our modern technological advances and our social, moral, and ethical responsibilities. This chapter discusses how partnerships with competing agendas can make a difference.

COMMUNITY HEALTH AND NURSING

WHAT IS COMMUNITY HEALTH?

In the spirit of learning about community, let us examine the definitions of *community*, *community health*, and *community health nurses*. The roles of the community health nurse are varied and challenging and have often depended heavily on the prevailing health problems of the time. However, the foundational principles of community health nursing remain the same. In Florence Nightingale's book *Notes on nursing: what it is, and what it is not* (1964, reprinted), she stated that the task of nursing was to "put the constitution in such a state as that it will have no disease, or that it can recover from disease." Nightingale outlined the following five essential points in securing the health of households and in promoting health: (1) pure air, (2) pure water, (3) efficient drainage, (4) cleanliness, and (5) light. She also identified proper nutrition, rest, sanitation, and hygiene as necessary for health. Today, community health nurses continue to focus on the role of health promotion, disease prevention, and environment as they deliver care.

The early nineteenth-century role of the community health nurse focused on environmental conditions such as sanitation, the control of communicable diseases, education in personal hygiene, and the care of sick persons in their homes. In the nineteenth century in the United States, the role of the community health nurse consisted of visiting nurses and settlement houses. Settlement houses were community-based houses where nurses lived among the "poor" people, with the philosophy that the most effective way to help people improve their health was for educated people such as nurses to live among them and teach by example (Kalisch and Kalisch, 1986). The first nurses to visit homes were in New York. In 1893 Lillian Wald organized a Visiting Nursing Service for the poor population of New York.

During the middle of the nineteenth century, the nation's attention focused on attacking community health problems and improving urban living conditions. The American Public Health Association began in 1872 and focused on interdisciplinary efforts, published a variety of health promotion and illness prevention materials, and lobbied for improved public health (Picket and Hanlon, 1990). Local health departments were established in cities at this time and targeted the elimination of environmental hazards associated with poor living conditions, crowding, and the close proximity of slaughterhouses to homes. In the twentieth century, community health nursing in the United States continued to evolve and adapt to meet the health care needs of a nation facing two major world wars and major economic depression. The 1960s witnessed a revolution in health care that affected community health and community health nursing. In 1964, the passage of the Economic Opportunity Act provided funds for neighborhood health centers, Head Start, and many other community action programs. Funding was also increased for maternal and child health, mental health and mental retardation, and community health training. In the latter part of the 1980s, *Healthy People 2010: a systematic approach to health improvement* was published to influence public health. The 1990s were a decade of debate about health care. The central issues have involved cost, quality, and access. The focus on cost suggests that many strategies are needed to reform medical care, not health care. The outburst of health maintenance organizations and other organized health care options have brought about an interest in maintaining the health of populations because these insurance groups often pay providers by population, not by fee-for-service of a single individual.

As the new millennium continues, the focus of the community health nurse centers around health promotion, disease prevention, and prevention of debilitating symptoms generated from chronic diseases. *Healthy People 2010* (*see* Boxes 13-1, 13-2, and 13-3) is about improving health—the health of each individual, the health of communities and the health of the nation. However, the goals and objectives of *Healthy People 2010* cannot by themselves improve the health status of the nation. Instead they need to be recognized as part of a larger approach to health improvement. Over the years, community health nursing has evolved from a home care service delivered by pioneers and philanthropists such as Lillian Wald to a broader-based population-focused discipline that considers individuals, families, groups, and communities as its scope of practice.

Population-based care has surfaced once more as a potential solution to the tremendous costs of the health care industry and in the hopes that individual citizens

BOX 13-1 *Healthy People 2010:* **A Systematic Approach to Health Improvement.**

The systematic approach to health improvement is composed of four essential elements:

❑ Goals
❑ Objectives
❑ Determinants of health
❑ Health status

Two overarching goals:

Goal 1: Increase quality and years of healthy life.
Goal 2: Eliminate health disparities.

The nation's progress in achieving the two goals of *Healthy People 2010* will be monitored through 467 objectives in 28 focus areas.

BOX 13-2 *Healthy People 2010*: **Top 10 of 28 Objectives for Improving Health**

1. Access to quality health services
2. Arthritis, osteoporosis, and chronic back conditions
3. Cancer
4. Chronic kidney disease
5. Diabetes
6. Disability and secondary conditions
7. Education and community-based programs
8. Environmental health
9. Family planning
10. Food safety

BOX 13-3 *Healthy People 2010:* **Determinants of Health**

Topics covered by the objectives in *Healthy People 2010* reflect the array of critical influences that determine the health of individuals and communities such as individual biology, behavioral influence on health, and the social-physical environment of the individual. Developing and implementing policies and preventive interventions that effectively address these determinants of health can reduce the burden of illness, enhance quality of life, and increase longevity.

Leading health indicators

Physical activity

(continued)

BOX 13-3 *Healthy People 2010:* Determinants of Health *(Cont'd)*

Overweight and obesity

Tobacco use

Substance abuse

Responsible sexual behavior

Mental health

Injury and violence

Environmental quality

Immunization

Access to health care

http://www.health.gov/healthypeople/

take an active role in their own health. *Empowerment*, both individual- and community-based, is a term often used in this conversation. The strategies proposed to improve the health of populations are many.

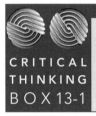

CRITICAL THINKING BOX 13-1

What are the activities in your community that improve the "community health?"

COMMUNITY-BASED APPROACH VS. COMMUNITY DEVELOPMENT APPROACH

Chavis and Florin (1990), in their work on community development in drug abuse prevention in San Jose, Calif, point out that community-based and community development approaches are opposite ends of a continuum. Elements of each can exist in programs, but the nursing focus is on empowering the community, organizations, and individuals within them. The community-development approach is the most effective.

WHAT IS THE COMMUNITY-BASED APPROACH?

The community-based approach focuses on solving problems by addressing deficits and, as such, tends to be oriented toward fixing existing weaknesses. This approach is very commonly seen in our health care system. Often politicians supported by health care organizations and professional lobbyists attempt to begin to solve community issues by doing what we call a *needs assessment*. By definition, this approach focuses on the weaknesses of those involved. Because a program may be physically located in the community, the tendency is to call it a "community program." Welfare assistance programs and other "community aid" programs instituted through public policies are common examples of programs based on need. Usually there is an application process and an identified need, which is usually financial, and that will guarantee inclusion in the program. An increase in need will most likely lead to more assistance, usually until the funding runs out or the state or federal budget is cut. In the meantime, there is no incentive for a "needy" individual or family to strengthen their situation. These services are usually located in local neighborhoods in cities throughout the country; there might even be one near your own home. Although initially these programs were designed to be of short-term assistance, they have turned into a big problem. The root of the issue is that there is money in serving the "poor." Politicians look good by serving the poor, cities get additional funding on the basis of how many poor they have, county and state health departments receive additional moneys to serve the poor, health professionals are employed to serve the poor, and so forth. The services provided for the "poor" are not usually community-based. If you were to explore the centers and clinics where services for the "poor" are rendered, you would find that the individuals that these health centers aim to serve are often not integrated into the neighborhood. The programs developed in this approach are most likely generated by health professionals and mandated by government agencies or entities not directly involved with the issues of the community.

WHAT IS THE COMMUNITY DEVELOPMENT APPROACH?

The community development approach allows individuals or organizations to identify their own strategies and issues by the building of coalitions and the assessment of the competencies and strengths of communities. This builds the capacity of the community. The essential decision-makers in this approach are community leaders identified by the community itself. This is empowerment. Empowerment in its simplest form is defined by Meredith Minkler (1989) as "the process by which individuals and communities gain mastery over their lives" (p. 17). To build the capacity of a community, let's consider an example of how an organization can build partnerships within an organization.

> In Tucson, Arizona, there is a group of interested organizations that came together to form what is called the Tucson KidsCare Coalition. As an initial step, two leading organizations working on increasing access to health care for children gathered with the idea that if organizations came together in their efforts, resources could be maximized and reaching efforts would be more effective. What was known from the beginning was that children's access to health care in the United States has consistently grown worse in the past decade (Box 13-4). In Arizona, more than one of every six children is uninsured, placing this state as the fourth worst in providing health care coverage for children. Millions more Americans and Arizonans are expected to join the ranks of those who are

uninsured. The recent recession-driven layoffs will further increase those numbers, making a serious problem even worse. It was this series of gloomy statistics that led this community to look at its strengths. We began to do an assessment of which organizations did what best. We found that although some organizations were excellent at outreach, they lacked much information on following up cases and documentation. We also found that many of the organizations had been to the same communities, replicating efforts with few results. Other organizations such as El Rio Community Health Center had unique relationships with the state system that allowed them to find services for those with urgent or unique circumstances. Therefore, we brought our efforts together through a series of conversations and a process of partnership-building. This process allowed each organization to see the others not as competing entities, but as collaborative members of a community engaged in building the capacity of organizations and the members they serve. The result was a strengthening of an already strong community.

BOX 13-4   Children's Access to Health Care

❏ Almost 11 million children in America are without health insurance.
❏ Approximately 280,000 children in Arizona are uninsured.
❏ Ninety percent of Arizona's uninsured children live with an employed main wage earner.
❏ State outreach efforts have failed to enroll the targeted number of children.

HOW DO YOU BUILD COMMUNITY CAPACITY?

This process of identifying the assets of a community or organization is called *asset mapping*. McKnight (1995) proposed that, from the identification of those strengths, we can influence a community identity of health and well-being, not illness, and hope that as a community we are better because we actually are and not because others tell us so. The work of building the strengths of the community is unlike the concrete tasks associated with providing traditional health care. When a community health nurse is involved in an immunization clinic, for example, there are certain concrete steps one must take to provide the immunizations. At the end of the clinic, everyone knows that there were a certain number of children who were vaccinated, a certain number of vaccines were given, and the process of administration was clear and concrete.

Building community capacity is a little more complex. There are some general guidelines that can be followed, but because of the nature of humanity and community life, the process is often a series of steps whereby the community alternately comes together and pulls apart. Only if certain processes are ensured can capacity be built.

HOW DO YOU PERFORM A COMMUNITY ASSESSMENT?

There are many ways of performing a community assessment. As mentioned earlier, a common way is to do a needs assessment. However, a needs assessment only provides half of the picture. A needs assessment will identify the deficiencies and weaknesses. If a community development approach is followed, the community assessment must include an evaluation of the assets of the community. As McKnight (1995) describes, looking at deficits is a valuable skill; however, as a "pervasive cultural value, it will inevitably blind communities to the capacities, assets, skills, and gifts that are essential to their power, wisdom, and health" (p. 76). So, although illnesses and needs are the essential components of growing medical systems, they are blinding for those interested in growing healthy communities.

WHAT IS GRASS ROOTS CAPACITY-BUILDING?

Building grass roots capacity is not very different from building capacity in professional settings. In a presentation to the American Academy of Nursing, Michaels and Luna (1998) list the following four principles of the development of community capacity:

1. *Entry ritual* is the response to a call for personal and community mission.
2. *Initiation ritual* is the personal disclosure in community settings such as a meeting or a gathering.
3. Expression is the active listening and sharing of diverse perspectives with face-to-face gatherings.
4. Consensus-building, honoring diversity, and personal mission allows us to come to decisions in face-to-face gatherings over time.

As defined by the community members, success in community means ownership of the process, more participation, an appreciation of diversity, and strengthened individual voices.

HOW DO WE BUILD A COALITION?

Let us begin by defining a coalition. A *coalition* as defined by Brown (1984) is an organization of different interest groups that combine their human and material resources to bring about a specific change that the members are unable to bring about independently. This definition contains two parts. First it notes that the coalition is made up of a group of diverse interest groups and second that the outcome of the coalition could not be produced by any one group independently. Coalitions by definition are not externally driven organizations but are rooted primarily in community. For coalitions to succeed, they must be deeply rooted in community and balanced with human service organizations.

It is within the work of the coalition that vision statements are created and implemented (Box 13-5). For this reason a continuous process of evaluation of the coalition operations and memberships must be carried out. Ongoing monitoring and evaluation of the coalition will produce the greatest results. The extent to which the activities of a coalition reflect empowerment outcomes is a critical differentiating point. Coalitions that claim to focus on empowerment but essentially provide services that support the status quo service-delivery model are not necessarily empowering coalitions.

BOX 13-5   Tucson KidsCare Coalition

Vision:

Through agency, neighborhood, and media collaboration, every child in Pima County will have health care coverage by the year 2003.

We will do that through the following different types of activities:

❏ Public education and outreach.

❏ Enrollment and follow-up of eligible children.

❏ Policy development.

Tucson KidsCare Coalition, 1999, Carondelet Health Network, Carondelet Community Trust.

The previous example of the Tucson KidsCare Coalition went through a series of changes when a private health network and a community health center came together. This coalition reflected the changes in the community and within the different member organizations. The vision continued as originally developed, and other strategies have changed with time. For example, the focus of enrollment strategies has changed from health fairs and communitywide activities to home visits by community lay health workers.

In enrolling thousands of children over the past 2 years, the members of the coalition have come to understand that it takes more than health insurance to keep a child healthy. It takes education, food, grandparents, parents, safe streets, and so forth to keep a child healthy. As the *Healthy People 2010* objectives indicate, healthy communities use a systematic approach to health improvement.

HOW DOES PUBLIC POLICY AFFECT THE HEALTH OF THE COMMUNITY?

We tend to explain many decisions affecting our health and quality of life in terms of "the system," and what "they" do to us, referring to government, politicians, financial institutions, corporations, religious leaders, and the media. Key concepts in public policy formation are tools that are used to understand and influence the health of the community. The Tucson KidsCare Coalition investigated and understood from the beginning that policies related to enrollment would have to be modified to make it feasible for individuals to enroll and stay enrolled in the KidsCare program. For purposes of completing the vision, the coalition determined that it would be to their advantage to get involved in politics.

First the organization defined within the coalition what was already being done. The Children's Action Alliance, a member of the coalition, had as its primary goal to provide advocacy for Arizona's children and families. The local state representative was invited to assist in educating the public and the coalition. This initial education session turned out to have very powerful effects for the coalition and fostered a strong relationship with state representatives. The coalition developed a list of three priority items that were important for policymakers to do; for example, change the policy that children who had been privately insured had to be without insurance for 6 months before they could enroll in the public assistance KidsCare program. This was successful. The coalition policymakers also wanted to release much-needed existing resources to be used for marketing and outreach; this action was also successful.

Following are some important questions to ask the group before becoming politically active:

- What is the national legislative agenda? Specifically, what do you want policymakers to do?
- Make a wish list of things that you would want policymakers in your area to do.
- Are you aiming to affect the upcoming elections? If not, have you endorsed a specific politician who supports your issues?
- Describe what you will give the policymakers in return for their support of your organization's mission.

A good place to begin is to learn how a bill becomes law. In the process you will find potential steps where you and your organization fit in. Finally as a spokesperson for your vision, it is important to learn how to articulate your interest and why it is important in a short but clear statement. Working with the media is an interesting way for nurses to get their message across. Letters to the editor and editorial boards and community bulletin boards are other means to send your message.

HOW DO YOU KNOW WHEN YOUR STRATEGIES HAVE BEEN SUCCESSFUL?

It is often said that communities measure their success through stories and health care systems through numbers and reports; perhaps a combination of both is particularly powerful. Stories often have a way of making numbers real, and numbers have a way of showing the strength of an issue. As part of the visioning exercise, together you should discuss and create the meaning of success for the coalition to achieve the best possible outcomes.

Nursing's unique role in improving health relies heavily on developing a systematic approach that is comprehensive and well planned. The role of community health nursing should reflect an in-depth knowledge of the community. This is assessed only by establishing relationships with leaders and members of the community. Establishing a coalition of true partnership is complex but possible. In our present times of conflicts and limited budgets, more and more organizations are looking to each other for support. Take advantage of this. To truly establish long-lasting change, you must get involved in the political process. Start with something as simple as finding out who your county supervisor is and what he or she does. Nurses can play a unique role in influencing government and its policies because of our engrained perspective of viewing our community and the world holistically.

REFERENCES

Chavis D, Florin P: *Community development, community participation*, San Jose, Calif, 1990, Prevention Office, Bureau of Drug Abuse Services.

Kalisch PA, Kalisch BJ: *The advance of American nursing*, ed 2, Boston, 1986, Little, Brown.

Lappe FM, Du Bois PM: *The quickening of America: rebuilding our nation, remaking our lives*, ed 1, San Francisco, 1994, Jossey-Bass.

Michaels C, Luna I: *Communities in action: shared principles guiding diverse efforts*, presented to the American Academy of Nursing 25th Convention, Acapulco, Mexico, 1998.

Minkler M: Health education, health promotion and the open society: an historical perspective, *Health Educ* Q 16(1):17-30, 1989.

Nightingale F: *Notes on nursing: what it is, and what it is not*, Philadelphia, 1964, JB Lippincott.

Picket G, Hanlon JJ: *Public health administration and practice*, ed 9, St Louis, 1990, Times/Mirror/Mosby College Publishing.

US Department of Health and Human Services: *Healthy People 2010: a systematic approach to health improvement*, US Department of Health and Human Services.

ADDITIONAL READINGS

Alinsky SD: *Rules for radicals: a practical primer for realistic radicals*, New York, 1971, Basic Books.

Brown C: *The art of coalition building*, New York, 1984, American Jewish Committee.

Jamieson M: *Grass roots efforts: nurses involved in political process, nurse case management in the 21st century*, St Louis, 1996, Mosby.

McKnight J: *The careless society: community and its counterfeits*, New York, 1995, Basic Books.

US Congress: *The US Congress Handbook*, 1993.

INTERNET RESOURCES

American Nurses Association
http://www.nursingworld.org

Community Health Status Indicators Project: Health Resources and Services Administration
http://www.communityhealth.hrsa.gov

Hardin MD
http://www.lib.uiowa.edu/hardin/md/publ.html

Health promotion
http://www.monash.edu.au/health/index.html

Health services and public health sites
http://www.lib.berkeley.edu/PUBL/internet.html

Health information resources
http://nhic-nt.health.org

Healthy People 2010
http://www.health.gov

Public Health Foundation
http://www.phf.org

CHAPTER FOURTEEN

Complementary and Alternative Therapies in Nursing and Health Care

MITZI A. FORBES, PhD, RN

I have an ear ache:
2000 BC—Here, eat this root.
1000 AD—That root is heathen. Here, say this prayer.
1850 AD—That prayer is superstition. Here, drink this potion.
1940 AD—That potion is snake oil. Here, swallow this pill.
1985 AD—That pill is ineffective. Here, take this antibiotic.
2000 AD—That antibiotic is artificial. Here, eat this root.

—*Author unknown*

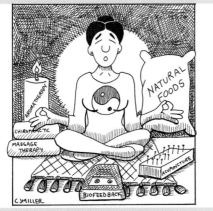

Complementary health care therapy is on the rise.

After completing this chapter, you should be able to:

■ Define complementary, alternative, and integrative health care.

■ Discuss the meaning of holism within complementary medicine.

■ Identify different types of complementary, alternative, and integrative therapies.

Y ou are a professional nurse, dedicated to giving excellent care. You work in the community, visiting patients in their homes, assessing their needs, and planning care to improve their health and well-being.

Today, you are visiting the home of Mrs. Woods, a 57-year-old patient who has been diagnosed with hepatic cancer. Chemotherapy is not working, so during your visit today you will encourage the patient, who is not expected to live another 6 months, to enroll in a hospice program. Mrs. Woods cries and tells you that she, her husband, and their friends are praying for her. "Can't we keep on praying?" she asks. You respond by

- Discouraging this activity so the patient does not cling to false hope.
- Telling the patient that prayer will not change the outcome.
- Telling the patient that you give care based on science, not superstition.
- Encouraging the patient and family to continue prayer, understanding that spiritual acts assist the patient and family to explore the meaning of life and may lead to a sense of peace and wholeness.

How would you respond? Would you choose any of the aforementioned options? Are you comfortable with your own feelings about the meaning of life and death, and health and illness? Would you choose to follow a healing path that is not considered conventional by modern Western medicine?

CONVENTIONAL AND INTEGRATIVE THERAPIES IN THE UNITED STATES

Conventional Western medicine has been called "allopathic." On the basis of a worldview strongly influenced by the Cartesian dualism and Newtonian physics of the seventeenth and eighteenth centuries, human beings are viewed as a collection of separate parts. Disease occurs when the parts break down. The body is viewed as separate from the mind. Patients have been treated by conventional medical practice as though they were broken machines. Like repairing a machine, fixing the broken body parts brings health. Many patients are dissatisfied with the paternalism of some physicians in the conventional medical system and the lack of control over their own health care. They believe that their psychological and spiritual well-being are being ignored. As a result, many people are turning to therapies that address them as whole beings rather than a collection of broken body parts.

Unconventional health-related therapies are often called *complementary or alternative*. The term *alternative* implies that a therapy is being used as a replacement for conventional medicine. The term *complementary* implies that a therapy is being used in addition to conventional medicine. Both terms convey an "us versus them" frame of reference. Dr. Andrew Weil, a physician noted for his leadership in bringing effective unconventional therapies into the mainstream of medical practice, prefers the term *integrative medicine*. The term *integrative* implies a blending or integration of systems into an approach that addresses the whole person.

Integrative therapies and a holistic philosophy of health are making major inroads into modern Western medicine. A recent search of the Internet revealed courses in alternative and complementary medicine available at 86 American medical colleges. Dr. Florence Selder (January 1999), a nurse psychotherapist who uses imagery in her practice, notes that therapies once considered alternative are becoming accepted in conventional practice. For example, imagery is becoming a common therapy in pain control. Some of your patients and their families already use integrative therapies in their health care. Many other patients will have heard of integrative therapy and want to know your opinion about how best to integrate unconventional therapies into their plan of care. You may use or practice some integrative therapy yourself. Research tells us that many Americans use at least one integrative therapy and the number is growing. In 1993 a landmark study published in the *Journal of the American Medical Association* reported that nearly 34% of Americans used at least one integrative therapy (Eisenberg, Kessler, and Foster, 1993). In response to this study, the National Institutes of Health established the Office of Alternative Medicine to fund research into the safety and efficacy of alternative and complementary therapies. In a recent update, the number of Americans who reported using integrative therapies had increased to nearly 47% (Eisenberg, Davis, Ettner, et al, 1998). Imagine that. Today, almost half of all Americans choose to include integrative therapies as part of their health regimen. The five integrative therapies most frequently reported by study participants were as follows:

- Massage.
- Chiropractic.
- Hypnosis.
- Biofeedback.
- Acupuncture.

WHAT ABOUT HEALING AND WHOLENESS?

Did you ever wonder how healers could work in hospice? Is healing possible for someone with a terminal illness? The word *healing* comes from a root that means "to make whole." Healing, then, is a journey toward wholeness (Dossey, 1989). Many patients desire to heal—and not just to cure disease. In fact some may feel a lack of wholeness in their lives and seek healing when there are no physical symptoms present. Healing can take place on many levels. Illness encompasses more than just the physical body. It also encompasses the mind, the spirit, the relationships and roles of the individual, and the community. If the final journey of life is a journey toward wholeness, then, yes, healing is occurring.

 What is wholeness? What does it mean to you?

Conventional medicine is starting to acknowledge wholeness when it addresses the body-mind connection. Nursing acknowledged wholeness when it addressed the person as body, mind, and spirit. The American Holistic Nurses' Association (AHNA), whose logo used to specify "body-mind-spirit," now speaks of the "physical, mental, emotional, social, and spiritual" aspects of patients (AHNA Standards, 2001). Recognizing that a person's psychological makeup encompasses both their mental (thinking processes) and emotional (feeling) nature further clarifies the psychological focus of holism. Eberst (1984) recognized six interactive dimensions of wholeness: mental, emotional, spiritual, physical, social, and vocational. The addition of the vocational dimension recognizes an important part of a patient's life that is often ignored when assessing the impact of illness.

ILLNESS AND CRISIS

During times of crisis, our sense of meaning and purpose in life are challenged. Health crises, whether acute, chronic, or developmental, are times when meaning and purpose may be challenged and often result in "distress of the human spirit." When this spiritual dimension is ignored, dissatisfaction with health care can result. According to the nursing literature, spirituality should not be confused with religiosity. *Religiosity* is the following of a particular religious form. Although many individuals express their spirituality through religious forms, religion is not a necessary ingredient of spirituality. Every person is a spiritual being (Newman, 1989). The nursing literature identifies spirituality as encompassing several things: a sense of meaning and purpose in life, a sense of connectedness, the potential for growth through adversity (Benzein, Saveman, and Norberg, 1998), and a sense of integrating wholeness (Burkhardt, 1989; Burkhardt, 1993; Conco, 1995; Nagai-Jacobson and Burkhardt, 1989; Reed, 1992).

Connectedness refers to individuals' sense of connection both within their own beings and with others. The "others" can include friends and family and can include feeling connected to something greater than the self (such as God, humanity, nature, the universe, and so forth). *Integrating wholeness* refers to the individual's sense that all the diverse aspects of life come together to create a whole. Within holistic philosophy, this whole is greater than the sum of the parts. Well-chosen integrative therapies, with their focus on the whole person, can assist patients in the healing process. Because many integrative practitioners include the spiritual aspect of individuals in their interventions, integrative theory is often associated with spirituality.

INTEGRATIVE THERAPY IN NURSING PRACTICE

Although many people think of integrative healers as belonging to other professions (e.g., chiropractic, massage therapy, naturopathy, acupuncture), many nurses are at the forefront of integrative health care (Box 14-1). Nursing theory has provided us with a strong theoretical base from which to practice integrative health. Dr. Martha Rogers, a nurse theorist who was intrigued by the cutting-edge theories of physics (such as general relativity and field theory), first published her theory of nursing in 1970, translating what was being discovered about the nature of the universe from physics to an understanding of the nature of human beings. Updated several times since 1970, Dr. Rogers' theory defined human beings as energy fields, greater than and different from the sum of their parts and characterized by pattern and wholeness. The environment was also characterized as a field; and patterns of human-environment interaction (later termed *processes*) were proposed. According to Dr. Rogers, we don't *have* energy fields, we *are* energy fields (Rogers, 1980) (Critical Thinking Box 14-1). Dr. Rogers' theory is further supported by the advances in physics. For example, string theory, an emerging view in physics that integrates both the theory of relativity and quantum theory, posits that all matter is composed of very small bits of energy.

BOX 14-1   Complementary and Integrative Therapies

Chinese therapies
- ❏ Acupuncture
- ❏ Acupressure
- ❏ Chinese herbal medicine

Natural healing
- ❏ Aquatherapy
- ❏ Aromatherapy
- ❏ Homeopathy
- ❏ Color therapy

Nutrition and diet
- ❏ Diet therapies
- ❏ Naturopathic medicine

Body work and movement therapies
- ❏ Yoga
- ❏ Rolfing
- ❏ Reiki
- ❏ Massage
- ❏ Qigong
- ❏ T'ai chi
- ❏ Reflexogy
- ❏ Shiatsu
- ❏ Therapeutic touch
- ❏ Healing touch
- ❏ Dance therapy
- ❏ Chiropractic
- ❏ Cranial osteopathy

Plant therapy
- ❏ Flower essence therapy
- ❏ Herbal medicine

Mind/body medicine
- ❏ Meditation
- ❏ Music therapy
- ❏ Visualization and imagery
- ❏ Hypnotherapy
- ❏ Biofeedback
- ❏ Light therapy

Ayurvedic medicine

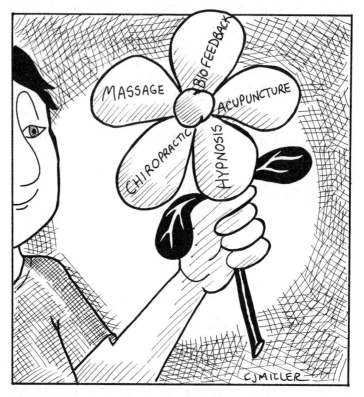

The five most reported integrative therapies.

The concept of human beings as energy is not really new. The idea is millennia old. Energy-based interventions are part of almost every indigenous healing system in the world. The human vital energy is known by many names in many cultures. The ancient Greeks called it *pneuma*. Among the Hindus of India, it is called *prana*. Among Asian cultures, it is known as *Qi* or *Chi*. All of these cultures developed practices that promote health by either teaching individuals to balance and revitalize their own energy or by assisting to balance and revitalize the energy of others. Energy interventions are increasingly supported by scientific research. In the 1970s, Dr. Valerie Hunt at the University of California Los Angeles used modified surface electromyography to research the outcomes of Rolfing, a deep-tissue massage (Hunt, 1977) and discovered that surface electrodes picked up a high-frequency, low-amplitude energy signature wherever they were placed on the body, including over resting muscles. Apparently developers of electromyography equipment were aware of this phenomenon, but they considered it error rather than data and so created filters to remove it. In fact, this high-frequency, low-amplitude energy appears to be the human energy field (or at least part of it because the field is postulated to extend beyond the physical confines of the body). (*See* Fig. 14-1.) Dr. Hunt spent many years continuing

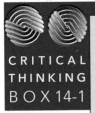

THINK ABOUT ... ENERGY FIELDS

Can you think of yourself as an energy field? It can be challenging. We don't usually perceive ourselves as energy fields. We perceive ourselves as solid beings. You are part of the environmental energy field of others, and they are part of your environmental energy field. Try to recall the last time you entered a room and felt that someone was angry. How did you know it? Were you feeling the angry energy being sent out by that person? Have you felt someone's sadness or someone's anxiety? What about someone's excitement and happiness? Have you ever been around someone and felt that they drained all your energy? Have you spent time with someone and felt energized? If everything you say, do, think, and feel is manifest in your energy field, what kind of effect do you have on patients? What difference does it make if you feel sad or distressed when you take care of someone else? If you ignore your own emotional and physical well-being, can you pass your negative energy on to others? Can you shield yourself from taking on the negative energy of others who are part of your environmental field? The American Holistic Nurses Association states that nurses must engage in self-care to be an instrument of healing for others (AHNA standards, 2001).

What implications does the aforementioned statement from the AHNA have on nursing students and on practicing nurses?

her studies, but at that period of time, the topic was marginally acceptable in scientific circles and was not readily funded. Her experience is summarized in her book, *Infinite mind: science of the human vibrations of consciousness* (Hunt, 1989). More recently, Dr. James Oschman, a cellular biologist and physiologist, has published a nice summary of the emerging field of bioenergy research in his book, *Energy medicine: the scientific basis* (Oschman, 2000). Dr. Oschman (personal communication, 2001) mentioned that the pulsing biomagnetic fields given off by the hands of healers when they are working are the same electromagnetic frequency that cells need to thrive. In his book, Dr. Oschman discusses various methods for measuring and studying energy interventions, including the use of a superconducting quantum interference device. You don't need expensive equipment to confirm the existence of the human energy field. Your hands should be enough (Critical Thinking Box 14-2).

WHAT ARE ENERGY-BASED THERAPIES?

If we understand ourselves to be energy beings, it is understandable that any crisis, injury, or illness will cause disruption in the balanced flow of the energy. Likewise, disruption in the flow of energy can result in symptoms of physical or psychological illness. Balancing and returning the optimal flow of energy facilitates healing.

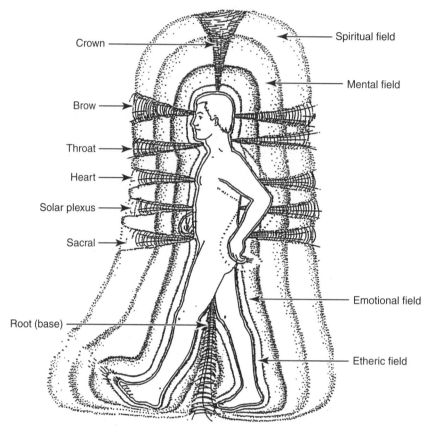

FIGURE 14-1
Model of the energy centers and energy fields.
(From Mentgen J: The healing touch level 1 program book, *Lakewood, CO, 2001, Colorado Center for Healing Touch.)*

Healing Touch

Introduced into nursing by Janet Mentgen, BS, RN, Healing Touch is taught internationally. Ms. Mentgen, like most practitioners of energy-based therapies, believes that all people are capable of practicing Healing Touch. We are all energy beings and are able to learn to use energy interventions to assist the healing process. Healing Touch requires no special equipment and can be done almost anywhere. Healing Touch uses the hands to assess, balance, and align the patient's energy field. Healing Touch may be done either with or without touching the patient's body. Before touching a patient, it is wise to ask permission. Although many patients enjoy the validation of physical touch, some feel threatened by it. This may be especially true of patients who have been abused or molested.

The American Holistic Nurses Association endorses Healing Touch, and certification as a Healing Touch Practitioner is available on completion of required

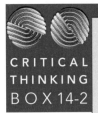

EXERCISE TO FEEL YOUR OWN ENERGY FIELD

1. Take a few deep breaths to let go of the mind chatter and get centered.
2. Rub your hands briskly together as if they were cold. When they are warm, separate your hands by a couple of inches. Allow your hands to assume a natural cupping position with the wrists relaxed.
3. Now move your hands apart by approximately 2 to 3 inches. Put them back together so they are not touching. Focus your consciousness on sensing anything that might be occurring between the palms of your hands.
4. Bring your hands approximately 4 to 6 inches apart and then bring them back together so they almost touch. Continue to play this imaginary accordion slowly, bringing your hands farther and farther apart and then back together. What are you feeling? Some people describe a sense of pulling like a magnet, a sense of heat or tingling. If you lost the sensation, start from the beginning again. If you feel something, you are feeling your own energy field or aura. If you do not feel anything, that is okay. At some point you probably will.

coursework and documentation of skill as a practitioner. Research has shown Healing Touch to be effective in reducing chronic pain (Darbonne and Fontenot, 1994), reducing pain and improving joint mobility after total knee replacement (Cordes, Proffitt, and Roth, 1997), and decreasing recovery time after abdominal hysterectomy (Silva, 1996). Research on Healing Touch is ongoing. To find out more about Healing Touch, contact Healing Touch International at 12377 W. Cedar Dr., Suite 202, Lakewood, CO 80228, or use the keyword "Healing Touch" to do a search on the Internet.

Therapeutic Touch

Therapeutic Touch is an energy-based intervention developed by Dora Kunz, a hands-on healer, and introduced into nursing by Dolores Krieger, PhD, RN (1979) of New York University. The Therapeutic Touch practitioner uses his or her hands to assess, modulate, and transfer energy to or from the patient to restore energy balance. The patient's body is not physically touched. All assessment and treatment is done with the hands placed several inches away from the patient's body but within the patient's energy field.

Research has shown that Therapeutic Touch is effective in treating many conditions. Therapeutic Touch has increased the speed of wound healing (Wirth, 1992); decreased the pain experienced by patients with arthritis while increasing their range of joint movement (Eckes, Peck, 1997), promoted relaxation, and improved immune function (Quinn, 1993). Research into Therapeutic Touch and other energy therapies continues.

Therapeutic Touch is taught in classes at the beginning and intermediate levels. Advanced classes are in the planning stage. To find out more about Therapeutic Touch and locate classes, contact Nurse Healers-Professional Associates, Inc. at 1211 Locust St., Philadelphia, PA 19107, or use the keyword "Therapeutic Touch" to do a search on the Internet. Of all the energy-based therapies, Healing Touch and Therapeutic Touch are unique in that they originated in nursing.

Reiki

The term *Reiki* is Japanese for "universal life energy." Although Reiki originated in Japan, many nurses practice it in the United States. Similar to some of the Healing Touch techniques, 30 minutes of Reiki therapy has been shown to increase salivary secretory immunoglobulin A (a measure of immune system function), reduce anxiety, and reduce systolic blood pressure (Wardell and Engebretson, 2001).

The International Society for the Study of Subtle Energies and Energy Medicine (ISSSEEM), an organization of scientists from many disciplines, has been formed to study the human energy field and energy-based medicine. For more information about ISSSEEM, contact the ISSSEEM Central Office, 356 Goldco Circle, Golden, CO 80403-1347.

Relaxation

It can be assumed that any hospitalized patient experiences some stress and anxiety. Individuals who are stressed experience activation of the autonomic nervous system (Guyton and Hall, 1995) and psychological discomfort. The physiologic manifestations of this activation include increased heart rate, respiratory rate, blood pressure, oxygen consumption, and muscle tone. In addition, the activity of the immune system is impaired. In short, the individual is ready for fight or fleeing. Such activation is useful if fighting or fleeing is necessary. However, activation of the fight-or-flight response when it is not needed can lead to a failure in the body's ability to repair itself and heal both physically and psychologically. Stress and anxiety beyond a mild level interfere with learning and judgment (Kneisl, 1995).

The fight-or-flight response can be counteracted by the relaxation response (Benson, 1975). In the relaxation response, the respiratory rate, heart rate, and blood pressure decrease, peripheral blood flow increases, epinephrine decreases, oxygen consumption decreases, sweat gland activity decreases, gastric acid secretion decreases, and killer cells of the immune system become more active. Nurses can use a number of integrative therapies to activate the relaxation response.

Breathing

Breathing patterns change in response to stress level. As part of the fight-or-flight response, breathing becomes rapid and shallow. However, deep, slow, rhythmic breathing elicits the relaxation response. It has also proved useful to clear the mind and increase the ability to focus and make judgments (Hendricks, 1995). Breathing exercises may be used alone or in combination with other therapies to promote relaxation. Breathing is also used to initiate entry into a quiet state of mind such as meditation and hypnosis.

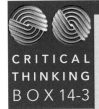

BELLY BREATHING

You may have heard about adbominal or diaphragmatic breathing. When many of us think about abdominal breathing, we focus on the upper abdomen because we know that is the area where the diaphragm expands and contracts. It is true that breathing occurs as the diaphragm pulls down into the upper abdominal area. However, if we are focusing on "breathing" into the upper abdominal area we are still breathing inefficiently. As the diaphragm contracts and lungs expand into the upper abdominal area, the upper abdominal tissues and organs push the lower abdominal tissues and organ outward. As this happens the belly pooches outwards. Because the lower abdominal area moves outward, it feels like the breath is going into the belly. If the abdominal muscles are tightened (as most of us try to do) it restricts deep breathing. Your body was not made to function with abdominal muscles tightly held. It is unhealthy.

1. Start by lying down. Take some deep breaths. Your breaths may already be causing your belly to move outward automatically.

2. Rest your hand on your belly (**below** the umbilicus). Do **not** tighten your muscles. Relax those lower abdominal muscles.

3. Now take a deep breath and imagine your hand drawing the breath down into your belly. As the air comes into the belly, it pushes your hand upward. The hand falls again as the breath flows out. (We know the breath is actually going into the lungs, but it **feels** like it is going way down into the belly. This sensation indicates we are breathing correctly.)

4. Continue breathing like this, in a slow relaxed way, for several minutes every day.

5. Next try standing up and placing your hand on your belly (below the umbilicus). Again breathe into the belly so that your hand is pushed outward. Is it harder to do standing up? Practice daily both lying and standing until you can easily do it standing.

6. Now try doing the same thing while sitting.

7. When you can take belly breaths lying, standing, and sitting, you have learned to breathe properly. Continue to practice daily.

This exercise is deceptively simple. As you start practicing this exercise, you may find that you can do it in a lying position and not in a sitting or standing position. Eventually, as your body becomes accustomed to belly breathing, you will be able to do it in almost any position. Don't become discouraged. I practiced it for a week before I could take a good belly breath while sitting or standing. Once you master the technique, you can use it to help reduce tension any time and any place. It is an excellent technique to teach to your clients.

As we grow up and become accustomed to a constant state of stress and anxiety, our typical breathing pattern may change to one that is shallow and rapid. Retraining oneself to breathe deeply and slowly increases our ability to handle stress without becoming "stressed out." Most adults breathe in the chest. Take a deep breath now. Notice what area of your body rises as you take the breath. Where did it go? Did it go into the upper chest area? For most people, this is what you will observe. Deep breaths should cause the belly to rise. Forget all those concerns you have about tight, flat stomach muscles. Tight stomach muscles interfere with deep, relaxing breathing. Try the breathing exercise in Critical Thinking Box 14-3 to learn how to breathe in a relaxed way. You can teach this technique to your patients in the hospital or in the community. Use it yourself when you notice tension.

Music

The use of music therapy dates back many millennia. Certain types of music are known to elicit the relaxation response. The most relaxing music is known to have between 60 and 70 beats per minute, simulating the relaxed resting heart rate (Alvin, 1966). When music has a beat faster than 70 beats per minute, it is stimulating rather than relaxing. Slower music (such as that used in the background of horror movies) can induce feelings of suspense. Music in the higher registers (flutes and strings) is more uplifting to mood than music in the lower registers (brass and woodwind). Appropriate choice of music is a useful adjunct in nursing practice (White, 1999).

Peaceful music may be used alone or in combination with other integrative therapies such as breathing exercises, guided imagery, and progressive muscle relaxation to reduce anxiety. Patients who were hospitalized for acute myocardial infarction have shown significant reduction in stress (as indicated by reduced heart rate, reduced respiratory rate, reduced myocardial oxygen demand, increased heart rate variability, and reduced state of anxiety) after 20 minutes of listening to relaxing music. A reduction in the stress level was still measurable 1 hour after the end of music treatment (White, 1999).

Meditation and Imagery

There are thought to be three types of meditation. The first type is concentrative meditation, in which the meditator focuses on an object. An example of concentrative meditation is Transcendental Meditation. The second type of meditation is mindfulness meditation, in which the focus is on the whole field. Mindfulness meditation is practiced at the behavioral level (the body in action), the physiologic level (the body in process), and the subjective level (the mind in action). Mindfulness meditation has the goal of maintaining attention rather than restricting attention to an object. The third type of meditation is a combination of the two aforementioned forms, Transcendental Meditation and mindfulness meditation. Although most meditation is done with the eyes closed to block out distractions, some meditation is done with the eyes open. Meditation has been shown to have significant relaxing effects on the body. A practice of daily meditation may lead to profound healing of emotions and increased feelings of connectedness and spirituality. An open-eyed meditation known as Heart-Math has increased the sense of well-being among persons hospitalized with schizophrenia without increasing their hallucinations (Davison, personal communication).

Imagery is the use of imagination to induce relaxation and encourage healing. Most people think of imagery as visualization. This is true when the image is a visual one. However, some individuals do not visualize when their eyes are closed. They can, however, imagine other sensations such as touch, smell, taste, and sound. Good use of guided imagery will invoke as many senses in the imagination as possible, allowing the patient to choose which sensation to include in their image. Asking patients to close their eyes and imagine a peaceful place from their past is a very easy way to elicit relaxation through imagery. Can they see the place, hear the sounds, smell the earth or the flowers or the water? Can they feel the warmth of the sun or the coolness of the breeze?

Studies on the use of imagery have been conducted in nursing. Patients who used imagery after surgery experienced reduced anxiety, reduced cortisol levels, and reduced inflammation at the surgical wound site (Holden-Lund, 1988). Imagery has been used to combat postoperative depression (Leja, 1989) and to reduce postoperative pain (Daake and Gueldner, 1989).

Hypnotherapy and Self-Hypnosis

Hypnosis is the process of being guided into a relaxed but focused state of awareness that, once established, allows the individual to be given subconscious suggestion to alter psychological and physiologic conditions or responses or reduce pain or stress in the subject. Self-hypnosis is when an individual learns to self-induce a relaxed, focused state of awareness while placing autosuggestions into their mind during the relaxed state to alter inappropriate mental or physical difficulties.

OVERVIEW OF SELECTED COMPLEMENTARY THERAPIES

WHAT IS AROMATHERAPY?

Aromatherapy consists of applying essential oils of plants that are highly concentrated plant and flower fragrance extracts to various locations on the body. It is said that the fragrances affect the limbic system, stimulating memory, emotion, and hormonal releases. Certain aromas can stimulate historical memory and by doing so cause a psychophysiologic response of well-being to occur in the body.

WHAT IS QUIGONG?

Qigong (pronounced *chee-goong*) focuses on breathing, meditation, and exercises that may be stationary or involve movement. The process is said to enhance and balance energy flow through the body. Some methods of Qigong qualify as energy therapies, as mentioned previously.

WHAT IS T'AI CHI?

T'ai chi (pronounced *tie chee*) is a type of Qigong that focuses on body movement and discipline and is considered a martial arts form because of the slow, meditative body movements and breathing techniques. The body movements are flowing, which in turn allows for unrestricted energy (*chi*) flow through the body. T'ai chi has been adapted by some teachers for use among those with arthritis and disability. T'ai chi practice has been shown to increase balance and is currently being studied as an intervention to decrease falls among the elderly.

WHAT IS YOGA?

Yoga is an ancient practice of slow, purposeful body movements, stretching, poses, and breathing techniques used to increase physical, mental, and spiritual well-being. It can be practiced by anyone but is dictated by an individual's physical limitations.

WHAT IS REFLEXOLOGY?

Reflexology is the use of direct manual thumb and finger pressure on various areas across the bottom of the foot. There are some reflexologies that include applying pressure to areas of the hands or ears. In reflexology the different areas on the bottom of the foot (palms or ear lobes) correspond to various organs of the body. By manual manipulation using mostly the thumbs and fingers, the reflexologist applies pressure to a spot on the bottom of the foot that corresponds to a certain organ in the body. The stimulus to that area of the foot is said to stimulate the healing and revitalization of the corresponding organ.

WHAT IS ROLFING?

Rolfing is the use of deep massage and movement exercises to realign the body to its original posture. Realignment is the outcome of the releasing of psychophysiologic stressors that take the form of adhesions in the fascia and the connective tissue covering the muscles. When deep massage (which can be painful) and movement exercises are used on the body, the muscles tend to relax, causing a release of muscle constriction, thereby allowing the body to realign itself naturally. The release occurs with the massage. Some people are said to have emotional responses such as crying and pictorial thought flashes when certain muscles are relaxed. It is said that these emotions are the result of psychologic stressors that originally caused the body muscles to stiffen, thus changing the outward structural alignment of the body.

WHAT IS SHIATSU?

Shiatsu is a Japanese form of acupressure. The thumb and fingers are used to apply pressure on certain pressure points on the body, which in turn increases the flow of energy throughout the body.

WHAT IS AYURVEDIC MEDICINE?

Ayurvedic medicine, which has been practiced in India for thousands of years, focuses on the whole person and their relationship to the outside world. It is believed that all diseases arise from stresses in the awareness or consciousness of the person. Treatment includes yoga, breathing exercises, meditation, herbs, emetics, enemas, oil massage, and specific diets.

APPLICATION TO NURSING PRACTICE

WHAT ARE IMPORTANT CONSIDERATIONS IN TAKING A HEALTH HISTORY?

When a nurse is taking a health history, either in the hospital or the community, the patient's use of integrative therapies needs to be recorded. Many patients use alternative medical therapies, such as chiropractic, homeopathy, Ayurvedic medicine, herbs, and vitamin therapies. It is important to note these. Some herbs interact with prescribed medications. Health providers need to know when this is occurring. By recording the use of integrative therapies, you may also learn what the patient does to relax. Plan the patient's care to take advantage of interventions with which they are already familiar. Remember to include a spiritual assessment in your health history. Patients may desire some spiritual support. Ask if they would like you to contact their minister, pastor, priest, or rabbi. Would they appreciate a visit from pastoral services? Do they wish to have privacy for prayer or meditation? Would they like instruction in relaxation and meditation techniques? Don't be afraid to ask these questions. In research studies, patients indicated that they appreciate being asked their preferences for holistic and spiritual care.

Although there are other forms of alternative medicine, the ones we have mentioned are some of the better known. Alternative medicine should be approached with an open mind and instinctual caution. The nurse and the patient should place importance on the credibility of the practitioner and research the pros and cons of the discipline. Any alternative practices that involve ingestion of a substance should be researched for side effects and compatibility with other medications. Careful consideration should be given when choosing conventional medicine over alternatives or combining the two approaches. Advise patients to discuss with the primary health care provider their thoughts about complementary medicine.

It is important for nurses to become aware and discuss these nontraditional, complementary therapies with their patients. Information should be given to patients on the basis of scientific research that would validate the usefulness and effectiveness of the therapy. One way to become familiar with these therapies is to try them for yourself. You may be pleasantly surprised at how a massage may lower your blood pressure and reduce stress or how yoga has improved your coordination and sense of well-being.

In summary, complementary and integrative therapies are increasingly becoming part of the regular health care regimen of the American public. Nursing has been at the forefront of this movement toward a more holistic approach to wellness and disease management. The thoughtful use of these types of therapies offers more choices for care that provide comfort and healing.

REFERENCES

Alvin J: *Music therapy*, London, 1966, J. Baker.

American Holistic Nurses' Association: Standards. In Dossey BM et al, editors: *Holistic nursing: a handbook for practice*, ed 2, Gaithersburg, Md, 1995, Aspen, pp. 25-36.

Benzein E, Norberg A, Saveman BI: Hope: future imagined reality, *J Adv Nurs* 28(5):1063-1070, 1998.

Benson H: *The relaxation response*, ed 1, New York, 1975, Morrow.

Burkhardt MA: Spirituality: an analysis of the concept, *Holist Nurs Pract* 3(3):69-77, 1989.

Burkhardt MA: Characteristics of spirituality in the lives of women in a rural Appalachian community, *J Transcult Nurs* 4(2):12-18, 1993.

Conco D: Christian patients' views of spiritual care, *West J Nurs Res* 17(3):266-276, 1995.

Cordes P, Proffitt C, Roth J: The effect of healing touch therapy on the pain and joint mobility experienced by patients with total knee replacements [unpublished research], 1997.

Daake DR, Gueldner SH: Imagery instructions and the control of postsurgical pain, *Appl Nurs Res* 2(3):114-120, 1989.

Darbonne MM, Fontenot T: The effects of healing touch modalities on patients with chronic pain [unpublished thesis], Northwestern State University, 1994.

Dossey B: Foreword, *Holist Nurs Pract* 3(3):vii-xi, 1989.

Eckes Peck SD: The effectiveness of therapeutic touch for decreasing pain in elders with degenerative arthritis, *J Holist Nurs* 15(2):176-198, 1997.

Eberst RM: Defining health: a multidimensional model, *J Sch Health* 54(3):99-104, 1984.

Eisenberg DM et al: Unconventional medicine in the United States. Prevalence, costs, and patterns of use, *New Engl J Med* 328(4):246-252, 1993.

Eisenberg DM et al: Trends in alternative medicine use in the United States, 1990-1997: results of a follow-up national survey, *JAMA* 280(18):1569-1575, 1998.

Guyton AC, Hall JE: *Textbook of medical physiology*, ed 9, Philadelphia, 1995, WB Saunders.

Hendricks G: *Conscious breathing: breathwork for health, stress release, and personal mastery*, New York, 1995, Bantam Books.

Holden-Lund C: Effects of relaxation with guided imagery on surgical stress and wound healing, *Res Nurs Health* 11(4):235-244, 1988.

Hunt VV: *Infinite mind: science of the human vibrations of consciousness*, Malibu, Calif, 1989, Malibu Publishing.

Kneisl CR: Stress, anxiety, and coping. In Wilson HS, Kneisl CR, editors. *Psychiatric nursing*, ed 5, Menlo Park, Calif, 1995, Addison-Wesley, pp. 66-84.

Krieger DK: *The therapeutic touch: how to use your hands to help or to heal*, Englewood Cliffs, NJ, 1979, Prentice Hall.

Leja AM: Using guided imagery to combat postsurgical depression, *J Gerontol Nurs* 15(4):7-11, 1989.

Mentgen JL: Healing touch, *Nurs Clin North Am* 36(1):143-158, 2001.

Nagai-Jacobson MG, Burkhardt MA: Spirituality: cornerstone of holistic nursing practice, *Holist Nurs Pract* 3(3):18-26, 1989.

Newman MA: The spirit of nursing, *Holist Nurs Pract* 3(3):1-6, 1989.

Oschman JL: *Energy medicine: the scientific basis*, Edinburgh, 2000, Churchill Livingstone.

Quinn JF: Psychoimmunologic effects of therapeutic touch on practitioners and recently bereaved recipients: a pilot study, *ANS Adv Nurs Sci* 15(4):13-26, 1993.

Reed PG: An emerging paradigm for the investigation of spirituality in nursing, *Res Nurs Health* 15(5):349-357, 1992.

Rogers ME: *An introduction to the theoretical basis of nursing*, Philadelphia, 1970, FA Davis.

Selder, F: Personal communication, January, 1999.

Silva MAC: The effect of relaxation (HT) touch on the recovery level of postanesthesia abdominal hysterectomy patients, *Alt Therap* 2(4), 1996

Wardell DW, Engebretson J: Biological correlates of Reiki Touch healing, *J Adv Nurs* 33(4):439-445, 2001.

White JM: Effects of relaxing music on cardiac autonomic balance and anxiety after acute myocardial infarction, *Am J Crit Care* 8(4):220-230, 1999.

Wirth DP: The effect of non-contact therapeutic touch on the healing rate of full thickness dermal wounds, *Subtle Energics* 1(1):1, 1992.

ADDITIONAL READINGS

Dossey L: *Healing words: the power of prayer and the practice of medicine*, ed 1, New York, 1993, HarperCollins.

Hover-Kramer D, Mentgen J, Scandrett-Hibdon S: *Healing touch: a resource for health care professionals* (part of the Nurse as Healer Series), New York, 1995, Delmar.

MacRae J: *Therapeutic touch: a practical guide*, ed 1, New York, 1987, Alfred A. Knopf.

INTERNET RESOURCES

American Holistic Nurses' Association
http://www.ahna.org

Healing Touch International
http://www.healingtouch.net

Holistic Alliance of Professional Practitioners, Entrepreneurs, Networkers, Inc. (HAPPEN)
http://www.therapeutictouch.com

National Center for Complementary and Alternative Medicine
http://nccam.nih.gov

The Alternative Medicine Homepage
http://www.pitt.edu/~cbw/altm.html

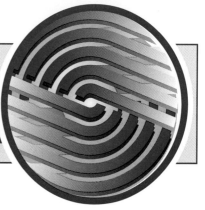

CHAPTER FIFTEEN

Trends and Economics in the Health Care Delivery System

JOANN ZERWEKH, EdD, RN, FNP, CS

By identifying the forces pushing the future, rather than those that have contained the past, you possess the power to engage with your reality.

—*Megatrends 2000, John Naisbitt and Patricia Aburden*

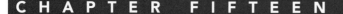

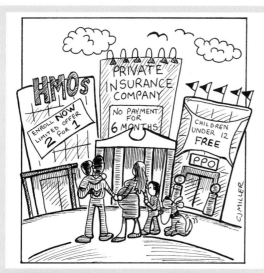

Health-care consumers are going to be shopping around to get the most for their health-care dollar.

After completing this chapter, you should be able to:

- Discuss how current trends will affect your future nursing practice.
- Identify social changes and their impact on nursing.
- Discuss how health care is financed.
- Identify basic concepts of budgeting.
- Discuss the impact that health care provider credentialing and quality improvement activities have on nursing practice.
- Describe how computers have affected nursing.

Dorothy was a little girl from Kansas who experienced another world and another time. That world was influenced and molded by the great Wizard. But the Wizard wasn't always there, nor would he perpetually control the culture of Oz. The same is true of our society. Individuals, trends, fads, and demands all influence the path and direction of our world. Our awareness of these demands and our responses to them allow us to direct our future. Remember, you do have a choice in creating the future.

The American health care system is one of the largest industries in the nation. Changes in the health care system are caused by consumer demands, technological advances, and governmental scrutiny. Nursing, as a large subsystem of the health care industry, will face the impact of the same dynamic forces on its theoretical viewpoint, its practice models, and its services to patients.

Today the nursing profession is relying on foresight, experience, and visionaries to pave a path toward nursing success. Your contributions will help make nursing an ever-more valued resource in the twenty-first century.

This chapter discusses the predicted trends that will influence the practice of nursing in the future. It also presents developments in quality improvement, practice models, health care financing, electronic information retrieval, communication by means of computerization, and the information superhighway that will have a major impact on nursing. Finally a review of key economic issues and health care system demands is presented to give you an idea of how cultural changes and external pressures will likely influence your practice.

TRENDS AFFECTING HEALTH CARE

The future holds many new social, political, and technological changes that will affect nursing directly and help shape our already powerful profession. The graying of America, technological advances, globalization, health care delivery system changes, and social evolution will dramatically change nursing roles and nursing delivery systems.

 Imagine activating your voice collar to record your nursing activities. (Beam me up, Scotty!) Picture yourself assuming a yoga position to teach meditation techniques to a cardiovascular patient.

HOW CAN NURSING RESPOND TO THESE TRENDS?

We must begin by understanding the impact these trends will have on nursing and then create a vision of where we want to be.

The mental image of shifting sands suggests a loss of control, an absence of stability, impermanence in the presence of permanence. Nursing's on-again, off-again courtship with surpluses and shortages is suited to that metaphor. "...Our forte has been to adapt, sometimes grudgingly, sometimes with panache for the victor, ameliorating the symptoms but avoiding the challenge of coming to terms with the underlying problem" (Joel, 1997, p. 7).

Creating this vision will allow us to develop educational and service strategies to guide nursing through the twenty-first century. Your contribution to creating this vision is crucial to the future and to the consumers of health care. The following trends are affecting nursing practice now and will continue to have a major impact throughout the twenty-first century:

1. Nursing will assume an undisputed dominant role in the health care delivery system, resulting in positions of high esteem with better salaries, incentives, responsibilities, and authority.
2. Care of the geriatric population will become an increasingly more prominent nursing specialty.
3. Nurses will play a major leadership role in determining and implementing health care policies.
4. Nurses will provide the expertise to integrate the multiple facets of health care— pharmacology, nutrition, preventive medicine, rehabilitation, and so forth— and thus to provide holistic care for an individual patient.
5. Technological advances will assist the nurse in providing high-quality care that is cost effective.
6. Specific outcome criteria will be important in determining the quality of care and will become health care facilities' overriding concern in the future.
7. Emphasis on case-managed care, as a replacement for the traditional sick-care approach, as prevention will be the key to reducing health care costs.
8. Increasing numbers of women and nurses will be making policy and governmental decisions affecting health care.
9. Education will become more user-friendly as the trend moves to a service economy in which knowledge is used.
10. Nursing professionals will begin sharing health care beliefs, cultural practices, resources, and the expanding body of nursing knowledge on an international level as globalization occurs.

Watching a war on television may sound farfetched, but as a result of advances in telecommunications, we all actually witnessed parts of Operation Desert Storm and the Gulf War, in addition to the horrific events of the September 11, 2001, terrorist attack. The world is rapidly moving toward a global information network. Eventually everyone will have their own personalized health status microchips that will match individual needs to health care service centers around the world. Naisbitt and Aburdene (1991) predict that the quality of life in rural areas will improve because of electronic and computer innovations. As we look around, we can see that their prediction is quite true. In this new world of information power, nurses will be recognized and rewarded for making use of their intelligence and creativity.

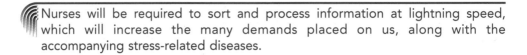

Nurses will be required to sort and process information at lightning speed, which will increase the many demands placed on us, along with the accompanying stress-related diseases.

With the development of nanotechnology, the expanding science of technology that examines or measures information at the molecular level (e.g., measuring at one billionth of a gram), nursing will be faced with new ethical concerns. To sum it up:

- New nursing care delivery systems must be developed to incorporate the demands of advanced technology.
- A shift must be made toward lower-technology, higher-touch therapeutic interventions to offset the technological boom.
- Therapies must be developed that combine conventional medical treatments with alternative care approaches (e.g., biofeedback, relaxation) to deal with stress (Curtin, 1990).

WHAT IS GLOBALIZATION, AND HOW DOES IT AFFECT NURSING?

The term *globalization* describes the spread of a common culture around the world, with a universal sharing of attitudes, products, industry, and stocks. With globalization, third-world countries will experience a developmental growth and make an even greater contribution to the global market. A religious and cultural resurrection will occur because of the blending of many cultural lifestyles (Miraldo, 1991). We will begin to service the world as one global economy.

- Nurses will need to learn about the health care beliefs and practices of other cultures in other nations and at home.
- International nursing forums will be required to meet the need for the sharing of nursing practices.
- Nursing and health care products, publications, and methods and the expanding body of nursing knowledge will find new possibilities in a global economy.

SOCIAL CHANGES AND NURSING

HOW DO SOCIAL CHANGES AFFECT NURSING?

Socially the entire world is evolving. With the demise of socialism and communism, there has been a rebirth of progress and growth. People are demonstrating a need as well as a desire for control over their lives, especially in the area of health care. This desire to create and grow will encourage a competitive market throughout the world.

According to Coile, "three driving forces—aging, technology, and costs—will reshape health in the future" (1991, p. 10). In the monthly labor review of November 2001, approximately 1.6 million new jobs are projected to be available in the health care industry from 2000 through 2010. Registered nurses are predicted to account for more than a third of these new jobs. With the growth in the job market, along with the shortage already occurring, the prediction is that there will be a shortage of more than 1 million nurses by the end of this decade (American Nurse, 2002).

Alternative Health Care. Consumers will make their own choices regarding health care—where they will obtain health care and in what type of setting. More unconventional healing alternatives will be available, such as getting in touch with one's own healing powers to mobilize the immune response. The practice of yoga for relaxation and the use of acupuncture, homeopathy, and chromotherapy are examples of this new wave of increased acceptance of healing therapies. See Chapter 14 for more discussion on alternative health care. Consumers are better-informed individuals who are taking more active roles in their health care.

Medicine and the Public Eye. The power that medicine holds over the consumer and society has been questioned, is continuing to be questioned, and is rapidly changing. What was once known as conventional medicine and the physicians who practiced in that arena no longer hold control over the patient. The patient is now being called a *health care consumer*. The general public is rapidly seeking more information and becoming more intelligent regarding their health care. This is causing unrest with the quality of service offered by many of the health care providers (e.g., health maintenance organizations [HMOs], preferred provider organizations [PPOs]). Health care information and services are expanding on the Internet at a phenomenal rate. As with any rapidly expanding service/technology, there are always problems. There is no effective control over the health information on the Internet. There are almost 15,000 Web sites that offer some form of medical advice. The Federal Trade Commission's Operation Cure All has found erroneous information and serious problems with medical information on the Internet (Tucker, 1999). Nurses are and will continue to be a resource for the consumer regarding how to find and evaluate medical information via the Internet. Nurses are in a position to be major players in the restructuring of the health care environment.

Quality of Care. Specific outcome criteria will be important as the public judges the value of health care. Health care will be viewed as a purchase, and the public will make sure it is getting its money's worth. Nurses will be in a position, as providers of health care, to offer the best services for the best price. The role of the nurse practitioner is an example of the increase in nurses as providers of health care. There has been significant increase in the number of graduates as well as the expansion of the role of the nurse practitioner. Into the next century, we will be continuing to develop mechanisms that measure the quality of the product. The bottom line in health care will be a focus on the value of the product. Quality measures will direct our activities at work and will require us to constantly maintain a level of excellence.

Aging Population. By the year 2010, there will be more than 40 million Americans age 65 or older. The portion of the population known as the "baby boomers" will be senior citizens and will represent the largest segment of the population. Hospitals that are currently struggling with survival will be ill equipped to provide health care to an aging population. The majority of people over 65 years of age have multiple-system health problems and chronic illnesses. For this group, the cost of health care will continue to increase. The statistical trends also indicate that the people in the nursing profession are aging faster than other professions. The average age of a nurse is now 44 years (Schreiber, 1999). The current nursing shortage crisis caused by decreased numbers of graduates, in addition to increased demands in the workplace, will be further complicated by the retirement of a large portion of the nursing workforce. In the health care industry, there have been minimal considerations for dealing with an aging nursing provider population. How to deal with the nursing shortage and how to fund and provide services for the elderly are two of the most sensitive political issues in the United States today.

New Wave of Technology. Computers, biosensors, implants, genetic therapies, and imaging devices are examples of the emerging technologies of the twenty-first century. Medical artificial intelligence in contexts such as computer-assisted surgery, electrocardiography and fetal monitoring interpretation, clinical diagnosis, and genetic counseling will have a major impact on our future. Telemedicine currently ranges from radiographic consultations across cities to telebiotic surgeries across hemispheres. Interactive disks already assist patients to make more independent medical decisions regarding their care. Devices for home use can help monitor blood pressure and blood glucose or perform a pregnancy test.

Health Care Information Superhighway. It is not unusual for a patient to visit a doctor, obtain a diagnosis for their problem, then go home and surf the Internet to find information related to the diagnosis. Another scenario is that the patient browses the Internet and finds a condition where the symptoms are closely related to what he is experiencing. He reads all he can find, and when he goes to the doctor he may be informed, misinformed, or overinformed, regarding the possible diagnosis of his problem. According to U.S. Census Special Studies reports (2001, September), 54 million households, or 51%, had one or more computers in August 2000. More than two in five households have Internet access—that's approximately 44 million households, or 42%, that had the Internet in 2000 (Fig. 15-1). This presents to the health care consumer a tremendous resource of information regarding their health care. The newsstands are full of periodicals that refer the consumer to Internet sources for answers to health care concerns. The public is and will continue to become more informed and will demand more preventive care, rather than focusing on the treatment of an illness once it has been diagnosed.

"Internet traffic will quadruple in 2001." Rich Karlgaard, *Forbes*, December 10, 2001, p. 22.

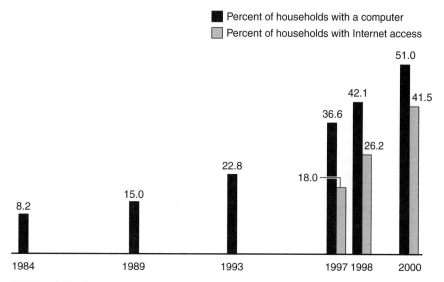

FIGURE 15-1
Computers and Internet Access in the Home: 1984 to 2000.

Work Psychology Changes. Organizations have revolutionized their view of workers from a dependent perspective to an independent perspective. Research and development of a body of knowledge related to work psychology has now established the concept of leadership as a facilitating role—assisting in moving work groups along the maturity continuum—rather than a role that calls for exerting control and making all decisions. Greater freedom and responsible interaction among employees and employers have encouraged work productivity, and this trend will continue into the next century.

We must make continued efforts to validate nursing's unique contribution to health care. Women are now considered a potential and an expanding labor source and, furthermore, a source of leaders in the business world. Can you believe that more than 5 million women are leading small to medium companies that are predicted to be the top companies in the future? Nursing is predicted to grow faster than the average for all occupations through the year 2006 (Bureau of Labor Statistics, 1999). Two population groups, women and the elderly, will continue to influence the work environment and cause a restructuring of work ethics and settings. The corporate world will recognize the need to balance personal, professional, and organizational goals.

HOW ARE COMPUTERS AFFECTING HEALTH CARE?

Telemedicine. In 1995 at the University of North Carolina, telemedicine was demonstrated to be very cost-effective for linking a neonatal cardiologist and other neonatal specialists to hospitals in the region which did not have these specialists on their staff. This provided a more rapid interpretation of neonatal cardiac problems. Previously the echocardiograms had to be sent to the University of North Carolina for interpretation with a 24- to 48-hour delay in the treatment of the infant. By evaluating the echocardiograms via telecommunication, there has been a significant decrease in length of stay for these infants. By this example, it is evident that telemedicine can be defined as the use of computer technology and telecommunications to provide contact between the health care provider and the consumer. As telehealth and telemedicine evolve, so do the definitions of their parameters. One of the primary goals of telemedicine is to provide access to rural and underserved communities. There are many different methods by which this can be and is being accomplished. There are partnerships between state agencies and rural health care organizations, between medical centers and prison health services, between major medical centers and rural health care providers, and between medical institutions that extend clinical expertise to physicians in rural areas. There are a multitude of approaches to the use of telemedicine, but the primary purpose is to fulfill a defined clinical need (Dakins and Kincade, 1997). There are also new resources for this emerging field of health care—*Telehealth Magazine* (http://www.telemedmag.com) and *Telemedicine Today* magazine (http://tie.telemed.org:80/).

Where Is Nursing in Telehealth/Telemedicine? Nurses are very actively involved in the delivery of nursing care through telemedicine or telenursing. As nurses become more involved in providing nursing care that extends across state lines, it becomes a question of what state is the nurse providing care or practicing. This was one of the considerations with the proposal and implementation of the Mutual Recognition Compact among states. Nurses are practicing triage from emergency care facilities, providing home care services, and assisting care for the terminally ill patients—all through telenursing. Nurses conduct video assessments, obtain vital patient information through telemonitoring, and determine whether someone needs to visit the patient in person.

A rapidly progressing trend is to use the resources a patient commonly has in their home. The telephone, television, and videocassette recorder are rapidly becoming vital links of health care information to and from the patient in their own home. The patient can have a video visit with a nurse or counselor through the television that can function over the cable television lines. A telephone voice mail system reminds her of her medication schedule. The patient has her electrocardiogram evaluated every day with the ambulatory electrocardiography monitor. The off-site nurse may call to review with the patient what is occurring when there is evidence of abnormal cardiac activity. Think about an electronic sensor pad that the patient will lay a hand on; it will transmit to the remote provider the patient's weight, blood sugar, vital signs, electrocardiogram readings, arterial blood gas parameters, and numerous other pieces of information. All this is provided to the patient, and the patient never sees or interacts with a computer.

FINANCING OF HEALTH CARE

ARE HEALTH CARE EXPENDITURES INCREASING?

The statistics continue to indicate an increase for expenditures on health care. The impact of managed care and a reduced economy wide inflation have assisted to control the health insurance costs. When the shift to managed-care plans occurred, the share of health insurance paid by the employee increased. This has reached a plateau, and there does not appear to be a continuing increase. This is certainly a change from the increases seen over the past few years. However, managed care has not reduced the growth of Medicare beneficiaries and overall spending. The results of managed care indicate a significant decline in the length of hospital stay, a shift from inpatient to outpatient procedures, but also an increase in coverage of procedures with more outpatient utilizations. The question remains—is this just a slowdown in the generally upward trend of health spending (Rubin, 1999)? There remain three basic reasons for the continued increase in health care costs: inflation, increased demand for services as a result of federal programs such as Medicare and Medicaid, and expensive technological advances in medicine. Cost containment still affects the groups at risk—the elderly, children from low-income families, and the indigent.

WHAT ARE THE NATIONAL HEALTH EXPENDITURE PROJECTIONS THROUGH 2005?

National health expenditures reached approximately $1 billion in 1995, and it is projected that they will be $1.5 billion in 2000 and $2.2 billion by the year 2005. This staggering projection of health care expenditures has tremendous importance not only for nursing but for all of us as consumers of health care. Personal health care expenditures—that is, all spending for health services received by individuals and for health products purchased at retail stores—are expected to reach $1.3 trillion in 2002 (from approximately $900 billion in 1995) and $2 trillion in 2005. These projections are consistent with the move from inpatient to ambulatory services. The shift away from institutional settings (hospitals) to outpatient and home health care, which is, in large part, financed by Medicare, will be the most dramatic, growing at a whopping 10% per year. In comparison, hospital spending grew less than 3% in 1994—the smallest increase on record, even smaller than the 1985 figure that coincided with the implementation of Medicare's prospective payment system (Burner and Waldo, 1995).

The projected growth in home health care services has occurred because technological changes have made it possible to deliver many services at home that were previously delivered in hospitals or institutional settings, such as intravenous antibiotics and physical therapy. However, Medicare reimbursements for services in the home health industry has experienced significant changes. There are tighter controls over the services that are approved for Medicare payment.

 Just what exactly are Medicare and Medicaid and how do we finance our health care?

WHERE DO THE HEALTH CARE FINANCING RESOURCES COME FROM?

There are basically three ways health care can be financed: self-payment, third-party payment (i.e., someone other than the individual pays the bill) through health care insurance, and health care assistance.

Self-Payment. An individual or family pays all of the costs for medical services. Before the 1930s this was the most-common method; now it is the least-common method.

Health Care Insurance. For the working individual, employer-provided health insurance is the most common form of insurance for individuals and their families. Health care costs have risen, and so have the cost of employers' contributions and, consequently, so have employees' contributions. Cost-containment strategies reported by the Health Care Finance Administration include reimbursement for generic prescriptions only, requirement of second opinions on surgery cases, preadmission testing to avoid hospital inpatient costs, and increased use of outpatient surgery. HMOs and managed care are offered as low-cost alternatives. More on HMOs later.

The Medicare program was initiated with the passage of Title XVII of the Social Security Act of 1965. This government-operated or public program is federally funded and financed through taxes on wages. Each of us who are currently employed pay a portion of our salary to the Medicare program. Currently covered under Medicare are individuals 65 and over who are eligible for Social Security benefits, disabled individuals, and individuals who have end-stage renal disease. Coverage consists of Part A, hospital insurance, and Part B, supplementary medical insurance that is voluntary and limited to those who have the premium deducted from their Social Security check. The majority of individuals, approximately 99%, subscribe to Part B (Smith and Maurer, 1995). It is projected that Medicare will pay for an increasing share of personal health care expenditures from 19.3% in 1993 to 22.6% in 2004 (Burner and Waldo, 1995).

The funding status of Medicare has become a national concern. If Medicare expenditures continue at the present rate of escalation, then Medicare will cease to be funded in the near future, depending on changes in the system and whose predictions you believe regarding when the Medicare resources will be depleted. In response to this, there is currently a bill before the legislature to overhaul the Medicare system. Whether this is passed, and what changes occur prior to passage, will have an impact on the integrity and the continuation of the Medicare system for payment of health care.

Health Care Assistance. Health care assistance is a type of third-party payment system in which payment is provided by a federal or state program or private charity. The most familiar is Medicaid, a grant program established under Title XIX of the Social Security Act. It was designed to provide medical assistance to the poor. It is a state and federal partnership. Most states provide coverage to families with children on welfare (Aid to Families with Dependent Children) and pregnant women. According to data from the Health Care Financing Administration (1994), almost 25% of all Medicaid recipients were enrolled in some type of managed-care plan. This trend is expected to continue, because third-party premiums are projected to be the fastest-growing component of the Medicaid program.

Private charity, such as nonprofit organizations that target special health needs (e.g., acquired immune deficiency syndrome) or special risk groups (e.g., pregnant teenagers), along with philanthropic gifts to hospitals and various agencies, assists individuals without insurance to obtain care. Overall this type of charitable contribution does not make up a significant portion of the health care budget.

WHAT ARE THE TRENDS IN REIMBURSEMENT?

The effects of rising health costs have stimulated significant changes in the reimbursement structure and delivery of health care services. In today's health care environment, more than ever, nursing is concerned about the cost and price of health care services. Such cost-based reimbursement, also called *retrospective*, was formerly the most common method used. A service was provided and then paid for after the fact. The physician and patient had almost unlimited autonomy in deciding what services were needed. Today's health care reimbursement relies on a *prospective* payment system that compensates the provider on an individual-case basis for health care services. According to most sources, this type of payment structure encourages efficiency and cost containment.

Diagnosis-Related Groups. With the prospective payment system, the health care agency and providers of care know in advance exactly how much they will receive for the services required to care for a patient with a particular diagnosis. An example of the diagnosis-related group (DRG) system might be a reimbursement of $1500 for a vaginal delivery, regardless of length of hospital stay or complexity of care. DRGs and prospective reimbursement have turned the delivery of health care around by 180 degrees. Giving quality care to patients in a timely and cost-effective manner has become essential in the present market.

Why do we have DRGs? In the 1980s several factors forced the government to find a new payment system for Medicare patients. These included:

- Spiraling health care costs
- Increasing use of hospital services
- A wide variation in cost of care among hospitals.

DRGs have been criticized for not adequately measuring the severity of illness or the different kinds of nursing resources used to care for patients. However, the current trend is demonstrating that discharging patients earlier not only doesn't compromise— but actually promotes—their well-being. The DRG system does offer an opportunity for nurses to use principles of research to predict nursing resource use by classification of patients. It should be possible to have patient-specific information in a form that will promote a comparison of quality and cost (Smith and Maurer, 1995). Before the implementation of DRGs, most nurse managers were not actively involved in the budget process. Now nurse managers are active in developing their unit's budget and maintaining operating costs within the budget. Performance evaluation and appraisal of employees depend not only on clinical expertise but, more and more, on the nurses' fiscal knowledge and responsibility.

HMOs. The year 1998 marked the second year in a row that more than half of the nation's HMOs lost money. Nationwide the HMOs in 1997 ended the year with 57% of them losing money. Consolidation of HMOs is occurring so rapidly that it is sometimes difficult for the patient to know where his health care financing is coming from. With the HMO, the member pays a flat fee. The member is expected to obtain care at the designated HMO facility, except in emergency cases. The organization provides both inpatient and outpatient care to families and individuals. With the consolidation in the HMOs, there is significant loss of continuity of patient care. With all of the changes and financial problems of the HMOs, it is predicted there will be significant increases in the respective health care premiums in the future.

PPOs. Another example of a prospective payment system, the PPO, is a group of health care providers that has negotiated a special reduced rate to attract health plan members. The PPO often offers individuals more freedom of choice in providers than the HMO, especially if the PPO network is large. Most PPOs operate independently and are not regulated by the government.

WHAT IS THE NURSE'S ROLE IN HEALTH CARE FINANCING?

Traditionally nurses have had limited power within the health care system. Information regarding the financing of health care was typically excluded from nursing curricula. Nurses increasingly are becoming part of the decision-making process involved in the reimbursement and financing of health care services. Nursing programs are stressing the importance of educating nurses as to the roles of patient/consumer advocate and change agent in our evolving health care delivery system. Nurses must start by becoming aware of the impact of finances through their own personal or professional experience. Understanding the basics of budgeting is imperative not only for the nurse manager, but also for the graduate entering the field.

 Providing high-quality patient care is no longer the only focus; achieving that goal of care with fiscally sound, effective financial methods is a priority.

BUDGETING BASICS

Before you start to skip over this section because it has to do with money, fiscal management, and budgeting, *stop!* Let's just look at the basics, the bottom line on the budgeting process. It doesn't have to be difficult.

WHAT IS FISCAL OR FINANCIAL MANAGEMENT?

Fiscal or financial management is derived from basic accounting principles. Learning them is a process just like the one that occurs when we learn medical terminology for the first time. There are some methods or measurements that follow specific rules that allow or permit a standard analysis when comparing one institution to another. For example, if we did not have specific medical terminology, we might just say, "The patient had something wrong with his belly and they took it out." To accurately describe the care required for this patient, we need to know that he had an appendectomy versus a subtotal gastrectomy. The language (medical terminology) helps us discriminate. Finance is the same. We just have to learn some basic terms (Box 15-1) and principles. For example,

 Assets = Liabilities + Owner's Equity (Net Worth)

 BOX 15-1 Fiscal Terminology

ACUITY LEVEL
A measurement that is used to describe the severity of illness in patients—usually four classifications

ASSETS
What is owned (equipment, property, cash in bank)

LIABILITIES
What is owned (accounts payable or amount of loans)

NET WORTH
Difference between assets and liabilities

VARIANCE
Difference between budgeted amounts and actual amounts—usually a negative (–) variance indicates a positive (+) bottom line.

WHAT MUST YOU KNOW ABOUT ACCOUNTING?

You don't have to know double-entry accounting to understand fiscal management and standard cost features. Make it a point to understand the accounting terms your nurse manager uses when working on the budget. Remember that your salary, benefits, working conditions, and patient load are all determined by someone's budget. Don't be afraid of appearing naive or foolish; you are *not* an accountant or auditor, so ask questions. Some key concepts to understand are related to budgeting, basic measures of costs, and budgetary indicators.

WHAT IS THE BUDGET PROCESS?

A *budget* is a plan or document that uses numerical data to forecast expenses of a usually fixed resource, such as money or time, during a given period (usually 1 year). The goal of budgeting is the optimal use of resources in the organization. There are three types of budgets that nurse managers frequently encounter:

Operating budget—daily costs involved in the day-to-day operation of a unit (usually excludes personnel costs). *Example:* medical supplies and equipment.

Capital budget—the outline or plan for buying large or fixed assets or types of equipment (that usually depreciate) associated with long-range planning, usually 3 to

5 years. *Example:* purchasing magnetic resonance imaging equipment or a computed tomography scanner or renovating a section of the building.

Personnel budget—often referred to as the *full-time equivalent budget* that plans the actual need for unit staffing 24 hours per day, 365 days a year; also involves estimating the acuity level of patients to determine the correct mix of nursing personnel needed to care for those patients.

Budgets can be classified according to how often they are done and the basis upon which they take place. The two most common types are *incremental budgeting* and *zero-based budgeting*. In incremental budgeting, the nurse manager prepares the budget on the basis of last year's expenditures. The advantages to this type of budgeting are that it is easy to prepare, it takes less time, and new programs and additional staffing are figured into the process. The disadvantage of incremental budgeting is that it is *not* cost effective, as there is little motivation to reduce expenses or prioritize programs and services. The zero-based budget is based on "rejustifying" the need for programs and services. In other words, the nurse manager must review the expected service, what resources that service will require, and the cost of each resource inclusion—a type of planning "from the bottom up." The major disadvantage is that it is a lengthy and complex process.

Following are four easy steps to budget planning:

1. *Determine the requirements of the budget.* Who develops the budget? It is usually best if top-level managers include unit managers in the process (i.e., involve the personnel who use the resources).
2. *Develop a plan.* What is the budgeting cycle? Twelve months? Six months? Selecting the optimal time is crucial to reducing predicted error (i.e., if the budget is predicted too far in advance, there is greater likelihood of error).
3. *Analyze and control the operation.* Ongoing analysis of monthly computerized statements that describe expenditures or any expected deviation is important. Although fluctuations occur, nurse managers are expected to be accountable for deviations.
4. *Review the plan.* Throughout the year the budget is reviewed and minor modifications are made as necessary. The nurse manager is in a key position to predict seasonal variations specific to the patients on the unit (Marquis and Huston, 1999).

How Do Budgets Fit Into the Cost-Control Picture? It is important to understand the different types of costs and how they are related to your unit. Effective cost control starts with keeping accurate, detailed records of costs, when they occur, and what they are for. A *unit cost* involves the cost of producing a single product or unit. Unit costs are expressed in terms such as per dollar of billing or per insurance policy issued. *Standard costs* include the normal or expected costs of an operation, product, or service, usually including labor, materials, and overhead charges. These costs become the standards against which you may judge your cost performance as good or bad. The *target* or *budget costs* are guidelines by which the nurse manager determines whether or not the unit has operated within allowable expenses. This is often called an *expense* or *operating budget*.

Usually a *cost variance report* (or budget variance report) is issued on a monthly basis to the nurse manager. This report is important in that it reports whether the unit has met its standard costs, exceeded them, or fallen below them. Other financial reports are the *payroll report* (employee earnings), *productivity report* (patient days compared with budget), and *supply variance report* (listing of all supply costs and variances compared to budget amounts).

WHAT ARE THE SOURCES OF COST PROBLEMS?

There are many reasons for cost problems. The old adage "If you are going to do something, do it right the first time" is applicable to the problems related to spiraling health care costs. Poor quality contributes significantly to increased cost (along with customer dissatisfaction) for the organization, as time is lost correcting problems and reworking the task. In addition, theft and carelessness contribute significantly.

The Italian economist Vilfrido Pareto's 80/20 Rule or law of maldistribution can be applied to practical cost containment and management. If 80% of the problems are caused by 20% of the employees, then most of the cost problems can be narrowed down to specific individuals or units rather than the entire organization. The important notion is that cost problems can be isolated and fixed in specific, identified problem areas.

The golden rule of cost-effectiveness is as follows:

When your costs are under or equal to your budget, they are in control— this is good. ☺ When your costs are over your budget, they are out of control—this is bad. ☹

WHAT DOES "COSTING OUT" NURSING SERVICES MEAN?

Nurse managers need to understand not only the total costs of running a unit, but also the costs by type of patient, especially within a managed-care system. As hospitals negotiate discounted arrangements with HMOs and PPOs, it becomes critical that the nurse manager understand the cost of treating a patient relative to the revenue received from treating that patient. There are various types of systems that can provide useful data. Even as a beginning nurse, you may be required to keep records related to time needed to complete various tasks. What type of system does your clinical facility use?

Remember, participating in fiscal management should be viewed as a fundamental and powerful tool for nursing!

COMPUTERIZATION AND THE "INFORMATION SUPERHIGHWAY"

HOW HAVE COMPUTERS AFFECTED NURSING?

Computer systems are rapidly evolving in the health care industry. You can open any nursing-oriented software buyer's guide and find programs to assist you in admission and discharge; nursing care planning and documentation; staffing, scheduling, and continuing education; costing out nursing services; and health care agency orientation. These programs are designed to facilitate your productivity by assisting you in managing the flow of information, problem solving, and accurately documenting.

Three distinct types of computers exist:

- Mainframe.
- Minicomputer.
- Microcomputer.

Mainframe computers, the fastest and largest computers available, are composed of many pieces of hardware (equipment). They have extensive memory capacity, are generally rented or leased because of their expense, and are usually located in a central area within a facility. They are used to collect, store, and process vast amounts of information. In health care agencies, they are used to organize patient databases, patient billing, budget reports, personnel files, and nursing management information such as staffing, scheduling, and incident reports. Smaller computers such as microcomputers can be linked within the mainframe to access information from many locations throughout a facility.

The minicomputer is a miniature version of the mainframe with a smaller memory capacity and a slower processing time. These computers may be found in smaller health care agencies or in special, more self-contained departments such as a pharmacy. There may also be multiple access terminals throughout a facility.

The microcomputer, also known as the *personal computer*, *home computer*, *laptop*, or *notebook computer*, has fewer hardware or equipment pieces than the mainframe, and its hardware components differ. These computers can unleash the staff nurse's or nurse manager's creativity. Even though these computers can process only one job at a time, they allow visualization of the input and output and can access a mainframe computer. The software and programs that enable you to use the personal computer are generally user friendly, meaning they guide the user in a step-by-step process. Access to this type of computer can encourage nurses to develop new charting or staffing ideas, record quality assurance findings, or develop patient education materials.

IS THE FUTURE IN THE PALM OF YOUR HAND?

Hand-held computer technology, through a PDA, or personal digital assistant, provides personal functions such as memos, calendars, address books, and e-mail. In addition, PDAs interface, or link, with personal computers and, by using special software, with hospital information systems. It is this linking that can reduce errors, save time, and increase revenue by streamlining recordkeeping. PDAs may be used a variety of ways in clinical settings, such as tracking patients and supervisors; determining the correct clinical pathway for a given diagnosis or plan of care; checking on drug dosages, interactions, and contraindications; and accessing a venerable list of resources and references. PDAs work in conjunction with a desktop computer through "hot synching," or "beaming," from one PDA to another. In other words, in order to hot synch you hook up your PDA to your computer so that they can work together to exchange data and software. Flexible, portable keyboards can be added to a PDA to make it easy to input data from a patient's bedside.

HOW WILL NURSING BALANCE COMPUTER TECHNOLOGY AND CARING?

Computers were initially introduced in health care agencies to assist with financial activities such as patient billing. Today computers are being used to directly facilitate nursing activities and patient hospitalization. The initial impact of computers in nursing came with the advent of technological systems developed to monitor patient health status (vital signs, electrocardiograms, and so forth). Now scheduling, staffing, and fiscal management activities are often computer-generated, as are programs designed to assist in the orientation and continuing education of nurses. Computers are promoted for their ability in saving nursing time, which is vitally important for cost containment. Some staff feel that computers are difficult to use, perhaps because of their unfamiliarity and their reluctance to accept them. Some experts feel that the increased use of computers may lead to decreased patient contact; however, others feel that bedside computers actually promote more patient-nurse interaction, because tedious tasks are increasingly handled at the bedside (Fig. 15-2).

In home care settings, having a notebook computer with a modem attachment can allow the nurse instant online access to patient records or resource information or the data can be input directly into a PDA. Computer literacy is becoming more important, because it enables nurses to use computer-generated information more efficiently and to incorporate such information into the patient's plan of care.

Patient privacy and confidentiality of health care records may pose an ethical issue. The disclosure of information takes on a new perspective with the increasing use of computers in health care. Nurses who are computer-literate are in a strategic position to safeguard a patient's right to privacy and confidentiality.

WHAT IS THE INFORMATION SUPERHIGHWAY? :-)

For those of you who haven't been online, turn your head sideways to see the smiley face. This is just one example for a "newbie," or newcomer to the Net, or Internet, of an *emoticon* that helps to let you know the mood of the person you are communicating with. Box 15-2 has some common emoticons listed. The *information superhighway* is a term used to describe the explosion of electronic information retrieval and communication taking place through computers and modems. So, how do you get involved in the information superhighway?

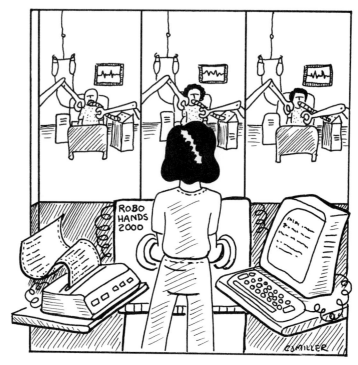

FIGURE 15-2

Advances in computer technology continue to assist the nurse, but technology cannot replace the humanistic aspect of nursing care.

 BOX 15-2   Emoticons

"Smiley" or "emoticons" are ways to punctuate your e-mail messages or online talk with textual symbols. They help clarify the sender's intention when it might otherwise be misinterpreted, since no eye contact or voice intonation is possible when you are online. Here are some emoticon examples:

:-)	Smile	:#	Lips sealed
;-)	Wink	:&	Tongue tied
:-(	Frown	:-[	Pout
:-/	Chagrin	:-*	Kiss
:-D	Laughing out loud	:-0	Yell
{ }	Hug or hugs {{{{}}}}	>:-(	Furious

The first things you will need are a computer, a modem, a commercial online system, and a willingness to do a little "surfing." Box 15-3 will help you with cyberspeak. The number of commercial online services available is growing at an incredibly fast rate throughout the world. Some examples of online services are America Online, CompuServe, Delphi, Prodigy, Microsoft, eWorld, AT&T, and

IBM. Most of these services can be purchased at computer software stores. These online services provide e-mail, breaking news stories, chatrooms, and access to the World Wide Web (WWW).

BOX 15-3 Cyberspeak

CYBERSPACE
An electronic "virtual" space that is not physically real, initially coined by William Gibson in a fantasy novel entitled *Neuromancer* to describe the world of computers and the society that gathers around them.

CYBERSPEAK
The language of people who communicate in cyberspace.

DOMAIN
A machine (often with an online service, such as America Online and CompuServe) that is connected to the Internet and is listed in the Domain Name System (the Internet's equivalent to a phone book). Common domains in the United States are as follows:

com—business and commercial
edu—educational institutions
gov—government institutions
mil—military installations
net—network resources
org—other (typically nonprofit).

ELECTRONIC MAIL (E-MAIL)
Mail prepared on a computer and sent to someone else who has a computer.

GOPHER
A way to search for information on the Internet by use of a program that allows you to access a remote computer's files.

INTERNET
An international communication "network of networks" that globally links or extends a web of independent domains interconnected with round-the-clock high-speed dedicated telephone lines.

INTERNET ADDRESS
The way to identify mail to and from the sender and receiver. Mail is sent to your domain. To identify an individual, the format is *username@domain name*, for example, tomlake@aol.com (Tom Lake at America Online).

URL (UNIFORM RESOURCE LOCATOR)
An address for each page or file available on the World Wide Web. Examples are http:/www/usatoday.com and http:/thorplus.lib.purdue.edu/reference/index.html

WORLD WIDE WEB (WWW)
A multimedia system of commercial activity that is set up to view colorful magazine-style "pages" containing text, photographs, and sound.

As Tom Lichty of America Online states, "The WWW is to the Internet what the automobile is to a freeway. You might say it's just another conveyance for information, but it's quickly becoming the dominant one, and it's the one that has captured the allegiance, imagination, and enthusiasm of millions of Net users worldwide" (1995, p. 20). *The Web is the primary medium for commercial activity.*

HEALTH CARE PROVIDER CREDENTIALING AND QUALITY IMPROVEMENT

WHAT IS THE JOINT COMMISSION ON THE ACCREDITATION OF HEALTHCARE ORGANIZATIONS?

The mission of the Joint Commission on the Accreditation of Healthcare Organizations (JCAHO) is to "enhance the quality of health care provided to the public" (JCAHO, 1992). To accomplish this mission, the JCAHO conducts systematic and intensive surveys of hospitals and other health care institutions to determine whether accepted standards of structure, process, and outcome are being met. The question being asked is "Can this health care organization provide quality health care to its patients?"

The survey and accreditation process the JCAHO uses is an intensive procedure, and the accreditation the JCAHO delivers is important to health care agencies. Many third-party payers, including Medicare, will only reimburse hospitals that are accredited by the JCAHO. The most favorable accreditation the JCAHO gives is valid for 3 years.

The arrival of the JCAHO survey team is a time of excitement and anxiety for health care providers. The presence of the survey team provides the hospital or health care agency an opportunity to display the programs and systems the institution has in place to deliver quality patient care. Accompanying this positive experience is the worry that the JCAHO may find a deficit in the health care program, which may result in failure to receive accreditation. Usually the hospital spends a year preparing for the visit by conducting mock surveys and reviewing and revising current practice. JCAHO maintains a free, direct consultation phone line to assist health care providers in clarifying and interpreting existing standards.

WHAT IS QUALITY ASSURANCE?

When asked, "Is nursing a profession?" most nurses will shake their heads up and down, emphatically responding "Yes" to the question. But inherent to professionalism is a dedication to providing quality service to a consumer (Walsh and Bernhard, 1981). Nursing efforts to monitor and improve patient care services are often recognized as *quality assurance*, *quality improvement*, or *quality evaluation*. Today these programs, whatever they are titled, are nursing's method of monitoring and improving consumer-oriented services, a giant step toward professionalism. Quality assurance is a process of evaluating outcomes of care and ensuring that each patient receives a predetermined high standard of care. This process is illustrated in Figure 15-3.

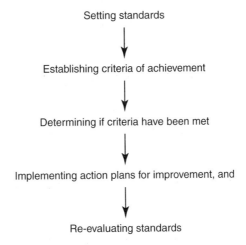

Setting standards

↓

Establishing criteria of achievement

↓

Determining if criteria have been met

↓

Implementing action plans for improvement, and

↓

Re-evaluating standards

FIGURE 15-3
Quality assurance.

Quality assurance is usually developed within an organization program unique to each institution. The program generally encompasses a philosophy of quality assurance, methods for accomplishing the process, time lines, and report format. However, the purpose of any quality improvement program must be focused on measuring and improving nursing care to patients.

To the recent graduate, the word *quality* can seem unconnected to measurement and void of any tangible context. But to consumers, *quality* means hospital cleanliness, accurate billing statements, courteous environment, nurse competency, available medical specialists, and low mortality rates. With health care consuming a larger percentage of the gross domestic product, health care professionals and consumers alike are becoming cost-conscious and quality-outcome–oriented (Miraldo, 1991).

The JCAHO has been a leader in demanding evidence of the provision of quality care. The current nursing standards address "the monitoring and evaluation of the quality and appropriateness of the patient care provided by all members of the nursing staff." This standard specifically requires nursing staff members to identify quality issues for each unit, methods for monitoring these issues, and methods for evaluating the outcomes. Such requirements have special implications for the recent graduate in terms of receiving adequate orientation to an agency's quality improvement program and expectations of the nurse concerning his or her participation in quality improvement methods. Today most quality improvement activities are unit-based and require intense staff nurse involvement. This situation is as it should be, because the nurse on the unit is the one who can best detect and quantify patient needs and outcomes.

Quality improvement approaches offer three perspectives from which to evaluate nursing care provided: structure, process, and outcome. Health care institutions' quality improvement methods usually contain a combination of all three perspectives to provide comprehensive quality care. The *structural* perspective encompasses evaluating the physical environment, organizational structure, and licensure of health care providers.

The *process* perspective examines what is actually being done for the patient. Standards of care as developed by the American Nurses Association, standardized plans of care, or written care plans represent what the nurse should be doing in collaboration with the patient and colleagues. These plans of care are necessary to ensure that each patient receives at least a minimum standard of the nursing product.

The *outcome* perspective highlights changes in the patient's health status. This perspective has gained momentum over the past few years, and quality improvement efforts are now being concentrated on documenting patient outcomes. Evidence of patient improvement, satisfaction, knowledge of health deviation, and compliance is a major focus of quality improvement methods. This perspective is purported to be difficult for nurses to measure because many patient outcomes are influenced by numerous health care professionals. However, creative nurses are constantly developing methods for examining the outcomes of their interventions.

WHAT ARE QUALITY IMPROVEMENT METHODS?

Quality improvement methods differ from institution to institution in terms of what is examined and how it is examined. However, the approaches are similar for determining quality nursing care efforts. Quality improvement manuals include the philosophy and objectives of the institution's program. Specific methods for reporting quality measurement results and feedback are also outlined in the manual. The results of quality assurance and the method used for obtaining feedback are dependent on the organizational framework and management philosophy. Indicators of care or problems associated with nursing care can then be identified, most often by the practicing nurse. Methods of determining the severity of the problem or indicators are devised. These methods include chart audits, questionnaires, surveys, and reviews. To ensure accuracy of measurement, efforts need to be directed at determining the reliability and validity of the measurement tools.

A threshold, or cutoff point, is determined for each indicator.

For example, if a unit or agency is measuring skin integrity, the threshold may be set at 3%, indicating that no more than 3% of the patient population at any given time will show evidence of skin breakdown; if patient knowledge of discharge medications is being examined, a high threshold, such as 96%, would be set to indicate that, at any time, 96% of the patient population will be knowledgeable concerning their medications prescribed on discharge.

In the past, auditing such indicators was done randomly; now, continuous evaluation is being advocated so that prompt action can be taken to identify the problem early and make plans to correct it. Once measurement has occurred and deficits have been identified, action plans are written and implemented to eliminate the problem. The creative genius of practicing nurses is once again called upon to develop methods for eliminating the problems and aligning the indicator measure to the preset thresholds.

In the future, an anticipated 70% of patient care will be given in the home. This means that nurses in the hospital will be seeing only the most critically ill patients. When those patients are ready to leave the intensive care units and the intermediate care units, instead of going to the general floor unit they may go to another facility, similar to what are called *nursing homes* in Great Britain. This part of the British model of care has been in place for many years and has been reviewed, not only by the United States but also by Canada, as an improved approach to providing care. Skilled-nursing facilities care for patients who are in various stages of recovery from injury or disease. Frequently these are the older patients with one or more conditions that may or may not be related to the primary acute condition. Approximately 65% to 75% of patients receiving care in a skilled-nursing facility are Medicare recipients. This is a less-expensive alternative to hospitalization in an acute-care hospital. Managed-care organizations are using these settings to control health care costs and continue to meet the needs of the patient (Levenson, 1998).

Preventive medicine and *preventive care* are the buzzwords of the future. Instead of waiting until someone is ill and needs hospitalization or emergency treatment, emphasis will be on preventing disease and keeping people in a state of wellness. Increased emphasis will also be placed on nutrition and exercise. Lifestyles will change. The graying of America is also going to continue to affect health care. The senior citizens of the future will probably be different from those we have cared for in the past. Many of them are the yuppies of today and the baby boomers, who are already very conscious of their health and interested in legislation related to their health care. As the elderly population grows, there will be fewer people to provide the tax dollars to sustain the kind of programs that we have today. Medicare, for instance, will have to change. Not only will we have DRGs, we may have something that goes beyond them. For example, there could be a penalty assessed to individuals who do not practice good health habits. That is, you may have to pay a higher premium for your insurance if you smoke.

CONCLUSION

Graduates of nursing schools today stand on the threshold of a whole new world, and it is a very good world. The only limiting barriers will be those we erect ourselves. Just as Dorothy in *The Wizard of Oz* found that the tools she needed to positively control her life were talent and knowledge from within, so must we find within ourselves the resources to proactively address a rapidly changing culture.

Significant economic and social trends are dramatically altering the forms of health care delivery in the United States and the roles played by nurses in the delivery of that care. Advances in technology, globalization of culture and communication, ever-widening computer applications, aging of the population, and dynamic changes in the health care industry are among major developments. Hospital and health care organization mergers, consolidation of major health plans, and growth of managed care have created a highly competitive environment (Friedman, 1995).

To cope with and to contribute to the future of health care, nurses must understand how computers are now being used in health care, and they must be able to work with computers in a cost-effective manner in their nursing practice. They must also understand how the JCAHO evaluates health care providers, and they must be familiar with HMOs and the prospective payment system using DRGs.

No matter what delivery system is in place in a particular institution, nurses will find that each is vitally involved with ensuring quality and in discovering measurable ways of monitoring that quality. Processes for instituting and maintaining quality differ widely, but what they must have in common are a clear method by which standards are adopted, a reliance on unit-based checks on quality, and an objective means of remedying deficits. For a bright future in the delivery of health care, nurses well acquainted with economic and social trends, the latest models of delivery, and the means of ensuring quality care are going to have a tremendous impact on the continuing evolution of trends in nursing and overall health care.

The good news: "Working together—physicians, nurses, other providers, and consumers of health care—we have all the resources we need here on Earth. Meaningful health care reform, including better primary care, needs common sense, not superhuman rescue fantasies" (Fagin, 1992, p. 543).

The bad news: "In times of rapid change, experience is your own worst enemy" (J.P. Getty).

REFERENCES

American Nurse: In brief, *Am Nurse* 34(1):5, 2002.

Bureau of Labor Statistics: *1998-99 Occupational Outlook Handbook*, Bureau of Labor Statistics, OOHInfo;cabls.gov. February, 1999.

Burner ST, Waldo DR: National health expenditure projections, 1994-2005, *Health Care Financ Rev* 16(4):221-242, 1995.

Coile RC: Health care's future: rising costs and concerns, *Healthc Trends Transit* 2(5):6-11, 1991.

Curtin LL: Designing new roles: nursing in the '90s and beyond, *Nurs Manag* 21(2):7-9, 1990.

Dakins D, Kincade K: The best in the US: programs of excellent 1997, *Telehealth Magazine* (telemedmag. com/topics/bus5.htm).

Fagin CM: The myth of Superdoc blocks health care reform, *Nurs Health Care* 13(10):542-543, 1992.

Friedman MA: Issues in measuring and improving health care quality, *Health Care Financ Rev* 16(4):1-13, 1995.

Joint Commission on the Accreditation of Healthcare Organizations: *Accreditation manual for hospitals*, Chicago, 1992, JCAHO.

Karlgaard R: Good, bad news for tech, *Forbes* 15:22, 2001.

Levenson S.A:. Subacute settings: making the most of a new model of care, *Geriatrics*, 53(7):69-74, 1998.

Lichty T: *America Online's Internet*, ed 2, North Carolina, 1995, Ventana Press.

Marquis BL, Huston CJ: *Management decision making for nurses: 124 case studies*, ed 3, Philadelphia, 1999, Lippincott-Raven.

Miraldo PS: The nineties: a decade in search of meaning, *Nurs Health Care* 11(1):11, 1991.

Naisbitt J, Aburdene P: *Megatrends 2000*, New York, 1991, Morrow, William & Co.

Nucifora A: Despite all of the hype, Internet numbers add up, *Business J* 19(42):29, 1999.

Rubin, RM: Good news for business: health care inflation is down, *Business Perspect* 11(3): 24, 1999.

Schreiber C: Thinning ranks, *HealthWeek* 1(14):15, 1999.

Smith CM, Maurer FA: *Community health nursing: theory and practice*, Philadelphia, 1995, WB Saunders.

Tucker C: Marcus Web-ly, MD, *Southwest Airlines Spirit*, October, 40, 1999.

US Census Bureau: *Home computers and Internet use in the United States, August 2000*, Washington, DC, 2001, US Department of Commerce, US Census Bureau.

Walsh M, Bernhard LA: *Leadership: the key to the professionalization of nursing*, ed 1, New York, 1981, McGraw-Hill.

ADDITIONAL READINGS

American Nurses Association, National League of Nurses, American Association of Nurse Executives: *Nurses national health care plan*, New York, 1991, ANA.

Bittel LR, Newstrom JW, Manning GL: *What every supervisor should know: supervision in action: an in-basket simulation by Reese and Manning*, ed 1, New York, 1990, McGraw-Hill.

Curran CR: IDN core competencies: Nursing's role, *Nurs Econ* 13(4):192, 249, 1995.

Emmett A: Health care trends that will reshape nursing, *Nursing* 24(4):50-53, 1994.

Gobis LJ: Computerized patient records. Start preparing now, *J Nurs Adm* 24(9):15-16, 60, 1994.

Kerfoot KM: Nursing report cards—the nurse manager's challenge, *Nurs Econ* 13(4):248-249, 1995.

Lucente B et al: Redesigning care delivery in the community hospital. *Nurs Econ* 13(4), 242-247, 1995.

Marrelli TM: *The nurse manager's survival guide: practical answers to everyday problems*, ed 1, St. Louis, 1993, Mosby.

Melchor C: Nurses go on-line: using computers and networks to advance the profession, *Am Nurse* 27(2):16, 1995.

Turner G: ANA creates new on-line computer network for nurses, *Am Nurse* 27(3):3, 1995.

INTERNET RESOURCES

Here are some suggested search engines and related Web sites:

Informatics

American Medical Informatics Association
http://www.amia.org

Stanford Medical Informatics
http://www-camis.stanford.edu

Medical Computing Today
http://www.medicalcomputingtoday.com

Joint Commission on the Accreditation of Healthcare Organizations
http://www.jcaho.org

Here is a Web site with resources on PDAs:
http://library.osfsaintfrancis.org/nursingpda.htm

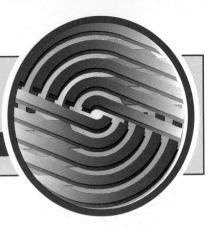

Nursing Informatics

JANET M. McLELLAN, RN, MSN, BC, NSA

"In all types of health care organizations, nursing is the hub of the information flow. Developing the science and technology of nursing informatics will enhance the information available to nurses for clinical practice, management, education, and research and will facilitate the role of nurses as communicators."

—*Patricia F. Brennan (1996), American Medical Informatics Association*

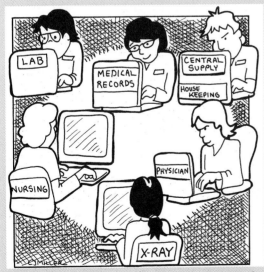

Nursing informatics—a specialty practice of nursing.

After completing this chapter, you should be able to:

■ Define nursing informatics.

■ Discuss the history of nursing informatics.

■ Describe several regulatory issues that affect the profession of nursing.

■ Discuss the necessity of using recognized taxonomies and nursing nomenclature in nursing documentation.

■ Describe what a nurse specializing in nursing informatics might do.

■ Discuss future trends in nursing informatics.

Computer automation is pervasive today. Everywhere we turn this technology is in evidence. The neighborhood grocery store has automated scanners and automated checkout lines. Your bank has automated tellers, check scanners, wire transfers, and online services. The local library has automated catalogs, interlibrary lending, and books online. From our homes, we can access the world through the Internet, researching any question, sending email, and purchasing just about anything through our personal computers (PCs). A litany of computerized marvels could fill volumes.

The explosion of new technology over the past twenty-five years that makes all this possible is truly phenomenal. What is even more incredible, and perhaps a bit frightening, is that this seems to be just the beginning. The time is coming, in the not-too-distant future, when the thoughts, communications, creations, manuscripts, learning material, and financial assets of the civilized world will exist primarily in electronic form. If the lights went out, civilization as we know it will cease to exist.

Health care is not immune. Some of the most complex automated systems and certainly some of the most complex requirements for these systems can be found in health care. Systems to serve the diverse needs of administration, patient management, finance, material management, billing and collections, decision support, managed care, nursing, operating room, emergency room, clinics, laboratory, imaging, intensive care, pharmacy, telemedicine, long-term care, home care, and physicians' offices need to be implemented and integrated across the continuum of care of modern health care organizations. As a result, the demand for health care professionals who are knowledgeable in the application of this technology is growing rapidly.

Even with technology all around us, we do not always feel comfortable with it. Technology is sometimes confusing, intimidating, and in large part because it changes so rapidly, downright bewildering. Despite these changes, there are some relative constants that make the field less confusing and easier to manage. One of the biggest challenges we face is how to properly harness and apply the available technology. The good news is that although the technology will continue to change and become more robust, the techniques used to apply the technology do not (Marreel and McLellan, 1999). The goal of this chapter is to explore how nursing is embracing, harnessing, and using this technology to increase the quality of patient care in all health care settings.

NURSING INFORMATICS

WHAT IS NURSING INFORMATICS?

In 1994, the American Nurses Association (ANA), recognized the field of nursing informatics (NI). The ANA has defined *informatics* as, "the activities involved in identifying, naming, organizing, grouping, collecting, processing, analyzing, storing, retrieving or managing data and information" (ANA, 1994). They have defined *nursing informatics* as a specialty that "integrates nursing science, computer science, and information science in identifying, collecting, processing, and managing data and information to support nursing practice, administration, education, research, and the expansion of nursing knowledge" (ANA, 1994). With the advent of clinical information systems, the electronic medical record has become the ultimate goal of health care organizations. The integration of 100% of all patient data in one record may not be realistic at present, but the nursing informatist plays an important part in moving the organization toward this goal.

Information is power. Lindberg and Humphreys (1995) stated that, "the effective practice of medicine is dependent on the ability of health professionals to locate relevant information quickly and to interpret it correctly." The study of nursing data, information, and knowledge—NI—is an integral part of the science of nursing and not a branch of computer science (Graves, Corcoran-Perry, 1996). Hannah, Ball, and Edwards (1994) defined NI as

> the use of information technologies in relation to those functions within the purview of nursing, and that are carried out by nurses when performing their duties. Therefore, any use of information technologies by nurses in relation to the care of their patients, the administration of health care facilities, or the educational preparation of individuals to practice the discipline is considered nursing informatics.

So, what does this mean? What does a nurse specializing in NI do on a daily basis? How does one become an expert in this unique field of nursing? What are the core competencies for NI?

WHAT IS THE BACKGROUND OF AN NI NURSE?

How does one begin? If a nurse were interested in computer technology, what would they need to know before they began looking into a NI position? Box 16-1 has a list of core competencies devised for a specialist in nursing informatics.

Qualifying for this list could be a bit overwhelming, but taken one step at a time, it is obtainable. There are a variety of journals, books, and seminars to assist in this endeavor. Local college classes may be available to expand knowledge of basic technology. Gaining the additional information and experience of a second profession makes the NI very valuable in the marketplace, because they have expertise in two unique environments.

WHAT ABOUT THE CERTIFICATION PROCESS?

In 1994 the American Nursing Credentialing Center provided a method for nurses to become certified in this specialty. A specialist in NI has a strong clinical background but usually has ceased giving direct patient care. Their focus is to improve patient care with healthcare automation that encourages caregivers and physicians to make more accurate and timely decisions. Box 16-2 lists the qualifications necessary to take the national NI Specialist certification examination.

The examination covers the following areas of expertise:

- System analysis and design.
- System implementation and support.
- System testing and evaluation.

- Human factors.
- Computer technology.
- Information/database management.
- Professional/practice/trends and issues.
- Theories.

A nurse interested in taking the Nursing Informatics certification examination should contact the American Nursing Credentialing Center. They will mail an application packet, providing an application form, sample questions, list of study sources, information on exam fees, and a list of approved proctored testing sites. This can be a fairly lengthy process as one must return the application and wait for processing; then an admission ticket is mailed back to the applicant if approved and only then can an appointment for testing be made. Depending on how busy the proctoring center is, it may take weeks to get an appointment. So, it is important to plan ahead.

This examination demands a good deal of preparation and research. The American Nursing Credentialing Center has compiled a list of books and literature from which the exam questions are taken. These are useful for study. Your hospital or specialty

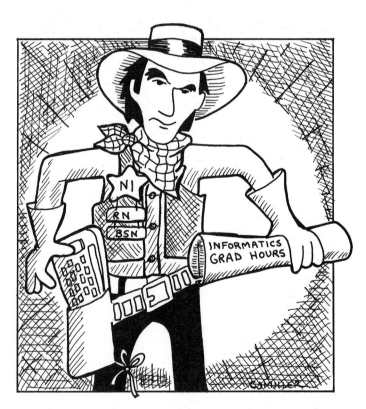

The new nurse entrepreneur in the competitive field of nurse informatics.

BOX 16-1   Core Competencies for a Specialist in Nursing Informatics

A nursing informatics specialist must have a good understanding of:

- ❏ The basic 'tools' and terminology of the trade; she must also have some experience with computers and information technology.
- ❏ How information technology can help with decision making and strategic planning at the executive level.
- ❏ How to actively and effectively participate in the evaluation, selection, implementation, and maintenance of a health care organization's information system.
- ❏ What information technology as an interdepartmental process means to the nursing department as a whole.
- ❏ The important role nursing data must play in the development or selection of a hospital information system.
- ❏ How computers and telecommunications technology can be used for staff development and clinical practice enhancement.
- ❏ How decision support systems can be used for strategic planning.
- ❏ The ethical issues regarding information technology, security, and confidentiality.
- ❏ How to evaluate, select, and manage the services of information technology consultants.
- ❏ How to use information technology for data collection for regulatory compliance.
- ❏ Market forces, vendor-marketing techniques, and emerging technologies for future decision making (Simpson, 1994, p. 18).

BOX 16-2   Qualification Criteria for Nursing Informatics Specialist Certification Examination

- ❏ Currently hold an active registered license in the United States or its territories and
- ❏ Hold a baccalaureate or higher degree in nursing: and
- ❏ Have practiced as a licensed registered nurse for a minimum of 2 years and meet the following in their current practice:
- ❏ Have practiced at least 2000 hours in the field of informatics nursing within the past 5 years or
- ❏ Have completed at least 12 semester hours of academic credits in informatics in a graduate program in nursing and have practiced a minimum of 1000 hours in informatics nursing within the past 5 years and
- ❏ Have had 20 contact hours of continuing education applicable to the specialty area within the past 2 years. Documentation of continuing education must be submitted. Author/presenter credits are allowable but can account for not more than half of the contact hour requirement. Author's work must be in a refereed publication. Combinations of continuing education and academic credit hours are acceptable. Contact hour credit will be allowed for attendance at professional meetings that include content appropriate to informatics nursing practice. Independent study, which has been approved for continuing education or academic credit, is also allowed (American Nursing Credentialing Center, 1995).

library should have a copy of these resources. If not most are available through Internet bookstores.

WHAT IS INVOLVED IN SYSTEM ANALYSIS AND DESIGN?

Health care first saw computer systems in the 1960s, which were introduced to assist in reimbursement concerns and primarily supported the financial department with charge capture and communication support. During the 1970s, the first hospital-wide information systems were offered. Although many products have evolved during the last 40 years, health care information systems continue to address the following issues and are striving to accomplish perfection in these areas:

- Support of clinical decision making with use of predetermined rules.
- Support of systems integration and external connectivity, sharing data throughout the institution, and having secure links with outside databases.
- Support of universal nomenclature and vocabularies.
- Support of theoretical frameworks specific to caregivers' scope of practice in the healthcare environment.
- Decrease or elimination of redundant data entry.
- Easy access to all archival data.
- Easy access to ergonomically safe workstations for data input.

NEEDS ASSESSMENT

Before a health-care organization can actually select a new software product they must decide what the needs of the organization are. There are several sources to consider. The main ones would include the following:

- The strategic plan of the organization.
- The information management plan.
- Departmental strategic plans.

An evaluation of current systems should be conducted. Documentation of strengths and weaknesses of the current methods and systems is necessary; in other words, "what are we currently doing well; what are we currently not doing well?"

In addition to strengths and weaknesses, organizational capabilities needed in the future should be considered. These capabilities are beyond the abilities of the systems and procedures currently in place. An extension of current capabilities may involve one or a combination of the following:

- Additions to existing systems.
- Interfaces between systems or software applications.
- Replacement of existing systems.
- Reorganization of personnel or physical workspace.
- Schedule changes.
- Forms redesign.
- Workflow modifications.

Once the capabilities and needs are identified, a document called the Request for Proposal (RFP) can be generated. This document is used to select the vendor, products, and services to be purchased. Although there are many formats, one that has proved effective contains eight sections (Box 16-3).

BOX 16-3   Request for Proposal

❏ Introduction
❏ Background information
❏ Future automation requirements
❏ General requirements for bidding
❏ System capability requirements
❏ Hardware and system software
❏ Vendor support
❏ System costs

Being familiar with clinical operations and information technology is essential to investigating and writing a good RFP. This document becomes the guide to the entire implementation process. The vendors must be held to their answers. The organization can use it to negotiate the system contract.

Once the RFP has been sent out, answered, received back, and scored, the finalists are revealed. Either off-site or on-site vendor demonstrations are conducted so users can view the functionality first-hand. It is imperative for the project team to control the demonstrations. Sending the vendor a list of questions or scenarios to demonstrate helps to guide them. Some vendors have been known to present a sales demonstration of 'vapor ware'—programs and functions that are in the minds of the programmers, but not on the shelf ready for use. Beware.

A NI specialist could facilitate any or all of this preparatory work: the needs assessment, the documentation of the RFP, and the coordinating of on and off-site demonstrations. It is imperative that a liaison be involved bringing the needs of both the clinical and technical sides of the healthcare organization to the attention of the administration and the vendor.

WHAT IS INVOLVED IN SYSTEM IMPLEMENTATION AND SUPPORT?

Planning the Project. The NI specialist may be responsible for the planning and implementation of a purchased clinical information system. It is important to follow the nine following steps in sequence when doing project planning:

- Define the project boundaries.
- Break project into manageable pieces.
- List activities.
- Identify important milestones.
- Estimate activity duration.

- Assign dependencies between tasks.
- List available resources.
- Define expectations of all involved.
- Never set target dates until all tasks have been estimated and assigned.

Organizing the Project. Implementation management involves much more than putting a plan together and monitoring its progress. A good project leader understands the principles of time management and is skilled in running an effective meeting. The mastery of several project management tools is necessary (Critical Thinking Box 16-1). Knowledge of basic system tools might include the following:

- A word-documenting tool.
- A project-management tool.
- An e-mail/communication tool.
- A slide-presentation tool.

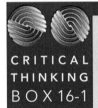

CRITICAL THINKING BOX 16-1

What experience have you had with management tools, such as e-mail, slide presentations, and so forth?

Managing the Project. Usually the project naturally falls out as smaller subprojects. Experts from the user community are useful on project teams. Within each of these smaller projects, team charters, meeting times, agendas and minutes, outstanding issues and next steps lists must be addressed and monitored by the team lead and the overall project leader. Meetings should be facilitated efficiently and on time. Each meeting should have objectives and goals to be met.

Milestones are identified and dates are monitored. It is necessary to be realistic in project timeframes, as there are always unforeseen issues that arise. If there is not a realistic time to start with, there is no chance at all of success.

System Testing and Evaluation. Each new or revised system must be tested to ensure that all data elements are processed correctly and that the outputs end up at the correct place. It is standard practice to do three levels of testing new software (Saba and McCormick, 2001). These are:

- Unit Testing—The actual programmers conduct this as the code is programmed. They are testing to make sure the programming protocols are being followed and the program does what is requested.
- Alpha Testing—This is the first testing of new software. It occurs within the development organization. It takes place in a development lab, and focuses on the correct execution of the application. It is common to use 'fake' patient data during this phase.

- Beta Testing—Occurs at the first patient site. The software is not yet ready for sale commercially, but it is necessary for the vendor production team to work with an actual real-life situation to test functionality. After the software 'passes' this testing, it is said to be 'ready for the shelf.'

You may have heard the term *beta testing* with regard to NCLEX developing a new generation of test items. It is very much the same process, checking software/test question before implementing them as part of the test plan.

After a software package is purchased, it is advised that the organization perform three more levels of testing, as follows:

- Functional Testing—Departments run tests to verify databases, files, and tables to ensure quality data. The department runs reports to check accuracy and validity. This testing may be repeated until the department has confidence that the data is 'coming across correctly.'
- Integrated System Testing—This occurs when all departments have completed their functional testing. During this phase, the total system is tested including interfaces between all 'standalone' systems and the new software. This testing mimics the actual 'live' environment in terms of volume of transactions, number of users, the interfaced systems, and the procedures to be used. In addition, the department policies and procedures and downtime procedures must be tested.
- End-user training—Because training occurs with all end-users, there will still be 'issues' that have not been found. Evaluation of these problems and correction is an ongoing process.

The NI specialist could be involved in all on-site testing. Developing meaningful testing scenarios is very important and should fall within their expertise. If the healthcare organization is engaged in beta testing, the NI may be called upon to do testing at that level also.

The Evaluation Phase. The evaluation phase reviews the new systems performance in detail. Utilizing the critical elements and functionality outlined in the RFP summarizes the expectations of the system. By conducting a thorough evaluation of the applications in detail, strengths and weaknesses are identified leading to system revisions and an ultimately better system (Marreel and McLellan, 1999).

WHAT HUMAN FACTORS NEED TO BE CONSIDERED REGARDING HEALTH CARE INFORMATION SYSTEMS?

Overall System Characteristics. The NI specialist must consider human factors when assisting with the purchasing and implementing a health care information system. Zielstorff, Hudgings, and Grobe (1993) developed the following list of important considerations:

- The system must be able to accommodate a variety of data-capture methods.
- Data-capture methods must be no more time-consuming than manual methods.
- Nursing process and vocabulary must be consistent across the health-care organization
- Interface design must be consistent across all legacy systems
- Connections to other existing systems—either internal or external to the agency—should appear 'seamless' to the user.

Ergonomics. Many of today's jobs are performed at a computer work area, often in a "shared" workstation. This is the case in a hospital setting, where nurses, physicians and every kind of ancillary caregiver use the nursing station 24 hours a day. This could number in the dozens of workers who use the same PC almost constantly. Change, variation, and adjustment to fit the individual are basic to the well-being of workers (Franchi and Fleck, 1994). Workstations should accommodate users of many different heights, weights, and individual needs. Computer vendors must keep in mind that the average age of a nurse is creeping toward the mid-40s, and letter size and font, proper lighting, and fewer shadows are vitally important to aid in viewing computer screens.

The successful ergonomic design of an office workstation depends on several interrelated parts. The task, the posture, and the work activities all interact (Marreel and McLellan, 1999). The three activities alone can be difficult to deal with, but these activities also must interact positively with existing furniture, equipment, and the environment. The combination makes the picture more complicated. Important parts of the workstation are as follow:

- The chair.
- The desk.
- The placement of the PC and keyboard.

The chair should be easily adjustable with strong lumbar supports. Usually wheels allow for easy movement and armrests may or may not be used, as they sometimes cause more problems than support.

The desk must be wide and deep enough to accommodate the PC footprint, keyboard, and mouse, with ample space around the machine to write, use the phone conveniently, and perform all other desktop activities.

The placement of the PC, keyboard, and mouse should be unique to every worker, but because this is highly unlikely, the monitor height should be approximately 18 to 22 inches above the desk surface, causing most users to view the screen with slightly lowered eyes. The keyboard should be placed directly in front of the user and the mouse on the user's dominant hand side of the machine. Some nursing stations designate some machines as 'left handed' mouse machines so as not to have to switch the mouse numerous times during a shift (Critical Thinking Box 16-2).

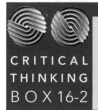

What is your workplace environment like? Does it take into consideration ergonomics? How could you make it better?

Poor workplace design is often the major source for cumulative trauma disorders. Cumulative trauma disorders have been associated with users who work for long periods of time at poorly constructed or poorly arranged workstations. Ergonomic design of work tasks can reduce or remove some of the risks. Other solutions may include the following:

- Information and training to workers about body positions that eliminate the opportunity for repetitive stress injuries to occur.
- Frequent switching between standing and sitting positions, reducing net stress on any specific muscle or skeletal group.
- Routine stretching of the shoulders, neck, arms, hands, and fingers has proved successful.

The NI specialist may be called upon to assist in the design and layout of a work area when installing a new system. Teaching and education of work area stretches and policies and procedures may fall to their area of expertise. It is necessary to understand the ergonomic principles to ensure the health of the staff working in this environment.

Computer Technology. The NI specialist must have a basic knowledge of how a computer works. Because this chapter has length limitations, the workings of a computer will not be covered in detail. It is important for the NI specialist to converse with the technology staff on an intellectual level. As an NI specialist gains experience with system implementation, training, testing, presenting, and facilitating knowledge in all these areas are important. There are many books available to gain basic computer technology information, in addition to a wealth of information on the Web (Critical Thinking Box 16-3).

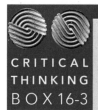

What has been your experience and exposure to the use of computer technology in the hospital? Your school? At home? Think of ways to become more familiar with the use of computer technology.

WHAT IS IMPORTANT TO UNDERSTAND ABOUT INFORMATION AND DATABASE MANAGEMENT?

In the past, the process of designing a database has been left to the information systems professionals. Why is it important for a NI specialist to understand information and database management? When reviewing the basic elements of an electronic medical record, it is important to be knowledgeable of all the places the data is stored and in what format it is accessible. Understanding database management allows for this.

The NI specialist would need to have an understanding of the two following types of databases (Hernandez, 1997):

- Operational databases—These are used wherever there is a need to collect, maintain, and modify data. This database stores dynamic data, which could change frequently. Examples would be inventory databases, order maintenance databases, and patient-tracking databases.
- Analytical databases—These are used to track historical and time-dependent data. This data would unlikely be modified. Examples would be chemical test databases and survey databases.

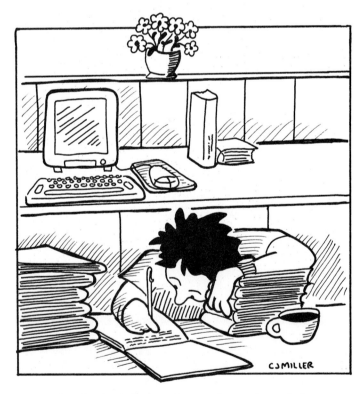

Even with technology all around us, we do not always feel comfortable with it.

The NI specialist would also need to be familiar with the following database models:

- Hierarchical database model.
- Network database model.
- Relational database model.

Although there is not space within this chapter to go into further detail, database management is imperative to understand the underlying design of the electronic medical record.

WHAT ARE SOME TRENDS AND ISSUES IN NURSING INFORMATICS?

Educational Opportunities. The acceptance of and urgent need for informatics preparation is evidenced by the dramatic increase in curriculum opportunities from universities and colleges around the country. These vary widely from graduate work to certification preparation and baccalaureate curriculum enhancements. There are still too few to meet the demand for this kind of education, but the ones that are well known are listed in Box 16-4.

BOX 16-4   Nursing Informatics Educational Programs

❑ University of Maryland
❑ University of Phoenix
❑ University of Utah
❑ New York University
❑ Duke University
❑ University of Iowa
❑ University of Arizona
❑ Northeastern University
❑ University of North Carolina–Chapel Hill

Regulatory and Accreditation Requirements. While there are many regulatory and governmental agencies instituting health care policy, Joint Commission on Accreditation of Healthcare Organizations (JCAHO) and Health Insurance Portability and Accountability Act (HIPAA) are two to take notice of. The NI specialist must have a clear understanding of these regulations to be able to guide the organization within these boundaries. To stay abreast of new regulations being signed into law and changes to existing regulations requires a constant effort.

HIPAA. In 1996 the HIPAA was developed. These standards are designed to ensure that health care organizations collect the right data in a common format so that they can share the data (Simpson, 2001). The major areas of impact from this regulatory legislation are as follow:

- Health Information Privacy Law.
- Data Security Standards.
- Electronic Transactions Standards.

Although some of the sections continue to be negotiated and final outcomes are yet to be determined, the privacy standards have been approved. Full compliance for these standards will be necessary by April 2003. Among many requirements, health care entities must adopt written privacy policies and procedures that define how they intend to abide by the highly complex regulation and protect individually identifiable health information. Each health care organization must ensure that all staff members who have access to patient information have an understanding of the consequences of noncompliance (Gale Group, 2001).

In 1998 the Department of Health and Human Services proposed that "All health plans, health plan providers, and healthcare clearinghouses that maintain or transmit health information electronically will be required to establish and maintain responsible and appropriate safeguards to ensure the integrity and confidentiality of the information" (Health Care Financing Administration, 1998) (Critical Thinking Box 16-4).

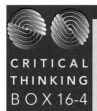

CRITICAL THINKING BOX 16-4

How has your clinical facility made changes to accommodate the Health Insurance Portability and Accountability Act (HIPAA) requirements?

JCAHO. The JCAHO wrote the Information Management (IM) Standards in the mid-1990s. The ten standards outline the need for Information Management regulation (Marreel and McLellan, 1999). These standards are as follows:

- IM 1—Planning: The planning process should include a thorough needs assessment. This standard states that the assessment should be comprehensive, but keep in mind, it should be appropriate to the needs and goals of the overall organization.
- IM 2—Security/Confidentiality: These standards deal with security, confidentiality, and integrity of data and information in the health care setting. With the advent of automated systems, networks, facsimile machines, photocopying machines, modems, answering machines, and so on, policies must be in place to ensure that the security and confidentiality of data are maintained.
- IM 3—Data Uniformity/Record Review: Consistency of data gathering and documentation throughout the organization is very important. Whenever possible, the same format and method of gathering should be maintained on forms, minimum data sets, histories and physicals, data definitions, and abbreviations. Cross-referencing software products with existing hard copies can be a maintenance issue, but it is necessary.

- IM 4—Training: This standard deals with the training of appropriate health care staff in the principles of information management. It is vitally important to recognize the strengths and weaknesses of the data being captured and analyzed.
- IM 5—Data Transmission: Data transmission deals with the consistency of forms, field definitions, codebooks, and standardization of things like interfaces, screen designs, data dictionaries, and data-entry policies and procedures.
- IM 6—System Integration: It is important to be able to combine information from several different systems in a meaningful way. Many hospitals have standalone systems for laboratory, radiology, pharmacy and so on. The systems integration standard makes this a priority.
- IM 7—Medical Record: The JCAHO is very interested in the medical record. It reviews what information is being kept in the record and also, who is putting it in, and whether the information serves the purpose of assisting in medical care decisions.
- IM 8—Aggregated Data: Basically, *aggregate data* refers to data from large numbers of medical records to support research, analyze trends, or support performance improvement activities. All health care organizations are required to submit information to state and federal agencies.
- IM 9—Library Services/Needs Assessment: Knowledge-based information includes journals, reference materials, and research data. Every health care organization is required to have access to current information. Every year a needs assessment is required to ensure that the correct information is available to health care providers, patients, and families.
- IM 10—Reference Databases: External databases are necessary for performance comparisons. The sharing of data for specific diseases or diagnosis, procedures, management, investigational drugs and devices, quality improvement, purchasers and payers, and state agencies is beneficial to all, but there must be policies and procedures ensuring safety and confidentiality of patient data.

The JCAHO sends out a team of experts every 3 years for a review of every health-care organization. This team inspects and reviews a variety of areas within each organization. The NI specialist may be called on to lead the effort for preparing the IM Standards for the JCAHO visit and for maintaining ongoing compliance (Critical Thinking Box 16-5).

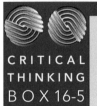

CRITICAL
THINKING
B O X 16-5

Have you had the opportunity to be in clinical during a Joint Commission on Accreditation of Healthcare Organizations visit? If so, what did you observe? How was the staff prepared for the visit?

Ethics.
Privacy and Confidentiality. Every health care organization has a responsibility to itself, to its patients, and to the community at large to have good control of its

information systems. Because the internal workings of healthcare rely on accurate and timely data and information, personal data about employees and patients must be kept safe and confidential. A corporate security plan is important to an organization.

Maintaining confidentiality implies a trust of the individuals that handle that data and information. These healthcare workers ensure the privacy of this information and use it only for the purpose for which it was disclosed.

Security policies must be explicit and well defined. Confidentiality agreements should be reviewed and signed upon hire and yearly there after. Breeches of security, confidentiality, or privacy should be dealt with quickly and the offender should be charged accordingly. Every lapse should be treated openly and made an example for others to note. The NI specialist may be involved in this process and the writing of the policies and procedures. Because this is outlined in both JCAHO and HIPAA standards, the NI specialist must be aware of the importance of these topics to the health care organization.

WHAT ARE SOME THEORIES—INFORMATICS NURSING CONCEPTS?

Nomenclature, Classification, and Taxonomy. Nursing nomenclature offers a recognized systematic classification and consistent method of describing nursing practice. Nomenclatures act as descriptors or labels, classifications groups, or class entities, whereas taxonomy is the study of the classifications.

In 1999 the American Nurses Association recognized the following nursing practice classification systems (Beyea, 1999):

- North American Nursing Diagnosis Association (NANDA) Approved List of Diagnostic Labels.
- Nursing Intervention Classification (NIC).
- Nursing Outcomes Classification (NOC).
- The Omaha Systems.
- Home Health Care Classification.
- Ozbolt's Patient Care Data Set (Critical Thinking Box 16-6).

If the unique nomenclature of these classification systems is used consistently, gathered data elements could be captured, stored, and manipulated accurately in the electronic medical record. Without a common language, data cannot be aggregated into useful language (Simpson, 2000). This need for consistency causes problems for software vendors as they attempt to produce unique and robust software packages but

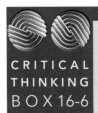

CRITICAL THINKING BOX 16-6

What has been your experience or exposure to these different practice classification systems? What does your clinical agency use?

need to use the recognized labels and groupings of nursing practice elements. So, what happens?

Currently each software vendor uses a unique patented naming convention for their specific functionality and then must "explain and define" these names and labels in their literature or presentations by relating them back to recognized nursing practice or data elements. This causes confusion to the user community.

The American Nurses Association Committee for Nursing Practice Information Infrastructure requires that classifications or languages meet certain criteria, including:

- The language provides a clinical useful terminology and rationale for development.
- The language consists of clear and unambiguous terms.
- The developer provides evidence of reliability, validity, and utility.
- The language includes a unique identifier for each item.

Each of these classifications or languages has made a unique contribution to the knowledge development in nursing. Learning about and working with standardized nursing languages will ensure nursing contributions are an integral part of any electronic medical record. Understanding those contributions through research and teaching will help to further define the scope of nursing practice. Standardized classifications or language, teaching, clinical practice, and research must be interrelated as nursing moves forward (Warren and Bickford, 1999).

Systems Theory. From the inception of NI during the 1990s, General Systems theory has served as a conceptual framework. The systems theory consists of the six following elements:

- Interdependent parts—Elements of the system that interact for processing.
- Input—Any outside element or factor that is brought into the system.
- Process—The activity within the system.
- Output—Any product that is produced from the processing activity.
- Control—Rules or procedures within the system.
- Feedback—Reusing output from the system as input back into the system for validation or correction.

This theory organizes interdependent parts working together to produce a product that none used alone could produce. Nursing Informatics uses this theoretical foundation for analysis and design, implementation and support, and testing and evaluation of automated systems. It is used as a basis for decision making, education curriculum needs, and system and project management.

Change Theory. Change is always occurring; sometimes it is planned and sometimes it happens quite unexpectedly. The effects of change range from positive to negative, from minor to major, from predictable to unpredictable. Our healthcare organizations are in constant change. With the advent of computers and new technology, nurses and caregivers are being forced to use this technology. By understanding the theory of change, it offers a foundation and approach to assist nurses and caregivers in the inevitable change that will occur with the implementation of a clinical information system. (See Chapter 5 for a discussion of the change process.) New methods always bring questions; what new responsibilities will there be? Will the education be enough to make the transition easy? Will there be additional pay, due to the increase in the necessary technology knowledge?

It is common for the NI specialist to be called upon to answer some of these questions. They act as a role model for the nursing and caregiver users, as they themselves have moved from a clinical background to being very comfortable in a technical environment. The NI specialist faces many challenges in daily activities, being in a position that might require the wearing of many hats and the bearing many responsibilities. This is a very exciting and rewarding nursing specialty that will continue to expand and grow well into the future.

SUMMARY

Computer technology is everywhere. The blending of computer technology with nursing science has developed this exciting, newly emerging field within health care. As a relatively new specialty, the American Nurses Association has developed a certification for nursing informatics. Core competencies include a good understanding of certain tools, the decision-making processes, and evaluation. Nursing needs to be actively involved in maintaining the information, establishing care standards, and working for better ways to improve quality care through technology.

> This is nursing's opportunity to have a positive impact on the way data are handled within the health care field.

REFERENCES

American Nurses Association: *The scope of practice for nursing informatics*, Washington, DC, 1994, ANA.

American Nurses Credentialing Center: *Informatics certification catalog*, Washington, DC, 1995, ANCC.

Beyea SC: Standardized language—making nursing practice count, *AORN J* 70(5):831-834, 837-838.

Franchi K, Fleck RA: Ergonomic improvements in the office environment, *Bus Horiz* 37(2):75, 1994.

Gale Group: HIPAA privacy rule takes effect, *Healthc Financ Manag* 55(6):9, 2001.

Graves JR, Corcoran-Perry S: The study of nursing informatics, *Image: Journal of Nursing Scholarship* 21:227, 1989.

Grohar-Murray ME, DiCroce HR: *Leadership and management in nursing*, ed 1, Norwalk, Conn, 1992, Appleton & Lange.

Hannah K, Ball M, Edwards M: *Introduction to nursing informatics*, New York, 1994, Springer-Verlag.

Health Care Financing Administration: *HHS proposes security standards for electronic health data* [press release]. August 11, 1998.

Hernandez MJ: *Database design for mere mortals*, Reading, Mass, 1997, Addison-Wesley.

Lindberg D, Humphreys B: *An emerging framework: data system advances for clinical nursing practice*, Washington, DC, 1995, American Nurses Publishing.

Marreel RD, McLellan JM: *Information management in health care*, New York, 1999, Delmar.

Saba VK, McCormick KA: *Essentials of computers for nurses: Informatics for the new millennium*, ed 3, New York, 2000, McGraw-Hill.

Simpson RL: Nursing informatics core competencies, *Nurs Manage* 25(5):18, 20, 1994.

Simpson RL: A systems view of information technology, *Nurs Adm Q* 24(4):80, 2000.

Simpson RL: Size up the big three, *Nursing Manage* 32(3):12, 2001.

Warren JJ, Bickford C: *ANA recognized nursing data sets, classification systems, nomenclatures.* Nursing Vocabulary Summit Conference, June 1999.

Zielstorff RD, Hudgings CI, Grobe SJ: *Next-generation nursing information systems: essential characteristics of professional practice*, Washington, DC, 1993, American Nursing Publishing.

ADDITIONAL READINGS

Azzarello J: Nursing informatics: could this new specialty be for you? *Home Healthcare Nurse,* Oct:634-641, 1999.

England DA: *Collaboration in nursing*, ed 1, Rockville, Md, 1986, Aspen.

White R: *How computers work*, Indianapolis, 1998, Que.

INTERNET RESOURCES

Computer-based Patient Record Standards
http://www.nursingworld.org/readroom/position/joint/jtcpri1.htm
Position paper from CPRI (the Computer-based Patient Record Institute, Inc.) endorsed by the American Nurses Association.

Authentication in a Computer-Based Patient Record
http://www.nursingworld.org/readroom/position/joint/jtcpri2.htm
Position paper from CPRI (the Computer-based Patient Record Institute, Inc.) endorsed by the American Nurses Association.

On Access to Patient Data
http://www.nursingworld.org/readroom/position/joint/jtdata.htm
Position paper from CPRI (the Computer-based Patient Record Institute, Inc.) and endorsed by the American Nurses Association.

American Nursing Informatics Association
http://www.ania.org

Online Journal of Nursing Informatics
http://cac.psu.edu/~dxm12/OJNI.html

Midwest Alliance for Nursing Informatics
http://www.maninet.org/index.asp

American Medical Informatics Association—Nursing Informatics Work group
http://www.amia-niwg.org

Nursing Informatics of the International Medical Informatics Association (IMIA)
http://www.imia.org/ni/index.html

Nursing World Informatics Links
http://www.nursingworld.org/rnindex/nit.htm

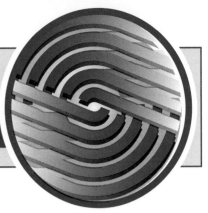

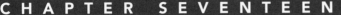

CHAPTER SEVENTEEN

Political Action in Nursing

BETTY J. SKAGGS, PhD, RN

One of the penalties for refusing to participate in politics is that you end up being governed by your inferiors.

—*Plato*

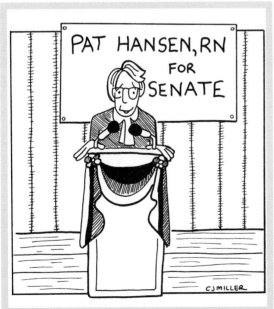

Nurses are playing a major role in the political process for planning the future of health care.

After completing this chapter, you should be able to:

■ Define *politics* and *political involvement*.

■ State the rationale for individual nurses' involvement in the political process.

■ List specific strategies needed to begin to affect the laws that govern the practice of nursing and the health care system.

■ Discuss different types of power and how each is obtained.

■ Describe the function of a political action committee.

■ Discuss selected issues affecting nursing:

   ■ Multistate licensure.

   ■ Nursing and collective bargaining.

   ■ Equal pay for work of comparable value.

Too often nurses feel the legislative process is associated with wheeling and dealing, smoke-filled rooms, and the exchange of money, favors, and influence. Many believe politics to be a world that excludes people with ethics and sincerity—especially given the controversies in past presidential administrations. Others think only the wealthy, ruthless, or very brave play the game of politics. It seems that the majority of nurses felt that the messy business of politicking should be left to others while they (nurses) did what they do best and enjoy most—take care of patients.

Today, however, more and more nurses are coming to realize that politics is not a one-dimensional arena, but a complex struggle with strict rules and serious outcomes. In a typical modern-day political struggle, a rural health care center may be pitted for funding against a major interstate highway. Certainly both projects have merit, but in times of limited resources not everyone can be victorious. Nurses now know that to influence the development of public policy in ways that affect the way we are able to deliver care, we must be engaged in the political process.

Cohen et al (1998) wrote that "the future of nursing and health care may well depend on nurses' skills in moving a vision. Without a vision, politics becomes an end in itself—a game that is often corrupt and empty" (p. 154). To demonstrate these skills, nurses must elect the decision-makers, testify before legislative committee hearings, compromise, and get themselves elected to decision-making positions. Nurses realize that involvement in the political process is a vital tool that they must learn to use if they are to carry out their mission (providing quality patient care) with maximum impact.

Depending on our political skills are "an estimated 14.0 percent of the population without health insurance coverage during the entire year in 2000" (US Government Census Bureau, 2001). These uninsured individuals (approximately 38.1 million) receive virtually no health care while countless other inadequately insured individuals receive health care only sporadically. Rural and inner-city residents have alarmingly high morbidity and mortality. Health care for rural citizens is virtually nonexistent. Although the situation is improving in some ways with managed care, even those fortunate enough to have insurance often experience problems accessing the care they need because of cost-cutting strategies.

Nurses' recognition of problems in the current health care system, combined with their commitment to the principle that health care is a *right* of all citizens, fuel their desire to become active in the political arena and to form a collective force to improve the health care system.

An example of the force and limitations of the nursing collective is evidenced in organized nursing's efforts to get a patient protection act through Congress. Similar legislation has been introduced yearly for the past several years; however, it has not yet passed. Several initiatives, such as allowing newly delivered mothers to stay in the hospital overnight if deemed necessary, have been successfully enacted in some states and local jurisdictions. However, to date, no major legislation has been passed on the federal level.

The legislation used in this example is S.B. 6 by Senator Daschle as presented in the 106th congressional session (1999-2000). This legislation, although oversimplified in this description, would, among other provisions, (1) provide access to individuals needing emergency care regardless of the specific terms of their health care coverage such as preauthorization, (2) require that quality-assurance measures be instituted to collect uniform quality data, and (3) establish certain parameters concerning the coverage information available to patients about the insurance plans and to ensure the privacy of individual health data.

In the course of this bill's progression through the Senate, the American Nurses Association President (at that time) Dr. Beverly Malone testified before the Senate Committee on Health, Education, Labor and Pensions (American Nurses Association, 2001). She eloquently addressed nursing's commitment to a broad-based patient protection act. Knowing that compromise language may need to be drawn, she spoke to nursing's support of specific points included in the bill and, at the same time, delineated our areas of disagreement. For example, she spoke of the importance of language that prohibited retaliation for health care professionals who advocate for their patients. Furthermore, she spoke of the importance of language that prohibits discrimination against any health care provider on the basis of type of licensure. That is, a patient protection bill must protect the consumers' right to choose any type of provider based on the service needed, not just medically provided care. On several occasions during the lobbying process, notices were sent through the association's legislative action network Nursing Strategic Action Team (N-STAT), instructing grass roots nurses to inform their senators of their views. Even though the bill did not garner the support necessary to be enacted that session, nursing was part of the process to shape the act and will see this policy enacted in the future. Note Figure 17-1, How Laws Grow—the final draft of the law may be totally different from the original intent.

Nursing will continue to lobby for new federal and state legislation that improves the quality and availability of nursing and health care.

WHAT EXACTLY IS POLITICS?

Politics, described as "influencing the allocation of scarce resources" (Leavitt and Mason, 1998, p. 9), is a vital tool that enables the nurse to "nurse smarter." Involvement in the political process gives an individual nurse a tool that augments his or her power—or clout—to improve the care provided to patients. Whether on the community, the hospital, or on the nursing unit level, political skills enable the nurse to identify needed resources, gain access to those resources, and overcome obstacles, thus facilitating the movement of the patient to higher levels of health or function. Let's look first at the nursing unit level:

> Your hospital is in the process of selecting a new supplier of widgets. You and the other nurses on your unit want to have input into that decision, because widgets are essential to the care of your patients and you have a definite opinion about the type of widget that works best. But the intensive care unit nurses, who are thought to be more important and valuable because the nursing shortage has made them as rare as hen's teeth, have the only nurse position on the review committee (and therefore, the director's ear!). You and the nurses on your unit strategize to secure input into this important decision.

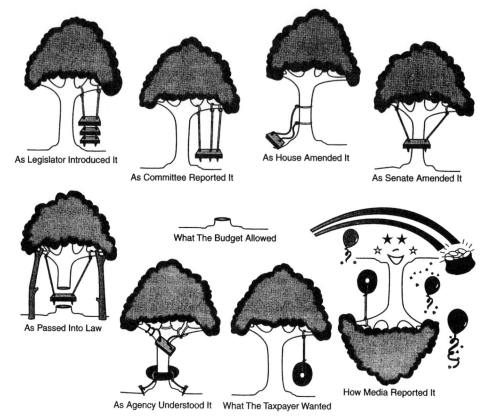

As Legislator Introduced It

As Committee Reported It

As House Amended It

As Senate Amended It

As Passed Into Law

What The Budget Allowed

As Agency Understood It

What The Taxpayer Wanted

How Media Reported It

FIGURE 17-1
How laws grow.

Your plan might look like this:

- Gather data about widgets—cost, suppliers, possible substitutes, and so on.
- Communicate to the head nurse and supervisor your concern about this issue and your plans to get involved in the decision (by using appropriate channels of communication).
- State clearly what you want—perhaps request a seat on the committee when the opportunity arises.
- Summarize in writing your request and the rationale, submitting it to the appropriate person(s).
- Establish a coalition with the intensive care unit nurses and other concerned individuals.
- Recall that the vice president for purchasing's mother was a patient on your unit and needed widgets in her care and be sure to include this example in your written request.
- Get involved with other hospital issues and contribute in a credible fashion (i.e., don't be a single-issue person).

WHAT OTHER STRATEGIES WOULD YOU SUGGEST?

This vignette illustrates what a politically astute nurse would do in this situation. Even though the example applies to a hospital setting, the strategies are comparable to those necessary for getting involved on a community, state, or even federal level. Practicing at the local level will provide good experience for larger issues—one has to start somewhere. Furthermore, a nurse involved on the local level will be able to hone her or his skills—gaining confidence in her or his ability to handle similar "exercises" in larger forums.

In the above example, the nurse was able to formulate several "political" actions to influence the outcome of the widget decision (Critical Thinking Box 17-1).

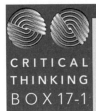

CRITICAL THINKING BOX 17-1

What are some issues in your school or hospital that are examples of political issues or the result of politics?

WHAT ARE THE SKILLS THAT MAKE UP A NURSE'S POLITICAL SAVVY?

Ability to Analyze an Issue (Those Assessment Skills Again!). The individual who expects to "influence the allocation of scarce resources" must do the homework necessary to be well informed. She or he must know all the facts relevant to the issue, how it looks from all angles, and how it fits into the larger picture.

Ability to Present a Possible Resolution in Clear and Concise Terms. The nurse must be prepared to coherently frame and present arguments in support of his recommendation. Preparation includes anticipating questions and objections so that a rebuttal will be logical and well developed.

Ability to Participate in a Constructive Way. Too often a person disagrees with a proposal being suggested to a hospital unit (or city council), but only gripes about it. The displeased individual seldom takes the time to study the problem or to understand its connection with other hospital departments (or city programs in a broader issue). Most important, the displeased person seldom suggests an alternate solution.

In short, if an individual's concern is not directed toward solving the problem, they will not be seen as a team player, but as a troublemaker. Constructive responses, perhaps something as simple as posing a single question such as "What solution would you suggest?" may help those involved think in positive terms and redirect energy to a more productive mode. Positive action can produce the kind of creative brainstorming that results in a solution.

Ability to Voice One's Opinion (Understand the System). Once the homework is done, let the *right* person know the determined opinion or solution. For example, the nurse might communicate concern and knowledge about the issue to the head nurse and supervisor. Of course, it is important to make an intelligent and well-informed decision about to whom it is best to voice one's opinion.

Having a confidant or mentor who knows the environment is one way to acquire this information. Another strategy is to use your listening skills. Simply standing back and listening are assets that will come in handy! Whatever the technique, studying the dynamics of the institution with all senses will help the nurse decide on the best person and the most appropriate way to communicate the proposed solution.

Ability to Analyze and Use Power Bases. While discussing issues with colleagues and studying the organization, be alert to the various power brokers. In the widget vignette, the nurse notes the VP of Purchasing is an obvious source of power in the hospital. She (the VP of Purchasing) will certainly concur with, if not make, the final decision. However, be aware that power does not always follow the lines on the organizational chart. The power of the nurse aide on the oncology unit who just happens to be the niece of the newly appointed member of the Board of Trustees may escape the notice of some. This person could be used to influence a decision if necessary. Similarly the fact that the VP of Purchasing's mother was on the unit should be filed in your memory for future use.

Facts may be facts, but where one gets information can sometimes make a statement as powerful as the information itself. Having the ability to use many different channels of information will give the nurse the power to choose among them.

WHAT IS POWER, AND WHERE DOES IT COME FROM?

Sanford (1979) describes five laws of power. She recommends that these laws be studied to identify strategies to develop power in nursing. The laws are as follows:

Law 1—Power Invariably Fills Any Vacuum. When a problem or issue arises, the prevailing desire is for peace and order. People are willing to give power to someone interested in restoring order to situations of discomfort. Therefore, someone will eventually step forward to handle the dilemma. It may be some time before the discomfort or unrest grows to heights sufficient for someone to take the lead. Even then, a poorly thought-out solution may be brought forward.

Nonetheless, a person exerting power will step forward to offer a solution. In some situations this person may be the previously identified leader, the head nurse, or the chair. More often there is an official power broker influencing the action. Know that there are opportunities to exert influence—for example, by taking the leadership role (i.e., stepping forward to fill the vacuum).

Law 2—Power Is Invariably Personal. In most instances, programs are attributed to an organization. For example, a fictitious program, *ImmunEYEs*, was proposed by the state and national children's and health associations. If one investigated, however, it might be found that the program began with a small group of friends talking over a pizza one evening, lamenting the number of infants still not immunized. In the course of their conversation, one might have said, "If we were to create a media blitz that would get the need for immunizations in the consciousness of parents—get the need for immunizations in their face!" And the next person might have said—in their eyes! "Yea, ImmunEYEs. Let's do it!"

Initiatives such as this start with one person creating a new approach to a problem. That person exercises power by providing the leadership or spark to create the strategy to carry out such an initiative, thus inspiring people to contribute to the effort.

Law 3—Power Is Based on a System of Ideas and Philosophy. Behaviors demonstrated by an individual as she or he exerts power reflect a personal belief system or a philosophy of life. That philosophy or ideal must be one that attracts followers, gains their respect, and rallies them to join the effort. Nurses have the opportunity to ensure that a patient's *right* to health care (versus privilege), access to *preventive* care, and similar values are reflected in policies and procedures.

Law 4—Power Is Exercised Through and Depends on Institutions. As an individual one can easily feel powerless and unable to deal with the complex problems facing a hospital, community, or state. But through a nursing service organization, a state nurse association, or a similar organization, that individual can garner the resources needed to magnify her power. The person-to-person network, the communication vehicle (usually an organization's newsletter or journal), and the organizational structure are established for precisely this function—to support and foster changes in the health care system.

Law 5—Power Is Invariably Confronted With and Acts in the Presence of a Field of Responsibility. Actions taken speak to the other nurses for whom nurses act and, most important, the patients for whom nurses advocate. The individual in the power position is acting on behalf of the group. Power is communicated to observers and is reinforced by positive responses. If the group thinks that its ideals are not being honored, the vacuum will be filled with the next candidate capable of the role and supported by the organization.

ANOTHER WAY TO LOOK AT POWER AND WHERE TO GET IT

In a classic much-referenced work, French and Raven (1959) describe five sources of power. They are (in order of importance): reward power, coercive power, legitimate power, referent or mentor power, and expert or informational power.

The strongest source of power is the ability to *reward*. The best example of making use of the reward power base is the giving of money. If, for example, one gives a decision-maker financial support for a future political campaign, the recipient will feel obligated to the donor and may from time to time "adjust opinions" to repay these obligations! Today, because caps have been placed on campaign contributions, the misuse of this type of reward has been reduced.

An additional source of reward-based political power is the ability to commit voters to a candidate through endorsements. This illustrates the importance of having a large number of members in an organization—in other words, a large voting bloc.

Second in importance is the power to *coerce* or "punish" a decision-maker for going against the wishes of an organization. The best example of this power, the opposite of *reward*, is the ability to remove the person from office at election time.

Third in importance is *legitimate* power, or the influence that comes with role and position. Influence derives from the status that society assigns individuals as a result of, for instance, old family money, membership in a respected profession, or a prominent position in the community. The dean in a school of nursing has a certain amount of influence just because of who she or he is. Right? A nurse's commitment to enhancing nursing's influence explains why we encourage and assist each other to achieve key decision-making positions—to build nursing's legitimate power base.

The fourth power base is that of *referent* or *mentor* power. This is the power that "rubs off" of influential persons. When representatives of the student body talk with the faculty about a problem they are having with a course and receive her or his support, the curriculum committee or dean is more likely to listen sympathetically than if the students were arguing only for themselves. The faculty, joining with the students to solve their problem, adds to the students' power. The wish to build this type of power encourages nurses to join coalitions, especially those including organizations with greater power than our own.

The last and weakest of the power bases is that of *expert* power. Nurses know about health and nursing care and are, therefore, able to impart knowledge in this area with great confidence and style. Typically nurses communicate this authority through letters written to legislators, testimonies presented in hearings, and through other contacts made on behalf of nursing and patients. Nurses do this well, but remember that this is the weakest source of power.

In summary, power is derived from various sources. Nurses use with the greatest frequency and ease the weakest of the power bases, that deriving from their expertise. Although this is an important power base, we must develop and exercise the other types as well. Only then will nurses realize the full extent of our potential (Critical Thinking Box 17-2).

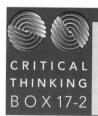

CRITICAL THINKING BOX 17-2

Who are the people in positions that reflect the different power levels in your school, hospital, and community?

NETWORKING AMONG COLLEAGUES

It has been said that one should never be more than two telephone calls away from a needed resource, whether it be a piece of information, a contact in a hospital in another city, or input into a decision one is about to make. The key to successful networking is consciously building and nurturing a pool of associates whose skills and connections augment your own.

As a recent graduate, one should begin the important task of networking by selecting an instructor from nursing school, one who is able to speak to your performance during nursing school. Ask this person if they would be willing to write a letter of reference for your first job. If she or he agrees, nurture this contact from now on. Keep this individual apprised of your whereabouts, your successes, and your plans for the future. This person will be an important link not only to your school, but also to your future educational and career undertakings. Then, at each future work site, find a head nurse or supervisor willing to write a reference and with whom to maintain contact. Keep building the network over your career.

Remember that this network must be nourished. Constant use of one's resources without reciprocation will exhaust them and make them unreliable sources of assistance in the future. But if properly cared for, this network will provide support for the rest of your career.

BUILDING COALITIONS

A coalition is a group of individuals or organizations that shares a common interest in a single issue. Groups with whom nurses might form coalitions are as diverse as the topics about which nurses are concerned. For example, nurses are concerned about and lobby for adequate, safe childcare, a safe environment, and women's issues. The numerous organizations interested in these diverse issues are potential candidates for a coalition with nursing organizations. It is not unusual, however, for two organizations to be in a coalition on one issue but adversaries on another. Indeed this is common in the political arena, where negotiations and compromises are the norm.

A warning: the selection of coalition partners should strengthen your cause or organization. Forming coalitions is a strategy to empower oneself. Therefore build coalitions with organizations enjoying greater power than nursing—not less (Critical Thinking Box 17-3).

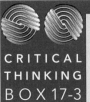

CRITICAL THINKING BOX 17-3

What are examples of nursing coalitions in your community or state?

WHAT ABOUT TRADE-OFFS, COMPROMISES, NEGOTIATIONS, AND OTHER TRICKS OF THE TRADE?

Politics is not a perfect art or science. In the heat of battle, nurses are often called on to compromise, but if they are unwilling to give on some principle, they sacrifice all.

To hold out for the ideal typically means that no progress toward the ideal will be realized. Often, changes in health care policies are achieved in incremental steps. However, the decision to compromise a value or principle must be carefully made with full realization of the implications—not an easy decision!

The political skills discussed so far apply to any situation, whether in a family, a hospital unit, or a community. The next part of the chapter will discuss skills that apply specifically to the governmental process.

HOW DO I GO ABOUT PARTICIPATING IN THE ELECTION PROCESS?

One key to successful political activity is involvement in the election process. This is the stage where one can get to know the candidates; they also get to know you. In addition, it is a time when one makes important contacts for that network (Box 17-1).

BOX 17-1   How Important Is One Vote?

In 1645 one vote gave Oliver Cromwell control of England.

In 1649 one vote caused Charles I of England to be executed.

In 1776 one vote gave America the English language instead of German.

In 1845 one vote brought Texas into the Union.

In 1868 one vote saved President Andrew Johnson from impeachment.

In 1875 one vote changed France from a monarchy to a republic.

In 1876 one vote gave Rutherford B. Hayes the presidency of the Nazi Party.

In 1941 one vote saved Selective Service—just weeks before Pearl Harbor was attacked.

Author unknown

From Goldwater, M., and Zusy, M. (1990). *Prescription for nurses: Effective political action.* St. Louis: C.V. Mosby, p. 31, with permission.

Getting involved in a candidate's campaign is simple. First study the positions to be filled. Then, with the help of the local nurses' association, the local newspaper, or the county or state Democratic or Republican Party, select the candidate whose views on health care most closely match yours. Next find the candidate's campaign headquarters. After this, contact the candidate's volunteer coordinator and see when volunteer help is needed. Most campaigns are crying for assistance with folding letters and stuffing envelopes, looking up addresses, and preparing bulk mailings. They will welcome you with great enthusiasm! Be sure to tell the campaign staff that you are a nurse and would be more than willing to contribute to the candidate's understanding of health care issues and to assist in drafting the candidate's positions on these issues (Critical Thinking Box 17-4).

Beware: involvement in campaigns and party organizations can lead to catching the political "bug." Victims of the political bug are overcome by a powerful desire to make changes in the system and see a multitude of opportunities to educate people

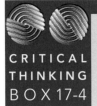

Who in your state government supports legislature that is pro-nursing and pro–health care?

about the health needs of a county, state, and nation. An example of two nurses who caught the bug: During a past national presidential election, the nurses at a state caucus volunteered to write the resolution for the party's position on health care, which, if passed, would become a plank in the platform. After much work drafting the statement and bringing it before various committees, they were ecstatic when it passed and became the health statement for their party! (Box 17-2)

BOX 17-2   Resolution Against Physician Abuse of Registered Nurses Passed by the 2001 Texas Nurses Association House of Delegates

Submitted by: Committee on Practice Issues
Category: Action
Rationale: Establishes action on issue of nursing shortage

Whereas, surveys and anecdotal information confirm that registered nurses experience verbal abuse as a routine part of their job and,

Whereas, of the thousands of nurses surveyed, it was found that 90% of nurses have experienced verbal abuse and most encounter an average of 5 incidents per month and,

Whereas, physicians are identified as regular perpetrators of verbal abuse and,

Whereas, registered nurses and the physician community recognize that it is a minority of physicians who engage in abuse of registered nurses and,

Whereas, the actions of this minority have negative consequences on the professional relationship between physicians and registered nurses and,

Whereas, verbal abuse is linked to increased turnover rates of nurses and,

Whereas, in professional work environments, registered nurses should not encounter such behavior and,

Whereas, in a nurse shortage environment, the profession cannot afford to lose even a single nurse to abuse and,

Whereas, nurses and physicians are called upon to be colleagues in the daily care of patients and communities and,

Whereas, the development of systems to increase patient safety, and manage chronic illness called for in the most recent Institute of Medicine Reports also require professional collegiality and,

(continued)

BOX 17-2   Resolution Against Physician Abuse of Registered Nurses Passed by the 2001 Texas Nurses Association House of Delegates (Cont'd)

Whereas, Texas Nurses Association is committed to Workplace Advocacy and the improvement of the workplace environment of registered nurses in Texas, therefore be it

RESOLVED, that the Texas Nurses Association make the elimination of physician abuse of registered nurses TNA's Eighth Commitment to Workplace Advocacy.

RESOLVED, that the Texas Nurses Association will advocate no less than a ZERO TOLERANCE of physician abuse of registered nurses.

RESOLVED, that the Texas Nurses Association work with employers of registered nurses in developing model policies against physician abuse of registered nurses.

RESOLVED, that the Texas Nurses Association work with the Texas Medical Association to promote adoption by the physician community of a ZERO TOLERANCE for registered nurse colleague abuse.

RESOLVED, that the Texas Nurses Association research and promote the use of strategies to support registered nurses who encounter abuse in the workplace such as:

✓ Code Nurse, a method that encourages nurses to drop what they are doing on a unit and come to silently support nurses who are experiencing physician abuse on the units.

✓ Conference calls, a strategy that provides witnesses when nurses make calls at night to physicians who are known to engage in abuse.

✓ The implementation of physician and nurse counselors who work with identified abusers of registered nurses.

✓ Education for registered nurses and physicians that provide strategies for identifying and managing abusive situations.

Moved by Sandy Oliver, passed. No opposition.

WHAT IS A POLITICAL ACTION COMMITTEE?

Another way that nurses can influence the elective process is through involvement in an organization's political action committee (PAC). Political action committees, or PACs, grew out of the Nixon/Watergate era, when Congress decided that candidates for public office were becoming too dependent on money supplied by special interests—individuals who give large political contributions and thereby exert undue influence over the elected official's decisions.

As a result, Congress limited the amount of money an individual may contribute to a candidate, established strict reporting requirements, and created a mechanism whereby individuals can pool their resources and collectively support a candidate.

The American Nurses Association's (ANA) national PAC is called ANAPAC. Through this vehicle, nurses across the country organize to collectively endorse and support candidates for national offices. Likewise, state nurses' associations have state-level PACs to influence statewide elections. There may be PACs in your area that endorse candidates in city elections. All PACs must comply with the state or federal election codes and report financial support given to candidates for public office.

Today PACs play an important role in the political process, since they provide a mechanism whereby small contributors can act as a collective, participating in the electoral process when otherwise they would feel outmaneuvered by the bigger players.

The ANA's Endorsement Handbook stresses four points regarding PACs:

- *Political focus.* The only purpose of any PAC is to endorse candidates for public office and then supply them with the political and financial support they need to win an election.
- *No legislative activities.* A PAC does not lobby elected officials; that is the job of the state nurse association and its government-relations arm. A PAC simply provides financial and campaign support for candidates whose views are generally consistent with those of its contributors.
- *Not "dirty."* A PAC does not "buy" a candidate or a vote; but the very nature of political life suggests that candidates who recognize an organization's ability to affect their electoral prospects will be inclined to listen to the group's views when considering specific pieces of legislation.
- Health concerns only. Nursing PACs evaluate the candidates on nursing and health concerns only. In other words, ANAPAC might solicit the candidates' ideas about how Congress might address the problem of elder abuse in long-term care facilities. But the organization as a nursing PAC should not include questions, for instance, about the source of funding for the new cabinet on foreign commerce. The organization speaks for members only on issues covered in its philosophical statements, resolutions, position statements, legislative platforms, or other documents that its members as an organization have accepted (Critical Thinking Box 17-5).

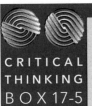

CRITICAL THINKING BOX 17-5

How has ANAPAC affected nursing on a national level? What have been the most recent activities of this organization? How does your state organization communicate or affect nursing and health care legislation in your state?

ANAPAC, The American Nurses Association's Political Action Committee.

AFTER GETTING THEM ELECTED, THEN WHAT?

Lobbying is the attempt to influence or sway a public official to take a desired action. Lobbying is also characterized as the education of the legislator about nursing and its issues. Educating officials, like educating patients, is an important part of the nurse's role.

As nurses we can lobby in several different ways. The first and best opportunity to lobby comes when the nurse first meets the candidate and evaluates her or him as a potential office-holder. This is the time to assess the candidate's knowledge of health care issues. Take the time to teach and to learn.

A second opportunity comes when the official needs information to decide how to vote on an issue. Depending on time constraints, the issue, and other considerations, a nurse might decide to lobby the official in person or in writing. If time and financial resources permit, the most powerful type of contact is a face-to-face visit. The only way to ensure time with your senator or representative is to make an appointment. Even then, one may not be successful.

If an unscheduled visit to the Capitol precludes an appointment, the best time to catch your senator or representative is early in the day, before the legislative sessions or committee meetings start—they rarely start before 10 or 11 AM. Contact with the legislator's aid or assistant can be just as effective as time with the official. Busy federal and state officials depend heavily on their staff. Treat staff members with the respect they deserve!

Finally, remember that contact should be made between legislative sessions and during holidays when the official is in her or his home district. The structure and content of the visit should be similar to that of a written contact. That is, know your issue, keep it short, identify the issue by its bill number and title, and communicate exactly what action you want the senator or representative to take. Here is a list of specific "Do's and Don'ts When Lobbying" (Box 17-3). As you begin lobbying, add your recommendations to the list.

If you cannot visit your representative because of time or travel restrictions, a well-written letter, electronic message (e-mail), or telephone call can communicate your message. Examine the sample letter in Box 17-4. Note that some pointers are listed at the foot of the page. Examples of the proper way to address a public official follow the sample letter in Table 17-1.

Letters are common methods of communicating with elected officials; however, a telephone call or e-mail is often necessary to relay your opinion when time is limited before an important vote. The suggested format and content of the electronic message and telephone message are similar to that of a letter or face-to-face interview.

Decisions about the type of contact to make with the decision-maker will vary depending on the situation. For example, if the bill is coming up the first time in committee, the strategy may be that 10 to 15 people write letters or e-mail messages or call the members of the committee. At this point, the number of contacts with the office is important. The reason is that the legislator's assistant typically answers the telephone or opens the mail, tallies the subject of the contact, and puts a hash mark in the "Pro HB 23" or "Con HB 23" column. Therefore, a greater impact will be realized if the contacts pertain to one bill. Bags of form letters, however, may have a negative impact on a lobbying effort. Make sure your callers/writers understand the issue and are able to individualize their contact with the elected official. People who contact the legislator's office with a script that they don't understand will not further the lobbying efforts of an organization.

BOX 17-3 Do's and Don'ts When Lobbying.

DO:

❏ Make sure your legislator knows constituents who are affected by the bill; suggest visits to programs in his/her area.

❏ Clearly identify the bill, using title and number, if possible.

❏ Be specific and know about the issue or bill before you write or talk.

❏ Identify yourself (occupation, hometown, member of ANA).

❏ Use your own words; if writing, use your own stationery. No form letters!

❏ Be courteous, brief, and to the point.

❏ Provide pertinent reasons for your stand.

❏ Show your legislator how the issue relates to his/her district.

❏ Respect your legislator's right to form an opinion different from yours.

❏ Present a united front. Keep our internal problems at home.

❏ Write letters of appreciation to your legislators when appropriate.

❏ Write letters at appropriate times, for example, when a bill is in committee request action that is appropriate for that stage in the legislative process.

❏ Establish an ongoing relationship with the public official.

❏ Know issues or problems your legislator is concerned about and express your interest in assisting him or her.

❏ Attend functions sponsored by coalition members. Be seen!

❏ Get involved in your legislator's campaign for reelection—or his or her opponent's, if necessary!

DON'T:

❏ Write a long letter or one on multiple points; deal with a single bill or concern per letter or contact.

❏ Use threats or promises.

❏ Berate your legislator.

❏ Be offended in the event of a cancelled appointment. Things are unpredictable during a legislative session.

❏ Demand a commitment before the legislator has had time to consider the measure.

❏ Pretend to have vast influence in the political area.

❏ Be vague.

❏ Hesitate to admit you don't know all the facts, but indicate you will find out—and do!

TABLE 17-1

How to Address Public Officials

The President
Writing*: The Honorable (Full Name)
President of the United States
The White House
Washington, DC 20500
Dear Mr./Madam President:
Speaking:
"Mr./Madam President"
"President (Last Name)"
The Vice President
Writing: The Honorable (Full Name)
Vice President of the United States
Executive Office Building
Washington, DC 20501
Dear Mr./Madam Vice President:
Speaking:
"Mr./Madam Vice President"
"Vice President (Last Name)"
A Senator
Writing: The Honorable (Full Name)
United States Senate
(will have office building and room address)
Washington, DC 20510
Dear Senator (Full Name):
Speaking: "Senator (Last Name)"
A Representative
Writing: The Honorable (Full Name)
U.S. House of Representatives
(will have office building and room address)
Washington, DC 20515
Dear Mr./Ms. (Full Name):
Speaking: "Representative (Last Name)"
"Mr./Ms. (Last Name)"
A Member of the Cabinet
Writing: The Honorable (Full Name)
Secretary of (Cabinet Agency)
(will have office building and room address)
Washington, DC 20520
Dear Mr./Madam Secretary:
Speaking: "Mr./Madam Secretary"
"Secretary (Last Name)"

*The correct closing for a letter to the president is "Very respectfully yours." The correct closing for all other federal officials noted here is "Sincerely yours."

BOX 17-4 Example of a Letter to a Public Official

Ima Nurse, RN
123 Main Street
Any Town, USA 12345-6789

The Honorable Y. R. Senator, Jr.
United State Senate
Washington, D.C. 20510

Dear Senator Senator:

I request your support of SB 101 regarding appropriations for nursing education and research. This bill is vital to the country's efforts to improve the number and quality of registered nurses. As you recall, the 1998 Verimportant Nursing Study demonstrated the growing demand for Advanced Nurse Practitioners to work with the increasing numbers of people over 65 years of age. This bill will provide funding to increase the number of faculty and student slots in the country's schools of nursing and to support nursing research in gerontological nursing. The expanding numbers of older people in our area of the country are not able to get the health care they deserve. During a trip home, I would like to take you to the Main Street Senior's Clinic. I know that you would be pleased with this service, as are the health care providers and the clients.

Will you support this bill? Do you have any questions about it? If so, please call me or the State Nurses' Association Headquarters.

Thank you for your concern with this issue and your continuing support of health care issues.

Sincerely yours,

Ima Nurse, RN

Points to note:
1. Neat, without typos or gramatical errors
2. Correctly addressed
3. Professional letterhead
4. Covering single topic
5. Refers to the bill by number and content
6. States request in first sentence
7. Brief rationale for request
8. Uses RN in inside address and salutation

The aforementioned efforts are sufficient early in the process; however, if a major, controversial bill is coming up for a final vote in the Senate, activating a statewide network and bombarding the senators with letters, e-mail messages, telephone calls, and telegrams—as many as possible—is a typical strategy. The bigger the issue, the bigger the campaign should be.

At several points in a lobbying season, but certainly after contacting the elected official for a major vote, a follow-up thank-you letter will strengthen your contact with the legislator and help establish you in her or his political network. In addition to reinforcing the reason for your original contact, thank the official for her or his concern with the issue and work in solving the problem by writing the bill or voting for it (or whatever) and for paying attention to your concern.

In summary, there are specific skills to learn for effective political involvement. But remember that many of the skills needed to be politically savvy are the very ones that will serve you well in everyday professional negotiations (Critical Thinking Box 17-6).

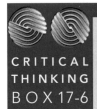

CRITICAL THINKING BOX 17-6

When are the bills that affect nursing and health care going to be presented to your state legislature?

As a recent graduate getting oriented to your first job and beginning to look around at what you and your colleagues need to improve, you will agree that political involvement is necessary to reach your goals. This author implores you *not* to wait to be "allowed" to make a difference, *not* to wait to be *invited* to join, and *not* to let someone else do the job. Please step forward! Act like the powerful, informed, influential nurse that you are. There is much that needs to be done—be a part of the action!

Margaret Mead said, "Never doubt that a small group of thoughtful, committed citizens can change the world. Indeed, it's the only thing that ever has." The nursing profession has much to accomplish; I'm pleased you will be joining us.

CONTROVERSIAL POLITICAL ISSUES AFFECTING NURSING

PROPOSED UNIFORM CORE LICENSURE REQUIREMENTS

What Is It? The National Council's Nursing Practice and Education Committee has proposed the development of core licensure requirements. This was in response to an increasing concern regarding the mobility of nurses and the maintenance of licensure standards to protect the public health, safety, and welfare. With the implementation of Mutual Recognition, it is important that health care consumers have access to nursing services that are provided by a nurse that meets consistent standards regardless where the consumer lives. The National Council (1999) defines competence as "the application of knowledge and the interpersonal, decision making, and psychomotor skills expected for the nurse's practice role, within the context of public health, welfare and safety" (p. 3).

The competence framework is based on the recommendations from the 1996 Continued Competence Subcommittee. This framework consists of the three following primary areas:

Competence Development—the method by which a nurse gains nursing knowledge, skills, and abilities. Competence Assessment—the means by which a nurse's knowledge, skills, and abilities are validated. Competence Conduct—refers to health and conduct expectations, including assurance that licensees possess the functional abilities to perform the essential functions of the nursing role (National Council of State Boards of Nursing, 1999, p. 3). These proposed requirements are going to cause controversy in the nursing community and will most likely require additional legislation in most states. An interesting question proposed by the committee was: *Do you really think nursing is that much different, that much safer on your side of the state boundary line* (p. 3)? The summary of the proposed competencies may be found in the *Book of Business* from the 1999 meeting of the National Council of State Boards of Nursing. Contact the National Council for the full paper that includes the rationales for the proposed requirements and discussion of how the committee developed the recommendations.

Organized nursing and state boards of nurse examiners have been working on a proposal to address some of the questions that is now ready to pilot. Agreements, known as *interstate licensure compacts*, are being created among several states that will specify the rights and responsibilities of nurses who choose or are required to work across state boundaries and the governing body responsible for protecting the recipients of nursing care (Thomas, 1999).

At press time, Arkansas, Arizona, Delaware, Idaho, Iowa, Maine, Maryland, Mississippi, Nebraska, North Carolina, South Dakota, Texas, Utah, and Wisconsin had enacted multistate compacts; however, legislation is pending in several states. New Jersey, Indiana, Tennessee, and North Dakota have enacted mutual recognition legislation; however, they will not implement the compact until a later date (http://www.ncsbn.org/public/nurselicensurecompact/mutual_recognition_state.htm).

States entering into interstate compacts agree to mutually recognize a nursing license issued by any of the participating states. To join the compact, states must enact legislation adopting the compact. The nurse will hold a single license issued by her or his state of residence. This license will include a "multistate licensure privilege" to practice in any of the other compact states (both physical and electronic). Each state will continue to set its own licensing and practice standards. A nurse will have to comply only with the license and license renewal requirements of her or his state of residence (the one issuing the license), but she or he must know and comply with the practice standards of each state in which she or he practices (http://www.ncsbn.org/public/nurselicensurecompact/nurselicensurecompact_index.htm) (Critical Thinking Box 17-7).

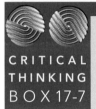

CRITICAL THINKING BOX 17-7

How will interstate licensure compacts affect the licensure and practice of nursing in your state?

As these agreements are established, experience with additional problems arising from the multistate practice of nursing will be identified and solved in amendments to state practice acts.

NURSING AND COLLECTIVE BARGAINING

March! There are no bunkers, no sidelines for nursing today. We find ourselves the center of attention. As the government and corporate America fight escalating health care costs, AIDS [acquired immune deficiency syndrome] is wreaking havoc and technology swells unchecked. Underpaid, overworked, and overstressed nurses are in the midst of a conflagration. Nursing is in greater demand than ever before. Remember Scutari. We must organize, unite, go on the offensive.
—Margretta Styles, 1988, as quoted in Hansten and Washburn, 1990, p. 53.)

The National Labor Relations Act is a federal law regulating labor relations in the private business sector (extended to voluntary, nonprofit health care institutions in 1974). This law grants employees the right to form, to join, or to participate in a labor organization. Furthermore, the law gives the employee the right to organize and bargain with his or her employer through a representative of his or her own choosing.

Collective bargaining continues to be a point of debate among nurses. Those supporting collective bargaining argue that it is a tool to force positive changes in the practice setting, a method of controlling the practice setting. Many positive changes in the clinical setting are attributed to advances made during contract negotiations. The major advantage of coverage under a collective bargaining agreement is that it is a contract negotiated and signed by duly authorized representatives of management and nurses and is, therefore, binding and enforceable. Opponents counter that such a written contract, although explicitly delineating terms of employment, can restrict the freedom, flexibility, and, as a result, the professional judgment of an RN.

In addition, opponents feel that as a profession, nurses should not use collective bargaining, but instead should influence the practice setting in ways that mean employee and employer working as a team and not as adversaries. They contend that a strike, the ultimate tool of any labor dispute, should not be used. Opponents further argue that practice standards are not negotiable. The points of disagreement between employer and employee are always economic: pay, vacation, sick leave, and similar issues.

What do you think? A paragraph in the ANA's publication *What you need to know about today's workplace: a survival guide for nurses* summarizes the challenge for us:

> In a work environment that is constantly changing, it is imperative that nurses are able to assess the true merits of various labor-management structures, to evaluate the real value of proposals to upgrade compensation packages, to determine appropriate levels of participation in workplace decision-making bodies, and to distinguish between long-range solutions and "quick fixes" to workplace problems (Flanagan, 1995, p. 5).

EQUAL PAY FOR WORK OF COMPARABLE VALUE OR COMPARABLE WORTH?

The concept of comparable worth or pay equity holds that jobs that are equal in value to an organization ought to be equally compensated, whether or not the work content of those jobs is similar. Pay equity relates to the goal of equitable compensation as outlined in the Equal Pay Act of 1963, and "sex-based wage discrimination" is a phrase that refers to the basis of the problems defined by Title VII of the Civil Rights Act of 1964.

As long ago as World War II, the War Labor Board suggested that discrimination probably exists whenever jobs traditionally relegated to women are paid below the rate of common-labor jobs such as janitor or floor sweeper. One of the first cases was that of the *International Union of Electrical Workers v. Westinghouse*. The union proved that male-female wage disparity existed and uncovered a policy in a manual that stated women were to be paid less because they were women. Back pay and increased wages were given in an out-of-court settlement in an appellate-level decision.

It was nurses who initiated the action, in *Lemons v. the City and County of Denver*. Nurses employed by the city of Denver claimed under the Civil Rights Act that they were the victims of salary discrimination, because their jobs were of a value equal to various better-paid positions throughout the city's diverse workforce. The court ruled that the city was justified in the use of a market pricing system (a form of pay based on supply and demand) even though it acknowledged the general discrimination against women. The court said that the case (and the comparable-worth concept) had the potential to disrupt the entire economic system of the United States. Because of this judgment and the fact that the nurses were unable to prepare a job evaluation program to substantiate their claim, the judge dismissed the case.

Another important concept in this area is "salary compression." That is, at the beginning of a nurse's career, she or he can expect to enter a beginning staff nurse position earning approximately $31,700. This same nurse can expect to earn a maximum salary of $49,100, or a 54.8% salary progression, over a career (Watson Wyatt Data Services, 2000/2001). Table 17-2 offers a comparison of nursing salary with that of other professions.

TABLE 17-2

Salary Data

United States: averages of all reporting hospitals (in thousands)			
Health Care Provider	Average Minimum	Average Mid	Average Maximum
Staff Nurse	31.7	40.4	49.1
Nurse Practitioner—General Care	47.3	59.6	71.8
Pharmacist	47.8	59.4	70.9
Physician's Assistant	47.8	60.3	72.6
Case Manager	36.8	46.4	55.9
LPN/LVN	21.7	26.9	32.0

LPN, Licensed practical nurse; *LVN*, licensed vocational nurse.
From Watson Wyatt Data Services: *ECS Hospital and Health Care Professional, Nursing & Allied Services Personnel Compensation Report*, Rochelle Park, NJ, 2000/2001, Watson Wyatt Data Services.

One explanation offered for the discrepancy is that the salary system for nurses is based on the assumption that most nurses are temporary workers. Therefore salary structures are relatively flat, with essentially no allowances for administrative responsibilities and almost no differential for experience.

Needless to say, much work continues to be done in this important area. Nurses and women in general must continue to strive for equitable compensation based on the inherent value or worth of the work performed, instead of on the basis of historically depressed pay levels or other discriminatory factors. Changes will be achieved as we educate others about inequities, initiate legal remedies in courts and state legislatures, and effect changes in the workplace.

REFERENCES

American Nurses Association: *State legislative trends*, 2000. Accessed November 28, 2001, at http://www.nursingworld.org/gova/state/hod99?intrstat.htm.

Cohen SS et al: Political analysis and strategy. A framework for action. In Mason DJ, Leavitt JK, eds. *Policy and politics in nursing and health care*, Philadelphia, 1998, WB Saunders.

Flanagan L: *What you need to know about today's workplace: a survival guide for nurses*, Kansas City, Mo, 1995, American Nurses Association.

French JRP, Raven B: The bases of social power. In Cartwright D, ed. *Studies in social power*. Ann Arbor, 1959, University of Michigan.

Hansten RI, Washburn M: *I light the lamp*, Vancouver, Wash, 1990, Applied Therapeutics, Inc.

Leavitt JK, Mason DJ: Policy and politics: a framework for action. In Mason DJ, Leavitt JK, eds. *Policy and politics in nursing and health care*, Philadelphia, 1998, WB Saunders.

National Council of State Boards of Nursing: *Map of state compact bill status*, 2001. Available at http://www.ncsbn.org/public/nurselicensurecompact/mutual_recognition_state.htm.

National Council of State Boards of Nursing: *Nurse licensure compact*, 2001. Available at http://www.ncsbn.org/public/nurselicensurecompact/nurselicensurecompact_index.htm.

National Council of State Boards of Nursing: Uniform core licensure requirements: a supporting paper. In *Book of Business*, Chicago, 1999, NCSBN.

Sanford ND: *Identification and explanation of strategies to develop power for nursing in power: nursing's challenge for change*, Kansas City, Mo, 1979, American Nurses Association.

Texas Nurses Association: Texas moves toward multistate nurse licensure legislation in 1999, *Tex Nurs* 72(10):4, 11, 1998.

Thomas K: A word from the Executive Director: multistate regulation moves forward, *RN Updates*, XXX(1), Austin, Tex, 1999, Texas State Board of Nurse Examiners.

US Government Census Bureau: *Health insurance coverage: 2000*. Accessed December 1, 2001 at http://www.census.gov/hhes/hlthins/hlthin00/hlt00asc.html.

Watson Wyatt Data Services: *ECS hospital & health care professional, nursing & allied services personnel compensation report*, Rochelle Park, NJ, 2000/2001, Watson Wyatt Data Services.

INTERNET RESOURCES

Nursing's federal-level governmental program American Nurses Association (you will find links to the state nursing organizations)
> http://www.nursingworld.org

Federal legislative information
> http://thomas.loc.gov

National Council of State Boards of Nursing, Inc.
> http://www.ncsbn.org/

National Library of Medicine
> http://www.nlm.nih.gov/
> *Many nursing specialty organizations have governmental affairs programs and Web sites. Check with the organization's Web site for additional links. See Appendix B for the Directory of National Nursing Organizations.*

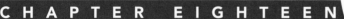
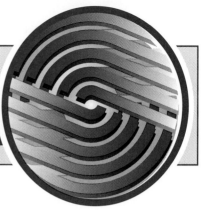

CHAPTER EIGHTEEN

A Collective Voice in the Workplace

MARY E. FOLEY, RN, MS

Compromise does not mean cowardice.

—*John F. Kennedy*

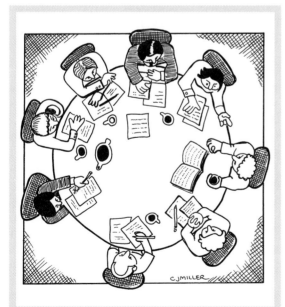

Is there a place for collective bargaining in nursing?

After completing this chapter, you should be able to:

- Describe the history of collective bargaining in nursing.
- Compare collective bargaining and other workplace governance structures.
- Identify the conditions that may cause nurses to seek collective bargaining representation.
- Identify the steps nurses would take to initiate collective bargaining representation.

Y|ou will soon be accepting your first position as a registered nurse (RN). You will not only be adjusting to a new role, but to a new workplace. Even in these times of dramatic change in health care, many of you will start your career in a hospital. In fact, the demographics about nurses show that more than two thirds of nurses in practice are providing care in hospitals.

It is understandable that your major concern may be your personal readiness to practice as an RN. Another legitimate—but often overlooked—concern of recent graduates and senior nurses is whether the workplace is prepared to let you practice as a professional! As you start your selection process for the first job or the last job of your career, your decision-making process can be made somewhat easier if you use some of the strategies recommended in materials like *Survival skills in the workplace: what every nurse should know* (Flanagan, 1990).

Hospital structures and governance policies can have a dramatic influence on how much a nurse fulfills her or his obligation to patients and families. Nurses have defined themselves as professionals and, as professionals, must have a voice in and control over the practice of nursing. When that voice and control are not supported by the work setting, a conflict will arise.

In some areas of the country, nurses have chosen to gain a voice in and assume control of their practice by using a collective bargaining model. This chapter is intended to give you an idea of why and how that has been accomplished. This chapter also honestly addresses some of the controversy that surrounds nursing and unions.

COLLECTIVE BARGAINING IN NURSING

IS THERE A PLACE FOR COLLECTIVE BARGAINING IN NURSING?

Should nurses use collective bargaining if they are professionals? Is nursing a profession or an occupation? These are questions nursing has debated throughout its history and continues to debate today.

A *profession* can be defined as a vocation that requires a long period of specialized education to prepare one for service to society. Because of their expertise and the value of their service, society grants professionals a measure of autonomy in their work. This autonomy permits professionals to make independent judgments and decisions on the basis of a theoretical framework that is learned through study and practice.

Conflict arises as nurse-employees advocate for their professional role in patient care and their health care institutions demand productivity and savings. In addition, nurses are no longer immune to job security issues. For example, as cost containment has become the watchword of the hospital industry, staff downsizing and increased nurse workloads have occurred at the same time that the patient population's acuity level has risen. In other words, the patients are sicker—and yet they are moved more quickly through the acute-care setting through such innovations as same-day surgery, same-day admissions, and early discharge. Add periodic shortages of nurses prepared for acute care, long-term care, and home care; the substitution of nurses with unlicensed assistive personnel; and chronic financial pressures on the health system, and tensions are understandably high.

A study conducted by a Kansas City, Kansas, labor-relations consulting firm defined why hospital employees and nurses joined unions and how union organizers garnered their support. Their conclusion confirms what has been suggested again and again:

> A myth widely subscribed to by hospital management is that big powerful unions organize professional nurses. In fact, unions do not organize nurses; professional nurses organize themselves. They do this because administrators and nursing supervisors fail to recognize and address nurses' individual and collective needs (Stickler and Velghe, 1980, p. 14).

A study from the University of California, Berkeley, found that nurses who engage in collective bargaining believe it is the only solution to a management-employee power struggle. They conclude that nurses decide to unionize because of their "inability to communicate with management and their perception of authoritarian behavior on the part of management" (Parlette, O'Reilly, and Bloom, 1980, p. 16).

Nursing has used collective action to its benefit, achieving professional goals while protecting and promoting public interest through lobbying efforts in the political arena. Many nurses support collective bargaining in the workplace as a way to control their practice by redistributing power within the health care organization.

"The power bestowed upon the nursing profession should derive not from the hospital administrator's benevolence, but rather from the public's view of the value of services provided by the practitioner" (Cleland, 1981, p. 17).

Ada Jacox (1980) has criticized nursing departments that fail to acknowledge that nurses are professionals. In her view (and this author's), the authority for nursing practice must rest within the profession. She suggests that collective bargaining through the professional organization may be a way for nurses to achieve collective professional responsibility.

IF I'M A NURSE, WHO SHOULD SPEAK FOR ME?

In choosing a job in a workplace that has or is about to select a union, consider what the choices have been for nurses. Meatpackers; Paperhangers; United Food and Commercial Workers; Longshoremen; Teamsters; Local 1199; the Service Employees International Union; the American Federation of State, County, and Municipal Employees; and the American Federation of Teachers are the unions that have competed for nurse representation. Union competition for nurses has become intense, especially as traditional union membership has declined. Some of these unions have offered nurses the prospect of endless resources and lengthy experience in labor relations.

At a time when competition for nurses was growing, the American Nurses Association (ANA) strengthened its own collective bargaining capacity by creating the United American Nurses in 1999, and in 2001, it was elected as a member of the American Federation of Labor and Congress of Industrial Organizations (AFL-CIO). Now nurses can enjoy the benefit of representation by nurses without the fear of distracting competition from other unions who are also members of the AFL-CIO. As Jacob, Cleland, and many other nursing leaders have stated, the professional association has the means and responsibility to represent nurses. The national professional organization for nursing is the ANA, with its constituent units, the state, and territorial nursing associations. Through its economic security programs, the ANA recognizes state nursing associations as the logical bargaining agents for professional nurses and has been the premier representative for nurses since 1946! These professional associations are indeed multipurpose; their activities include economic analysis, education, nursing practice, research, collective bargaining, lobbying, and political action.

LEGAL PRECEDENTS FOR STATE NURSING ASSOCIATIONS

The legal precedent that determined that state nursing associations are indeed qualified under labor law to be labor organizations is the 1979 Sierra Vista decision. I contend that these associations are not only proper and legal, but also the preferred representatives for nurses in this country for purposes of collective bargaining.

> The state nursing association is really the only safe ground, what I could call the neutral turf, on which professional nurses can meet and discuss issues as colleagues, issues that are of a generic and important nature to all nurses, regardless of title.

It is in the nursing associations that staff nurses, educators, advanced-practice nurses, and administrators are able to talk as nurses. Issues associated with clinical ladders, staffing, unlicensed assistive personnel, patient acuity, reimbursement climate, and regulatory matters affect all nurses and benefit from our collective thinking and the application of our collective resources.

NURSE PARTICIPATION IN COLLECTIVE BARGAINING

If the ANA and state nursing associations are logical bargaining agents for professional nurses, why are so few nurses joining associations and even fewer pursuing collective bargaining? A little known fact is that almost 80% of nurses belong to no association and have no professional affiliation. Most persons join an organization only in response to a particular incentive or when coerced. Otherwise, people will "free ride," or-enjoy whatever collective goals are obtained without helping to pay for them (Olson, 1971).

Collective bargaining for nurses usually occurs in states where there is also significant union activity. About half of the state nursing associations engage in collective bargaining. The climate is very volatile across the country, and unions are trying to organize new categories of workers, with special emphasis on the growing health care sector in states that have not traditionally been active in the labor movement. Some state nursing associations had previously left the arena because of external pressures: challenges from competing unions, excessive resistance by employers, or state policies that make unionization difficult, such as right-to-work laws. (In states with right-to-work laws, it is illegal to negotiate an agency shop requirement; membership and dues collection can, therefore, never be mandatory even if the workers are covered by a collective bargaining agreement.) Philosophical conflicts regarding the benefits and risks of professional association bargaining have also led nurses in some states to abandon or avoid union activities.

Rabban (1991) has concluded that when "substantial" and "unambiguous" support for professional values is included in collective bargaining agreements, unionization and professionalism are compatible. How will collective professional goals be achieved if so many nurses depend on the time and finances of so few? There are 2.2 million working nurses, but only a few hundred thousand are organized for collective bargaining. Some, including me, believe that the ANA's efforts to address workplace concerns will result in larger membership numbers in the near future, but for now, there are too few nurses involved in the nursing associations.

WHERE DOES COLLECTIVE BARGAINING BEGIN?

Nurses in the private sector are guaranteed legal protection, as stated in the National Labor Relations Act, if they seek a collective bargaining agent. Once a drive for such representation is under way and 30% of the employed nurses in an institution have signed cards signaling interest in representation, both the employer and the union are prohibited from engaging in antilabor action. Employers are prohibited from firing the organizers, refusing to allow dissemination of union information in the workplace, and ignoring the request for a vote for union representation. After the organizing campaign, a vote is taken; a majority made up of 50% plus one of those voting selects or rejects the collective bargaining agent.

Your employer may choose to bargain in good faith on matters concerning working conditions by recognizing the bargaining agent before the vote. This approach usually occurs only if management believes a large majority supports the foundation of a union. In other cases, your employer may appeal requests for representation to the National Labor Relations Board (NLRB). Before and during the appeal, other unions may intervene and try to win a majority of votes.

Arguments are made before the NLRB regarding why, by whom, or how the nurses are to be represented. For example, the hospital may raise the question of "unit determination." The original policy interpretation of the labor law simultaneously limited the number of individual units an employer or industry would have to recognize, yet allowed for distinct groups of employees, like nurses, to have separate representation. Nurses historically had been represented in all-RN bargaining units, and most bargaining units throughout the country reflected that pattern.

MILESTONES IN COLLECTIVE BARGAINING

During the late 1980s, the demand among nurses for representation was growing; yet efforts to organize nurses for collective bargaining were being stymied by the precedent set in what was called the St. Francis II case. That precedent stopped approving all-RN bargaining units. The ANA decided that this NLRB decision had to be challenged. The chief opposition to nursing was the American Hospital Association (AHA). A legal battle then ensued, with the ANA and other labor unions against the AHA. The ANA was able to convince the NLRB to hold national hearings on this controversy. The NLRB issued a ruling that reaffirmed the right of nurses to be represented in all-RN bargaining units. That ruling was challenged by the AHA in an Illinois federal court, and an injunction was imposed at that time. The ANA deemed it essential to take this issue to the highest court in the country so it could be finally settled. Hence the ANA, with the NLRB, appealed the case to the U.S. Supreme Court. In May 1991, to the satisfaction of nurses throughout the United States, the U.S. Supreme Court confirmed that the NLRB had ruled properly and correctly in determining that nurses in this country have a right to be represented for purposes of collective bargaining in all-RN bargaining units.

Nurses represented by a bargaining agent have the right to drop or change (decertify) that agent by a similar campaign of signatures (30%) of the affected members, followed by a vote, again requiring 50% plus one (a simple majority) in a unitwide election. Although the election process may ensure fair representation and an agent's accountability, election campaigns can be destructive and diversionary when initiated for frivolous reasons (those of little or no weight or importance, not worthy of serious notice). An example could be a competing union that promises it can "do better" for the membership if only the nurses will decertify their current union and elect the competitor. Such campaigns have occurred in Washington, Florida, and New York. It is anticipated that some of this competition for the already organized will stop now that the United American Nurses/ANA are part of the AFL-CIO, and there are protocols that discourage such struggles. Another form of potential conflict will be for the right to organize new bargaining units, but again, the AFL-CIO provides some guidelines for those campaigns as well. Some unions remain outside the protective rules of the AFL-CIO and may present themselves as nurse advocates, so not all competitions are over.

CONTRACTS

WHAT CAN A CONTRACT DO?

Generally speaking, what can a union contract do in a hospital setting? A study of 36 hospitals nationwide, all of which had extensive experience with collective bargaining, illustrates the positive effects a union can have:

1. Unions stimulate better hospital management by fostering formal, central, and consistent personnel policies with better lines of communication.

2. Unions "force" improvements in the workplace so that recruitment and retention become easier (Juris and Maxey, 1981).

Wages. Wages are the foundation of a contract. Wages are the remuneration one receives for providing a service and reflect the value put on the work performed. In a 1990 article on the history of nursing's efforts to receive adequate compensation, Brider reaffirmed the need to continue efforts on behalf of nursing salaries. The author correctly stated that ". . . from its beginnings, the nursing profession has grappled with its own ambivalence: how to reconcile the ideal of selfless service with the necessity of making a living" (p. 77). The article cited the nurses who recorded both their joy in productive careers and their disappointment with the way their work was valued. Nursing has certainly come a long way from the $8 to $12 monthly "allowance" in the the early 1900s, but the challenge remains to bring nursing into line with comparable careers.

During the late 1980s, nursing wages experienced dramatic increases as a direct result of the highly publicized shortage of nurses. Collective bargaining agreements from New York to the Northwest reflected wage gains that were hoped would place nursing wages and benefits in a competitive position to attract women and men making choices about their careers. However, health care compensation studies, nurse surveys, and national salary studies all confirm a slowing of wage gains for nurses, and many studies have demonstrated that when adjusted for inflation, nurse salaries from 1980 to 2000 have remained flat in real dollar terms (US DHHS, 2000). As we enter the twenty-first century, it is beginning to become clear that there is another shortage of nurses looming that is already being felt in specialty areas, such as critical care and the operating room. Whenever the supply and demand favors nursing, wages are evaluated and there is usually an adjustment of entry level wages (to address recruitment) and wages paid for nurses who remain in practice (for retention).

The larger issues of nurse compensation involve the challenge of addressing the negative effects of "wage compression." This economic concept means that nurses who have been in practice for 10 and 12 years may make less money than recent graduates in their first nursing jobs! Bargaining goals of the 1980s sought to shift some of the dollars available for nursing wages away from the novice, or entry-level nurse, to the experienced nurse in the form of higher maximum wages. Subsequent salary surveys have confirmed some success in this area. The long-term impact on nursing as a whole is improved when wage levels are addressed comprehensively, with permanent adjustments that value the contributions of nurses. Unfortunately, it is not uncommon during times of shortages to see hiring bonuses, or relocation bonuses, to attract nurses into new positions. It would be preferable to see those dollars redistributed for the purposes of building the base. Other innovative approaches would be to use those dollars to support nurses while they learn new skills or advance their career.

Many studies have documented that, sometimes after 5 years, a nurse begins to practice with a level of intuition and expertise that is beneficial to the patients and the practice environment (Benner, 1982). As a result many contracts now include tenure steps that reward nurses who have been in practice for many years in the same institution (longevity). This provision helps ensure the salary growth over what is now a lifetime of employment, or career growth. Salary increment steps now continue to the 10th, 15th, and even the 25th year in some hospitals. Compensation for other indicators of achievement, such as certification and degree completion, may be seen in contract settings, and often vary from the East Coast to the West Coast. These pay practices are also not limited to contract settings exclusively, because many institutions realize the positive effect these professional pay practices will reap.

Job Security Versus Career Security. It is probably not news to any student enrolled in a nursing program that he or she has entered a field that is undergoing many challenges—both from within and outside nursing. The economic environment in the health care industry, coupled with rapid technological progress and a renewed interest in primary and preventive care, has dramatically shifted a great deal of health care away from the hospital setting. The Division of Nursing Sample Survey (U.S. DHHS, 1992) reported a rise of 66% in the number of nurses providing care in outpatient settings between 1988 and 1992 and a rise of 30% in the number of nurses working in public/community health during the same time. The 2000 Division of Nursing Sample Survey (U.S. DHHS, 2000) again confirmed that nurses have professional opportunities across a diverse continuum, but it also validated that large numbers of nurses, 59% of the 2.2 million working nurses, are still employed in hospital-based care. The health care environment is ever-changing. Managed care, managed care reform, shorter lengths of stay, new technologies and pharmaceuticals, limited resources, and a growing demand on all health services by our growing aging population are just a few of the factors that affect the world in which nursing care is delivered. These new paradigms have challenged nurses and their representatives to modify bargaining strategies and turn attention to issues of sustaining quality nursing care in the face of shortages, to overcome negative practices such as mandatory overtime, and to advocate for health and safety initiatives like safer needle devices and ergonomics.

The ANA, through its affiliated members, has committed significant time and resources to simultaneously maintaining the essential role of the RN in the acute-care setting through bargaining agreements and workplace advocacy *and* ensuring that nurses are prepared for changing settings and roles and are supported as new settings emerge. Strategies include promotion of a national program to support workforce retraining in cooperation with the U.S. Department of Labor and collective bargaining language and workplace strategies to provide retraining and transfer opportunities to the experienced nurse moving into the nonhospital setting. The Division of Nursing Sample Survey in 2000 confirmed that more nurses are working than ever before, and these diverse settings provide an opportunity for nurses to leave traditional jobs but remain active in their chosen profession (U.S. DHHS, 2000).

Seniority Rights. Nurses who remain on staff at an institution accrue seniority rights. These rights derive from the idea that permanent employees should be rewarded for their service and viewed as assets. In nursing employment contracts there are provisions (seniority language) that give senior nurses the right to accrue more vacation time and be given preference when requesting time off, new positions, or relief from shift rotation requirements. In the event of a staff layoff the rule that states "the last hired become the first fired" protects senior nurses. Seniority rules may be applied to the entire hospital nursing staff or be confined to a unit. Transfers and promotions must reward the most senior qualified nurse in the institution.

Resolution of Grievances. Methods to resolve grievances, which are sometimes explicitly spelled out in a contract, are an important element of any agreement. A grievance can arise when provisions in a contract are interpreted differently by management and an employee or employees. This difference often occurs when issues related to job security (a union priority), job performance, and discipline (a management priority) arise. *Grievance mechanisms* are used in an attempt to resolve the conflict with the parties involved. The employer, the employee, or the union may issue a grievance. Nurses who are covered by contracts should be represented at any meeting or hearing that they believe may lead to disciplinary action being taken against them. Such representation can be provided by a co-worker, an elected nurse representative, or a member of the labor union's staff.

If the grievance mechanism does not lead to resolution of the issue, some contracts allow for referral of the issue to arbitration. A knowledgeable—but neutral—arbitrator acceptable to both parties (union and hospital) will be asked to hear the facts in the case and issue a finding. In preagreed, binding arbitration the parties must accept the decision of the arbitrator. For example, some hospital contracts require that when management elects to discharge (suspend or terminate) a nurse, the case must be brought to arbitration. The case is presented to an arbitrator chosen from an established list of arbitrators. On the basis of the arbitrator's finding, the nurse may be reinstated, perhaps with back pay, remain suspended, or be terminated. If the contract states that the arbitrator's decision is final and binding, there is no further contractual avenue for either party to pursue.

Arbitration. Arbitration has also been used to resolve issues involving the "integrity of the bargaining unit." Arbitrators have been asked to decide whether nurses remain eligible for bargaining unit coverage when jobs are changed and new practice models are implemented.

Mediation, arbitration, and fact-finding have all been used to resolve conflicts in union contracts. There is strong support for use of these methods, but hospital management personnel often resist using them. Nurses usually fare well when contract enforcement issues are submitted to an arbitrator and facts, not power or public relations, determine the outcome.

WHAT ARE THE ELEMENTS OF A SOUND CONTRACT?

Membership. The inclusion of union security provisions is an essential element of a sound contract and one of the defined goals of collective bargaining (union integrity). *Security provisions* include measures such as enforcement of membership requirements (collection of dues and access by the union staff to the members). A legal modification of the closed shop is the *agency shop*, in which new employees are required to join the union within a given period of time.

Objection to an Assignment. The right and means for a nurse to register objection to a work assignment are considered an essential element in a union contract with professional values. Professional duty implies an obligation to complete an assignment despite the nurse's disagreement with it. Nurses cannot abandon their post without risking disciplinary action. Some contracts and national proposals endorse objection (support nurses who disagree in writing with an assignment) when the assignment could violate the patient protection language of the state nurse practice act. An *assignment-despite-objection* report is submitted to the nursing administrator and the bargaining agent simultaneously, thus officially registering the complaint.

Inadequate staff, poorly prepared staff, high patient acuity, and excessive use of registry personnel are all problems that motivate nurses covered by union contracts to submit assignment-despite-objection reports.

Constructive follow-through by management may improve the situation in the future, just as inaction could serve as a basis for a grievance or negotiated change in the contract. Ideally the professional performance or professional practice committee (one that is mandated by contract) at the facility will work with nursing administrators to address nurses' complaints and decide whether they reflect a pattern or remain unresolved. A nurse who registers a complaint alerts management to a problem. This act can be constructive in that it can help a nurse vent frustration and anger and help him or her turn a bad experience into a positive one. Better care standards result.

Staffing. Staffing requirements are mandated by various agencies. For example, Medicare, state health department licensing requirements, and the Joint Commission on the Accreditation of Healthcare Organizations each publish staffing standards. However, standards that outline nurse-to-patient ratios do not address the issue of what qualifications the nurse must have. For example, a standard that requires one nurse per patient in the intensive care unit does not mandate that the nursing staff needs to have had certain education and experience to work in the intensive care unit.

Staffing concerns are foremost in the minds of nurses during this period of cost-cutting, restructuring, design, downsizing, and general confusion in the health care arena. The ANA has undertaken a nationwide campaign to call attention to the quality and safety concerns associated with health care changes that in any way reduce the role of the RN in the acute-care setting, although that concern can be extended to all settings in which patients depend on nurse expertise. The "Every Patient Deserves a Nurse" campaign has provided an effective vehicle for state nursing associations to communicate with the public and policy makers about the essential role of the RN (Himali, 1995a). As an extension of that program, the ANA has set the goal of developing and implementing a "Nursing Care Report Card" to measure health care settings by using nursing measurements. Key elements of the report card will include characteristics of the nursing staff and patient outcomes, both positive and negative. As a result of this essential work in the early 1990s, the ANA funded the Nursing Outcome Indicator Project in six states to evaluate outcomes of "nursing sensitive" patient care. (ANA, 1996). This body of scientific research has enriched the field of measurement for safe staffing and can now be used as a scientifically valid foundation to guide nurse staffing standards and ensure the safe care of the public.

National issues that are addressed by nurses involved in workplace advocacy include the reduction of overall staff numbers and substitution of other health care workers, or unlicensed assistive personnel, for RNs. Other common areas of concern that often appear on the bargaining table are issues that arise from scheduling, such as 10- and 12-hour shifts, floating, use of agency/registry personnel, and RN responsibility for supervising other personnel. Mandatory overtime first began to be reported in late 1999; by 2000 it was an epidemic. Three major strikes occurred in 2000 in state nursing associations (Worcester, Mass; Nyack, NY; and Washington, DC) and in Youngstown, Ohio, in 2001. Mandatory overtime and efforts to limit the use of such a practice was the primary reason for the strikes by the registered nurse bargaining units. Registered nurses reject mandatory overtime on a number of fronts. It diminishes the sense of control nurses, or any employees, have over their personal work lives. Nurses with family or other personal obligations found that the inability to plan their work schedule added to their stress—and dissatisfaction—with their work life (ANA, March/April 2001).

Retirement. The usual pension or retirement programs for nurses have been either the Social Security System or a hospital pension plan. Individual retirement accounts, which are transferable from hospital to hospital in case of job change, are relatively rare and should be a topic of negotiations. The ANA has entered an agreement with a national company to provide a truly portable national plan, unrestricted by geographic location or employment site. Although this plan could be complicated by conflicting state laws governing pension plans, a precedent was set as long ago as 1976, when California nursing contracts mandated employer contributions to individual retirement accounts for each nurse with immediate vesting (eligibility for access to the fund) and complete portability for the participants (meaning that the nurse could take the pension to another hospital and continue to add to it).

One of nursing's most attractive benefits has been a nurse's mobility, the opportunity to change jobs at will. A drawback of this mobility, however, is the loss of long-term retirement funds. Pension programs should be looked at not as a reward for continued service, but as a basic protection earned by employees as part of their benefit program. With financial cutbacks in the hospital industry, retirement plans are in danger of being targeted as givebacks in negotiations rights or benefits to be traded away in lieu of another issue or benefit that may be more pressing at the time. Health insurance coverage persists as a key concern of employees and has been at the root of the majority of labor disputes in all industries in the last few years. It is not inconceivable that nurses may be asked to trade off long-term economic security (pensions) for short-term security (e.g., health benefits, wages).

Other Benefit Issues. All employees in the United States have been experiencing a dramatic reduction in their health benefits packages. This trend is reflective of the crisis of the health care system and the escalating costs of health care. Nurses have not been immune to the reduction in health benefits, and access to health care benefits will continue to be a major issue for nurses and all employees until substantial reform is accomplished.

Other issues that have affected nurses as employees are family-leave policies, availability of daycare services, long-term disability insurance, and access to health insurance for retirees. An issue of special concern to nurses involves the scheduling of work hours. Although some men have been joining the nursing profession, nursing remains a 97% female occupation. That reality must be addressed by benefit packages that provide flexibility for women who assume multiple roles in today's society. Women, and nurses in particular, provide care to both children and parents. Nurses are asking nursing contract negotiators to secure leave policies that permit use of sick time for family needs and scheduling that is both flexible and allows part-time employment and work-sharing.

The urgency of the emerging nursing shortage has stimulated some employers to offer attractive schedules, and even dry cleaning and oil-changing services are being introduced by some employers as they struggle to recruit and retain staff. Nurses can appreciate these extra services just like any employee, but what they really want is an environment that supports their goal of providing quality nursing care. Multiple surveys and publications document the stress and perceived deterioration of nurse satisfaction and, potentially, the quality of patient care. The ANA conducted an online survey in late 2000, released in February 2001, that reflected the depth of despair nurses are feeling (ANA, March /April, 2001). One of the most discouraging findings was that 52% of nurses stated they would not recommend nursing to a relative or friend.

Health Hazards. Nurses are using collective action to protect themselves against health hazards and unsafe working conditions and to advocate for positive health and safety programs. Right-to-know provisions (knowledge of where and what a hazardous substance is and how to use it safely) and job security in the case of reassignment can be written into contracts. Such agreements have been included in contracts in the District of Columbia and Illinois. Nationally the ANA is urging the Occupational Safety and Health Administration to provide hazardous-substance information to health workers. Nursing associations and unions have advocated for inclusion of strict infection control guidelines for health care facilities to protect workers from blood-borne pathogens including hepatitis B and human immunodeficiency virus. An aggressive safer needle campaign started to move state to state, and in November 2000, the ANA and other health care worker advocates were able to celebrate the passage of national legislation that expanded protection from blood-borne diseases through the use of safer needle devices. Nursing has also played a major role in designing and advocating stringent ongoing education and training on universal precautions, postexposure protocol, and latex allergies. Additional health and safety concerns include the reemergence of tuberculosis and a high incidence of violence in health care settings.

Some state nursing associations have introduced legislation to rectify worker's compensation policies once an exposure has occurred in the workplace. The ANA and other unions have used collective bargaining agreements, aggressive government relations campaigns, and nursing practice networks to educate nurses about workplace risks.

The Minnesota Nurses Association conducted a study that illustrated an alarming trend that appears to connect the dramatic staffing changes with the near-doubling of RN workplace injuries (Himali, 1995b). These findings indicate the need for the bargaining representative to be able to make the connection between practice trends and health and safety issues.

COLLECTIVE BARGAINING AND NURSING PRACTICE

HOW CAN NURSES CONTROL THEIR OWN PRACTICE?

Hospital management representatives often ask staff nurses what they mean when they say their goal is to control nursing practice. These managers seem unclear about what it is we consider appropriate practice issues, and they react negatively to the concept of *control*. The essence of the professional nurse contract is control of practice. For example, nurse councils or professional performance committees provide the opportunity for nurses within the institution to meet regularly. These meetings are sanctioned by the contract. The elected staff nurse representatives may, for example, have specific objectives to

- Improve the professional practice of nurses and nursing assistants.
- Recommend ways and means to improve patient care.
- Make recommendations to the hospital management when, for example, a critical nurse staffing shortage exists.
- Identify and recommend the elimination of hazards in the workplace.

The importance and relevance of such professional practice committees was documented by a 1986 review of state nursing association contracts. When 381 agreements were analyzed, 424 references to professional practice committees were identified.

Nurse Practice Committees. Nurse practice committees should have a formal relationship with nursing administration. Regularly scheduled meetings with nursing and hospital administrators can provide a forum for the discussion of professional issues in a "safe" atmosphere. Many potential contract conflicts can be prevented by discussion before contract talks begin or grievances arise. Ideally physicians should be a part of these forums; joint-practice language has been proposed in some contracts. Current nursing concerns continue to focus on staffing ratios, patient acuity, patient classification systems, training, and appropriate use of nursing assistants.

Trends have see-sawed between a climate of shortage to one of record layoffs of RNs, and now there are reports of a shortage that by every indication may be severe and prolonged.

Environments that reduce the number of direct-care nurses, midlevel management nurses, nurse educators, and clinical staff specialists will jeopardize patient care. Numerous studies have confirmed the relationship between the staffing level of RNs and the quality of patient outcomes (Prescott, 1993; Kovner and Gergen, 1998)

Because a principle of professional nursing practice requires nurses to be involved in making decisions that will affect their working conditions and quality of the care, it is reasonable to expect nurses to use their union contract to assist them in dealing with issues such as staff mix. When nurses refer to *control of nursing practice*, they are not talking about infringing on the rights or responsibilities of managers to ensure financial stability and administrative order. Rather nurses are referring to the elements that affect professional practice for which they, as licensed professionals, are responsible.

In the 1980s the American Academy of Nursing started to work on the topic of "magnet hospitals" (American Academy of Nursing, 1983), which described professional practice environments that had a reputation of recruiting and retaining nurses and welcomed staff involvement in unit and hospital decision making that positively influenced practice. In 1994, the American Nurses Credentialing Center, a subsidiary of the ANA, developed the Magnet Nursing Services Recognition Program for Excellence in Nursing Services (ANA, 1998). On the basis of the quality indicators and standards as defined in the ANA's Scope and Standards for Nurse Administrators (ANA, 1996) the program measures qualitative and quantitative factors of nursing services. Since 1994, almost 40 hospitals and one long-term care facility have been awarded a magnet credential. Almost 20% of the facilities awarded the recognition have a collective bargaining agreement with the nurses.

The significance of this program has been the recognition that an environment that ensures that nursing will be one of the organization's highest priorities, professionally and clinically, will succeed on many planes. These "forces of magnetism" have been shown to result in lower nurse turnover, higher patient satisfaction, higher nursing satisfaction, and even fewer needlestick injuries by the nursing staff (Aiken, Smith, and Lake, 1994). And most importantly, those facilities that have achieved this status confirm that with a conscious effort, optimal nursing settings can, and do exist!

Concept of Shared Governance. Many facilities are implementing a variety of practice models that they call *shared governance*. *Shared governance* is defined as an arrangement of nurses (staff and managers) that attempts to emphasize the principles of participatory management in those areas related to both the governance and practice of nursing (Porter-O'Grady and Finnigan, 1984). Also labeled *self-governance, participative decision making, staff by-laws*, and *decentralized nursing services*, these are structural activities meant to address nurse participation in control of practice. The concept of shared governance has worried unions that represent nurses in collective bargaining. The historical precedents of shared governance in an academic setting mandate caution when applied to health care settings. It is necessary to avoid a legal finding that the nurses, who are part of a shared governance model, have become so involved in the governance activities of the facility that they are no longer eligible for representation by a bargaining agent. That is exactly what happened in the Yeshiva University faculty precedent (Yeshiva, 1980).

Some shared-governance models make no effort to hide the fact that their express purpose is to involve nurses in decision making and yet retain the unilateral decision-making authority of managers. That certainly would violate the principles of professional participation in decision making. It is also a major disadvantage to nurses employed by institutions if shared-governance models are adopted in lieu of collective bargaining agreements. In an environment in which collective bargaining already exists, it is probably unnecessary to adopt a totally new model to achieve shared governance if, in fact, the professional practice committee is involved, as it should be, in providing staff nurse input into decisions that affect the professional practice of nursing. To preserve bargaining rights, the model must be compatible with collective bargaining rights and must clearly define the demarcation between professional and management issues.

Clinical or Career Ladder. The clinical ladder (Huey, 1982; Wieczorek, Weissman, and Hiatt, 1982; Wieczorek, Weissman, and Savino, 1982), or career ladder, has a place in collective bargaining agreements. The clinical ladder was designed to permit recognition of the long-term career nurse who wishes to remain clinically oriented. The notion to reward the clinical nurse with pay, and status, along a specific track or "ladder" is the result of the great contributions of a nurse researcher, Dr Patricia Benner. Her descriptions of growth and development of nursing knowledge and practice provided the basis for a ladder model that can be used to identify and reward the nurse along the steps from novice to expert (Benner, 1982). Reports issued by the Institute of Medicine (1983) and the U.S. Department of Health and Human Services Secretary's Commission on Nursing (1988) all cited the career ladder as an effective tool for use in the retention of career-minded nurses.

Negotiations. The principles of successful negotiations are difficult to articulate. Nurse negotiators are elected by their peers and must represent a diverse population (a multiple of specialty areas, educational backgrounds, and practice needs). Nurses have little or no introduction to labor practices or procedures in nursing education programs, so they must learn on the job. Foreign nurses are at a greater disadvantage because they are unfamiliar with cultural factors that affect negotiations, such as power, politics, economics, and competition (Critical Thinking Box 18-1).

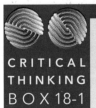

CRITICAL THINKING BOX 18-1

Does information regarding labor practices need to be in the nursing curriculum?

Negotiations are held before a contract is agreed on and again just before it expires. Nurses in the bargaining unit will elect a negotiating team to represent them.

These nurses may be assisted by labor union staff, skilled negotiators, economists, and/or legal staff.

Professional goals and practice needs should be discussed in negotiations, but personnel directors, hospital administrators, and hospital lawyers often seem to have difficulty relating to discussions of nursing practice concerns. Nursing directors usually remain in the wings, only joining the discussion when invited by the hospital administrators. The resolution of disagreements about professional issues necessitates a long and thoughtful process. Complex issues such as recruitment, retention, staffing, and health and safety, can be better addressed in a more collegial setting.

What nurses want and what they can achieve during negotiations may be worlds apart. Although a survey of the nurses may produce a "wish list," it must be pared down to only those issues that are of greatest importance to the whole and have the most chance of surviving the give-and-take of collective bargaining. If nurses are not helped to understand the negotiation process, they could begin to feel that their individual needs are not being attended to.

Strikes and Other Labor Disputes. Just what can nurses do in the face of a standoff during contract negotiations? Nurses' options are quite different than they were before 1968, when nurses felt a greater sense of powerlessness. At that time, despite nurses' threats of sickouts, walkouts, picketing, or mass resignations, the employer maintained an effective power base. Threats of group action attracted public attention, but nurses' threats had little effect on employers because nurses represented through the ANA had a no-strike policy. As negotiations became more difficult, it was apparent that nurses were in a weaker bargaining position because of the no-strike policy. The ANA responded to the state nursing associations and, in 1968, reversed its 18-year-old, no-strike policy.

Strikes are used only after every other alternative fails. Nurses who strike take their appeals to the "street," hoping for positive public response. Strikes remain rare among nursing units, but, as was mentioned previously, when patient care and safety are at risk, nurses may have to strike, as they started to in 2000 to address mandatory overtime. Many nurses are uncomfortable with the idea of striking, believing that they are abandoning their patients. This image may conflict with the service ideal. It is important for nurses who contemplate striking to discuss plans for patient care with nurses who have previously conducted strikes so that they will be assured that plans to care for patients are adequate.

When an impasse is reached in hospital negotiations, national labor law requires nurses to issue a ten-day notice of their intent to strike. Every effort must be made to prevent a strike in the public's interest. Mediation is mandated by the NLRB, and a board of inquiry to examine the issue may be created before a work stoppage. The hospitals are supposed to use this time to reduce the patient census and to slow or halt elective admissions. In the meantime the nurses' strike committee will develop schedules for coverage of emergency rooms, operating rooms, and intensive care areas. This coverage is to be used only in the case of real emergencies. Planning patient care coverage should reassure nurses troubled by the strike scenario. Nurses who agree to work in emergencies or at other facilities during a strike often donate their wages to funds set up for striking nurses.

Employer Strategies. According to one definition, *collective bargaining* is a struggle for power in which the opposing parties, the employer and the collective bargaining agent, rival and manipulate each other to improve and advance their respective positions. In the health care setting the broadly defined bargaining objectives include the following:

- To protect the economic position and personal welfare of the worker.
- To protect the union's integrity as an ongoing institution.
- To recognize the outer limits imposed on collective bargaining outcomes by the economic conditions of the industry and the employer and by the climate of opinion (Stern, 1982, p. 11).

The National Labor Relations Act governs labor practices and prohibits certain unfair practices once an organizing campaign has been initiated. An employer cannot engage in interference, domination, discrimination, or refusal to bargain and cannot unjustly discipline an employee simply for union activities.

Before 1983, Medicare allowed hospitals to include antiunion expenses in their bills. Hospitals, like private industry, have hired expensive antiunion industrial relations firms to coach management in techniques to quickly detect prounion sentiment. However, this practice demonstrates the fine line between legal and illegal activities. One wonders why that same money could not be used to compensate nurses, to improve patient care and nurses' working conditions, or to introduce positive approaches to conflict resolution.

An important employer-initiated legal action had the potential for broad negative implications for all RNs—both those who are and those who are not represented by collective bargaining. In a troubling decision by the U.S. Supreme Court in May 1984, any nurse who "directs other employees" could be fired for protesting job conditions or questioning management decisions that placed the quality of patient care at risk. Nurses inevitably supervise a wide range of ancillary personnel, such as assistants and clerks, and, for RNs, licensed practice and vocational nurses. This ruling overturned a 20-year-old decision of the NLRB that a nurse is *not* a supervisor when acting in the best interest of the patient in seeing that the work of aides is done right. This change could have been a staggering setback for nurses, as they become advocates for patient safety and quality in the current climate (*NLRB v. Health Care & Retirement Corp. of America, 1994*). NLRB circuit court opinions after the 1994 opinion continued to be split on the question of registered nurse status as employees or supervisors, so the U.S. Supreme Court considered another case in late 2000 (*NLRB v Kentucky River Community Care Inc* et al, 2000). The ANA submitted an amicus brief in support of the NLRB, in coordination with the four other AFL-CIO unions who represent large numbers of nurses.

The critical issue, again, revolved around the following question: "When a registered nurse exerts professional judgment in performing her professional duties and often has to assign and direct junior colleagues and nonprofessional assistants, is she doing so as guided by her status as a licensed professional or in a management/ employer role as an employer?" It was with great disappointment when it was announced in May 2001, that the Supreme Court had voted five to four to strike the NLRB interpretation of what constitutes supervisory independent judgment (ANA,

July/August, 2001). Although this may further complicate which nurses will be eligible for collective bargaining, the court did note that it might be possible to distinguish employees who direct the manner of others' performance of discrete tasks from employees who direct other employees.

Business and labor are both in search of more positive ways in which to work together. National grants have been sponsored by the Department of Labor and the Federal Mediation and Conciliation Service to undertake alternatives to traditional bargaining. At least two Midwestern nursing organizations used "win-win" bargaining techniques and found them to be constructive methods of negotiation.

FUTURE TRENDS

WHAT LIES AHEAD?

The nursing community was struck in the late 1980s with a deeply entrenched, widespread, and possibly permanent imbalance between the demand for nurses and the ability of nursing education to supply adequately prepared RNs to meet future public needs. For about 2 years, it was common to pick up publications or turn on a national talk show, whether on radio or television, and find coverage of the shortage of nurses. As we continue through the twenty-first century, we are at a similar crossroads, and as the public demand for nurses continues to rise, there may be enduring shortages of nurses prepared for future roles.

The public should be concerned about an inadequate supply of nurses. Building on that concern, and the recent terrorist attacks on America, there is increased interest by the press and the policy-makers to be sure nurses are prepared in adequate numbers, and that their working environment supports quality nursing care. That attention is helping nurses achieve better wages and working conditions and must also lead to support for nursing faculty and loans and scholarships to address the educational pipeline for nursing. The question of job satisfaction, however, must not be overlooked.

In survey after survey, the no. 1 reason nurses are unhappy with their nursing practice environment is their dissatisfaction with the care that they are able to give in that environment.

Nurses throughout the country have felt firsthand the effects of cost containment. Those effects have been detrimental to the quality of care that professional nurses are charged to provide. From a professional practice perspective, mandatory overtime and short staffing are some of the factors that may be contributing to the preponderance of medical errors documented in the Institute of Medicine report on medical errors, "To Err is human: building a safer health system" (Institute of Medicine, 2000). The ANA was the sole voice in recognizing these as potential contributing factors, and have led the way in pushing research agendas that further quantify what are safe hours of work, and how patient safety can be ensured (ANA testimony, 2000). And just as occurred during the whistleblower issue, the ANA and the state nursing associations are in the lead in federal and state legislative efforts to address overtime and state staffing in the context of safe patient care.

What lies ahead for collective bargaining and all forms of collective action for nurses must be viewed within the context of the larger changes occurring in the health care system and in the financing mechanisms.

> There is still a heightened awareness among both the politicians and the public that something is grievously wrong with not just how we pay for our health care, but what we are receiving at that high cost.

This issue of health access is one that will probably be with us for the rest of our professional lives. As nurses advocate for improved access to health services, we believe those services will, by necessity, be delivered in environments and by providers that have not traditionally been a part of our medical care system. Just as cost containment of the 1980s brought emphasis on home care, early discharge, and alternatives to institutional care, remedies to improve access will include school-based care, workplace-based care, community care, and broader access to nursing care.

The concepts embodied in the *Nursing Agenda for Health Care Reform* (ANA, 1991), as follow, should be the collective vision of nurses throughout the country as the struggle continues to achieve true health care reform:

- Guaranteed access to care for all residents of the United States.
- Emphasis on primary, preventive care delivered in a continuum of care.
- Enhanced use of nurses in advanced practice (nurse practitioners, certified nurse midwives, and clinical specialists).
- Expanded community-based care.
- Use of acute-care facilities for briefer, more-intensive care.
- Cost-containment efforts to deliver quality care at the lowest cost and more efficiently.
- Health care institution mergers, closure, and integration of services and product lines to meet varying community needs.
- An increasing reliance on the skills and voice of nurses to ensure quality care.

The workplace advocacy goals for nursing during this transition will be focused on quality of care and assisting nurses as they expand their skills into community settings.

Nurses who are not organized for collective bargaining purposes should examine their work settings. If collective bargaining could improve the lines of communication, management authority, benefit packages, or practice controls, then explore the possibility of an organizing campaign. Organizing and retaining nurse interest is a serious and strenuous undertaking. The benefits and protections that accrue when nurses act collectively strengthen nursing and help nurses everywhere improve patient care.

By committing to paper the status of current affairs, I condemn this chapter to obsolescence! The very nature of nursing supply and demand defies prediction. I am convinced that the profession of nursing will ensure that adequate numbers of nurses are properly prepared and that the public will demand that nurses are part of any, and all, care structures they use.

I am more convinced than ever that multipurpose state nursing associations affiliated with the ANA provide the preferred structure for all nurses to address their workplace concerns. The ANA is evaluating how it will relate to the larger labor community and is internally discussing options for structural changes that will ensure support for both the bargaining and the nonbargaining goals of the association.

> Nursing has a unique contract with society to promote good health care and, as a natural outcome, promote the health and welfare of the nurse and the profession of nursing.

The multipurpose nature of the professional nursing association will preserve the future of nursing. This chapter cannot stand alone, nor can the nurses in the workplace stand alone if they are to offset the forces that negate the contributions of nurses. Political action and lobbying, research, and education are necessary to further the cause of nursing and to meet the public's health care needs. Although nursing works to change the health system and improve citizens' access to care, nurses will continue to depend on collective action and a collective voice to advocate for optimal working conditions and standards of practice. Welcome to nursing! Join us in our efforts to unify our skills, knowledge, and voices as we create our vision.

REFERENCES

Aiken LH, Smith HL, Lake ET: Lower Medicare mortality among a set of hospitals known for good nursing care, *Med Care* 32(8):771-787, 1994.

American Academy of Nursing: *Magnet hospitals: attraction and retention of professional nurses*, Washington, DC, 1983, American Nurses Association.

American Nurses Association: *Am J Nurs* 9:1223-1231, 1989.

American Nurses Association: *Nursing agenda for health care reform*, Washington, DC, 1991, ANA.

American Nurses Association: *Scope and standards for nurse administrators*, Washington, DC, 1996, ANA.

American Nurses Association: Looking for quality patient outcomes: The American Nurses Credentialing Center's magnet program recognizes excellence. *Nurs Trends Issues* 3(4):1-6, 1998.

American Nurses Association: ANA poll: RNs say poor working conditions affect care, *Am Nurse* 33(2):1-2, 2001.

American Nurses Association: ANA not dissuaded by Supreme Court decision on 'supervisors,' *Am Nurse* 33(4):1-2, 2001.

Benner P: From novice to expert, *Am J Nurs* 82(3):402-407, 1982.

Brider P: Professional status. The struggle for just compensation, *Am J Nurs* 90(10):77-80, 1990.

Cleland V: Taft-Hartley amended: implications for nursing. The professional model, *Am J Nurs* 75(2):288-292, 1975.

Flanagan L: *Survival skills in the workplace: what every nurse should know*, Kansas City, Mo, 1990, ANA.

Himali U: ANAW sounds alarm about unsafe staffing levels: PR campaign sheds light on RN replacement trends, *Am Nurs* 27(2):1, 7, 1995a.

Himali U: An unsafe equation: fewer RNs = more workplace injuries, *Am Nurse* 27(5):19, 1995b.

Huey F: Looking at ladders, *Am J Nurs* 82(10):1520-1526, 1982.

Institute of Medicine, Health Care Services, Nursing and Nursing Education Committee: *Nursing and nursing education: public policies and private actions.* Washington, DC, 1983, National Academy Press.

Institute of Medicine: To Err is human: building a safer health system, ed 1, In Kohn LT, Corrigan J, editors. Washington, DC, 2000, National Academy Press.

Jacox A: Collective action: the basis for professionalism, *Superv Nurse* 11(9):22-24, 1980.

Juris H, Maxey C: The impact of hospital unionism, *Mod Healthc* 11:36, 1981.

Kovner C, Gergen PJ: Nurse staffing levels and adverse events following surgery in U.S. hospitals. *Image* 30:4, 1998.

NLRB v Health Care & Retirement Corp of America, 114 Supreme Court 1778 (1994).

NLRB v Kentucky River Community Care Inc. et al, 532 Supreme Court (2001).

Olson M: *The logic of collective action: public goods and the theory of groups,* Cambridge, Mass, 1971, Harvard University Press.

Parlette GN, O'Reilly CA, Bloom JR: The nurse and the union, *Hosp Forum* 23(6):16-17, 1980.

Porter-O'Grady T, Finnigan S: *Shared governance for nursing: a creative approach to professional accountability,* Gaithersburg, Md, 1984, Aspen.

Prescott PA: Nursing: an important component of hospital survival under a reformed health care system, *Nurs Econ* 11(4):192-199, 1993.

Rabban D: Is unionization compatible with professionalism? *Industrial Labor Relations Rev* 45(1):97-110, 1991.

Stern EM: Collective bargaining: a means of conflict resolution, *Nurs Adm Q* 6(2):9-20, 1982.

Stickler KB, Velghe JC: Why nurses join unions, *Hosp Forum* 23(2):14-15, 1980.

US Department of Health and Human Services, Secretary's Commission on Nursing: *Final report,* Washington, DC, 1988, US DHHS.

US Department of Health and Human Services, Division of Nursing: *Sample survey, Bureau of Health Professionals,* Washington, DC, 1992, US DHHS.

US Department of Health and Human Services, Division of Nursing: *Sample survey, Bureau of Health Professionals,* Washington, DC, 2000, US DHHS.

Wieczorek RR, Weissman GK, Hiatt H,: A clinical career pathway: the Mount Sinai experience part 1, *Nurs Health Care* 3(10):533-535, 1982.

Wieczorek RR, Weissman GK, Savino A: A clinical career pathway the Mount Sinai experience part 2, *Nurs Health Care* 4:318, 1982.

Yeshiva, supra, 103 LRRM at 2553 (1980).

ADDITIONAL READINGS

American Nurses Association: *Am J Nurs* 46: 728, 1946.

American Nurses Association: *Collective bargaining and the nursing profession,* Kansas City, Mo, 1983, ANA.

Becker ER, Sloan FA, Steinwald B: Union activity in hospitals: past, present, and future, *Health Care Financ Rev* 3(4):1-13, 1982.

Moore JD Jr: Labor looks to lead counter-revolution, *Mod Healthc* 25(42):46-48, 1995.

McKibbin RC: *The nursing shortage and the 1990s: realities and remedies,* Kansas City, Mo, 1990, ANA.

News and background information, *Labor Relations Rep* 116:11, 1984.

Nurse membership in unions, *Am J Nurs* 37:766, 1937.

Shramm C: Economic perspectives on the nursing shortage. In Aiken L, editor, *Nursing in the 1980s: crises, opportunities, challenges,* Philadelphia, 1982, JB Lippincott.

US Department of Health and Human Services, Division of Nursing: *Sample survey, Bureau of Health Professionals,* Washington, DC, 1996, US DHHS.

US Department of Labor: *Labor bulletin,* Washington, DC, October 1993, US Department of Labor.

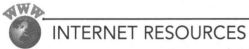

INTERNET RESOURCES

American Nurses Association
http://www.nursingworld.org

Critically analyzing information sources
http://www.library.cornell.edu/okuref/research/skill26.htm

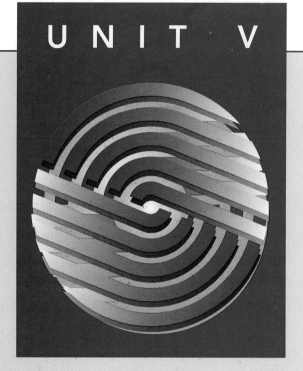

ETHICAL AND LEGAL
ISSUES IN NURSING

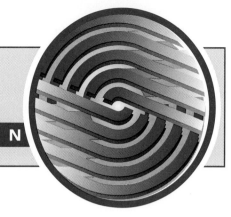

CHAPTER NINETEEN

Ethical Issues

ALICE B. PAPPAS, PhD, RN

People of Orphalese, you can muffle the drum, and you can loosen the strings of the lyre, but who shall command the skylark not to sing?

—*Kahlil Gibran, The Prophet*

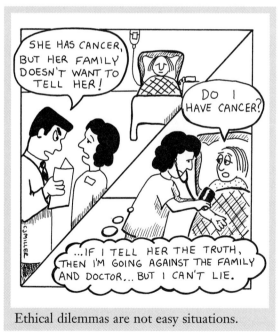

Ethical dilemmas are not easy situations.

After completing this chapter, you should be able to:

- Define terminology commonly used in discussions about ethical issues.
- Analyze personal values that influence approaches to ethical issues and decision making.
- Discuss the moral implications of the American Nurses Association and International Council of Nurses codes of ethics.
- Discuss the role of the nurse in ethical health care issues.

Concern about ethical issues in health care has increased dramatically in the last 2 decades. This interest has soared for a variety of reasons, including advances in medical technology; social and legal changes involving abortion, euthanasia, patient rights, end-of-life care, and reproductive technology; and growing concern about the allocation of scarce resources, including a shortage of nurses. Nurses have begun to speak out on these issues and have focused attention on the responsibilities and the possible conflicts that they experience as a result of their unique relationship with patients and their families and their role within the health care team.

UNDERSTANDING ETHICS

Let's begin by defining commonly used terms (Box 19-1).

BOX 19-1   Definition of Terms

Advance directive: A written statement of a person's wishes about how he or she would like health care decisions to be made if he or she ever loses the ability to make such decisions independently.

Bioethics: Ethics concerning life.

Bioethical issues: Subjects that raise concerns of right and wrong in matters involving human life (e.g., euthanasia, abortion).

Durable power of attorney for health care decisions: A document that allows a person to name someone else to make medical decisions for him or her if he or she is unable to do so. This spokesperson's authority only begins when the patient is incompetent to make those decisions.

Ethics: Rules or principles that determine which human actions are right or wrong.

Ethical dilemma: 1. A situation involving competing rules or principles that appears to have no satisfactory solution. 2. A choice between two or more equally undesirable alternatives.

Living will: A document that allows a person to state in advance that life-sustaining treatment is not to be administered if the person later is terminally ill and incompetent.

Moral or ethical principles: Fundamental values or assumptions about the way individuals should be treated and cared for. These include **autonomy, beneficence, nonmaleficence, justice, fidelity,** and **veracity.**

Moral reasoning: A process of considering and selecting approaches to resolve ethical issues.

Moral uncertainty: A situation that exists when the individual is unsure which moral principles or values apply in a given situation.

Values: Beliefs that are considered very important and frequently influence an individual's behavior.

WHAT ARE YOUR VALUES?

Clarification of your values is suggested as a strategy to develop greater insight into yourself and what you hold dear. Values clarification involves a three-step process: choosing, prizing, and acting upon your value choices in real-life situations (Steele and Harmon, 1983). Opportunities to make choices and improve your decision making are included in the following pages. As you consider your values, you will, I hope, gain more understanding about the underlying motives that influence them. It is not intended as a "right" or "wrong" activity, rather, it is a discovery about the "what" and "why" of your actions. Don't be surprised if your peers or family hold different views on some topics. And remember: the values that are "correct" or "right" for you may not always be the "right" values for others. Your values may also change over time as you face different life experiences.

Evaluate the critical-thinking questions, write down your responses to them, and consider the possible reason or reasons for your choices. The critical-thinking exercise (Critical Thinking Box 19-1), Listing Values, is suggested as a means of clarifying your values. Discuss your answers with peers and decide how comfortable you are in discussing and defending your values, especially if they differ from the values of your peers. Critical Thinking Box 19-2 involves reproductive issues and has been included here because of the proliferation of reproductive technology, including genetics, and the ongoing moral and political debate regarding abortion.

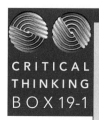

CRITICAL THINKING BOX 19-1

LISTING VALUES

List ten values that guide your daily interactions.

1. _____
2. _____
3. _____
4. _____
5. _____
6. _____
7. _____
8. _____
9. _____
10. _____

Choose a partner (if available).
1. Discuss with a partner each of the values you listed and how they guide your interactions.

(continued)

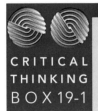

CRITICAL THINKING BOX 19-1

LISTING VALUES *(Cont'd)*

2. Compare your list of values with your partner's and discuss similarities and differences in the two lists.

3. Prioritize your list and discuss why you feel some are more important than others.

From Steele, S., and Harmon, V. (1983). *Values clarification in nursing* (2nd ed.) East Norwalk, CT: Appleton-Century-Crofts, p. 90, with permission.

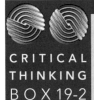

CRITICAL THINKING BOX 19-2

REPRODUCTIVE EXERCISE

Identify your degree of agreement or disagreement with the statements by placing the number that most closely indicates your value next to each statement.

1. = Strongly Disagree
2. = Disagree
3. = Ambivalent
4. = Agree
5. = Strongly Agree

_____ 1. Contraception is a responsibility of all women.

_____ 2. Some types of contraception are more valuable than other types.

_____ 3. Abortion as a form of contraception is completely unacceptable.

_____ 4. Abortion decisions are the responsibility of the pregnant woman and her physician.

_____ 5. The birth of a "test tube baby" is a valuable medical advance.

_____ 6. Genetic screening should be done frequently.

_____ 7. Genetic counseling should provide information so that clients can make informed choices about future reproductive decisions.

_____ 8. Amniocentesis should be required as part of prenatal care.

_____ 9. Genetic engineering should be advanced and promoted by federal funding.

_____ 10. Artificial insemination should be available to anyone who seeks it.

_____ 11. Sperm used in artificial insemination should come from all strata of society like blood transfusions do.

_____ 12. Fetal surgery should be done even when it places another fetus at risk (i.e., a twin).

_____ 13. Surrogate mothers play an important role in the future of families.

CRITICAL THINKING BOX 19-2

REPRODUCTIVE EXERCISE *(Cont'd)*

_____ 14. Fetuses who survive experimentation should be raised by society.

_____ 15. Women should be encouraged to participate in fetal research by carrying fetuses to desired dates and then giving the fetus to the scientist for research.

_____ 16. Contraception is reserved for women of legal ages.

_____ 17. Adolescents should require a parent's signature for abortion.

_____ 18. Information about genetically transmitted diseases should be provided to all pregnant women.

_____ 19. Women at high risk for genetically transmitted diseases should be encouraged to have amniocentesis.

_____ 20. Infants born with severe defects should be allowed to die through a natural course.

From Steele, S., and Harmon, V. (1983). *Values clarification in nursing* (2nd ed.) East Norwalk, CT: Appleton-Century-Crofts, p. 169, with permission.

MORAL/ETHICAL PRINCIPLES

What Is the Best Decision? And How Will I Know? Despite different ideas regarding which moral or ethical principle is most important, ethicists agree that there are common principles or rules that should be taken into consideration when an ethical situation is being examined. As you read through each principle, consider instances in which you have acted on the principles or perhaps felt some conflict in trying to determine what was the best action to take.

Autonomy—A Patient's Right to Self-Determination Without Outside Control. Autonomy implies the freedom to make choices and decisions about one's own care without interference, even if those decisions are not in agreement with those of the health care team. This principle assumes rational thinking on the part of the individual and may be challenged when the rights of others are infringed upon by the individual.

■ CONSIDER THIS:

What if a patient wants to do something that will cause harm to himself or herself? Under what circumstances can the health care team intervene?

Beneficence—Duty to Actively Do Good for Patients. For example, deciding what nursing interventions should be provided for patients who are dying when some of those interventions may cause pain. In the course of prolonging life, harm sometimes occurs.

■ CONSIDER THIS:

Who decides what is good? Patient, family, nurse, or physician? How do you define good?

Nonmaleficence—Duty to Prevent or Avoid Doing Harm Whether Intentional or Unintentional. Is it harmful to accept an assignment to "float" to an unfamiliar area that requires the administration of unfamiliar medications?

■ CONSIDER THIS:

Is it acceptable to refuse an assignment? When does an assignment become unsafe?

Fidelity—The Duty to be Faithful to Commitments. Fidelity involves keeping information confidential and maintaining privacy and trust (e.g., maintaining patient confidentiality regarding a positive human immunodeficiency virus test or "blowing the whistle" about unscrupulous billing practices).

■ CONSIDER THIS:

To whom do we owe our fidelity? Patient, family, physician, institution, or profession? Who has the right to access patient medical records? When should we "blow the whistle" about unsafe staffing patterns?

Justice—The Duty to Treat All Patients Fairly, Without Regard to Age, Socioeconomic Status, or Other Variables. This principle involves the allocation of scarce and expensive health care resources. Should uninsured pregnant patients have access to epidural anesthesia for childbirth, or is this a luxury reserved for those who have insurance or who pay out of pocket?

■ CONSIDER THIS:

What is fair, and who decides? Why are some patients labeled very important persons? Should they receive a different level of care? Why or why not? What kind of access to health care should illegal immigrants receive: preventive or just more costly emergency room care?

Veracity—The Duty to Tell the Truth. The principle of veracity may become an issue when a patient who suspects that her diagnosis is cancer asks you "Nurse, do I have cancer?" Her family has requested that she not be told the truth because their culture believes bad news takes away all hope for the patient.

■ CONSIDER THIS:

Is lying to a patient ever justified? If a patient finds out that you have lied to them, will they have any reason to trust you?

Each of the aforementioned principles sounds so right, yet the "consider this" questions indicate that putting them into practice is sometimes easier said than done. Reality does not always offer textbook situations that allow flawless application of ethical principles. As Oscar Wilde, an Irish playwright, once said, "The truth is rarely pure, and never simple." You will encounter clinical situations that challenge the way in which you apply the principle or that cause two or more principles to be in conflict, creating moral uncertainty, which is often referred to as an *ethical dilemma*.

Which Principle or Rule Is Most Important? Current thinking on the part of ethicists favors autonomy and nonmaleficence as preeminent because they emphasize respect for the person and the avoidance of harm. However, there is no universal agreement and many individuals rely on spiritual beliefs as the cornerstone to ethical decision making. Traditional and contemporary models of ethical reasoning offer worldviews from which these principles can be derived, interpreted, and comparatively emphasized. Nevertheless, they are not without their critics, including nurses. In recent years, nursing ethicists have advanced a new approach to ethical issues emphasizing an ethic of caring as the moral foundation of nursing. The nursing profession is being encouraged to consider all ethical issues from the central issue of caring. Because caring implies concern for preserving humanity and dignity and promoting well-being, the awareness of rules and principles alone may not adequately address the ethical issues that nurses confront, such as suffering or powerlessness. Research regarding the application of caring to ethical issues is under way, but a practical model for applying this ethic of caring to clinical situations does not yet exist. At the present time the most care-centered approach to ethical dilemmas is to consider the relative "benefits versus burdens" that any proposed solution offers to the patient.

So How Do I Make an Ethical Decision? At the present time, there are a number of approaches to ethical decision making. Here is a brief overview of the three most commonly applied models of ethical reasoning. The first two types are considered normative because they have clearly defined parameters or norms to influence decision making. The third type is a combination of the other two models.

Deontological. Derived from Judeo-Christian origins, the deontological normative approach is duty-focused and centered on rules from which all action is derived. The rules represent beliefs about intrinsic good that are moral absolutes revealed by God. This approach reasons that all persons are worthy of respect and thus should be treated the same.

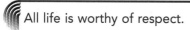

All life is worthy of respect.

As a result of the rules and duties that the deontological approach outlines, the individual has clear direction about how to act in all situations. Right or wrong is determined on the basis of one's duty or obligation to act, not on the consequences of one's actions. Therefore abortion and euthanasia are never acceptable actions because they violate the duty to respect the sanctity of all life, and lying is never acceptable because it violates the duty to tell the truth. The emphasis on absolute rules with this approach is sometimes seen as rigid and inflexible, but its strength is in its unbending approach to many issues, emphasizing intent of actions.

Teleological. Derived from humanistic origins, the teleological approach is outcome focused and places emphasis on results. *Good* is defined in utilitarian terms: That which is useful is good. Human reason is the basis for authority in all situations, not absolutes from God. Morality is established by majority rule, and the results of actions determine the rules. Because results become the intrinsic good, the individual's actions are always based on the probable outcome.

 That which causes a good outcome is a good action.

Simplistically this view is sometimes interpreted as "the end justifies the means." Abortion may be acceptable because it results in fewer unwanted babies. Euthanasia is an acceptable choice by some patients because it results in decreased suffering. Limiting hospitalization coverage after delivery is acceptable because it saves money and does not adversely affect outcome for most mothers and newborns. The rights of the individual may be sacrificed for the majority utilizing this approach.

Situational. Derived from humanistic and Judeo-Christian influences and most commonly credited to Joseph Fletcher, an Episcopalian theologian, the situational view holds that there are no prescribed rules, norms, or majority-focused results that must be followed. Each situation creates its own set of rules and principles that should be considered in that particular set of circumstances. Emphasizing the uniqueness of the situation and respect for the person in that situation, Fletcher appeals to love as the only norm. Critics of this approach argue that this can lead to a "slippery slope" of moral decline.

 Decisions made in one situation cannot be generalized to another situation.

Abortion is the best choice for an unmarried 16-year-old because it gives her the opportunity to finish school and mature, but it may not be the best answer for all girls in such a situation. "Pulling the plug" on a terminally ill patient who does not want any more extraordinary care is an act of love. Withholding or withdrawing treatment is ethically correct from the individual patient's perspective if the burden of treatment outweighs the benefit of merely extending life. Defining "burden" has to be approached from the patient's perspective, not from others who may feel burdened by the patient's need for care. Coming from the perspective of benefit versus burden can assist patients and families to make difficult decisions on the basis of the patient's clear or intended wishes discussed over a period of time. Nurses and other health care providers need to be patient advocates, speaking out for those who are disadvantaged and cannot speak for themselves.

Table 19-1 compares the relative advantages and disadvantages of each approach. Remember that there is no perfect worldview. If there were, debate would stop and the need for continued ethical deliberation would cease. The ethical models presented

TABLE 19-1

Three Approaches to Ethical Decision Making: Comparison of Advantages and Disadvantages

Ethical approach	Advantages	Disadvantages
Deontological	Clear direction for action. All individuals are treated the same. Does not consider possible negative consequences of action.	Perceived as rigid. Does not consider possible negative consequences of actions.
Teleological	Interest of the majority is protected. Results are evaluated for their good, and actions may be modified.	Rights of individual may be overlooked/denied. What is a good result? Who determines good? Morality may be arbitrary.
Situational	This approach mirrors the way most individuals actually approach day-to-day decision making. Merits of each situation are considered. Individual has more control/autonomy to make decision in his or her own best interest.	What is good? Who decides? Morality is possibly arbitrary. Lack of rules of generalizability limits criticism of possible abuse.

here are not intended to be all-inclusive or exhaustive in depth. Rather they should whet your appetite for further content. Many journals and texts are devoted to the topic, and you are encouraged to see how ethicists apply these and other models to issues that affect your area of practice. Surveys of nurses indicate an ongoing interest and expressed need for ethical discussion and support in practice.

How Do I Determine Who Owns the Problem? The decision to choose a particular model of ethical reasoning is personal (Table 19-1) and based on your own values. Familiarize yourself with various models to decrease your own moral uncertainty and gain some understanding of the values of others. The following guidelines are suggested as a means of analyzing ethical issues that will confront you in nursing practice. You may not be a pivotal decision-maker in all situations, but these guidelines can assist you.

First, Determine the Facts of the Situation. Make sure you collect enough data to give yourself an accurate picture of the issue at hand. When the facts of a situation become known, you may or may not be dealing with an ethical issue.

As an intensive care unit (ICU) nurse, you believe that the wishes of patients regarding extraordinary care are being disregarded. In other words, resuscitation is performed despite expressed patient wishes to the contrary. You need to

■ Determine whether discussion about extraordinary care is taking place among patients, families, and attending physicians.

■ Clarify the institution's policy regarding cardiopulmonary resuscitation (CPR) and do-not-resuscitate orders.

■ Determine what input the families have had into the decisions (i.e., whether the families are aware of the patient's wishes).

■ Explore the use of advance directives documentation at your institution, and determine whether patients are familiar with the use and possible limitations of living wills.

■ Share your concerns with the attending physicians to obtain their views of the situation. Discuss the situation with your clinical manager to clarify any misconceptions regarding policy and actual practice.

Second, Identify the Ethical Issues of the Situation. In the ICU scenario, if competent patients have expressed their wishes about resuscitation, this should be reflected in the chart. If a living will has been executed and is recognized as valid within your state, its presence in the chart lends considerable weight to the decision. The patient should be encouraged to discuss his or her decision with family to decrease the chances for disagreement if and when the patient can no longer "speak" for himself or herself. If immediate family members disagree with the living will, the physician may be reluctant to honor the will, at least in part because of concern regarding possible liability. If a living will is executed without prior or subsequent discussion with the attending physician, there may be reluctance to honor the will because the physician was not informed of the patient's decision. The physician may feel that the patient did not make an informed decision. However, a durable power of attorney for health care (DPAHC), combined with a living will and completed before the patient's present state of incapacitation, would stand as clear and convincing evidence of the patient's wishes, preventing such a problem. The example of extraordinary care in the ICU illustrates the existence of some values and principles in possible conflict.

Patient: Values autonomy, including right to decide when intervention should stop.

Family: May value life at all cost and be unwilling to "let go" of the patient when a chance exists to prolong life regardless of life quality.

Physician: May feel that the patient has a fair chance to survive and that the living will was executed without being "fully informed." The duty to care/cure may outweigh the physician's belief in the exercise of patient autonomy and fidelity.

Nurse: Values patient autonomy and the need to remain faithful to the patient's wishes. Concern for the needs of the family, in addition to respect for the physician-patient relationship, may cause some conflict.

Institution: Examination of institutional policy may reveal a conflict between stated policy (e.g., honoring living wills) and actual practice (e.g., code all patients unless written physician orders indicate otherwise).

In this situation, the ethical components of this second step involve autonomy and fidelity versus beneficence.

Third, Consider Possible Courses of Action and Their Related Outcomes.
Having collected data and attempted discussion on the issue with all involved parties, you are faced with the following options:

1. Advocate for the patient with physicians and the family by facilitating communication.
2. Encourage the patient and family to share feelings with each other regarding desires for care.
3. Encourage the family, patient, and attending physicians to discuss the situation more openly.

If the advocacy role does not bring about some change in behavior, consider the possible input and assistance of an interdisciplinary ethics committee (IEC). In the last decade such committees have evolved in response to the growing number of ethical issues faced in clinical practice. At present, more than 65% of hospitals have such a committee, and it may become an integral aspect of every institution if Medicare reimbursement is linked to the presence of an ethics resource. The IEC is typically composed of physicians, clergy, social workers, lawyers, and, increasingly, nurses. Any health team member can access the committee with the assurance of receiving at least a helpful, listening ear. If necessary, the committee will convene to review a clinical case and will offer an unbiased opinion of the situation. Committee members may be helpful in clarifying issues or offering moral support; they may also be persuasive in suggesting that involved parties (i.e., family, physician, patient, and nurse) consider a suggested course of action. The authority of an IEC is usually limited, because the majority of IECs are developed with the understanding that the advice and opinions offered are not binding to the individual. However, it can serve as a potent form of moral authority and influence if used.

Taking the initiative to express your values and principles is not necessarily easy. As a recent graduate, it may seem safer to "swallow hard," remain quiet, and invest your energies into other aspects of your role. You may risk ridicule, criticism, and disagreement when you speak out on an ethical issue, especially if your view is different or unpopular. However, you risk something far more important if you do not speak out. Silence diminishes your own autonomy as a person and as a professional. Depending on the situation, it may raise eyebrows, but it is important to make your concerns known because some values may be imposed on the patient or you in the clinical setting and those values may not be morally correct. You may not agree with these values or feel that they are in the best interest of the patient.

Fourth, After a Course of Action Has Been Taken, Evaluate the Outcome.
In the ICU scenario, did improved communication occur among patients, families, and physicians? Were your efforts to advocate met with resistance or a rebuff? What could you try differently the next time? What values or principles were considered most important by the decision-makers? What kind of assistance did you receive from the IEC? What role did nursing play in this situation, and was it appropriate?

What Other Resources Are Available to Help Resolve Ethical Dilemmas?
Professional resources are also available to provide direction about ethical issues and
behavior. The first of these is the American Nurses Association (ANA) *Code of ethics
for nurses* (2001). The code is a statement to society that outlines the values, concerns,
and goals of the profession. It should be compatible with individual nurses' personal
values and goals. The code provides direction for ethical decisions and behavior by
repeatedly emphasizing the obligations and responsibilities that the nurse-patient
relationship entails.

The provisions of the *Code of Ethics* allude to the ethical principles mentioned
earlier in this chapter and certainly imply that fidelity to the patient is foremost.
A copy of the code with interpretive statements is available from the ANA. If you
did not purchase a copy as a reference for school, consider buying it for your own use
in practice.

Critics of the *Code of ethics for nurses* cite its lack of legal enforceability. This is a
valid criticism because the code is not a legal document like licensure laws. However,
it is a moral statement of accountability and can add weight to decisions involving legal
censure. Many practicing nurses claim ignorance of the *Code of ethics for nurses* or
believe that it is a document for students only. However, the *Code of ethics for nurses* is
for all nurses and was developed by nurses. Take the opportunity to become familiar
with its contents. Box 19-2 lists the International Council of Nurses *Code for Nurses*.

BOX 19-2   International Council of Nurses *Code for Nurses*

ETHICAL CONCEPTS APPLIED TO NURSING
- ❏ The fundamental responsibility of the nurse is fourfold: to promote health, to prevent illness, to restore health, and to alleviate suffering.
- ❏ The need for nursing is universal. Inherent in nursing is respect for life, dignity, and rights of man. It is unrestricted by considerations of nationality, race, creed, color, age, sex, politics, or social status.
- ❏ Nurses render health services to the individual, the family, and the community and coordinate their services with those of related groups.

NURSES AND PEOPLE
- ❏ The nurse's prime responsibility is to those people who require nursing care.
- ❏ The nurse, in providing care, promotes an environment in which the values, customs, and spiritual beliefs of the individual are respected.
- ❏ The nurse holds in confidence personal information and uses judgment in sharing this information.

NURSES AND PRACTICE
- ❏ The nurse carries personal responsibility for nursing practice and for maintaining competence by continual learning.
- ❏ The nurse maintains the highest standards of nursing care possible within the reality of a specific situation.
- ❏ The nurse uses judgment in relation to individual competence when accepting and delegating responsibilities.

BOX 19-2 International Council of Nurses *Code for Nurses* (Cont'd)

❏ The nurse when acting in a professional capacity should at all times maintain standards of personal conduct which reflect credit upon the profession.

NURSES AND SOCIETY
❏ The nurse shares with other citizens the responsibility for initiating and supporting action to meet the health and social needs of the public.

NURSES AND CO-WORKERS
❏ The nurse sustains a cooperative relationship with co-workers in nursing and other fields.
❏ The nurse takes appropriate action to safeguard the individual when his care is endangered by a co-worker or any other person.

NURSES AND THE PROFESSION
❏ The nurse plays the major role in determining and implementing desirable standards of nursing practice and nursing education.
❏ The nurse is active in developing a core of professional knowledge.
❏ The nurse, acting through the professional organization, participates in establishing and maintaining equitable social and economic working conditions in nursing.

From International Council of Nurses, (1973), *ICN Code for Nurses: Ethical concepts applied to nursing*, Geneva, Switzerland: Inprimeres Populaires, with permission.

In 1973, the American Hospital Association published a *Patient's bill of rights*. Now revised and known as *Your rights as a hospital patient* (Box 19-3), this document reflects acknowledgment of patients' rights to participate in their health care and was developed as a response to consumer criticism of paternalistic provider care. The statements detail the patient's rights with corresponding provider responsibilities. Read over each statement and consider whether they seem reasonable. When first developed, many of the statements were considered radical. This document reflects the increasing emphasis on patient autonomy in health care and defines the limits of provider influence and control. Earlier beliefs that the hospital and physician know best (paternalism) have been challenged and modified. This document is likely to be further refined as joint responsibilities between patients and health care providers (Critical Thinking Box 19-3).

BOX 19-3 Your Rights As a Hospital Patient

We consider you a partner in your hospital care. When you are well-informed, participate in treatment decisions, and communicate openly with your doctor and other health professionals, you help make your care as effective as possible. This hospital encourages respect for the personal preferences and values of each individual.

(continued)

BOX 19-3   Your Rights As a Hospital Patient *(Cont'd)*

While you are a patient in the hospital, your rights include the following:

❑ You have the right to considerate and respectful care.

❑ You have the right to be well-informed about your illness, possible treatments, and likely outcome and to discuss this information with your doctor. You have the right to know the names and roles of people treating you.

❑ You have the right to consent to or refuse a treatment, as permitted by law, throughout your hospital stay. If you refuse a recommended treatment, you will receive other needed and available care.

❑ You have the right to have an advance directive, such as a living will or health care proxy. These documents express your choices about your future care or name someone to decide if you cannot speak for yourself. If you have a written advance directive, you should provide a copy to the hospital, your family, and your doctor.

❑ You have the right to privacy. The hospital, your doctor, and others caring for you will protect your privacy as much as possible.

❑ You have the right to expect that treatment records are confidential unless you have given permission to release information or reporting is required or permitted by law. When the hospital releases records to others, such as insurers, it emphasizes that the records are confidential.

❑ You have the right to review your medical records and to have the information explained, except when restricted by law.

❑ You have the right to expect that the hospital will give you necessary health services to the best of its ability. Treatment, referral, or transfer may be recommended. If transfer is recommended or requested, you will be informed of risks, benefits, and alternatives. You will not be transferred until the other institution agrees to accept you.

❑ You have the right to know if this hospital has relationships with outside parties that may influence your treatment and care. These relationships may be with educational institutions, other health care providers, or insurers.

❑ You have the right to consent or decline to take part in research affecting your care. If you choose not to take part, you will receive the most effective care the hospital otherwise provides.

❑ You have the right to be told of realistic care alternatives when hospital care is no longer appropriate.

❑ You have the right to know about hospital rules that affect you and your treatment and about charges and payment methods. You have the right to know about hospital resources, such as patient representatives or ethics committees, that can help you resolve problems and questions about your hospital stay and care.

❑ You have responsibilities as a patient. You are responsible for providing information about your health, including past illnesses, hospital stays, and use of medicine. You are responsible for asking questions when you do not understand information or instructions. If you believe you can't follow through with your treatment, you are responsible for telling your doctor.

(continued)

BOX 19-3   Your Rights As a Hospital Patient (Cont'd)

This hospital works to provide care efficiently and fairly to all patients and the community. You and your visitors are responsible for being considerate of the needs of other patients, staff, and the hospital. You are responsible for providing information for insurance and for working with the hospital to arrange payment, when needed.

Your health is dependent not just on your hospital care but, in the long term, on the decisions you make in your daily life. You are responsible for recognizing the effect of life-style on your personal health.

A hospital serves many purposes. Hospitals work to improve people's health; treat people with injury and disease; educate doctors, health professionals, patients, and community members; and improve understanding of health and disease. In carrying out these activities, this institution works to respect your values and dignity.

Reprinted with permission of the American Hospital Association, copyright 1992.

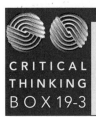

CRITICAL THINKING BOX 19-3

What is the current standing of the "Patient's Bill of Rights" in Congress?

Consider the settings in which you have had clinical experiences and decide how well these rights have been acknowledged and supported. In your future practice keep these rights in mind. Observing them is not only the "right thing to do," it is enforceable by law.

Another document was developed in 1992 and revised in 1996 as a response to the rapidly growing home health care area of community nursing. The National Association for Home Care established a *Home Care Bill of Rights* for patients and families to inform them of the ethical conduct they can expect from home care agencies and their employees when they are in the home. This document is widely used and addresses the rights of the patient and provider to be treated with dignity and respect; the right of the patient to actively participate in decision making; privacy of information; financial information regarding payment procedures from insurance, Medicare, Medicaid, and so forth; quality of care; and the patient's responsibility to follow the plan of care and notify the home health nurse of changes in his or her condition. Surprising as it may seem, there are instances of nurses who have lost their license as a result of unethical behavior toward patients in their homes. These abuses include financial and sexual exploitation—major violations of professional boundaries.

Home care nurses often face difficult ethical dilemmas about the delivery of care to patients. For example, a patient will require or desire more care or visits than Medicare or private insurance will pay for. All home care agencies have policies written to guide them through the decision-making process when they can no longer receive reimbursement for a patient's care. Often it is the responsibility of the home care nurse to find another community agency that can meet the patient's needs at a cost the patient can afford (Critical Thinking Box 19-4).

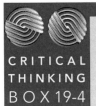

CRITICAL THINKING BOX 19-4

How does the *"Home Care Bill of Rights"* differ from *"Your rights as a hospital patient"*? How are they similar?

A fifth document that you should be familiar with is the *Nuremberg Code* (Box 19-4). This code grew out of the blatant abuses perpetrated by Nazi war criminals during World War II in the name of science. Experiments were conducted by health care professionals without patient consent and resulted in horrific mutilations, disability, and death. The *Nuremberg Code* identifies the need for voluntary informed consent when medical experiments are conducted on human beings. It delineates the limits and restrictions that researchers must recognize and respect. Because of the preponderance of research in many clinical settings, nurses have a responsibility to understand the concept of voluntary informed consent and support the patient's rights throughout the research process. After reading this code, you should have increased awareness of the patient's right to autonomy and the health care provider's responsibility to be faithful to that right.

 BOX 19-4   The Nuremberg Code

The great weight of the evidence before us is to the effect that certain types of medical experiments on human beings, when kept within reasonably well-defined bounds, conform to the ethics of the medical profession generally. The protagonists of the practice of human experimentation justify their views on the basis that such experiments yield results for the good of society that are unprocurable by other methods or means of study. All agree, however, that certain basic principles must be observed in order to satisfy moral, ethical, and legal concepts:

1. The voluntary consent of the human subject is absolutely essential. This means that the person involved should have legal capacity to give consent; should be so situated as to be able to exercise free power of choice, without the intervention of any element of force, fraud, deceit, duress, overreaching, or other ulterior form of constraint or coercion; and should

(continued)

BOX 19-4   The Nuremberg Code (Cont'd)

have sufficient knowledge and comprehension of the elements of the subject matter involved as to enable him to make an understanding and enlightened decision. This latter element requires that before the acceptance of an affirmative decision by the experimental subject there should be made known to him the nature, duration, and purpose of the experiment; the method and means by which it is to be conducted; all inconveniences and hazards reasonably to be expected; and the effects upon his health or person which may possibly come from his participation in the experiment.

The duty and responsibility for ascertaining the quality of the consent rests upon each individual who initiates, directs, or engages in the experiment. It is a personal duty and responsibility which may not be delegated to another with impunity.

2. The experiment should be such as to yield fruitful results for the good of society, unprocurable by other methods or means of study, and not random and unnecessary in nature.

3. The experiment should be so designed and based on results of animal experimentation and a knowledge of the natural history of the disease or other problem under study that the anticipated results will justify the performance of the experiment.

4. The experiment should be so conducted as to avoid all unnecessary physical and mental suffering and injury.

5. No experiment should be so conducted where there is an a priori reason to believe that death or disabling injury will occur; except, perhaps, in those experiments where the experimental physicians also serve as subjects.

6. The degree of risk to be taken should never exceed that determined by the humanitarian importance of the problem to be solved by the experiment.

7. Proper preparations should be made and adequate facilities provided to protect the experimental subject against even remote possibilities of injury, disability or death.

8. The experiment should be conducted only by scientifically qualified persons. The highest degree of skill and care should be required through all stages of the experiments of those who conduct or engage in the experiment.

Reprinted from Trials of war criminals before the Nuremberg Military Tribunals under Control Council Law No. 18, Vol. 2. (1949). Washington, D.C., U.S. Government Printing Office, p. 181.

CONTROVERSIAL ETHICAL ISSUES CONFRONTING NURSING

Situations that raise ethical issues affect all areas of nursing practice. The following is a sampling of issues that consistently cause controversy.

Abortion. This issue has raged in the United States since the 1973 *Roe v. Wade* Supreme Court decision. The resolution of this case struck down laws against abortion but left the possibility of introducing restrictions under some conditions. Efforts toward that end continue today with mixed results for both pro-choice and pro-life factions. Increasing efforts are focused on the need for parental notification/consent.

Historical references to abortion can be found as far back as 4500 BC (Rosen, 1967). It has been practiced in many societies as a means of population control and terminating unwanted pregnancies, yet sanctions against abortion are found in both ancient biblical and legal texts. Interestingly, the ancient sanctions against abortion generally related to fines payable to the husband if the pregnant woman was harmed. This form of sanction derived from the concept of woman and fetus as male property. Greek philosophers, including Aristotle and Plato, made a distinction between an unformed fetus and a formed fetus. A fine was levied for aborting an unformed fetus, whereas the aborting of a formed fetus required "a life for a life." The number of gestational weeks that determine whether a fetus was formed was not stated, although the time of human ensoulment was understood: Aristotle believed that a male fetus was imbued with a soul at 40 days' gestation (*quickening*), versus 90 days for a female (Feldman, 1968). The subject of ensoulment became part of the ongoing debate regarding the time when the developing fetus becomes human. In other words,

---

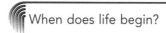 When does life begin?

Judeo-Christian theologians generally came to identify the beginning of life at conception or the time of implantation. Yet, even within this tradition, the Jewish *Talmud* and Roman law stated that life begins at birth because the first breath represents the infusion of life. These varied views continue to the present.

Social customs and private behavior regarding abortion have frequently differed from theological teaching. The first legal sanctions against abortion in the United States began in the late nineteenth century. Before that time, first-trimester abortions were not uncommon and in fact were advertised, supporting the idea that abortion before quickening was acceptable.

The ethical debate about abortion today is a continuing struggle to answer the question of when life begins and to determine an answer to the following questions:

- Does the fetus have rights?
- Do the rights of the fetus (for life) take precedence over the right of the mother to control her reproductive functions?
- When is abortion morally justified?
- Should minors have the right to abortion without parental consent or awareness?

The struggle to answer these questions has polarized individuals into "pro-life" or "pro-choice" camps. Yet opinion polls on the subject have found very few people to be against abortion in all circumstances or to favor abortion as a mandatory solution for some pregnancies. The majority of Americans express views anywhere between these extremes and the legal battle to maintain or restrict abortion access continues. The controversy has escalated into violence in some areas of the country, with abortion clinics and personnel subjected to attack; some abortion providers have even died. This violence has resulted in the decreased availability of abortion services in a number of areas.

The Roman Catholic Church has been the religious group most frequently identified with the pro-life movement, but there are other groups—religious and otherwise—that support a ban on abortion. Pro-life proponents generally condone abortion only to save the life of the mother. These antiabortion groups are criticized by pro-choice as extremists, antiwoman, and repressive.

The pro-choice movement is vocal in championing the woman's right to choose and promoting the safety of legalized abortion. They cite the tragedy of past "back-alley" abortions and compare restrictions on abortion to infringements on the civil liberties of women. Within the pro-choice movement are many individuals who favor restrictions on abortions after the first trimester and oppose the use of abortion as a means of birth control. Pro-life proponents view pro-choice supporters as antifamily extremists who do not represent the views of the majority of Americans.

How Does the Abortion Issue Affect Nursing? Nurses are involved both as individuals and professionals. Some general guidelines to consider are as follow:

- Consider what your values and beliefs are in relation to abortion and how you can best apply these values to your work and possible political action.
- If you choose to work in a setting in which abortions are performed, review statement one of the ANA's *Code of Ethics for Nurses:* "The nurse, in all professional relationships, practices with compassion and respect for the inherent dignity, worth and uniqueness of every individual, unrestricted by considerations of social or economic status, personal attributes, or the nature of the health problems" (ANA, 2001).

This statement outlines your responsibility to care for all patients. If you do not agree with an institution's policy or procedure regarding abortion, the patient still merits your care. If that care (i.e., assisting with abortions) violates your principles, you should consider changing your job or developing an agreement with your employer regarding your job responsibilities. If you cannot provide the care that the patient requires, make arrangements for someone else to do so.

- You do not have to sacrifice your own values and principles, but you are barred by the ANA *Code of ethics for nurses* from abandoning patients or forcing your values on them. Such abandonment would also constitute legal abandonment, and you would be subject to legal action.
- Some hospitals have developed conscience clauses that provide protection to the hospital and nurses against participation in abortions. Find out if your institution has such a clause.

Consider your response and possible conflict in the following situations:

You are a labor and delivery nurse working on a unit that performs second-trimester saline abortions in a nearby area. You are not a part of the staff for the abortion area, but today, because of short-staffing, you are asked to care for a 16-year-old who is undergoing the procedure.

You work in a family-planning clinic that serves low-income women. Because of escalating violence against abortion providers, the nearest abortion clinic is 100 miles away. You are restricted from giving information regarding abortion services because of federal guidelines.

A 41-year-old mother of five has expressed interest in terminating her pregnancy of 6 weeks' gestation. She confides that her husband would beat her if he knew she was pregnant and contemplating abortion.

You are teaching a class on sexuality and contraception to a group of high school sophomores. Two of the girls state that they have just had abortions. In response to your information regarding available methods of contraception, one of the girls states, "I'm not interested in birth control. If I get pregnant again, I'll just get an abortion. It's a lot easier."

You have a history of infertility and work in the neonatal ICU. You are presently caring for a 24-week-old baby born to a mother who admits to taking "crack" as a means of inducing labor and "getting rid of the baby." The mother has just arrived in the unit and wants to visit the baby.

These sample scenarios are meant to illustrate the conflicts that personal values, institutional settings, and patients may create for the recent graduate. In your responses consider how you might lobby or participate in the political process to change or support existing policies regarding abortion and access to such services.

Euthanasia. *Euthanasia* refers to "mercy killing." It is a Greek word that means "good death" and implies painless actions to end the life of individuals suffering from incurable or terminal diseases. Euthanasia has been closely tied to a "right-to-die" argument, which has gained a good deal of attention in the past decade. Euthanasia is classified as *active, passive,* or *voluntary. Active euthanasia* involves the administration of a lethal drug or another measure to end life and alleviate suffering. Regardless of the motivation and beliefs of the individuals involved, active euthanasia is legally wrong and can result in criminal charges of murder if carried out. In recent years, incidents of active euthanasia have become periodic news events as spouses or parents have used measures to end the suffering of their mates or children (from, for example, advanced Alzheimer's disease or vegetative coma). *Passive euthanasia* involves the withdrawal of extraordinary means of life support (e.g., ventilator). *Voluntary euthanasia* involves situations when the dying individual expresses his or her desires regarding the management and time of death to a sympathetic physician who then provides the means for the patient to obtain a lethal dose of medication.

As technology has advanced, patients are routinely kept alive today who would never have survived a few short years ago. Concerns regarding prolonging life and suffering for those individuals have resulted in a movement to have "right-to-die" statutes and living wills accepted (Fig. 19-1). In those states that have such statutes and recognize living wills, termination of treatment in such cases has become easier. Right-to-die statutes free health care personnel from possible liability for honoring a person's wishes that life not be unduly prolonged (Rudy, 1985).

Another document, the DPAHC, helps ensure that a living will is carried out. The DPAHC identifies the individual who will carry out the patient's wishes in the event that he or she is incapacitated and also informs health care providers about the specific wishes of the patient regarding life-support measures.

A major impact on the availability of living wills and the DPAHC (which are referred to as *advance medical directives*) resulted from the introduction of the Patient Self-Determination Act in December 1991. Passed as part of the Consolidated Omnibus Budget Reconciliation Act (COBRA), advance directives are federally mandated for all institutions receiving Medicare or Medicaid funds. On admission all competent adults must be offered information about advance directives. This means that all adults are told about the purpose and availability of living wills (*treatment directive*) and DPAHCs (*appointment directive*). They are then offered assistance with completing these documents if desired. After 10 years of having advance directive information available to patients, the impact of this document on decision making is varied. It certainly has influenced the communication patients have with their families, physicians, and other health care providers regarding their wishes at the timing of signing, but patients often change their minds when their health care status changes, frequently opting for the prolongation of life. A problem has surfaced regarding the timing of information to patients regarding advance directives. If patients first hear about advance directives on admission to acute-care settings, anxiety regarding their admission and the separate concept of advance directives may seriously affect informed decision making at that time. Advance directives should ideally be discussed before serious illness and at the very least in a noncrisis environment to encourage nonpressured decision making. Cultural, religious, and racial issues regarding DPAHC have also surfaced and need to be researched to determine the best approaches for a culturally diverse society. Patients and families need reassurance that declining extraordinary care does not mean the abandonment of caring and palliative care when needed.

Decisions to withdraw or withhold nutrition and hydration from patients is complex and the subject of ongoing debate by ethicists, health care personnel, and the legal system. In response to the issues of hydration and nutrition, the Ethics Committee of the ANA developed guidelines in 1988. These guidelines state that there are few instances when withholding or withdrawing nutrition and hydration are morally permissible. Although intended only as a guideline, this document provides direction for nurses who face such issues. Its wording has been both praised for its clarity and criticized for possible ambiguity. The primary exception to hydration and nutrition withdrawal is when harm from these measures can be demonstrated. This document is available from the ANA.

Futile Care and Physician-Assisted Suicide. Futile care (futility) and physician-assisted suicide (PAS) are two ethical and human rights issues that have drawn a great deal of attention and debate. In a survey conducted by the ANA's Center for Ethics and Human Rights in June 1994, respondents were asked to identify 10 of the most frequently occurring ethical issues. Approximately 55% identified "end-of-life

ADVANCE DIRECTIVE
Living Will and Health Care Proxy

Death is a part of life. It is a reality like birth, growth and aging. I am using this advance directive to convey my wishes about medical care to my doctors and other people looking after me at the end of my life. It is called an advance directive because it gives instructions in advance about what I want to happen to me in the future. It expresses my wishes about medical treatment that might keep me alive. I want this to be legally binding.

I cannot make or communicate decisions about my medical care, those around me should rely on this document for instructions about measures that could keep me alive.

I do not want medical treatment (including feeding and water by tube) that will keep me alive if:
- I am unconscious and there is no reasonable prospect that I will ever be conscious again (even if I am not going to die soon in my medical condition), *or*
- I am near death from an illness or injury with no reasonable prospect of recovery.

I do want medicine and other care to make me more comfortable and to take care of pain and suffering. I want this even if the pain medicine makes me die sooner.

I want to give some extra instructions: *[Here list any special instructions, e.g., some people fear being kept alive after a debilitating stroke. If you have wishes about this, or any other conditions, please write them here.]*

The legal language in the box that follows is a health care proxy.
It gives another person the power to make medical decisions for me.

I (name) _____ , who lives at _____

_____ , phone number _____ ,

to make medical decisions for me if I cannot make them myself. This person is called a health care "surrogate," "agent," "proxy," or "attorney in fact." This power of attorney shall become effective when I become incapable of making or communicating decisions about my medical care. This means that this document stays legal when and if I lose the power to speak for myself, for instance, if I am in a coma or have Alzheimer's disease.

My health care proxy has power to tell others what my advance directive means. This person also has power to make decisions for me, based either on what I would have wanted, or, if this is not known, on what he or she thinks is best for me.

If my first choice health care proxy cannot or decides not to act for me, I (name) _____

_____ , address _____ ,

phone number _____ , as my second choice.

(over, please)

I have discussed my wishes with my health care proxy, and with my second choice if I have chosen to appoint a second person. My proxy(ies) has(have) agreed to act for me.

I have thought about this advance directive carefully. I know what it means and want to sign it. I have chosen two witnesses, neither of whom is a member of my family, nor will inherit from me when I die. My witnesses are not the same people as those I named as my health care proxies. I understand that this form should be notarized if I use the box to name (a) health care proxy(ies).

Signature _____

Date _____

Address _____

Witness' signature _____

Witness' printed name _____

Address _____

Witness' signature _____

Witness' printed name _____

Address _____

Notary [to be used if proxy is appointed] _____

Drafted and Distributed by Choice In Dying, Inc.—the National Council for the right to Die. Choice In Dying is a National not-for-profit organization which works for the rights of patients at the end of life. In addition to this generic advance directive, Choice In Dying distributes advance directives that conform to each state's specific legal requirements and maintains a national Living Will Registry for completed documents.

CHOICE IN DYING INC.—
the national council for the right to die
(formerly Concern for Dying/Society for the Right to Die)
200 Varick Street, New York, NY 10014 (212) 366-5540

5/92

FIGURE 19-1

Advance directive.
(From Choice in Dying [formerly Concern for Dying/Society for the Right to Die], 200 Varick Street, New York, NY 10014-4810.)

decision" as one of the top four issues, and 37% identified "providing futile care" as an important priority issue facing nursing (Scanlon, 1994).

What Is Futility? *Medical futility* refers to the use of medical intervention (beyond comfort care) without realistic hope of benefit to the patient. *Benefit* is defined as improvement of outcome. A concrete example of futility would be the continuation of ICU care for a patient in a persistent vegetative state who would, on discharge from the hospital, return to a nursing home incapable of interacting with the environment. The futility debate concerns the very nature of the definition of *benefit*, in addition to who defines it. The economic pressure to control health care costs is also causing a focus on ways to eliminate "unnecessary" intervention.

On paper, futility can be defined, but its application to diverse clinical situations remains a challenge. The debate involves multiple parties whose interests and values are not always compatible. For example, patients and families have argued both for the right to refuse care that they believe is futile and the right to receive all possible care in the face of a medical opinion of futility. This argument raises two related questions, as follow:

- Do patients or families have the right to demand and receive treatment that health care providers believe to be futile?
- Do physicians have the right to refuse treatments that they believe to be futile despite patient or family desire to initiate or continue such treatment?

Ethics committees have researched the issue and struggled to agree on a working definition to provide direction and support for clinicians and patients and families who are faced with difficult decisions regarding care. Many institutions have developed guidelines for the withdrawal of treatment (except for comfort care). These guidelines emphasize the importance of clear, ongoing communication among all health care team members and with the patient and family. Accurate, compassionate discussion is essential to convey a unified approach to the realities and limitations of possible medical care. The guidelines should never be used as a threat or to imply abandonment. They are, as their name implies, guidelines. Lack of agreement among the patient, the family, and the health care team is likely to delay or prevent withdrawal of treatment, primarily because of the fear of liability, even in cases of brain death. Supporting the patient or family decision may be difficult because of personal values and professional opinions. It is crucial to clarify where professional loyalties should lie.

Pressures to eliminate unnecessary costs also influence the futility debate. Insurers, clinicians, and health care institutions increasingly question medical expenditures that produce futile outcomes and prolong the inevitability of impending death. Insurance reimbursement is likely to further limit and deny payment for treatment judged to be of no benefit. A possible risk is that beneficial treatment may be eliminated or denied solely because of economic concern in cases having an uncertain outcome. Nurses need to keep informed on institutional guidelines regarding medical futility and communicate clearly with patients, families, and physicians regarding expected goals and likely outcomes of care. The patient's welfare—and not economic concerns—should be the primary driving force for withdrawal of treatment.

Physician-Assisted Suicide. PAS has gained national attention because of Dr. Jack Kevorkian's persistent efforts to publicize and bring legitimacy to a formerly taboo topic. He has assisted or attended in the deaths of more than 130 terminally and chronically ill patients (Hyde, 1999). His work caused the state of Michigan to pass legislation barring PAS. Proponents of PAS have managed to put the issue on the ballot in three Western states since 1991, with passage occurring in the November 1994 Oregon election. PAS was immediately challenged in the Oregon court by right-to-life advocates but finally went into effect October 27, 1997. A first-year review of the law's impact indicated that 15 people had died as a result of prescriptions for lethal medications. Reasons cited for the use of a lethal dose include concern with loss of control over autonomy. Fear of uncontrolled pain or financial pressure was not mentioned (Chin et al, 1999). In 1997 the U.S. Supreme Court considered the "right to die" in the Burt Case, ruling that no constitutional right exists. This ruling gave considerable attention to the many issues and unmet needs regarding end-of-life care in this country.

PAS has been debated for years, and opinions on both sides among physicians and the public are very strong. The American Medical Association opposes PAS because it violates the most basic ethical principle: "Physician, do no harm." Physicians have traditionally taken care of the living patient, and support for PAS threatens to destroy this fundamental relationship. Many individual physicians have, however, changed their minds in recent years because of their work with terminally ill patients. More than a few of these clinicians have come to believe that the only option for the relief of some persons' pain and suffering is death, although continued progress in the management of physical pain in recent years may eliminate that reason.

Although the legalization of PAS is tied up in the courts, the practice goes on— generally in private without headlines. Both critics and supporters of PAS state that secrecy is because of the fear of arrest for homicide. Estimates by the Hemlock Society are that one in four acquired immunodeficiency syndrome deaths are from assisted suicide, including PAS (Conner, 1994). There have been some court rulings supporting the right to PAS by terminally ill patients on the basis of the Fourteenth Amendment's guarantee of personal liberty. These decisions have been assailed by the right-to-life groups as an antilife philosophy, which dishonors the intrinsic value of life.

PAS affects nursing practice because a decision to perform PAS may involve the nurse. The term *PAS* implies that the physician is the active agent, but a lethal dose may be ordered by the physician for the nurse to administer. Nurses need to be aware of the legal and ethical implications of such an order. The administration of a lethal dose for the explicit purpose of ending a patient's life is an illegal act that can be prosecuted as homicide. Yet, from an ethical point of view, many would consider this the ultimate act of mercy. In coming years, clinicians, ethicists, the public, and the courts will continue to struggle with how best to respect the life and wishes of terminally ill patients without "doing harm." Nurses need to remain aware of their nurse practice acts, and the *Code of ethics for nurses*, as they balance patient needs with their conscience and value systems.

Ethicists generally agree that although the prolongation of life by extraordinary means is not always indicated, clarifying the circumstances when such care may be stopped (withdrawn) or possibly never begun (withheld) frequently creates controversy, particularly when the quality of life (coma, persistent vegetative state) is likely to be questionable.

Opponents of the right-to-die movement believe that it represents the erosion of the value of human life and may encourage a movement toward the acceptance of suicide as part of a "culture of death." They caution that the lives of the weak and disabled may come to be devalued as society concentrates on the pursuit of "quality life." If passive euthanasia achieves societal acceptance, who will speak out in favor of protecting incompetent or dependent individuals who are not living society's view of a *quality life?*

Proponents of the right-to-die movement believe that it provides a more natural course of living and dying to the individual and family by avoiding the artificial prolongation of life through technology. The availability of technology to prolong life often raises the question "we can, but should we?"

Surveys of medical and nursing school curricula in the United States reveal minimal content on end-of-life care issues. Schools continue to focus curricula more on the curative approach to illness and disease, neglecting to address the palliative, comfort-directed needs of individuals who require care in the last months and days of their lives. This fact, combined with the aging of our population, points out the need for improvement in the education of both current clinicians and students in health care institutions. A growing number of proactive clinicians and educators concerned with the quality of care provided to dying patients and their families have created an educational movement called *End of Life Care.* The specific program targeted for nursing is called End of Life Nursing Education Consortium Project. This project is a partnership between Los Angeles City of Hope Medical Center and the American Association of Colleges of Nursing targeting nursing faculty across the country in an effort to expand both the quantity and quality of curriculum dealing with end-of-life care. Studies of patients facing end-of-life issues indicate that pain and symptom management, communication with one's physician, preparation for death, and the opportunity to achieve a sense of life completion are the most consistently important issues (Steinhauser et al, 2000). Most health care providers are not adequately prepared to manage these issues with their current educational preparation. It will be interesting to see the impact of these efforts on patient care over the next decade. Perhaps we will be better prepared to accept the reality that everyone does die. As nurses, we are challenged to make this last event of life a better experience for all.

Consider your response and possible conflict in the following critical-thinking situations:

A 22-year-old quadriplegic repeatedly asks you to disconnect him from the ventilator. His family rarely visits, and he believes that he has nothing to live for.

The spouse of an advanced Alzheimer's patient states that he can no longer watch his wife of 43 years suffer. "She would not have wanted to live this way." His wife is presently being treated for dehydration, malnutrition, and a urinary tract infection. She is confused and is frequently sedated to manage her combativeness. The use of a feeding tube is being contemplated because of her refusal to eat.

The attending physician for a patient with terminal acquired immunodeficiency virus refuses to order increasing doses of pain medication because of her concern that it may cause a repeat episode of respiratory depression. The patient's pain is unrelieved, and he begs you for medication. "Please help me. I know I'm dying."

The parents of a 29-week-old premature infant with Down syndrome and tracheoesophageal fistula request that no extraordinary care be provided. They want the baby kept warm and nurtured but refuse to sign the consent form for surgery.

For each of these scenarios, consider both what your reaction would be and the possible resources you would use to resolve the conflicts.

The Use of Reproductive Technology. Depending on the source, data indicate that 10% to 20% of all couples in the United States are identified as infertile. Because of this and the legalization of abortion, the development and use of reproductive technology is a subject of considerable interest and controversy.

What Is the Ethical Consideration in Artificial Insemination? Artificial insemination (AI) involves the use of husband or donor sperm in cases of infertility or when a single woman wishes to be artificially impregnated. The ethical arguments surrounding the issue involve beliefs about the use of reproductive interventions both inside and outside of marriage. For example, the Roman Catholic Church opposes AI, including the use of husband sperm, under all circumstances because it is an unnatural act and reduces people to objects (Berger, 1987).

Proponents of AI cite the ability of a woman to achieve pregnancy with a relatively simple intervention. The use of husband sperm allows a woman to achieve pregnancy with her own husband's genetic material and is generally supported because it is within a committed relationship. The issue is more controversial when donor sperm is used and the woman is single. The way in which we define *family* and *parenthood* may be challenged, particularly when lesbian couples are involved.

What Are the Ethical Issues Surrounding Surrogate Motherhood? The flip side to AI is surrogate motherhood. Unlike simple AI, there is no anonymity of the donor uterus. The surrogate mother is known, having been selectively chosen and contracted for the purpose of carrying a fetus for another couple to claim as their own. To date, some genetic fathers and artificially inseminated surrogate mothers have fought bitter legal and emotional wars to gain custody of the offspring.

Concern for the well-being and rights of the newborn, genetic father, and surrogate mother have been discussed at great lengths in the courts, the media, and ethical circles. Efforts have been made to remove the financial incentives for surrogate motherhood (New York Advance Legislative Service, 1992) because carrying a pregnancy for the purpose of making money has been likened to selling a human being. Contracting for the "sale" of a human being has raised disturbing issues, including the refusal of the biological mother to relinquish the child despite a "contract" (Baby M) and the birth of a grossly deformed child to a surrogate mother, resulting in the refusal of anyone to accept the child as his or her own. The latter case was most damning because the child was likened to "damaged goods," abandoned by both the buyer and seller.

What Is the Ethical Issue Regarding the Use of Fetal Tissue? Fetal tissue from elective abortions has been identified as potentially beneficial in the treatment of Parkinson's disease and other degenerative disorders because of its unique embryonic qualities. Proponents argue that it is available tissue that can be put to some beneficial use in patients who at present do not have any other hope of significant improvement or cure.

Critics who assail the use of fetal tissue as a further erosion of respect for the unborn were successful in spurring a federal ban on the use of fetal tissue for research in the United States during the 1980s. They believe that the limited research that has already occurred regarding fetal tissue has created the mentality that pregnancy can be used as a means of providing parts and tissues for others. This ban was removed in early 1993 after President Clinton took office and has recently (2001) received narrowly defined approval by the Bush administration for genetic research. A similar line of thinking has been used regarding the use of anencephalic infants as organ donors. Does the good (beneficence) achieved from the use of fetal tissue for patient's with Parkinson's disease outweigh the harm inflicted by viewing a fetus as a source of parts?

What Are the Ethical Issues Regarding In Vitro Fertilization? This procedure involves the fertilization of a mother's ovum with the father's sperm in a glass laboratory dish followed by implantation of the embryo in the mother's uterus. Since the birth of the first successful in vitro fertilization baby in 1978, the procedure has gained popularity as a last-chance method for some infertile couples to have a child. The availability of the technique has created a new subspecialty practice in obstetrics and raised ethical issues for consideration. Opponents of the procedure argue that it is an unnatural act and removes the biologic act of procreation from the intimacy of marriage. The cost of the procedure is also a source of criticism, calling into question whether it should be covered by insurance and whether the procedure should be available to all couples, regardless of ability to pay. Many couples are now lobbying to select the sex of their baby, choosing the desired embryo for implantation and destroying the undesired embryos. If technology can be made to meet our desires for a 'designer baby," does that make it a morally correct course of action?

Questions concerning informed consent for the procedure merit attention as well. Many infertility clinics offer this service but have not been upfront about their success rates or qualifications. Standardized methods of reporting this information have just recently been established. To be ethical, all such clinics should define success the same way; for example, success equals pregnancy or success equals live birth. The two definitions are very different. Information about the qualifications of the staff should be available to patients, and the subspecialty should lobby for standards of practice that are enforceable and available to the public. Possible side effects from the drugs used to induce hyperovulation and from anesthesia or surgical injury during the laparoscopy should be explained.

Should anyone who desires the procedure have access, or should the procedure be limited to those in a heterosexual marriage? Most clinics have limited their services to heterosexual couples to avoid adverse publicity, but this policy is starting to change as single and lesbian women seek out avenues of becoming biological parents.

Most importantly, to whom does the embryo belong and what are his or her rights? There have been court cases involving marital disputes regarding the custody of frozen embryos. What are the rights of the embryos in such instances? Can a parent choose to destroy the embryos over the objection of the estranged spouse, or should one parent be able to obtain custody of the embryos when his or her spouse wants them to be thawed out and destroyed? What responsibility does the staff have for maintaining parental ownership of the embryos?

How Should the Ability to Diagnose Genetic Defects Prenatally Be Used? At present, genetic disorders such as Tay-Sachs disease, cystic fibrosis, Huntington's chorea, and retinoblastoma can be diagnosed early in pregnancy. As this technology advances, how should it be used? Should screening remain voluntary, or, as some have suggested, should it be mandatory to detect fetal disorders that could be aborted or possibly treated? Should the results of such genetic screening be made available to insurance companies? Critics argue that this information could be used as a means of coercion for couples regarding reproductive decisions if future insurance coverage is then limited. As this technology advances, safeguards need to be applied to prevent invasion of privacy and any societal movement toward eugenics. As the human genome project allows us to become capable of knowing our genetic code and possibilities for disease, it raises the question of who should have access to that information.

Allocation of Scarce Resources. When the subject of scarce resource allocation is mentioned, justice is the core issue. What is fair and equal treatment when health care financing decisions are made? Who should make such decisions and on what basis? Critics argue that health care is not a scarce resource in this country, but that the access to such care is scarce for many. They believe that this scarcity of access could be eliminated if our priorities in governmental spending were altered. However, as of 1998, 13.4% of our gross national product was spent on health care (National Center for Health Statistics, 2001), an alarming amount because the cost of health care has continually skyrocketed. Managed care put a temporary brake on runaway costs, but that brake seems to have failed in the last year. Yet 14% of individuals living in the United States (almost 1 in 7) are without health insurance or a reasonable means of accessing anything but stopgap emergency care (U.S. Census Bureau, 2001). The solution to this issue remains unclear. Thus far, any form of national health insurance has been soundly defeated. In the meantime, managed care is influencing a larger and larger share of the insured population, raising related issues of restricted access to specialized care and loss of patient and physician autonomy.

Allocation also raises a number of questions. For example, do all individuals merit the same care? If your answer is an immediate "yes," would you change your mind if the patient were indigent, with no chance of paying the bill? If you still say "yes," should this same indigent patient receive a liver transplantation as readily as someone who has insurance or cash to pay for it? Should taxpayers be responsible for the medical bills for organ transplants, cardiac bypass surgery, or joint replacements for incarcerated felons? These and other questions are being asked by individuals, government, and ethicists, in addition to health care providers. Perhaps at the core of this subject is a more fundamental question: Is health care a right or a privilege that comes with the ability to pay? If access to health care is a right that should be provided to all citizens, are we as a society prepared to pay the bill? And is there a level of health care that is essential for all, beyond which financing becomes a private matter?

The type of care that is provided and supported is another aspect of the debate. For example, should health promotion and prevention be emphasized as much as or more than illness-oriented and rehabilitative care? It is widely acknowledged that each dollar spent on preventive care (e.g., prenatal care) saves three or more dollars in later intervention (e.g., neonatal ICU), yet our national and state health care expenditures (Medicare and Medicaid) are traditionally weighted in favor of an illness model for reimbursement. Managed care is an effort to apply the brakes to health care costs, yet it is increasingly criticized as prioritizing the financial bottom line over the quality of care.

What Are Some of the Possible Solutions Being Debated? In recent years some individuals, including the former Colorado Governor Richard Lamm, have proposed the idea of health care rationing for the elderly, specifically as it relates to the use of expensive technology that often prolongs the last few weeks of life and suffering (Lamm, 1986). He believes that such eleventh-hour expenditures are unwanted by many elderly and consume disproportionate amounts of health care resources. He has been criticized for his views but defends his ideas as an example of acknowledging the finite resources of society.

Lamm believes that other more vulnerable groups, such as uninsured children, should be given a more equitable portion of health care services (e.g., well-baby clinics). Others argue that health care is already being rationed and that we should recognize this fact and articulate our priorities.

The state of Oregon has gone one step further, imposing guidelines on the type of care that its Medicaid funds will cover. Deciding that preventive care affects a majority of its citizens, Oregon made funding for such measures as immunizations and prenatal care a priority, whereas extraordinary care that benefits only a few individuals, such as a bone marrow transplantation, will not be covered (Rooks, 1990). This utilitarian approach, emphasizing the greatest good for the greatest number, is not without its critics, but it is an effort to provide direction for health care priorities. Oregon's plan was initially vetoed by the federal government and has undergone some revision, still emphasizing preventive care and treatment for disorders that affect a majority of citizens. Other states are now looking at the Oregon model as they plan health care reform.

Health Care Rationing. You may have already experienced situations of health care rationing or limited access. As a nurse you may, on one hand, feel powerless and frustrated when patients do not receive care because they cannot afford it or, on the other hand, feel angry because indigent patients are placing heavy burdens on both private and public facilities. Consider your values and professional responsibilities as you think through this issue. As an individual and a nurse, you need to take a stand regarding health resource allocation and support efforts to improve access, while determining in your mind what type of health care you believe to be ethically justifiable.

As medical technology advances, ethical issues and concerns will play an ever-increasing role in your nursing practice. The general public, the health care professions, religious traditions, and the legal system will all have influence in the attempts to resolve the ethical issues affecting health care in the twenty-first century. Keeping an open mind in these controversial dilemmas is difficult, but it is hoped you will examine your personal values and continue to make decisions that are based on the welfare of the patients.

REFERENCES

American Nurses Association: *Code of ethics for nurses*, Kansas City, Mo, 2001, ANA.

Berger J: Vatican official assails method of fertilization, *New York Times*, Oct 8, 1987:B6.

Chin AE et al: Legalized physician-assisted suicide in Oregon—the first year's experience, *N Engl J Med* 340(7):577-583, 1999.

Conner D: Assisted suicide ban in Washington struck down. *Los Angeles Times*, May 4, 1994:A, 17:1.

Feldman DM: *Marital relations, birth control and abortion in Jewish law*, New York, 1968, Schocker.

Fletcher JF: *Situation ethics*, Philadelphia, 1966, Westminster.

Hyde J: Prosecutors drop assisted suicide charge against Kevorkian, 1999. http://detnews.com/1999/metro/9903/13/031301.htm

Lamm RD: Rationing of health care: the inevitable meets the unthinkable, *Nurs Pract* 11(5):57, 61-64, 1994.

National Center for Health Statistics: http://www.cdc.gov/nchs/fastats/hexpense.htm

New York Advance Legislative Service: *Regular session*, Ch 308, SB 1906, 1992.

Rooks JP: Let's admit we ration health care—then set priorities, *Am J Nurs* 90(6):38-43, 1990.

Rosen H, editor: *Abortion in America*, Boston, 1967, Beacon Press.

Rudy EB: The living will: are you informed? *Focus Crit Care* 12(6):51, 1985.

Scanlon C: Ethics survey looks at nurses' experiences, *Am Nurse* 26(10):22, 1994.

Steele SM: *Values clarification in nursing*, ed 2, East Norwalk, Conn, 1983, Appleton & Lange.

Steinhauser KE et al: Factors considered important at the end of life by patients, family, physicians, and other health care providers, *JAMA* 284(19):2476-2482, 2000.

Trials of War Criminals before the Nuremberg Military Tribunals under Control Council Law No. 18. Vol. 2. (1949). *Nuremberg Code*. Washington, DC: U.S. Government Printing Office.

US Census Bureau: *Health insurance coverage: people without health insurance for the entire year by selected characteristics: 1999 and 2000*, http://www.census.gov/hhes/hlthin00/hi00ta.html. Accessed Oct 15, 2001.

ADDITIONAL READINGS

Alaniz J: Death and dying: nurses recognize need for better training to deal with end of life issues, *NurseWeek 2001*.

Bandman EL, Bandman B: *Nursing ethics through the life span*, ed 3, East Norwalk, Conn, 1995, Appleton & Lange.

Banja JD: Nutritional discontinuation: active or passive euthanasia? *J Neurosci Nurs* 22(2):117-120, 1990.

Botes A: A comparison between the ethics of justice and the ethics of care, *J Adv Nurs* 32(5): 1071-1075, 2000.

Congressional Digest: President Clinton's Address to Congress, October, 225, 1994.

Costello J: Truth telling and the dying patient: a conspiracy of silence, *Int J Palliat Nurs* 6(8):398-405, 2000.

Curtin LL:. Euthanasia: a clarification, *Nurs Manage* 26(6):64-67, 1995.

Daly G: Ethics and economics, *Nurs Econ* 18(4):194-201, 2000.

Deloughery GL: *Issues and trends in nursing*, ed 3, St Louis, Mo, 1998, Mosby.

Edwards BS: Does the DNR patient belong in the ICU? *Crit Care Nurs Clin North Am* 2(3):473-480, 1990.

Erlen JA: Anencephalic infants as a source of organs: the need for caution, *Child Health Care* 19(3):187-189, 1990.

Ferrell B et al: Beyond the supreme court decision: nursing perspectives on end-of-life care, *Oncol Nurs Forum* 27(3):445-455, 2000.

Fiesta J: The Cruzan case—no right to die, *Nurs Manage* 21(9):22, 1990.

Goodman E: Death on the ballot, *Boston Globe*, Nov 3, 1994:19, 1.

Hall JK: *Nursing: ethics and law*, Philadelphia, 1994, WB Saunders.

Hudson T: Are futile-care policies the answer? Providers struggle with decisions for patients near the end of life, *HospHealth Netw*68(4):26-30, 32, 1994.

Kemp C: Culture and the end of life, *J Hospice Palliative Nurs* 2(3):109-200, 2000.

Leutwyler K: A healthy mess. Congress won't bite the cost-control bullet, *Sci Am* 271(4):28-31, 1994.

Mathes MM: Withholding and withdrawing artificial nutrition and hydration—a legal perspective, *Medsurg Nurs* 9(5):270-273, 2000.

Mitty EL: Ethnicity and end-of-life decision-making, *Reflect Nurs Leadersh* 27(1):28-31, 46, 2001.

Mohr WK, Horton-Deutsch SD: Malfeasance and regaining nursing's moral voice and integrity, *Nurs Ethics* 8(1):19-35, 2001.

National Association for Home Care: *What are my rights as a patient?* 1996, http://www.nahc.org/Consumer/wamraap.html.

Noddings N: In defense of caring, *J Clin Ethics* 3(1):15-18, 1992.

Oberle K, Hughes D: Doctors' and nurses' perceptions of ethical problems in end-of-life decisions, *J Adv Nurs* 33(6):707-715, 2001.

Pederson C et al: Using structured controversy to promote ethical decision making, *J Nurs Educ* 29(4):150, 1990.

Seroka TA: Values clarification and ethical decision-making, *Semin Nurse Manag* 2(1):8, 1990.

Shannon TA: Ethical issues involved with in vitro fertilization, *AORN J* 52(3):627-631, 1990.

Siveira MJ et al: Patients' knowledge of options at the end of life: ignorance in the face of death, *JAMA* 284(19):2483-2488, 2000.

White KR, Coyne PJ, Patel UB: Are nurses adequately prepared for end-of-life care? *J Nurs Scholarsh* 33(2):147-51, 2001.

INTERNET RESOURCES

Ethics Links
http://www.mic.ki.se/Diseases/k1.316.html

Medical Ethics Readings
http://www.uwc.edu/fonddulac/faculty/rrigteri/biomed.htm

MedWeb
http://www.medweb.emory.edu

National Center for Health Statistics
http://www.cdc.gov/nchs

University of Buffalo Center for Ethics & Humanities in Health Care
http://wings.buffalo.edu/faculty/research/bioethics/other.html

Human Genome Project
  http://www.ornl.gov/hgmis/

Hospice

Hospicecares.org
  http://hospice-cares.com

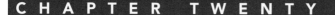
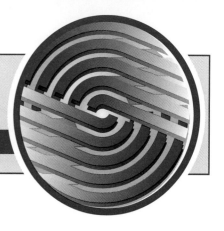
Legal Issues

ROBIN L. PERIN, RN, BS, JD

"The law is good, if a man use it lawfully."
—*The First Epistle of Paul the Apostle to Timothy 1:8*

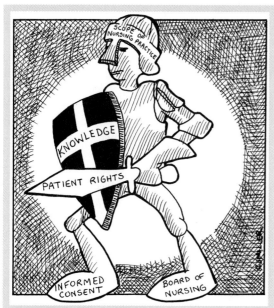

Knowledge regarding legal aspects is the best defense a nurse can have.

After completing this chapter, you should be able to:

- Discuss various sources and types of law.
- Relate the nurse practice act to the governance of your profession.
- Understand the functions of a state board of nursing.
- Describe your responsibilities for obtaining and maintaining your license.
- Be able to identify the elements of nursing malpractice and how they are proven in a malpractice claim.
- Incorporate an understanding of legal risks into your nursing practice and how to minimize these.
- Take an active role in improving the quality of health care as required by legal standards.
- Participate as a professional when dealing with nurses who are impaired or functioning dangerously in the work setting.
- Discuss the concerns surrounding at least two controversial legal issues.

When you graduate and become a registered nurse, you will also be achieving a new status under the law. An example of this change is that after meeting certain criteria, you will have a license to practice nursing. This license sets certain standards that you must follow as a nurse in the state. Should you not live up to these standards, your state can take away your ability to practice as a nurse. Also as a professional, you may be sued. Of course a person can always be sued if his behavior is negligent (unreasonable) and someone gets harmed. However, when you are working as a professional, the expectations for your behavior are higher than simply being a reasonable person. You are expected to perform as a reasonable nurse. If your actions are not what a reasonable nurse would do, and this causes someone to be injured, you can be sued in malpractice.

People react to these changes in legal status differently. Some nurses see the law as a big monster that is unpredictable, very frightening, and out to do them harm. They tend to act like ostriches and stick their heads in the sand whenever a legal subject is raised. If they become involved in a legal action, they are terrified and presume that terrible things will happen to them. Other nurses find the law to be quite interesting and attempt to learn all they can about how it may affect their practice. These nurses often find the law to be a very helpful tool to ensure safe practices. They also are much better able to protect themselves when they are dealing with legal issues. I hope that this chapter will be a start in your becoming a legally educated nurse. Remember, though, that the law is always changing, and to keep up with it requires continuous vigilance.

Before beginning a discussion of legal aspects in nursing, there is some practical advice that you can always use in any situation in which you wonder whether what you are doing or proposing to do is legal. It is called the "Mother Rule." When such a question about the legality of an action comes to you, ask yourself if you would feel comfortable telling your mother about what you are doing or propose to do. If your answer to this question is "no," then it probably is not legal. Why?

If you are uncomfortable with what you are doing, it may involve lying in some manner, which is involved in a claim for *fraud* or *defamation.* Perhaps you are doing something outside your scope of practice or something that is unsafe for the patient and could cause injury. These types of actions are involved in *malpractice. Invasion of privacy* and breach of *confidentiality* are claims that involve gossip or talking about patients unnecessarily.

In addition to the aforementioned, mothers are on juries. As jurors, they are instructed about laws, but they often cast their "votes" for what they think is "right" or "wrong." In every lawsuit, jurors are faced with evidence for both sides. In some respects, this forces them to simply make a human decision regarding the events. If you can feel comfortable when telling your mother (a jury) about what happened— truthfully and without hiding anything—then it is likely that you can do the same confidently with a jury. It is also likely that you will be believed and found to have acted reasonably. Simplified, that is all you need to do. Now let's address the more formal aspects of this thing called "law."

SOURCES OF LAW

WHERE DOES "THE LAW" COME FROM?

People will often tell you that you can't do something because it's illegal. Or they will make a statement that the law is this or that. Some nurses, who are afraid of laws, will simply believe what they are told. Other nurses will ask, "What law?" This is an important question because there is often much misinformation regarding the law floating around institutions where nurses work.

The most common type of law affecting nurses is **statutory law** or **statutes** or **laws.** These are the documented rules for living in your state (state laws) or the United States (federal laws) that are passed by state legislatures and by Congress. Statutory laws cover the rules for our relationships with each other and can be viewed as the ethics of our society written down. The section on definitions is one of the most important parts of a statute. There you can find what the authors of the statute mean when they use a certain word. Of course this is helpful because we all use words differently, but when reading laws, a more precise understanding is necessary. (Box 20-1 has a listing of definitions of common legal terms.)

Nurse practice acts are examples of state statutory laws and can be easily found online, in a public library, or obtained from the state board of nursing. (See the listing

---

BOX 20-1   Common Legal Terms

Advance directive: A document made by a competent individual to establish desired health care for the future or to give someone else the right to make health care decisions if the individual becomes incompetent; examples include living wills and medical power of attorney.

Defamation: A civil wrong in which an individual's reputation in the community, including the professional community, has been damaged.

Defendant: The person who is being accused of wrongdoing. The person then must defend himself or herself against the charges. In a malpractice claim, the nurse or other provider.

Deposition: An oral investigation done under oath and taken in writing. The purpose is to answer questions related to a specific issue. The deposition may include expert witnesses or those directly related to the case. It may be included in the trial phase of the case.

Diversion program: A program for treatment and rehabilitation of substance abusers. Such programs may be used by boards of nursing for encouraging treatment but are independent of such boards.

Expert witness: A person who has specific knowledge, skills, and experience regarding a specific area and whose testimony will be allowed in court. An expert witness may be asked to provide information regarding the standards of care.

(continued)

BOX 20-1   Common Legal Terms *(Cont'd)*

Good Samaritan law: Provides civil immunity to professionals who stop and render care in an emergency. Care provided must be within the expertise of the individual.

Interrogatory: A process of discovering the facts regarding a case through a set of written questions exchanged through the attorneys representing the parties involved in the case.

Jurisdiction: The court's authority to accept and decide cases. May be based on location or subject matter of the case.

Malpractice: Improper performance of professional duties; a failure to meet the standards of care that resulted in harm to another person.

Negligence: Failure to act as an ordinary prudent person when such failure results in harm to another.

Plaintiff: The person who files the lawsuit and is seeking damages for a perceived wrongdoing. In medical malpractice, the patient.

Reasonable care: The level of care or skill that is customarily used by a competent health care worker of similar education and experience in caring for an individual in the community or state in which the person is practicing.

Standard of care: Standards based on various types of evidence as to what is reasonable and prudent behavior for a health care professional.

Statute of Limitations: Laws that set time limits for when a case may be filed. Differ from state to state.

Telemedicine: Using telecommunication technology, usually interactive, to provide medical information and services.

Torts: Civil (not criminal) wrongs committed by one person against another person or property. Includes the legal principle of assault and battery.

Whistleblower: Individual "on the inside" who reports incorrect or illegal activities to an agency with authority to monitor or control.

Whistleblower statute: Law that protects a whistleblower from retaliation. Usually involves specific criteria about how whistle was blown.

---

at the end of this chapter.) It would first be important to see how a "registered nurse" is defined in your state to see whether there is a clue there about what nurses can or cannot do. Usually, however, these laws are quite general and might not answer your specific question about whether registered nurses in your state can administer intravenous (IV) conscious sedation.

■ HYPOTHETICAL CASE STUDY #1:

You are working in a hospital where a very well-known actor is admitted with a diagnosis of pneumocystic pneumonia. You know that this is usually associated with acquired immunodeficiency syndrome. During the patient's stay, you are asked by a physician to give an IV drug to sedate this patient while she does a procedure. The patient becomes oversedated, has a respiratory arrest, and dies. You are so upset about this that you call your best friend, who is also a nurse, to talk about the incident. You mention the actor's name and the fact that he had acquired immunodeficiency syndrome. Your friend says that it was "illegal" for you to be giving what he calls "IV conscious sedation" and you are in deep trouble. Where might you be able to search to determine whether this is true? What type of legal trouble might you have?

The next type of law is *constitutional law*. This type of law refers to the rights, privileges, and responsibilities that were stated in, or have been inferred from, the U.S. Constitution, including the Bill of Rights. States may not pass laws or institute rules that conflict with constitutionally granted rights or rules because the Constitution is the highest law of our country. Freedom of speech and religion are such rights. The right to privacy is an example of a right inferred from the Constitution (Critical Thinking Box 20-1).

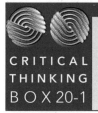

CRITICAL THINKING BOX 20-1

In hypothetical case study #1, can you identify where a constitutional law might have been broken?

The third type of law to consider is *administrative law*. This body of law is made by administrative agencies that have been granted the authority to pass rules and regulations and render opinions, which usually explain in more detail the state statutes on a particular subject. Examples of this type of law are the rules and regulations passed by boards of nursing to control nursing practice in each state. This might well be a source for finding out specifically about nurses giving IV conscious sedation in your state. There may also be an "advisory opinion" given by the state board of nursing on this topic. Your state board of pharmacy may also have other regulations that describe their rules for administering medications and who may do this.

Another type of law is *common law*, which includes decisions made by judges in court cases or is established by rules of custom and tradition. *Case law* is composed of the decisions rendered in court cases by appeal courts. Often, nurses will hear about something happening in a court case and think that there must be a document somewhere talking about that case. This is not necessarily true, because not all cases reach the level of an appeal court, where a record of the court's opinion and reasoning is recorded. Cases are usually appealed to higher courts because there is an issue of statutory law involved. Many cases do not have such issues and are, therefore, not appealed or recorded.

Once there is a recorded court opinion, the result is the legal principle of *stare decisis*, which means that if an issue has been decided, all other cases concerning the same issue should be decided the same way. Another word for this is *precedent.* Although you may hear of a case in which a nurse was found negligent in administering IV conscious sedation, there may not be case law on this issue to set a legal precedent in your state. Each state has its own case law. Each state's body of case law differs because it is based on the decisions of individual judges, who often do not resolve issues in the same way as judges in another state and who base their decisions on differing state statutes.

COURT ACTIONS BASED ON LEGAL PRINCIPLES

There are two major classifications of court of common law legal actions that can occur as a result of either deliberate or unintentional violations of legal rules or statutes. In the first category are *criminal* actions. These occur when you have done something that is considered harmful to society as a whole. The trials will involve a prosecuting attorney, who represents the interests of the state or the United States (the public), and a defense attorney, who represents the interests of the person accused of a crime (defendant). These actions can usually be identified by their title, which will read "State vs. [the name of the defendant]" or "US vs. [the name of the defendant]. Examples include murder, theft, drug violations, and some violations of the nursing practice acts such as misuse of narcotics. Serious crimes that can cause the perpetrator to be imprisoned are called *felonies.* Less-serious crimes resulting in fines are *misdemeanors.* The victim, if there is one, is considered only a witness in the criminal trial and does not receive any of the money from fines. In the hypothetical case study #1, your actions would not likely result in a criminal action. Recently, however, there have been instances in which a nurse was thought to have recklessly caused a patient's death, and a case was brought in criminal court for negligent homicide. The issues involved in such criminal actions will be discussed later in this chapter.

In the second category of legal claims are *civil* actions. These actions concern private interests and rights between the individuals involved in the cases. Private attorneys handle these claims, and the remedy is usually some type of compensation that restores the injured party to their earlier position. Examples of this type of action include malpractice, negligence, and informed consent issues. The victim (patient) or victim's family (patient's family) brings the lawsuit as the *plaintiff* against the *defendant* who may be the individual (nurse) or company (hospital) who is believed to have caused harm. In the situation presented, you might be sued for malpractice by the actor's spouse if it is felt that you acted below a standard of care and caused the actor's death.

Sometimes an event can have both criminal and civil consequences. When that happens, two trials are held with different goals. The amount of evidence required to support a guilty verdict is different for each type of trial. The criminal case requires that the evidence show that the defendant was guilty beyond a shadow of a doubt. The civil case requires only that the evidence show that the defendant was more likely guilty than not guilty. That is why you may see situations where someone such as O.J. Simpson can be found not guilty in the criminal trial, and guilty in the civil trial.

LEGAL CONTROL OVER NURSING PRACTICE

Having a license to practice nursing brings you into close contact with laws and government agencies. The nurse practice act is the statute governing nurses in your state. The board of nursing is the agency designated to apply the laws to individuals.

There are nurses who do not understand their responsibilities in relationship to their licensing board. Do not become one of these. State Boards act under the police power granted each state from the federal government to protect the safety of its residents. Persons serving on such boards take this responsibility seriously. They expect that you will also.

■ HYPOTHETICAL CASE STUDY #2:

After your incident with the actor, you decide to leave the state. You have to answer detailed questions on your licensure application for the new state about any previous malpractice claims. You had heard something about a claim being filed against the hospital but had left shortly after that. Now you have received a notice from the State Board of Nursing of your previous residence inquiring about the incident with the actor and asking for a response within two weeks. The letter has taken a long time to be forwarded to you, and you have passed the deadline given to you. What should you do?

WHAT ARE THE LEGAL ASPECTS OF LICENSURE?

Receiving a license to practice nursing is a privilege, not a right. Even the successful completion of an educational program in nursing and/or passing the National Council Licensure for Examination for Registered Nurses (NCLEX-RN) does not guarantee that a license will be granted. A license is granted by a state after a candidate has successfully met **all** the requirements in that particular state. Examples of these requirements may include high school education, successful completion of a nursing education program, application to the appropriate national and state agencies, fee payment, not being a felon (i.e., not having a criminal record), and passing the national exam for the appropriate level of licensure (NCLEX-RN or PN). Because the license is intended to guarantee public safety, the level of expertise necessary to pass the test is the minimum level needed to provide safe care. The state also continues to monitor your practice and to investigate complaints regarding this practice.

When you move to a new state, you need to make certain decisions with regard to your license. You may want to continue being licensed in the state of past residence. It is important to keep your past state board informed of your current residence so you receive important documents in a timely fashion that can affect your future ability to practice. You also need to be informed of licensure and practice requirements of a new state of residence before you begin to practice there.

Each state's practice act may be different from any other state's act. In the past, this has posed many hurdles for nurses who traveled or had practices across state lines. States have attempted to resolve these issues by developing a licensure model that will allow participating states to recognize licensure of another state. This works in the same manner as your state driver's license being recognized in other states, but your having to adhere to that state's driving laws. As of January 2002, 16 states had passed laws to accept the Nurse Licensure Compact, or the *Mutual Recognition Model* (NCSBN, 2002). You can practice in those states if your home state is part of the model.

If you travel to another state, or cross state lines in the normal course of your practice, either with a specific patient or to perform some nursing services in another state, you need to check with the board of nursing in the states in which you are performing nursing care to determine their rules about practice within their borders. An example of this would be telephone triage or telemedicine programs with patients outside of your state. You can obtain copies of a state practice act from the board of nursing or licensing agency for nurses in that state (see Appendix A for addresses of state boards of nursing).

Some practice acts regulate nursing by controlling who may use the titles registered nurse and licensed practical nurse or licensed vocational nurse. Others regulate by controlling the scope of practice and determining the specific activities for each level of nursing—that is, who can perform what functions. In most states, the nurse practice act does the following:

1. Describes how to obtain licensure and enter practice within that state.
2. Describes how and when to renew your license.
3. Defines the educational requirements for entry into practice.
4. Provides definitions and scope of practice for each level of nursing practice.
5. Describes the process by which individual members of the board of nursing are selected and the categories of membership.
6. Identifies situations that are grounds for discipline or circumstances in which a nursing license can be revoked or suspended.
7. Identifies the process for disciplinary actions, including diversionary techniques.
8. Outlines the appeal steps if the nurse feels the disciplinary actions taken by the board of nursing are not fair or valid.

Some practice acts are very specific and detailed, others simply grant the board authority to declare the rules and regulations (administrative law) and to establish the details. To understand the scope of practice within a specific state in which you are practicing or wish to practice, you must obtain a copy of the state nurse practice act that includes the law, rules, and regulations that the board or administrative agency has established in that state.

Because you have gone to a great deal of expense and work to obtain your nursing license, you should guard it carefully. Never ignore or take lightly any document received from your state board of nursing. Even if you think you have received a notice in error, contact the board of nursing immediately (Box 20-2).

The power of the board to discipline is the power, which can have an adverse effect on the nurse's ability to practice. It is important that each nurse carefully review the power of the Board within the state of their practice Several levels of disciplinary actions can occur based on the severity of the problem. Boards of nursing have the authority to censure, to suspend, to revoke, or to deny licensure. Each of these actions can be temporary or permanent. It would be prudent to consult an attorney who is

> ### BOX 20-2 Protect Your License
>
> ❑ Do not let anyone else borrow it.
> ❑ Do not let anyone copy it unless you write "copy" across it. In some states it is illegal to copy your license.
> ❑ If you lose it, report it immediately and take the necessary steps to obtain a duplicate.
> ❑ Be sure that the board of nursing knows whenever you change your address, whether you move across the street or across the nation.
> ❑ Practice nursing according to the scope and standards of practice in your state.
> ❑ Know your state law so you will not do anything that could cause you to be disciplined by the removal of your license.
> ❑ Meet all renewal requirements on time.

versed in health care law if you should receive notice of any possible action against your license. Such a person can be your advocate and explain your rights and how best to deal with the state board. Seeking legal advice is an investment to protect your investment. Some institutions assist nurse employees in these instances, and some nurse insurance policies will also defend nurses in these "administrative actions."

WHAT ABOUT THE IMPAIRED NURSE?

Impaired nurses are nurses who are unable to function effectively because of some type of substance abuse (i.e., alcohol, prescription drugs, or illegal drugs.). More attention is currently being given to this area because of the heightened awareness of substance abuse in our society as a whole, in addition to the increasing recognition of the severity of the problem among health care workers (Haack, 1989). One of the most common reasons for state board action against nurses involves the taking of hospital medications for personal use (Fiesta, 1998). Boards of nursing are increasingly concerned about this issue, because it has significant impact on rendering safe, effective patient care (Deloughery, 1998). Some states will also discipline a nurse who knows about but fails to report an impaired nurse. You are never doing a colleague a favor by not reporting impairment. A dead patient at the hands of an impaired nurse is a terrible outcome if it could have been prevented.

Do not ever assume that you or your colleagues are immune from impairment. High stress and easy access to drugs seem to contribute to this common problem for health care providers (Haack, 1989). There is a slippery slope that occurs when a nurse first takes any medication, even an aspirin, that does not belong to him or her. It is best to see that first wrong as a start to many future wrongs and never do it. If you do find yourself in trouble with drugs or alcohol, it is far better to voluntarily report this to your state board of nursing, rather than to be caught or to harm other persons. Most boards react favorably to the nurse who seeks assistance, rather than one who is reported by law enforcement agencies or a hospital as required by law.

Many states have taken a rehabilitative approach to this problem, rather than a punitive one, particularly to those who self-report (Youm and Haack, 1996). These states have programs set up to allow nurses to meet specific behavioral criteria, such as blood or urine testing, ordered evaluations, and attendance at rehabilitation programs, either while disciplinary action is being taken or instead of bringing formal proceedings. The primary concern is to assist the impaired nurse back to full and appropriate nursing practice. If a nurse is involved in a voluntary rehabilitation program through a contract with a state board and backslides or has additional problems, the board may bring formal action against the nurse that will negatively affect licensure for the rest of his or her life and can also involve criminal sanctions.

WHO KNOWS ABOUT THE DISCIPLINARY ACTIONS AGAINST NURSES?

When an action is taken by a state board against a nurse, states have differing methods of reporting such action to health care providers and others to protect the public. **NURSYS** is a comprehensive electronic information system that includes the collection and warehousing of nurse licensing information and disciplinary actions. Previously called NIS and ELVIS, as it underwent different stages of development, the term "NURSYS" is a derivative of nurse and system. NURSYS contains data on a nurse's personal information (identity, residence), license information, education information, disciplinary action information, verification and fee tracking requests, and historical information (any changes to the aforementioned data). NURSYS is the information system that supports the mutual recognition of nurses' licenses. It is a locked system at present and only Member Boards of Nursing and the National Council of State Boards of Nursing (NCSBN) have access to the information stored there. Future development may include limited access by government agencies, potential employers, and consumers (*Forum*, 1999).

Another national storehouse of information is **The National Practitioner Data Bank,** which was part of a federal law under Medicare called *The Health Care Quality Improvement Act* (Denega, 1993). Although primarily set up to identify physicians who had committed malpractice and/or who had licensure problems across state lines, nurses also may be reported to the Data Bank for adverse licensure actions and certain malpractice claims (Kelly and Joel, 1999).

TORTS

Civil, as opposed to criminal, actions are also called *torts*. Remember that civil actions occur when a plaintiff files a lawsuit to receive compensation for damages he or she suffered as a result of a perceived wrong. The economic reason for filing the suit should never be forgotten. This is important to keep in mind should you or a colleague become involved in a tort action. Try not to interpret everything in terms of a personal insult and/or an intentional desire to cause you personal and professional harm. This is not a criminal action and the terms "guilty" or "innocent" are not appropriate, nor are words such as "killed" that can sometimes be heard in the gossip mill or read in the media.

There are two categories of tort actions. Unintentional torts are those that usually involve an inadvertent, unreasonable act that causes harm to someone. We might call these acts "incidents" or "accidents." Intentional torts are those acts done deliberately by a defendant. Although sometimes occurring in the heat of a moment, they are not considered accidental in nature.

NURSING MALPRACTICE

The most common unintentional tort action brought against nurses is a malpractice claim. Let's explore what this means.

■ HYPOTHETICAL CASE STUDY #3:

You are a nurse working in a hospital. The physician tells you that you need to give an injection of vistaril. You make sure that the order is documented in the medical record. The medication comes up from the pharmacy and you check it against the physician's order and find it to be correct. You walk into the patient's room and check the patient's identification to make sure it is the right patient. You give the injection in the patient's right upper outer quadrant of the buttocks and document this in the medical record. The patient leaves the hospital. A year later you are told that a lawsuit has been filed against the hospital by the patient. It seems the patient is claiming that the injection you gave him caused sciatic nerve damage and his whole leg is numb (Critical Thinking Box 20-2).

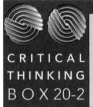

CRITICAL THINKING BOX 20-2

Who may have malpractice liability in this situation and why? You? The physician? The hospital? What defenses might be available to you?

LEGAL COMMENTARY

Many times nurses worry about being sued for something when, in the eyes of the law, no malpractice has occurred. Not all poor outcomes are malpractice. A nurse also may legitimately make an error in judgment. Therefore it is important for a nurse to know the basic elements that must be proved before malpractice can occur. Then the nurse can evaluate incidents realistically.

BASIC ELEMENTS OF MALPRACTICE

What Are The Basic Elements Of Malpractice?

1. You must have a duty. In other words there must be a professional nurse-patient relationship.
2. You must have breached that duty. In other words you must have fallen below the standard of care for a nurse.
3. Your breach of duty must have been a foreseeable cause of the patient's injury.
4. Damages or injury must have occurred.

These four elements need to be present in each malpractice case. The job of the patient's (plaintiff's) attorney is to prove to a jury that each element has occurred. Your attorney, on the other hand, defends you by proving that all or even just one element did not happen. This is not always a black and white process, which can often be frustrating and confusing. Still, it is important for the nurse to evaluate events in light of these elements and to know how they are proved in court.

Do You Have A Professional Duty? To make a claim of malpractice against a nurse, the plaintiff must establish that there is a nurse/patient relationship, or in legal terms, that you had a professional duty to a patient. A duty is implied if you are employed by and render services at a health care institution such as a hospital or nursing home. This would also be true if you work as a registered nurse for a home health agency in the home, or in a school, or in a physician's office.

In the case studies, you are working as a nurse in a hospital and the nurse-patient relationship is implied. Therefore the first element can easily be proved. What if you are giving medical advice in your home informally as a friend, relative, or neighbor? In this setting, it is not implied that you are acting as a nurse; and proving that you owed your friend a duty as a professional might be difficult. There is no payment, or institution, or formal contract. Therefore, although nurses are continually warned about being sued in this situation, it is unlikely that a plaintiff's attorney would easily prevail on the element of duty for such casual comments to others outside your employment.

What if you stop at an accident to assist someone who is injured? Because most states want to encourage medical professionals to help people at accidents without fear of a lawsuit, *Good Samaritan Statutes* have been passed. These laws give immunity from malpractice to those professionals who attempt to give assistance at the scene of an accident. In essence you do not have any professional duty to stop, although you may feel an ethical duty to do so. If you do, know that in most—if not all—states you cannot be sued in malpractice for what you might or might not do. That is, you do not have a professional standard of care to adhere to unless you are a professional at the scene as part of your employment. All persons, of course, are expected not to leave the victim in a position that is more dangerous than when you found them.

Sometimes nurses volunteer to give nursing assistance at sports events or other activities in which it is foreseen that professional services may be needed. In thinking about this, you may see that such a situation is not quite as clear as other situations. If you are at a first aide station and/or wear a badge indicating you are a nurse, then you have an appearance that you are a professional and people may rely on that when seeking advice or assistance. Some states give immunity to professionals under these circumstances by statute (Arizona Revised Statutes §32-1472). *It is important to know your status under such circumstances in your state, and/or if you have immunity and/or are covered by malpractice insurance.*

What is the Professional Duty Owed? Once it is established that you owe a duty to the person, the question becomes what is that duty? How does a plaintiff's attorney establish what the duty might be? A nurse's duty owed is different than that of a physician or nursing assistant. The duty of a nurse will be to act as a reasonable nurse under the same or similar circumstances. The duty or standard of care for the physician will be to act as a reasonable physician. You can see that the two will be different. Of course the most interesting question in any malpractice case will be how will my attorney prove that I acted as a reasonable nurse? The following will be considered when attempting to establish through evidence what the standard of care for the nurse might be.

What About the Nurse Practice Act? Perhaps the most important guideline for nurses will be the Nurse Practice Act in the state in which you are practicing. Most acts describe in fairly general terms what a nurse may do. Prohibitions, or things that are considered unprofessional conduct, are usually more specific. A violation of such a license prohibition means that you have fallen below a standard of care set by the state for nurses. It also may mean that you risk an action against your license. If you don't know what these prohibitions are, then you are putting yourself in jeopardy. As stated previously, and applied here to the standard of care, be sure to keep up with your licensing standards.

What Is An Expert Witness? The most common way to establish the duty owed by a nurse is by the testimony of a registered nurse usually, but not always, with training and background similar to yours. This expert witness will then testify regarding what a reasonable nurse in the same or similar circumstances would be expected to do, and that you did not do it. If a plaintiff's attorney cannot find an expert nurse to testify that you did not act reasonably, then in most instances the case cannot go forward. In general, a patient cannot simply claim professional malpractice without having a professional witness to prove this.

In the same manner, if the plaintiff has an expert witness to prove you fell below the standard of care, you will need an expert witness to testify that you did not. Some nurses enjoy being expert witnesses either for the defense of a nurse, or as part of the plaintiff's claim against a nurse. Either role requires both integrity and professionalism to be effective and believed by a jury.

There is a type of malpractice case in which an expert is not required. This type of claim is called *res ipsa loquitur,* or "the thing speaks for itself." This claim is very difficult to prove because the patient must have enough evidence to show that (1.) the injury would ordinarily not occur unless someone were negligent, (2.) the instrumentality causing the injury was within the exclusive control of the defendant, and (3.) the incident was not owing to any voluntary action on the part of the plaintiff (Fiesta, 1998). If a patient can prove that all of these exist, the burden then shifts to the defendant nurse to prove that malpractice did not take place. Incidents such as operating on the wrong body part or leaving a surgical sponge in a patient fall into this category of claims.

What are Established Policies and Procedures? Policies and procedures established by the institution in which you work are most crucial pieces of evidence for establishing a standard of care. Most good plaintiffs' attorneys will request a set of hospital policies as soon as a lawsuit is filed. For instance, in hypothetical case studies #1 and #3, a lawyer might ask for the hospital's policies on documentation and administration of medications. If you did not follow that policy, then you fell below a standard of care set by your institution.

You can see why you need to know and read the policies within your health care facility or corporation. These policies should also be a resource when you have questions about how to do certain procedures, or what your rights are in a certain situation. Policies are the laws under which you must live. It is also important for you as a professional to participate in making or changing policies so that they accurately reflect what nurses are doing in your institution. In addition, the policies set standards for giving quality and consistent patient care. If you have followed a policy, it can also be used proactively to prove that you followed the standard of care set by your institution.

What About Accreditation and Facility Licensing Standards? Most health care facilities and other health care organizations such as Health Maintenance Organizations (HMOs) must go through a process whereby they become licensed and/or accredited. The Joint Commission for Accreditation of Healthcare Organizations (JCAHO) and the National Committee of Quality Assurance are two such organizations that set standards for health care organizations. These standards can often be used as evidence of the standard of care for nurses working in such facilities. For instance, the JCAHO requires that the preparation and dispensing of medication(s) adhere to law, regulation, licensure, and professional standards of practice (JCAHO, 2000). There is also a standard that prescriptions or orders are verified and patients identified before medication is administered (JCAHO, 2000). A state facility licensing requirement might be that the facility develop policies and procedures that govern the safe administration of drugs and that "each dose of medication administered shall be recorded in the patient's medication record and shall show the date, time, dosage and method of administration and a method of identifying the person who administered the dose" (Arizona Administrative Code R4-23-660).

What About Textbooks and Journals? If you become a defendant in a lawsuit, you may be asked about texts used in the workplace such as the *Physician's Desk Reference*. You may also be asked whether you subscribe to a nursing journal. Articles or portions of such publications may be used as evidence of the standard of care for nurses to follow. For instance, if a nursing journal has published a recent article on correct administration of intramuscular injections, that may be used to demonstrate what you should have done. The fact of having a *Physician's desk reference* on a nursing unit might be used to demonstrate that a source for the correct dose of any medication and its correct administration was/is immediately available to you where you work.

What Are Professional Standards for Organizations? Professional organizations such as the American Nurses Association or the Association of Perioperative Registered Nurses may publish certain standards or practice guidelines. These may also be used as evidence for what a reasonable nurse should do under certain circumstances. If you are ever part of a group that sets professional standards, be sure that the standards are practical and reasonable. Knowing they can be used against nurses in malpractice claims explains why using unattainable ideals for standards, although sounding nice, can be harmful. Such standards can also be used to demonstrate that the nurse did or did not follow the standard of care.

In summary, there are many different types of evidence used by plaintiff attorneys to demonstrate an expected standard of care. The nurse needs to remember that these same documents can be used to demonstrate that you did follow the standard of care. Let us see how.

Applying the Standard of Care to the Case Study. In the hypothetical case study #3, the plaintiff will have to find a nurse that will testify to the correct method of giving intramuscular injections. If you did not give the injection in such a manner, then the jury can infer that you did not act reasonably. However, if the correct method is to give the injection intramuscularly in the upper, outer, quadrant of the buttocks and you have documented that you did this, an expert's testimony will not help prove anything. Also, if you can show that you followed hospital policies in the administration of the medication, again, there will be no proof of falling below a standard of care.

What if the patient attempts to claim a case using the theory of *res ipsa loquitur?* Again, the patient's lawyer must prove that the claimed injury could not have happened unless there was negligence. As demonstrated earlier, you would be able to prove through your documentation that you were not negligent. In addition, your attorney would also be demonstrating your lack of liability through the third element of malpractice. Do you remember what that is?

Was There A Breach of Professional Duty? Not only must a plaintiff prove what the standard of care is in a given situation, the plaintiff must prove that you did not meet the standard of care. Other legal terms used regarding this needed element might be that you "fell below the standard of care" or you "breached the duty owed the patient." In other words the plaintiff must demonstrate through the evidence listed earlier that you did not act as a reasonable and prudent nurse under the circumstances. Please remember that even if you did not act reasonably, there are other elements that must be proved to have a malpractice claim.

Did the Breach of Duty Cause the Injury? Causation is an element often overlooked by the nurse, and yet is most often hotly argued by attorneys. Did the difficult birth cause the child to have cerebral palsy or did a genetic birth defect cause the baby to have a difficult delivery? Was the injury caused by the auto accident or by the medical care? Did the patient have the physical problem before the medical care or after? Was the injury caused subsequently by the patient's lack of compliance with the treatment plan, or did the patient subsequently injure herself after the medical care was rendered?

The causation requirement must be proved by the plaintiff's attorney, and as you can imagine, this may not be easy. Certain well-documented observations will make such proof impossible.

1. Document clearly the patient's physical and mental condition upon admittance to and discharge from your health care facility or unit. Both of these observations can be used to demonstrate that either the patient had the symptom when she came and/or did not have the symptom upon leaving.

2. After any incident, such as a patient fall, the patient's physical and mental condition must be documented. This will help demonstrate that subsequent complaints cannot be attached or caused by the incident.

3. Document clearly any actions of a patient that demonstrate noncompliance with medical directives. When a patient states or clearly demonstrates that he is not taking medications as ordered or is not following a prescribed physical therapy regimen, this can cause therapeutic failure, rather than the treatment itself. A documented "no show" at an outpatient clinic can dispel later claims that you ignored complaints and so caused the injury.

4. Document clearly when a patient complains and does not complain. If, in the case study, it is documented that the patient has been up and walking after the injection and has no complaints, it will be very difficult to prove that the injection caused the problem.

5. Be very careful when documenting what a patient *states* as opposed to what you think may have happened. If a patient states that an injection caused a problem, it is best to document clearly "Patient states, 'My leg has felt numb since I received an injection in the hospital,'" rather than document, "Hospital injection caused patient's leg to be numb." The latter documentation may inadvertently be condemning a health care provider who has done nothing wrong.

6. Document the patient's own admissions. "I knew I shouldn't have gotten out of bed so soon" can be helpful if a patient falls and then later tries to blame the nursing staff. "My wife tried to remove the stitches, but she could not get that deep one" can raise doubt regarding what caused the incision to become infected. Infection is very rarely considered to be malpractice unless it can be proved to have been caused by negligence such as not using good aseptic technique.

7. Document clearly discharge instructions. In today's managed-care environment, many acutely ill patients are sent home to care for themselves. If they and/or their families have not been given clear instructions on not only their care, but also symptoms to watch for that may need attention, they may attempt to blame health care professionals for what occurs at home. A clear, documented discharge

plan after any procedure that can have adverse outcomes is imperative, not only to prevent law suits, but for good patient care. A warning to a patient to call a specific number if adverse symptoms occur can save a life and prevent a lawsuit. Emergency departments have long understood the importance of such instructions and the age of specialized computer software programs makes them easily accessible to everyone. Even veterinarians are able to do computerized discharge planning for pets (Fig. 20-1).

8. A patient's allergies or lack thereof is another way of preventing a malpractice claim. Neither nurses nor physicians cause patient's to have allergies. They do have a duty to not give medications to patients when prior experience has demonstrated that the medication has caused an allergic reaction. "No known allergies" can completely eliminate a claim involving an allergic reaction.

APPLYING "CAUSATION" TO THE CASE STUDY

Returning to the case example, the patient will have to prove that your injection caused the numbness in his leg. There are many intervening factors that could have caused this numbness. You do not have to prove anything because you, as a defendant, do not have a "burden of proof." The plaintiff may have a very difficult time, especially if there are no documented complaints by the patient of problems at the time of the injection or shortly thereafter.

Just remember that a patient's claim that you or another provider caused some particular injury or problem should not automatically be assumed to be true. Although you do not have to argue the point with the patient, you also do not have to agree. Injuries have many causes and many stories behind them.

- Document the facts.
- Document what you see and do.
- Your role is to render nursing services, not to judge.
- Leave the determination of fault to the courts.
- Your actions and truthful documentation will be your best defense.

Did the Patient Suffer Damages or Injury? The last element that must be proved is that your breach of duty caused injury to the patient. This last element of malpractice can also be overlooked, as the nurse becomes embroiled in the fact that a mistake has been made. For instance, in many cases of medication error, the patient is not permanently harmed, because a single dose of most medications will not cause a permanent change. This does not mean that medication errors should be taken lightly or that some medications cannot cause death with a single mistake. They can. It only means that it is very unlikely that a malpractice claim will be brought for a medication error that does not cause injury.

Damages can be viewed as the sum of money a court or jury awards as compensation for a tort action. *General damages* are those given for intangibles such as pain and suffering, disfigurement, interference with ordinary enjoyment of life, and loss of consortium (marital services). *Special damages* are the patient's out-of-pocket expenses such as medical care, lost wages, and rehabilitation costs (Campion,

SAGUARO CANYON PET CLINIC

8959 E. Tanque Verde
Tucson, Arizona 85777
520/999-9999
Client Number: 975

Invoice Nbr: 011365
Date: February 14, 1996
Doctor: Kitty Friend
Home telephone: 999-9999

Iam A. Goodguy
1234 N. Paseo
Tuscon, AZ 85777

Animal: Lexie
Species: Feline
Altered: Yes
Breed: Manx
Age: 1 Year
Sex: Male

HEALTH CARE MESSAGES

February 14, 1996

Your pet has had an operation that requires special precautions and follow-up care at home under your supervision. These are covered in the instructions below. A decreased appetite for one or two days may be normal. However, if any of the following symptoms should occur, please contact our office:

(1) Loss of appetite for over two days.
(2) Refusal to drink water for over one day.
(3) Depression.
(4) Elevated or sub-normal temperature.
(5) Diarrhea.
(6) Vomiting.

It is very important, and your responsibility as the owner, to follow the instructions below to ensure a satisfactory recovery for your pet.

DIET: Feed your pet his/her regular diet.

ACTIVITY: Restrict activity for 10 days to inside the house or on other clean, dry, confined area. Replace litter in catbox with thin strips of shredded newspaper to protect paws.

CARE OF PAWS: Check paws twice daily for any signs of excessive licking or separation of surgery incision sites. Keep claws clean and dry. Call us if you are unable to discourage chewing or if the paws are excessively tender or your cat is lame.

MEDICATION: Give antibiotic medication as directed on perscription label twice daily.

POST-SURGERY: We suggest that the declawed cat be kept indoors for its protection; although the escape mechanisms are still functional, your pet may not be able to defend itself adequately outdoors.

If you have any questions or problems, please call us at 999-9999.
Thank you.

FIGURE 20-1

Even veterinarians are able to do computerized discharge planning for pets.

1990). Some states have limited the amount of damages that a plaintiff can receive (Critical Thinking Box 20-3).

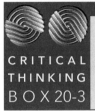

CRITICAL THINKING BOX 20-3

Does your state limit the amount of damages a plaintiff can receive?

For a malpractice plaintiff's attorney to take a claim to trial, it may cost that person more than $100,000 (Lobe, 1995) Because malpractice claims are brought on a contingency fee basis, the attorney will get paid only if he/she wins the claim. In this situation the damages must be greater than the costs to make the claim worthwhile. When worrying about an incident and whether or not a suit will result, it is helpful to understand what factors make claims worthwhile.

1. The most important factor involved with damages is the age of the patient. The younger the patient with a permanent injury, the longer will be the time of suffering, the costs of future medical care, the loss of wages or income, and the emotional loss to the family. Therefore, to assess damages, the first question an attorney asks is the age and status of an individual. An 83-year-old widower who has a numb leg will not have a large claim for damages. He will not lose wages. He does not have to support a family. It is likely that he has other illnesses or physical problems that might contribute to difficulty with ambulating. His life expectancy is not great. A 30-year-old single mother with three dependent children who has made her living as a waitress might well have costly damages if a numb leg hinders her ability to walk and provide for her family.

2. The nature of the injury is also a consideration in evaluating damages. Is the injury permanent? Is it one for which a jury will have great sympathy, as when there is a huge disfiguring facial scar? Is it one that demonstrates a blatant mistake such as surgery performed on the wrong limb?

3. Does the claim involve any act of malicious misconduct or an intentional cover up? Such acts inflame juries and cause them at times to award what is called ***"punitive damages."*** These damages seek to punish those whose conduct goes beyond normal malpractice. Claims in which this might occur are rare, but they involve issues such as changed medical records, lies being told to patients, or intentional misconduct while under the influence of alcohol or drugs. Such punitive awards can add millions of dollars to an otherwise low-damage claim.

Again, the principles of good documentation can make the damages of a claim not worth pursuing. It is particularly important that there is accurate evidence of damages at the time the injury occurred. Any time there is an incident involving a patient, such as a fall, an immediate and thorough exam can greatly assist in substantiating the patient's condition and thus, damages. The exam and findings need to be accurately documented. Subsequent exams and evaluations should be completed. Documentation of the patient's complaints, or lack of complaints, at the time of an incident can prove extremely beneficial. A simple, "no complaints" or "denies pain," will refute a patient's later claim that I was terribly injured by the fall.

Sometimes when a clear mistake has been made that falls below the standard of care and has caused an injury, your attorney will admit negligence. This is often a relief to the nurse who does not wish to try and defend a mistake and/or not tell the truth. The case is then brought solely on the amount of damages. Often the patient's perception of the injury is greatly augmented. Usually the patient will have to go through what is called an independent medical examination to substantiate injury.

Damages Applied to the Case Study. In the case study, numbness of a limb may be difficult to prove. Nerve conduction studies may be performed in an independent medical examination to demonstrate that the injection could not have caused the neurological injury of which the patient complains. Numbness also does not mean lack of function and would not usually prevent any activity of daily living. Again, the age and status of the claimant would play an important role, as would your documentation of the patient's lack of complaints and ability to ambulate.

WHO MIGHT HAVE LIABILITY (RESPONSIBILITY) IN A CLAIM?

■ HYPOTHETICAL CASE STUDY #4:

You are a nurse working on a surgical unit in a hospital. One evening you are asked to float to pediatrics. The only experience you have with children happened when you were a student. A physician asks you to give digoxin to an infant and writes an order for 2 cc. This seems like a lot of medication to you, so you ask the head nurse on the unit about the dose. The head nurse assumes you are speaking about an oral dose of the medication and states that this is normal. You give the medication by injection and shortly thereafter the child's heart stops beating and he is coded. When you attempt to use an ambu bag, it is not on the crash cart. The child eventually recovers. Twenty one years later you receive notice that a young man is suing you for giving him the wrong dose of digoxin when he was an infant.

Personal Liability. There is often confusion about who can be held accountable for your actions as a nurse. You may hear things such as, "Don't worry, I'll take responsibility for this." Understand that in the eyes of the law, each individual is accountable for their own actions. There is no defense called "She made me do it." Even if you are not personally named in a lawsuit, you will be asked to give evidence regarding your involvement and will have to be able to defend your actions under oath. "I was just following orders" does not explain why you as a professional made a medication error. You are held to a professional standard of care to know about the medications you are administering, including the correct dose. In hypothetical case study #4 you may be named and would most likely have liability.

Physician and Other Independent Practitioner Liability. For many years, physicians were seen as "The Captain of the Ship" and thus ultimately responsible for everything that happened to the patient (Richards and Rathbun, 1983). This doctrine is no longer true. Unfortunately, some physicians still mislead nurses by ordering them to do things and then assuring them that they will assume any risk involved. Although nurses do have a duty to follow physician's orders under most circumstances, this is never true if the nurse believes or has reason to believe that the order is unsafe for the patient, or not within the nurse's scope of practice. In hypothetical case study #1, giving an order for the nurse to give IV conscious sedation does not relieve the nurse of a duty to determine whether this is within his or her scope of practice. If not, the order must be refused. In hypothetical case study #4, if the nurse did not know the correct dose of digoxin, there was a duty to look up the correct dose. It is also true that if the physician's order is wrong, or done in a negligent manner such as in the hypothetical, it does not relieve the physician from having liability in addition to the nurse.

In instances when a nurse is hired directly by a physician to work in an office practice, the physician, as the employer, can be held vicariously liable on a theory of respondeat superior. This is a Latin term meaning that the master is responsible for acts of the servant, translated in modern day to "the employer is responsible for the acts of the employee." The physician, then, rather than the nurse may be named in the lawsuit. Remember, though, that you will still have to answer for your actions.

Another issue is what the nurse should accept as delegated or ordered by other independent health care practitioners such as nurse practitioners, and physician assistants. States may have different rules about who can give orders to the RN. The general rule is that the RN can accept orders from other licensed health care workers who are working within their scope of practice. To be sure about your state, contact the board of nursing. When accepting delegated duties, remember that you should only accept duties you are competent to carry out and that are within your scope of practice.

Supervisory Liability. Questions often arise regarding the nurse's responsibility for acts of those working under him or her. The standard of care for a supervisor is to act as a reasonable supervisor under the same or similar circumstances. A supervisor can be expected to ensure the following:

- The task was properly assigned to a worker competent to safely perform it.
- Adequate supervision was provided to the worker if needed.
- The nurse provided appropriate follow-up and evaluation of the delegated task.

As in hypothetical case study #3, a supervisor could be expected to more closely supervise a float nurse or a recent graduate than someone who is an experienced nurse on a pediatric unit. It is also incumbent upon a person being supervised to ask for assistance if they are faced with a problem for which they lack the necessary skills to resolve. In hypothetical case study #4 this was done, but the nurse administering the medication and the supervisor miscommunicated on the method or route of administration. Do you think this can happen?

Delegation of nursing duties to unlicensed health care workers presents supervisory nurses with some special risks. Changes in health care delivery systems and financing are resulting in some unfamiliar categories of unlicensed caregivers with a wide variety of skills and expertise. Some boards of nursing have informed their licensees that each nurse remains personally liable for any task delegated to an unlicensed worker on the theory that the delegated task is considered the nurse's responsibility, rather than within the scope of practice of the unlicensed worker. Other boards of nursing have stated that they will apply to delegation the traditional standards for supervising any health care worker as described earlier.

Certain nursing responsibilities, such as nursing diagnosis, assessment, some portions of planning, evaluation, and documentation, and teaching, should not be delegated to unlicensed staff. Contact the board of nursing in your state to better understand your responsibilities in the delegation of nursing duties.

Institutional Liability. As in the aforementioned case involving physician liability, health care institutions such as hospitals are usually sued under a theory of *respondeat superior* for the actions of their employees. An institution cannot really do or not do any act that can cause a lawsuit except through its employees or agents. That is why most all health care institutions carry insurance to cover the acts and omissions of their employees. Otherwise, a corporation could go bankrupt if sued. For the most part, institutions and not individual nurses are named defendants in a lawsuit, but again this does not relieve the nurse from having to formally answer to the court for his or her own actions or inaction. An institution's policies or lack thereof is also a common claim in a lawsuit. For instance, there can be a claim in hypothetical case study #4 that the institution should have had a policy on floating nurses to other units in the hospital, and that such persons should never be given the responsibility of taking off physician's orders.

Student Liability. Nursing students have responsibility for their own actions and can be liable (Guido, 2000). Again, the adage that students practice under their instructor's license is not true. As a student you may have an instructor supervising you closely in the early stages of your education, but at the end of your program, it is likely that you will have less supervision. Student nurses at all times will be held to the standard of an RN for the tasks they perform (Guido, 2000). It is, therefore, important that students never accept assignments beyond their preparation and that they communicate frequently with their instructors for assistance and guidance.

Instructors are responsible for reasonable and prudent clinical supervision, a standard that may be higher than other worker supervision because of the student's lack of experience. Nurses performing as preceptors for students have the same supervisor liability they have for any other worker. Instructors and preceptors need to remember that the level of expertise of individual students may vary, and the standard used to evaluate the student's performance usually requires more supervision than some more experienced workers may need.

WHAT DEFENSES MIGHT BE AVAILABLE IN MALPRACTICE CLAIMS?

If the plaintiff in a malpractice claim does not prove each of the elements previously discussed, the defense can ask for a dismissal of the claim by making various *motions* (formal requests) to the court. There are several other issues that may have an effect on the outcome of a malpractice claim.

A *Statute of Limitations* is a law that sets a time period after an event during which a lawsuit must be filed. States have different statutes and case law surrounding this time limit. Usually the time is measured from the time of the event or incident, last date of treatment, or from the time the event was or should have been discovered. For minors, some states allow the time to be counted from the time they reach *majority* (usually 18 years old), unless a suit has already been brought on their behalf by parents or others. Therefore in hypothetical case study #4, a suit could be brought two or three years after a person turns 18 years (majority) for an injury occurring as an infant. Other states do not permit this delay. Lack of mental competence will also delay the time requirements in some states.

Failure to file the lawsuit within the statute of limitations time results in the loss of the right to sue. This can be considered a defense, because filing after the date allows the defendants to have the case dismissed. It is important to know, however, that in most states, the statute starts running when the patient knows of the injury. If there is any type of cover-up regarding an incident, the statute will not run. Recent developments by JCAHO now make it mandatory that patient's be told if there is an unanticipated outcome (American Society of Healthcare Risk Management, p. 6; JCAHO, RI.1.2.2, 2000). How this new requirement will be implemented in each accredited institution is still unknown.

Proving that the patient assumed the risk of harm, or that the patient contributed to the harm by his or her actions provides another type of defense. *Assumption of the risk* states that plaintiffs are partially responsible for consequences if they understood the risks involved when they proceeded with the action (Guido, 2000). An example would be a mentally competent patient who has been warned to use a call light but who insists on crawling out of the bottom of the bed and, thus, injures herself.

Contributory negligence is an older doctrine that used to be an all or nothing rule. Patients who had any part in the adverse outcome were barred from compensation. Today, most jurisdictions use a *comparative negligence* theory and reduce the money award by the injured party's responsibility for the ultimate harm done (Guido, 2000). One case found that a patient could be negligent and thus be at least partially responsible by (1.) refusing to follow advice or instructions; (2.) causing a delay in treatment or not returning for follow-up; (3.) furnishing false, misleading, or incomplete information to a health care provider; or (4.) causing the injury that causes a need for medical care (*Harvey v. Mid-Coast Hospital*, 1999).

WHAT EVIDENCE CAN HELP ME IN A LAWSUIT?

The Medical Record. In many instances, you can become a nurse hero or in deep trouble, having to do simply with your accurate and timely documentation in the medical record. One of the most important tools for all providers in a malpractice claim is the medical record. This is the first piece of evidence asked for by the attorney for the plaintiff. The nurses' notes are often the first part of the record to be examined. Their integrity, accuracy, and completeness will make a claim defensible or indefensible. Good documentation, therefore, is one of the best defensive actions a nurse can take. By recording the care administered, the specific time it was administered, the patient's response, and the overall status of the patient's condition, the nurse can demonstrate that the standard of care was met.

Your defense attorney will use the medical record extensively and will very early in a claim make a time line of events that surrounded the incident. The most effective defense is to put on a play to a jury regarding what occurred to demonstrate all that was done for the patient. A good educational exercise is to take any patient's chart and see whether you can present a play regarding what happened to that patient during your care.

Some nurses have advocated the maintaining of personal notes regarding the circumstances of a particular incident. The rationale for this is so they can carefully review the notes; it will also assist them to more clearly recall the situation should they be required to do so. However, another consideration is that these notes are also discoverable by the other side and may be extremely dangerous. These notes are frequently written on an emotional level. In most states what you write, unless to your attorney or under a peer-review privilege, will have to be produced. Personal documentation about what others did or did not do or what you think they did wrong or should have done will always come back to haunt the nurse. Documentation regarding an incident should be thoroughly and factually done in the medical record and not in personal records or a diary.

There is an adage that "If it is not documented, it wasn't done." In reality, it is simply difficult to prove it was done if there is no documentation and the plaintiff claims it wasn't done. It is then a "He said, She said" type of argument. A more accurate statement might be "If it is documented, it was done." Once it is documented at the time of the event, there is a strong presumption that the documentation is accurate and whatever a patient says to the contrary is simply self-serving. That is why it is so important to document extensively, accurately, and very factually in the medical record (Box 20-3). This is especially true when there is an adverse event.

 BOX 20-3 Tips for Being at Your Best When Administering Medications

❑ Be very careful if you have been interrupted during a task. This is very common in nursing. Many accidents happen because the nurse did not remember what he or she had been doing or where he or she was in a task. Shift change is also a common time for mistakes.

❑ If you are fatigued, you are more likely to make mistakes. Follow all the steps thoroughly when you are tired. This is one of the reasons that double or long shifts may not be wise.

(continued)

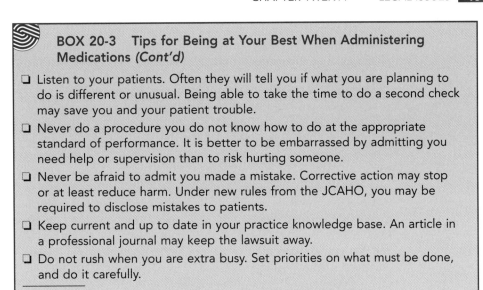

BOX 20-3   Tips for Being at Your Best When Administering Medications (Cont'd)

❑ Listen to your patients. Often they will tell you if what you are planning to do is different or unusual. Being able to take the time to do a second check may save you and your patient trouble.

❑ Never do a procedure you do not know how to do at the appropriate standard of performance. It is better to be embarrassed by admitting you need help or supervision than to risk hurting someone.

❑ Never be afraid to admit you made a mistake. Corrective action may stop or at least reduce harm. Under new rules from the JCAHO, you may be required to disclose mistakes to patients.

❑ Keep current and up to date in your practice knowledge base. An article in a professional journal may keep the lawsuit away.

❑ Do not rush when you are extra busy. Set priorities on what must be done, and do it carefully.

JCAHO, Joint Commission for Accreditation of Healthcare Organizations.

HOW CAN I AVOID A MALPRACTICE CLAIM?

There are certain situations that contain a high risk for a lawsuit against nurses. These situations most often relate to patient safety, improper treatment, problems with monitoring, medication errors, and failing to follow proper procedures and policies.

Medication Errors. One study claims that 770,000 hospital patients experience an adverse drug event yearly and that almost half are preventable, such as those attributable to miscalculations, drug interactions, or drug allergies (Guido, 2000; Clinical News, 1997). Increased hospital costs for inpatients may be $2 billion for the nation as a whole (Kohn, Corrigan, and Donaldson, 2000). The most common errors include the failure to administer the right drug to the right patient, in the right amount, by the right route, and at the right time. Claims involving medication errors are augmented when the nurse fails to record the medication administration properly, fails to recognize side effects or contraindications, or fails to know a patient's allergies.

The nurse's ability to listen to a patient or family member who notices that a medication is new, or recheck when anything such as color or amount seems unusual, may prevent a serious error. Many nurses feel rushed by the amount of work they are expected to accomplish and do not want to take extra time for anything. Making this check a priority will prove to be time well spent. Dealing with an error and the consequences to the patient will be longer and more painful.

Although many medication errors do not cause permanent or serious damage to patients, there are certain medications that can. Medications, such as chemotherapy, should be attached to protocols that help ensure safe administration. In addition, whenever a medication error occurs, the source of the error and the system failure should be carefully investigated. Most institutions are now attempting to ensure that punitive measures are not attached to medication errors. This is to facilitate reports to be made and systems involving the team of ordering practitioner, dispensing pharmacy, and administering nurse to have checks and balances to prevent any team member from causing harm to a patient (Kohn, Corrigan, and Donaldson, 2000) (Box 20-4).

BOX 20-4   Guidelines for Defensive Charting

❑ All entries should be accurate and factual.

❑ Make corrections appropriately and according to agency or hospital policies. Do not ever obliterate or destroy any information that is or has been in the chart.

❑ If there is information that should have been charted and was not, the nurse should make a "late entry" noting the time the charting actually occurred and the specific time the charting reflects. Example: 10/13/03, 10:00 late entry, charting to reflect 10/13/03 . . .

❑ All identified patient problems, nursing actions taken, and patient responses should be noted. Do not describe a patient problem without including the nursing actions taken and the patient response.

❑ Be as objective as possible in charting. Rather than charting "the patient tolerated the procedure well," chart the specific parameters checked to determine that conclusion. Example: "ambulated, tolerated well" would be more effective if charted "ambulated complete length of hall, no shortness of breath noted, pulse rate at 98, respirations at 22."

❑ Each page of the chart should contain the current date and time. Frequently chart forms are stamped ahead of time. Each time you enter information on a new page, make sure it reflects the current time of charting.

❑ Each page of the chart should include the full name and professional designation of every person making an entry on that page.

❑ Follow through with who saw the patient and what measures were initiated. Particularly note when the physician visited; if you had to call a physician for a problem, record the physician's response, the nursing actions, and the patient's response. If orders were received, be sure they are signed according to policy. This is especially important if you had to make several calls to the physician.

❑ Make sure your notes are legible and clearly reflect the information you intended. It is a good idea to read over your nurse's notes from the previous day to see if they still make sense and accurately portray the status of the patient. If the notes do not make sense to you the next day, imagine how difficult it would be to decipher the information at a later date.

❑ Pertinent notes from other providers should also be reviewed. The medical record is for communication. A jury will never understand if team members are not coordinating efforts and thought.

Provide a Safe Environment. Patient safety is being more and more recognized as a duty of health care institutions (JCAHO, 2001). Ensuring patient safety has many aspects. Nurses sometimes do not recognize the multiple roles that they must play in this area. They are responsible for knowing how equipment should work and not using it if it is not functioning correctly; removing obvious hazards such as chemicals, which might be mistaken for medications; and making the environment free of hazards such as inappropriately placed furniture or equipment, and spills on the floor. An additional preventative measure is knowing how to document correctly if an incident occurs, so that there cannot be a doubt regarding the facts of what happened and all you did to protect the patient.

Patient Falls. Patient falls represent one of the primary risks in this category and second to medication errors in numbers of untoward events (Guido, 2000). This may include falls out of bed, falls on something spilled on the floor, or falls because a nurse has not provided adequate supervision for the patient. Falls, particularly repeated falls, are a major source of both physical and psychological injury to elderly patients (Tideiksaar, 1998). They are therefore among the most common sources of claims against nurses.

Many people have spent much time and effort in attempts to change patient care so that falls do not occur. Proposals coming out of such efforts range from total lack of restraints (Walker, 1992) to environmental modifications (Tideiksaar, 1998).

If a patient falls, the nurse's first duty is to the patient. This involves the following:
- Notifying a physician to assess and treat the patient.
- Making sure that the patient is protected from a second fall.
- Notifying the family so that they are not surprised by a patient's injury.
- Documenting what occurred.

Nurses are best able to defend themselves in these cases when their institution has a policy regarding protecting vulnerable patients against falls, sometimes called a "fall protocol." These policies establish levels of risk in patients such as age, confusion, sedation, and steps the nurse must take to protect the patient such as side rails, soft restraints, or bed position. If the nurse follows such a protocol, then it is difficult for a plaintiff to prove that the nurse fell below a standard of care (Critical Thinking Box 20-4).

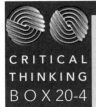

CRITICAL THINKING BOX 20-4

What fall protocols have you observed in your clinical settings? How are they the same, and how are they different?

Documentation is extremely important when a patient falls. The following should be considered:

- Document factually how the fall was discovered, where the patient was found, what facts surrounded the fall. An example is to document that patient was found beside the bed, with the side rails up, and the bed in the low position.
- Document what the patient says in regard to the fall. A statement such as "I know you told me to put on the call light, but you all seemed so busy that I didn't want to bother you," can be of great benefit to the nurse. "I put on the call light, but nobody came" can of course have the opposite effect.
- Document whom you notified such as the physician, the family.
- Document what was done for the patient such as an exam, x-rays, orientation to surroundings, monitoring after the incident, restraints, and assistance with further ambulation.
- Document your adherence to any policies of the hospital regarding vulnerable patients or those at risk for falls.

Equipment Failure. Today many nurses feel that they spend more time nursing equipment than the patient. This can be true. What nurses do not understand is that there is a certain standard of care connected with equipment. It must be used as directed by the manufacturer, and the nurse has a duty to know what that is and follow such directions. There is also a duty to make sure that the equipment is properly maintained and that records are kept of this maintenance. The equipment needs to be working properly and not used when a known defective condition exists. Lastly the device must be available for use. In hypothetical case study #4, the fact that the ambu bag was not available can be viewed as liability for either the nurse responsible for checking crash carts, or the institution for not seeing that the carts are checked.

In a lawsuit the nurse will need to prove that equipment failure, rather than human error caused the injury. Part of that proof will rest in the piece of equipment itself. Therefore one of the most important aspects of the defense will be not to lose or let go of the equipment or device before it is thoroughly evaluated by a neutral party after an incident. Often the manufacturer will ask for the equipment, but their interests might be adverse to yours to prove user error rather than equipment failure. In addition, the nurse should adhere to any institutional policies regarding incidents involving equipment failure.

Nurses may also have a duty to be sure their institution complies with the Safe Medical Device Act of 1990. This federal law requires that all medical device-related adverse incidents be reported to manufacturers and in the case of death, to the Food and Drug Administration, within 10 days. The purpose of this act is to protect the public from devices that may be defective (Guido, 2000).

■ HYPOTHETICAL CASE STUDY #5:

Mrs. Hayes, 67, with chronic obstructive pulmonary disease, is having increasingly difficult respirations, increased cyanosis, and increased anxiety. She tells you she just can't breathe. You have done all the measures for which you currently have orders, without her getting relief. It is 2 AM. You call the physician. She orders Valium 10 mg intramuscularly now. Even as a recent graduate you know that Valium is contraindicated by the respiratory status. You call your supervisor, who tells you that Dr. Jones is a good physician and must know what she is doing. What should you do?

Failure to Adequately Assess, Monitor, and Obtain Assistance. Most often the nurse should not delegate to another the responsibility of assessing and evaluating patient care and progress. If some portions of this duty are done by others (e.g., another RN, licensed practical nurse, unlicensed personnel), the nurse primarily responsible for the care of the patient must still be aware of the findings and confirm them when they indicate a change in patient condition or progress. Documentation of the changes and events surrounding the changes is critical. Rapidly increasing numbers of cases are occurring when there is an inadequate nursing assessment, or a failure to monitor and obtain *needed medical assistance* for a patient whose condition is changing. In relationship to the latter there may also be liability for failure *to challenge an inappropriate order.*

These areas are uncomfortable for many experienced nurses, not just for the recent graduate. Frequently these areas involve challenging a physician or other health care professional. They require that the nurse have current and accurate information. They also require that the nurse use assertiveness techniques well. It is not enough to identify problems. The nurse must identify the problems and contact the physician or other individuals to get appropriate care.

Of most help in situations such as hypothetical case study #5 is a policy that clearly delineates the chain of command for the institution. With a policy in place, the nurse can be clear about who must be notified about a potentially problematic order, and it can be documented appropriately. It is important that the nurse be protected from any retaliation in such instances by the institution that stands to lose if the patient's safety is not put first.

Accurate documentation of the nursing assessment and of frequent monitoring will be required to prove what you have done. Flow charts and forms can be timesaving devices in this area. Electronic communications now make such time consuming documentation more readily available. This documentation is especially important in the critical care setting and in the obstetrical suit. The attachment of accurate times to such monitoring activities will be your best defense tool in many malpractice claims.

Failure to Adequately Communicate. Perhaps the most important role of everyone on the health care team is to adequately communicate. The patient's total care rests on this whether it is communication in the medical record or through verbal communication. The most frequent claim against nurses in this area is the failure to communicate changes in the patient's condition to a professional with a need to know. This is especially true in acute-care settings during the night hours as in hypothetical case study #5. Communication is not always welcomed in the middle of the night and is impaired because it is not face to face, and the receiver may not be fully awake and alert. At such times, it is incumbent upon the nurse to repeat information if he or she does not believe it is being understood and/or taken seriously. Thorough documentation of the communication will protect the nurse, but it should not be done defensively or thought of as a substitute for proper care.

Communication with certain hearing- and speech-impaired patients and with ethnically and culturally diverse patients will often provide a challenge to good nursing care. The Americans with Disabilities Act is a federal statute that has requirements for institutions rendering health care to have certain translators available for key health care interactions. The failure to do so may put the institution at risk for fines, and penalties *(Freydel v. New York Hospital, 2000)*.

Failure to Report. States have many statutes that require health care providers to report certain incidences or occurrences. If the provider fails to report as required and a person is injured, there can be negligence *per se*, and no expert testimony will be needed to prove a case (Prosser, 1971). In addition, both institutional and professional licensure can be affected. It is important that nurses are aware of the reporting statutes in the state in which they are practicing. In some states, it is not only a duty, but also the law to report certain incidences. The following are examples of such statutes involving a duty to report.

- A duty to report other health care professionals whose behaviors are unprofessional and/or could cause harm to the public.
- A duty to report evidence of child or adult abuse.
- A duty to report certain communicable diseases.
- A duty to report certain deaths under suspicious circumstances.
- A duty to report certain types of injuries that are or could be caused by violence.
- A duty to report evidence of Medicare fraud.
- Emergency Medical Treatment and Labor Act violations.

The nurse must know what areas must be reported, who should report, how the report should be accomplished, and to whom a report should be made. Institutional policies and nurse practice acts on these topics are invaluable.

Many nurses are afraid to report their employers, other professionals, or other agencies because of the possibility of retaliatory action against them. Most mandatory reporting statutes give immunity to those who report in good faith. Some states have specific ***Whistleblower Statutes*** that not only protect nurses from retaliatory action, but may reward them. The content of these statutes differs from state to state, so the nurse must know whether one exists in the state of practice, and what protection is provided. A federal statute, the ***False Claims Act,*** provides protection under certain situations for reporting Medicare fraud (Critical Thinking Box 20-5).

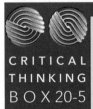

CRITICAL THINKING BOX 20-5

Which states have "whistleblower" protection?

INTENTIONAL TORTS

Intentional torts are civil claims that are closely related to criminal acts in that they involve intent to do the wrong. Instead of seeking to put the bad actor in jail, however, these wrongs attempt to right the wrong by compensating the plaintiff. These claims are less common than malpractice claims, but the following can be brought against a nurse.

Assault and battery are the legal terms that are applied to nonconsensual threat of touch (assault) or the actual touching (battery). Of course in health care there is a lot of touching. Permission to do this touching is usually implied when the patient seeks medical care. Sometimes, however, a patient refuses to have certain procedures done, or has certain procedures done without giving an informed consent. Also, a patient may wish to leave an institution against medical advice and nurses use physical restraint or touching to keep them from leaving. All of these actions can lead to a civil claim of assault and battery.

False Imprisonment means making someone wrongfully feel that he or she cannot leave a place. It is often associated with assault and battery claims. This can happen in a health care setting through the use of physical or chemical restraints, or the threat of physical or emotional harm if a patient leaves an institution. Threats such as "If you don't stay in your bed, I'll have to sedate you" constitute false imprisonment (Ellis and Hartley, 2001). This tort might also be telling a patient that he or she may not leave the emergency department until the bill is paid. Another example is using restraints or threatening to use them on competent patients to make them do what you want them to do against their wishes. Unless you are very clearly protecting the safety of others, you may not restrain a competent adult (Guido, 2000) (Critical Thinking Box 20-6).

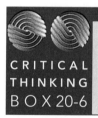

CRITICAL THINKING BOX 20-6

In what situations would it be acceptable to restrain a patient?

Even in the psychiatric case in which someone is thought to be a danger to self or others, there are many very specific state and federal laws to follow (Ellis and Hartley 2001). There are also many restrictions on the appropriate use of both hard and soft restraints and elevated scrutiny on their use in long term care facilities (Tideiksaar, 1998). Sometimes there can be a claim of elder abuse for the misuse of restraints. You must be aware of policy in your agency and state statutory restrictions.

Defamation (Libel and Slander) refers to causing damage to someone else's reputation. If the means of transmitting the damaging information is written, it is called libel; if it is oral or spoken, it is called slander. The damaging information must be communicated to a third person. The actions likely to result in a defamation charge are giving out inaccurate information from the medical record such as in hypothetical case study #1 or speaking negatively about your co-workers (supervisors, doctors, other nurses).

Two defenses to defamation accusations are truth and privilege. If the statement is true, it is not actionable under this doctrine. However, it is often difficult to define truth, because it may be a matter of perspective. It is better to avoid that issue by not making statements about other people unnecessarily. An example of privilege would be required good faith reporting to Child Protective Services of possible child abuse.

Recovery in defamation claims usually requires that the plaintiff submit proof of being injured, i.e., loss of money or job. Some categories, such as fitness to practice one's profession, do not require such proof, as they are considered sufficiently damaging without it. Comments about the quality of a nurse's work or a physician's skills in diagnosing illness would fit in this category. You can avoid this claim by steering clear of gossip and/or writing negative documents about others in the heat of the moment and without an adequate factual basis.

THE INVASION OF PRIVACY AND BREACHES OF PRIVILEGE AND CONFIDENTIALITY

A good general rule in relationship to torts involving the sharing of patient information is the following. Always ask yourself, "Do I have the patient's consent to share this information, or is it necessary to the health care services for this patient?" If the answer to either is "no," then the information should not be communicated.

The public's attention has been recently focused on privacy because of a new privacy regulations under an older federal law called the Health Insurance Portability and Accountability Act of 1996. These specific privacy regulations will become effective in April 2003 and have an elaborate system for ensuring privacy for individually identifiable health information. Even information used to render health care services must have the patient's specific consent for their use in health care operations such as billing and utilization review. Notice must be given to the patient of how the information will be used. All nurses working in health care must be aware of this new law and how their institutions propose to comply with it.

Many states have physician-patient privilege laws that protect communications between caregivers and their patients. This enables information to pass freely between physician and patient without concern that it will be shared with those who do not need to know it. This includes law enforcement. The privilege usually extends to information about a patient in the medical record or obtained in the course of providing care. Most states extend physician-patient privilege to nurses and sometimes to other health care givers as well. This privilege belongs to the patient, not the health care giver, which means that only the patient can decide to give it up.

As a professional it is important to observe *confidentiality* when talking about patients at home and at work (Fig. 20-2). Nurses must be very careful to keep information about the patient or from the patient to themselves and to share it only with health care workers who must know the information to plan or give proper care. This is often difficult to do as seen in hypothetical case study #1.

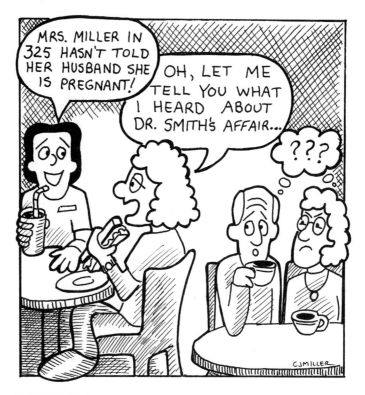

FIGURE 20-2
Maintaining confidentiality is both an ethical and a legal
consideration in nursing.

Computer documentation and national clearing houses for health information present significant confidentiality issues. Such technologies offer many advantages, including easier and broader access to needed information ands more-legible documentation. These same advantages also present concerns because it is more difficult to ensure confidentiality. Many hospitals and agencies already have policies and procedures in place such as access codes, limited screen time, and computers placed in locations that promote privacy. Security standards under the Health Insurance Portability and Accountability Act of 1996 will have to be followed once these are finalized. The nurse is still responsible for the protection of confidentiality when computers, faxes, E-mail, or other rapid communication techniques are used.

A similar cause of action is for ***invasion of privacy.*** This cause of action can apply to several behaviors, like photographing a procedure and showing it without the patient's consent, going through a patient's belongings without consent, or talking about a patient's private life publicly.

MISCELLANEOUS INTENTIONAL TORTS AND OTHER CIVIL RIGHTS CLAIMS INVOLVED WITH EMPLOYMENT

The aforementioned torts and others can be relevant to nurses in regard to their employment. These intentional torts can be brought personally against the nurse, and are not usually covered by any insurance. *Tortious Interference with Contract* is a claim that someone maliciously interfered with a person's contractual (often employment) rights. This can occur, for instance, if a nurse attempts to get another nurse fired through giving false or misleading facts to a supervisor. *Intentional Infliction of Emotional Distress* is described in its title, and can also be attached to malicious acts in the employment setting. These and certain civil rights claims such as *Sexual Harassment* and *Discrimination* are both rights and potential liabilities for every person in the work force. Although beyond the scope of this text, policies and information regarding these issues demand further investigation by each health care employee to ensure that their rights and the rights of others are not violated.

WHAT IS A DEFENSE TO INTENTIONAL TORTS?

Informed Consent. Consent is usually a complete defense to all of the aforementioned intentional torts. You cannot have a claim for assault and battery, if the patient has given consent for the procedure. Likewise, there can be no invasion of privacy if the patient has given consent to share confidential information with someone else such as their lawyer.

There is much confusion about informed consent in that many people believe it to be a piece of paper with "informed consent" written on it. This is not true. Informed consent in the health care setting is a process whereby a patient is informed of the risks, benefits, and alternatives of a certain procedure, and then gives consent for it to be done. The piece of paper is simply evidence that the informed consent process has been done.

The nurse's role in the consent process is often confusing. Remember that it is ultimately the responsibility of the person doing the procedure to provide the basic explanation of its risks, benefits, and alternatives. In regard to most procedures and operations, this responsibility ultimately belongs to the physician. However, in some settings the nurse is part of an educational process involving videos, booklets, handouts, and other aids to the patient's understanding. In addition, as nurses perform more procedures, the process of informing the patient of what is to occur is the nurse's.

For surgeries and other physician performed procedures, nurses may be asked, "to get the consent." Be clear what this means. In essence it means to witness the patient's voluntary signature on a form that should be filled out by the person performing the procedure. That is all. However, as a witness to a signature, documentation of the patient's level of understanding, or the patient's refusal to receive information, or reluctance to have the procedure done is critical to the witnessing role.

Consent forms must be signed when a patient is considered able or competent to make informed decisions and before the procedure is done. This means that the form must be signed before the administration of preprocedure medications, which often contain narcotics or other mind-altering drugs. The patient is the only person who may give consent if he or she is competent. Competency is defined differently from state to state and the nurse should be aware of how it is defined in his or her state of practice. Competency is presumed and therefore any claim of incompetence would have to be proved.

States differ with regard to how consent can be given if the patient is incompetent. ***Advanced directives*** such as a ***medical power of attorney*** or a ***living will*** may give information about the patient's wishes. These documents allow individuals to prepare for possible incompetence in advance by formalizing their wishes about their further health care decisions in writing. The living will is used to allow a competent adult to direct what he or she wishes in regard to health care upon becoming incompetent. This may include that he or she does not want any unusual medical procedures or life-saving equipment used to prolong life.

Often used in conjunction with the living will is the durable or medical power of attorney. This document allows the competent adult to appoint a specific person to authorize care if he or she becomes incompetent. The durable power of attorney does not usually become effective until a person loses competency. This document may be used in conjunction with or without a living will (see Chapter 18 for more information on advance directives). Congress has passed the Patient Self-Determination Act of 1990 requiring hospitals to inform their patients of the availability of advance directives. State law defines the required wording for these documents and any other formalities necessary in their preparation.

If a family challenges a living will, a nurse will need to go through the administrative chain of command, where, it is hoped, a lawyer will be involved. A general rule is for nurses to follow the directives in a living will unless or until there is a court order to do otherwise. This means that families need to obtain legal services and go to court to overturn or challenge this document. All persons, no matter what their age, should complete advanced directives and a medical power of attorney or a living will.

When a patient does not have an advance directive and is incompetent, there are also state laws that give guidance regarding who can act as a ***surrogate decision-maker.*** Parents must usually sign for minor children. Spouses or immediate family members may usually sign for unconscious patients. In other instances, if no one is available or designated, a court can appoint someone for the purpose of medical decisions in a very short time. Informed consent is not required if the procedure is necessary to save a life and is done during an emergency.

Competent patients may always decline to give consent for a procedure, even if doing so may have serious consequences for their health status. In certain instances, pregnant women may not be permitted to refuse a treatment if doing so will result in serious harm to the fetus. Such a case should be referred to risk management and resolved before the procedure is done. Consent may be withdrawn at any time before the procedure. Documentation of events surrounding such incidents should be accurate and complete.

CRIMINAL ACTIONS

Nurses who violate specific criminal statutes, such as those having to do with illegal drug use, negligent homicide, and assault and battery, risk criminal prosecution. Conviction of certain types of crimes must be reported to the state board of nursing and will usually result in a review of licensure status. You must be aware of the rules in the state in which you practice.

WHAT CRIMINAL ACTS POSE A RISK TO THE NURSE?

Theft and Misappropriation of Property. Sometimes nurses fail to adequately protect a patient's property and thus open themselves up to claims of theft. Many patients bring valuables to health care facilities or think that they do. Clear notice to the patients before admittance to leave valuables at home is helpful. A thorough and documented list of property upon admittance is imperative to prevent such claims, as is the locking up of valuables. When dentures and other property have not been adequately stored or monitored, the nurse may be held responsible.

Another aspect of this problem is theft from the employer. Because of the extensive and costly nature of this problem, many employers have developed elaborate systems to try to discourage theft. With an ever-increasing focus on lowering health care costs, those related to employee theft will not be tolerated. Occasionally nurses accidentally leave the job with tape, bandages, or other supplies in their pockets. These should be returned. Better yet, establishing a routine of checking your pockets before leaving for home will help reduce this risk. No employer's property should ever be intentionally taken by a nurse.

Nursing Practice Violations. Scope-of-practice violations that result in the death of a patient may be the result of nurses doing tasks or procedures that have not been accepted by the state board of nursing as within the appropriate scope for nurses, or doing actions that have been approved for advanced practice nurses only. In some states these violations and other possible violations of the nurse practice act are misdemeanors, but in other states they may be felonies. In rare cases, charges of murder or negligent homicide may be filed against the nurse (Kowalski and Horner, 1998). This fairly new trend should be of concern to all nurses as mistakes will always occur in medicine. To err is human (Kohn, Corrigan, and Donaldson, 2000). "Making an error that endangers the patient is terrifying; making one that kills a patient can be career-ending because of the guilt, regret, and self-blame." If fear of criminal prosecution and prison are added to these personal responses, how can we believe thoughtful, caring people will continue in the profession? As Curtin (1997) asks, "What conceivable social good will be achieved by putting these nurses in jail?" (Kowalski and Horner, 1998).

Violations of the Food and Drugs Act. Participating in any activity with illegal drugs or the misappropriation or improper use of legal drugs may result in criminal action against the nurse. Conviction for a crime in this area will almost always result in action against a nurse's license. As described earlier, there is a high incidence of substance abuse in the medical profession, so nurses need to be aware of the risks and avoid them. Writing prescriptions for drugs without the authority to do so is a criminal activity. Obtaining drugs illegally for friends and/or family needs, even if they seem legitimate, will still have criminal consequences.

RISK MANAGEMENT AND QUALITY IMPROVEMENT

HOW DO I PROTECT MYSELF AND MY PATIENT FROM ALL THESE RISKS?

The safety of patients often involves two separate formalized processes in institutions. One involves quality and goes by many names such as "quality assurance" "continuous quality management," or "continuous quality improvement." In relationship to nursing practices, *peer review* is the process of using nurses to evaluate the quality of nursing care. This means that you, as a professional nurse, will be continuously involved in evaluating the care that you and other nurses provide. In the past this was only done through retroactive review of care using such techniques such as nursing audits to evaluate care already given. The current focus is on looking for ways to do better all the time. Currently Texas is the only state that has passed legislation requiring peer review as a part of the nurse practice act (http://www.bne.state.tx.us/prp.htm). Examples of activities that may be involved in this process include the following:

1. Evaluation of what nurses are doing for patients.
2. Policy and procedure development.
3. Staff preparation, competency and skill documentation.
4. Continuing education and certification.
5. Employee evaluations.
6. Ongoing monitoring such as infection control and risk-management systems.

Accreditation of hospitals now requires that the activities chosen for peer review be documented and demonstrated within the agency (JCAHO, 1998). This is a very positive development in nursing as it ensures that nursing practice is being scrutinized and evaluated and that guidelines for nursing care delivery are being evaluated and enforced by nurses, for nurses.

Risk management is a newer process and is most often involved when incidents or untoward events occur that may pose a financial risk or risk of lawsuit to the institution. This department, through a risk manager, will first often gather evidence surrounding the event in "anticipation of litigation." Such evidence will include interviews with those involved and physical evidence such as relevant documents (Figs. 20-3 and 20-4}. It will then evaluate how to prevent a reoccurrence by changing systems that have broken down to allow an adverse occurrence. This might mean setting a new standard that can then be evaluated and ensured through a quality assurance process.

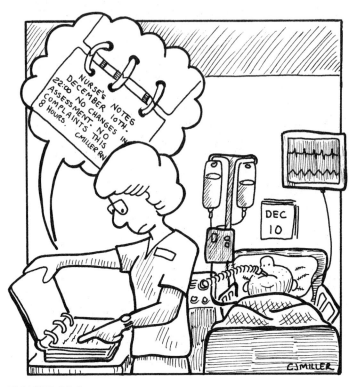

FIGURE 20-3
It is critical that the nurse's notes reflect the current condition of the patient.

One tool often used by risk management is the incident report. Incident reports generate many legal concerns as in most states they must be produced in a lawsuit and can be used as evidence against individuals and the institution (Guido, 2000). Therefore extreme caution should be used when completing one, and only the person directly involved should objectively document the facts. Conclusions, opinions, defensiveness, and judgment or blame of others have absolutely no place in this document or process. In addition, the form should never be used for punitive reasons, as this will almost certainly increase the possibility that it will not be filled out honestly if at all (Kohn, Corrigan, and Donaldson, 2000).

Although you would not mention that you filled out an incident report in the medical record, the same objective, factual documentation of an incident should be made in the medical record by the person involved in the incident. Lack of documentation in the face of a known occurrence will always be considered a cover-up and thus will be extremely detrimental to any subsequent legal action. Never speculate about who or what caused an incident, as this may inadvertently give the plaintiff their causation argument, which may not be true.

An example of risk management and quality assurance working together would be the following. A fire breaks out in the operating room and a patient is burned.

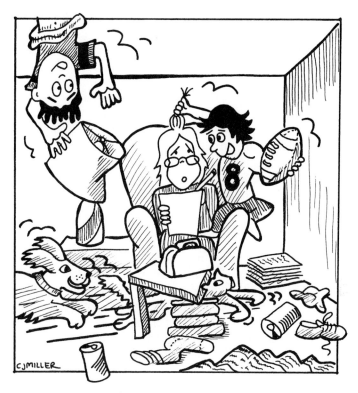

FIGURE 20-4
Charting in the home setting can be challenging.

Immediately after this event, a risk manager might be notified through a telephone call and then later an incident report. The risk manager would come immediately to the scene and collect all items and or equipment involved in the fire (evidence) to determine the cause of the fire. He or she would also interview those who saw the fire (witnesses) to determine facts involved. The risk manager may also take specific actions to assist the patient and/or family, in addition to giving advice to those involved regarding documentation of the event and/or communications. Sometimes financial settlements are made very early to avoid the costly process of a lawsuit. Risk management might also identify ways to prevent another occurrence, such as removal of all alcohol-based skin preparations from the operating room. This standard may then be periodically evaluated by the quality assurance department to ensure the continued safety of a patient.

Risk managers usually work very closely with insurance companies that cover institutions and their employees for all types of financial risk including malpractice and general liability. The defense and prevention of many claims starts with good risk management. Yet such efforts must also be made by every individual on the health care team who identifies a risk to patient safety and does something constructive to correct it. Several simple risk-management actions by nurses can often prevent a lawsuit. These include the following:

1. Approaching angry patients with an apology and an offer to help (Fiesta, 1988; Gutheil, Bursztajn, and Brodsky, 1984). Moving toward the patient who has experienced an unexpected outcome rather than away is always the best policy. Isolation and a feeling of abandonment in the face of an untoward event only augment the feeling that a wrong was done.

2. Sharing uncertainties and bringing patient's expectations down to a realistic level during the informed consent process also prevent claims based upon disappointment that an outcome is not perfect (Gutheil, Bursztajn, and Brodsky, 1984).

3. Refusing to participate in hospital gossip, jousting in the medical record, or judging others on the medical team will contribute to an atmosphere of teamwork and compassion, rather than competition, blame, and retaliation. The latter can ultimately contribute to unsafe patient care.

MALPRACTICE INSURANCE.

One of the more controversial topics for nurses involves the need for nurses to purchase individual malpractice insurance policies (Guido, 2000; Kelly and Joel, 1999; Simpson, 1998; Murphy, 1998). There is often misinformation about what these individual policies will do or cover and there is little substantiation for what most authors say. Part of the problem is that lawyers, rather than insurance professionals, talk about what the policies mean. In addition, sometimes insurance companies use scare tactics to induce nurses to purchase their products. An informed nurse should at least know what questions to ask.

WHAT ABOUT INDIVIDUAL MALPRACTICE INSURANCE?

Some individual nurse policies claim that you can prevent settlement of a claim if you wish to do so (have a consent clause). However, a close reading of the policy might demonstrate that should the case then be lost at trial or settled for more than the insurance company wished to offer, they have the right to collect that difference and the cost of defense from you. Therefore the consent you have a right to withhold has very little meaning.

The fact that registered nursing insurance costs have not changed much since introduced on the market, although all other malpractice insurance costs have risen drastically, is an indication of its lack of use (Campion, 1990). In addition, you can buy an individual nursing malpractice policy for $80, whereas a policy for physicians ranges from $80,000 to $120,000, and for extended-practice nurses, who often function independently, it is around $1200. This also is an indication of how often the registered nursing insurance policy is actually used.

WHAT IS INSTITUTIONAL COVERAGE?

Most all health care corporations or institutions carry very large insurance policies that specifically cover acts or omissions of their employed nurses. This includes both when the institution only is named under the previously described *respondeat superior* doctrine, or when an individual nurse employee is named. Most all individual personal nursing malpractice policies are ***secondary*** to this policy. This means they cannot be used in any manner if the institutional policy is used to cover the claim. It is not correct to assume that you can have your personal attorney present to represent your personal interests in addition to the institutional attorney. Even if you could, having two attorneys will often divide the defense and augment the claim (Simpson, 1998).

A representation that the institutional attorney will only look out for the institution's interests and not yours is questionable in that attorneys ethically must represent both your interests and the institution's. In addition, the institution's interests are rarely, if ever, adverse to yours. Both of you wish to settle claims that have liability and defend claims when there is no liability.

The claim that an institution will insure you, but then turn around and sue you is belied by the fact that one cannot find statistics to verify this common claim. Institutions spend millions of dollars on insurance to specifically cover the acts of nurses. In addition, if institutions sued the nurses working for them, they would not keep nurses. Recently one case is cited in the literature as demonstrating that an institution sued its nurse (*St. Anthony's Hospital v. Whitfield*, 1997), and yet a reading of that case as reported does not disclose the reasons for the claim (Murphy, 1998).

It is true that if an employee commits a criminal act that by its nature is outside the scope of their employment, such as forced sexual intimacies with a patient, an institution may not defend the employee, nor cover costs. In this regard, though, criminal acts are not insurable under laws in most all states and therefore are not covered by any policy (Simpson, 1998).

WHAT SHOULD I ASK ABOUT INSTITUTIONAL COVERAGE?

There are certain things that a prudent nurse concerned about coverage should do. All nurses should request and have a right to a document, which gives them the following information regarding their employer's insurance coverage for them:

1. The name of the institution's insurance carrier, the limits of the policy, and the rating of the insurance company (Best Rating A+++ is the highest).
2. Whether they are covered for all acts occurring within the scope of their employment and during the time they are employed.
3. The acts for which they do not have coverage.
4. If the hospital will cover them if they need to appear before the state board of nursing in relationship to a malpractice claim. If not, an individual insurance policy that clearly does may be valuable.
5. If the nurse is an independent practitioner and/or in an extended practice role, he or she should be absolutely certain how they are covered by their institutional employers.
6. If a nurse does utilization review for an insurance company that is involved in an employee benefit plan, there may be individual exposure (Murphy, 1998).
7. If the nurse is working in a physician's office that has limited coverage.
8. If the nurse is self-employed, then of course individually purchased coverage is essential.

You may obtain individual policies from all companies selling insurance to nurses. If you are concerned about your institutional coverage, obtain such policies and determine whether they truly offer more or additional coverage. As stated earlier, the cost is very low, and even though the protection may also be limited, some nurses feel more secure owning these policies.

WHAT HAPPENS WHEN I GO TO COURT?

Sometimes, despite all your efforts, you find yourself in litigation as a defendant. Know that very few claims go to trial. Therefore you do not need to picture yourself in a setting from *The Practice* or *Law and Order* with a prosecutor tearing you apart. Ninety-five percent of personal injury lawsuits are either dismissed or settled out of court, usually after an investigatory process called "discovery." (Fish, Ehrhardt, and Fish, 1990). This involves written questions about situations surrounding a case, *interrogatories,* and a recorded oral questioning process called a ***deposition.***

Depositions are oral statements given under oath and are extremely important in any malpractice claim. They are used to evaluate the merits of the case, the credibility of the witnesses, and the strength of the defendants. Cases are won or lost in this process. Therefore, with the help of your attorney, you must be very prepared. If you have not been offered the chance to meet with your attorney well before your deposition, request the time to do so. This is your right and an ethical obligation of the attorney. Being prepared ahead of time can have a significant effect on your performance under stress. Many attorneys will role-play situations with you so you will get the feel of the process. There are also good books, videos, and other aids that should be considered. Ask your attorney, or check with your hospital Risk Management Department, in addition to the public library and Web sites.

Depositions occur in a less formal setting than the courtroom. Attorneys for both sides will be present, but this is not the time to tell your story. The attorney questioning you will be either the attorney for the plaintiff or for the other defendants whose interests may be adversarial to yours. Your attorney can object to certain questions, but on the whole you will have to answer them anyway because in the deposition there is no judge to rule on the objections. Remember that you are there to answer questions in a truthful manner, but not to teach or inform.

The following are tips for how a nurse should act in a deposition.

1. You need to look and act like a professional. That means that you must be prepared. Know the case; and review your documented record ahead of time.
2. Be clear, accurate, and very concise. It is often said that if you say more than seven words, it is too much. If you do not know an answer, say so—do not guess.
3. Never give opinions unless asked for them. Stick to the facts!
4. Speak slowly and in a well-modulated tone of voice. Do not allow yourself to be rattled by the opposing attorney.
5. If you do not remember a question or do not understand it, ask for it to be repeated or clarified. Many attorneys use long, multipart questions to confuse you. Do not get caught in this trap.
6. If you have made a statement and later realize it is not correct, do not be afraid to say so, rather than to skirt issues or contradict yourself.
7. Do not allow yourself to be goaded into an angry or emotional response. You can always ask for a break during a deposition to collect yourself and your thoughts.

8. Avoid the use of "always" and "never" and vague comments like "maybe," "I think," or "possibly."

9. Do not answer more than is asked for by the question. This helps maintain focus and clarity. The attorney desires to catch you in contradictory statements. The shorter your statements, the less likely that is to happen.

A lawsuit is a very disconcerting and disheartening process to everyone involved. Your ability to realize this and not feel alone in the process is extremely important. Often institutions mandate that persons involved in litigation receive counseling to help them resolve the anger and depression that most everyone feels at some point. Be sure to use resources available to you including your lawyer. Remember that the old adage of "this too will pass" is true.

CONTROVERSIAL LEGAL ISSUES AFFECTING NURSING

Because developments and advances in medical and nursing care occur constantly, there are many areas of practice that do not have firm rules to follow when making decisions. Changes in health care delivery and society's values have sparked controversy about a variety of issues.

HEALTH CARE COSTS AND PAYMENT ISSUES

One example is third-party reimbursement, or the right of an individual nurse, usually a nurse practitioner, to be paid directly by insurance companies for care given. Recently Medicare has passed rules that allow nurse practitioners to bill independently under their own provider number. This is a very important step in the field of independent practice for nurses, as many health care insurers follow the lead of Medicare in billing issues.

In relationship to the right to bill, all nurses do need to understand billing and reimbursement rules so that they cannot ever be accused of participating in fraudulent billing schemes. For instance, although RNs can bill for certain follow-up care in the outpatient clinic as services rendered "incident to" what the physician does, there are strict requirements of physician involvement that nurses must understand. Nurse practitioners need to be careful that their services are not also being illegally billed for by physicians with whom they collaborate.

From another perspective, the high cost of health care is also driving the proliferation of health care workers with less training and education than nurses, who can be hired for less money. Often these unlicensed workers have no laws circumscribing their practice and are doing tasks that have traditionally been done by RNs or LPNs, such as administering medications and giving injections. This is an important issue for nurses, especially when asked to supervise such workers and/or compete for positions in the health care market.

Legislative changes are necessary to alter these and other policies. Your support will be important when your state decides such issues. Professional behavior includes concern with and participation in the direction health care and particularly nursing care will take in the future.

HEALTH CARE DELIVERY ISSUES

Changes made in the types of systems used to deliver health care and in the techniques used by the systems have created many concerns for nurses. Hospitals and other expensive acute-care settings are giving way to outpatient clinics and same-day surgery centers. This means that people are being sent home while still acutely ill to take care of themselves or relatives without the benefit of hospital nursing services. This makes the nurse's role in discharge planning and patient education an extremely important one to prevent deterioration of certain health or surgical conditions in the home. In addition, it means that home health care nurses are routinely organizing care that used to be only rendered in hospitals. For example, respirators in the home are not unusual. With this change, however, come more independent responsibilities for nurses. Responsibility can translate into liability.

Telephone nursing triage and telemedical nursing care present new and unusual legal concerns because of the difficulties of providing accurate long-distance care, and the independent nature of these tasks. Although these nurses bring nursing care to many areas that have not had access to this care in the past, selecting appropriately prepared individuals to provide the care and educating them to function effectively when they cannot see the patient are challenging tasks.

HMOs and other forms of prepaid health care have helped reduce the rapidly growing costs of health care through a process called *utilization review*. Nurses hired to do this review are often asked to make judgments regarding whether or not a patient should be discharged. Early discharge of patients and limits on insurance reimbursements for certain allowable medications, equipment and external services have sometimes caused ethical and legal problems for health care professionals (Deloughery, 1998).

Past laws protecting the HMOs from malpractice claims when patients were harmed because of flawed utilization review practices are now being challenged. There is a growing public concern that managed-care organizations are making large profits while patients covered under their programs are not receiving adequate care. Both Congress and state legislatures are attempting to pass statutes to curb this practice (Kongstvedt, 2001).

The many changes occurring in the workplace often create levels of confusion and frustration, which make it more difficult to focus on the quality of the care being given on a day-to-day basis. These issues are examples of how legal issues interweave with all the other events in your professional life. Nurses must remain involved in these matters to stay aware of how their legal responsibilities are influenced by them.

ISSUES ABOUT LIFE-AND-DEATH DECISIONS

Controversial ethical issues surrounding life and death also, of course, present controversial legal issues. Scientific research and new technologies can blur the line between life and death. As a nurse, you can often find yourself in the center of such controversies, so you need to be very aware of what your state's laws are on at least the following subjects.

Abortions. Where can abortions be performed? Who can perform them? When can an abortion be performed? Under what conditions? Under what if any conditions can teenagers obtain an abortion?

Fetal Rights. If a fetus is born alive, what rights does it have? What rights do the parents have? What rights do health care workers have? What are the laws surrounding fetal death and/or the cessation of life preserving treatments?

Human Experimentation or Research. What can be legally done with the products of conception? What types of consent are necessary to enroll a patient in research studies? What types of Boards and oversight must be involved to approve and monitor human research studies?

Patient Rights. What rights do patients have in your state in relationship to medical records, medical information, giving consent, participating in their care, suing providers, dictating issues surrounding their death, donating organs, being protected from abuse, receiving emergency treatment, being protected from the practice of unlicensed providers, transplantation of organs, accessibility of the disabled to health care, privacy and confidentiality?

CONCLUSION

As time goes on, laws will be changing and new areas will arise that nursing will have to address. Continuing education, critical thinking, and an open mind will help you to learn about and deal with the legal issues that will touch your professional life daily. Get involved whenever possible with safety, quality, and risk-management processes in your institutions. Be someone who has an educated opinion about conflicts inherent in medicine and nursing. Take the opportunity to visit the hearings conducted by your state's board of nursing and by the state legislature. By becoming involved with the legal and disciplinary process, you will be much more aware of how you can protect yourself and your patients and influence the direction of health care issues. By concluding this chapter, it is hoped that you also feel more confident when faced with "the law."

REFERENCES

American Society for Healthcare Risk Management: *Perspective on disclosure of unanticipated outcome information*, Chicago, 2001, ASHRM.

Campion FX: *Grand rounds on medical malpractice*, Milwaukee, 1990, American Medical Association.

Curtin LL: When negligence becomes homicide. . ., *Nurs Manage* 28(7):7-8, 1997.

Deloughery G: *Issues and Trends in Nursing*, St Louis, 1998, Mosby

Denega D: National Practitioner Data Bank impacts nursing practice, *Am Nursing* 25(7):10, 1993.

Ellis JR, Hartley CL: *Nursing in today's world*, Philadelphia, 2001, Lippincott-Raven.

Fiesta J: *The law and liability: a guide for nurses*, ed 2, New York, 1988, Delmar.

Fish RM, Ehrhardt ME, Fish B: *Malpractice: managing your defense*, New Jersey, 1990, Medical Economics Books.

Freydel v. New York Hospital, No. 97 Civ 7926 (SHS), Jan 4, 2000

Guido GW: *Legal and ethical issues in nursing*, Upper Saddle River, New Jersey, 2000, Prentice Hall.

Gutheil TG: On apologizing to patients, *Risk Management Foundation of the Harvard Medical Institutions Inc* 6:3-4, 51, 1987.

Gutheil TG, Bursztajn H, Brodsky A: Malpractice prevention through the sharing of uncertainty. Informed consent and the therapeutic alliance, *N Engl J Med* 311(1):1:49-51, 1984.

Harvey v. Mid-Coast Hospital, 36 F. Supp. 2d 32, D. Maine, 1999.

Haack MR, Hughes TL: *Addiction in the nursing profession: approaches to intervention and recovery*, New York, 1989, Springer.

Hogue E: *Nursing case law reporter: cases and commentary*, Owings Mills, Md, 1983, National Law Publishing.

Joint Commission on the Accreditation of Healthcare Organizations: *Nursing care scoring guidelines: 1991 standards*, Oakbrook Terrace, Ill, 1990, JCAHO.

Joint Commission for the Accreditation of Healthcare Organizations: *Sentinel event statistics*, Oakbrook Terrace, Ill, 1998, JCAHO.

Joint Commission on the Accreditation of Healthcare Organizations: *Comprehensive Accreditation Manual for Hospitals: The Official Handbook*. Oakbrook Terrace, Ill, 2000, JCAHO.

Kelly LY, Joel JA: *Dimensions of professional nursing*, New York, 1999, McGraw-Hill.

Kohn LT, Corrigan JM, Donaldson MS: *To err is human: building a safer health system*, Washington, DC, 2000, National Academy Press.

Kongstvedt PR: *Essentials of managed health care*, ed 4, Rockville, Md, 2001, Aspen.

Kowalski K, Horner MD: A legal nightmare. Denver nurses indicted, *MCN Am J Maternal Child Nurs* 23(3):125-129, 1998.

Lobe TE: *Medical malpractice, A physician's guide*, New York, 1995, McGraw-Hill.

Murphy EK: Individual malpractice insurance decisions revisited *AORN J* 67(6):1234-1236, 1998.

Prosser WL: *Law of torts*, Minnesota, 1971, West Publishing Co.

Raleigh Fitkin-Paul Morgan Memorial Hospital v. Anderson, 42 NJ 421, 201 A. 2nd 5 37, 1964.

Richards EP, Rathbun KC: *Medical risk management*, Rockville, Md, 1983, Aspen.

St. Anthony's Hospital v. Whitfield, 946 SW2d 174 (Tex App 1997).

Simpson KR: Should Nurses Purchase Their Own Professional Liability Insurance? *Am J Maternal Child Nurs* 23(3):1998.

Tideliksaar R: *Falls in older patients: prevention and management*, Baltimore, 1998, Health Profession Press.

Walker RS: *Falls and serious injuries before, during and after a nursing home became restraint free* [thesis], Arizona: University of Arizona, 1992.

Yocum CJ, Haack MR: *Interim report: a comparison of two regulatory approaches to the management of chemically impaired nurses*, Chicago, 1996, NCSBN.

ADDITIONAL READINGS

Aiken T, Catalano JT: *Legal, ethical and political issues in nursing*, Philadelphia, 1994, FA Davis.

Cruzan v. Director, Missouri Department of Health, 110 S. Ct. 2841, 1990.

Edge RS, Krieger JL: *Legal and ethical perspectives in health care*, New York, 1998, Delmar.

Forum: Nursing Practice and Education Committee: *National Council's Business Book—1999*, Chicago, 1999, NCSBN.

Marrelli TM: *TM Marrelli's home care nurse news*, Marrelli and Associates, Inc.

Marrelli TM: Manager's corner: telemedicine in a rural setting, *TM Marrellis Home Care Nurse News* 5(11):1998.

Milstead JA: *Health policy and politics*, Rockville, Md, 1999, Aspen.

Perin RL: *Risk management for physicians*, Arizona, 1996, Health Science Media for The Arizona Board of Regents.

Polston MD: Whistleblowing: does the law protect you? *Am J Nurs* 99(1):26-32, 1999.

Schwirian P: *Professionalization of Nursing*. Philadelphia, 1998, Lippincott.

Yocum CJ: *Job analysis for newly licensed registered nurses*, Chicago, 1996, NCSBN.

INTERNET RESOURCES

Federal Web Locator
http://www.infoctr.edu/fwl

U.S. Federal Government Agencies
http://www.lib.lsu.edu/gov/fedgov.html

Agency for Healthcare Research and Quality (formerly the Agency for Health Care Policy and Research)
http://www.ahcpr.gov

Centers for Disease Control
http://www.cdc.gov

Association of Perioperative Registered Nurses
http://www.aorn.org/clinical/default.htm

Department of Health and Human Services
http://www.os.dhhs.gov

FedWorld
http://www.fedworld.gov

Food and Drug Administration
http://www.fda.gov

Health Care Financing Administration
http://www.hcfa.gov

Indian Health Service
http://www.ihs.gov

National Council of State Boards of Nursing
http://www.ncsbn.org

National Institutes of Health
http://www.nih.gov

Occupational Safety and Health Administration
http://www.osha.gov

Social Security Administration
http://www.ssa.gov

United Nations
http://www.un.org

Veterans Administration
http://www.va.gov

World Health Administration
http://www.who.ch

Joint Commission on the Accreditation of Healthcare Organizations
http://www.jcaho.org

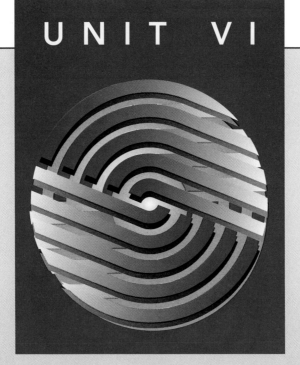

UNIT VI

IN SEARCH OF EMPLOYMENT: FINDING YOUR NICHE IN THE WORLD

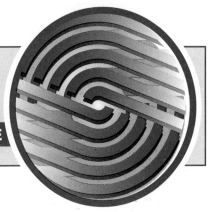

CHAPTER TWENTY-ONE

Employment Considerations: Opportunities and Résumés

JO CAROL CLABORN, MS, RN, CNS

GAIL M. COLLIER, RN

Success is getting what you want. Happiness is wanting what you get.

—*Dale Carnegie*

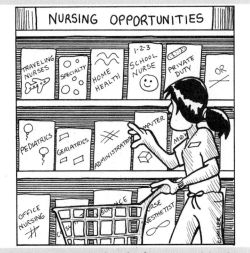

There is a smorgasbord of opportunities in nursing. You can always go back and make another selection.

After completing this chapter, you should be able to:

- Assess trends in the job market.
- Describe the important parts of a résumé.
- Review the primary aspects of obtaining employment.

Early in 2000, evidence of a nursing shortage began to become evident. Government as well as scholastic research began to predict an oncoming crisis in nursing. Nursing shortages are not new—they have been cyclical in the profession for years; however, the current shortage may be more critical than any previous shortage. There are significantly more lucrative options available to those individuals who in past years would have chosen nursing. Because of these increased opportunities, there has been a significant decline in students enrolling in nursing school. The decline in enrollments is further compounded by the aging of nurse educators and the aging of the nursing workforce. These trends in the ranks of nursing are further complicated by an aging population. The demand for nurses is going to far outreach the resources for years to come. It is projected by the year 2020, there will be 20% fewer nurses than the projected workforce requirements (Valentine, 2002). It is very important for you as a recent graduate to carefully assess the market and find a position that fits what you need and want.

JOB MARKET

WHAT IS HAPPENING IN THE JOB MARKET?

Over the past 10 years, there have been many ups and downs in the job market for nurses. In the mid-1990s there was downsizing, increased employment of unlicensed assistive personnel, and a tight job market for nursing. This was especially true of the job market for the recent graduate. Early in 1997 there were again signs of change. Some hospitals were beginning to claim nurse shortages, especially in the specialty areas. The twenty-first century begins with critical issues for health care: nursing education, practice, and safe health care for the public.

The changing picture of nursing employment was very aptly described by Lucille A. Joel in an editorial in the *American Journal of Nursing* in 1997.

> The mental image of shifting sands suggests a loss of control, an absence of stability, impermanence in the presence of permanence. Nursing's on again, off-again courtship with surpluses and shortages is suited to that metaphor.
>
> Our forte has been to adapt, sometimes grudgingly, sometimes with panache for the victor, ameliorating the symptoms but avoiding the challenge of coming to terms with the underlying problem (Joel, 1997).

The graying of the American population is going to have a tremendous impact on the health care industry. There will be a substantial increase in the number of geriatric patients, and they will also have increased needs for multilevels of health care. Not only is there a significant graying of the population, there is also a graying of the nursing corps as well. The experts indicate that the average age of a nurse in the United States is now over 44 years (Schreiber, 1999). There is an increasing number of subacute settings and the development of long-term care facilities (Levenson, 1998).

What is going to happen with nursing employment and the job market when a large percentage of nurses become part of the older generation? Who will mentor the new nurses? What will the job market be for the graduate nurse over the next 5 years? What changes will be forced on nursing and health care? There is only one thing for sure—it is going to continue to change (Critical Thinking Box 21-1).

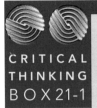

CRITICAL THINKING BOX 21-1

What changes have you already observed as a result of the nursing shortage? What impact has the shortage had on salaries and staffing in your community? If the signs of a nursing shortage were beginning to surface in 1997, why are we (nursing, education, hospitals, government) just now responding to the problem?

SEEKING EMPLOYMENT

HOW TO FIND A JOB THAT'S RIGHT FOR YOU

As you are preparing for graduation, it's time to focus on your interests and set your sights on your first job as a graduate nurse. What are your career goals? Don't worry if you are not too sure; frequently you need to immerse yourself in the world of nursing to determine where you really want to go. You will need to take time to select the job that will not only offer you immediate satisfaction, but allow you to practice in an environment you are prepared for as well as give you the opportunity to grow. Because nursing offers so many options, it is exciting to think of all the possibilities that can occur along your career path. So, the first thing to do is to "think big." That's right, let yourself dream. Envision yourself moving in any direction in a career that fascinates you with possibilities that you can hardly imagine to exist.

> I am walking in the door of the corporate office of the UCLA Medical Center. I feel a
> sense of energy and vitality as I see my name on the door—Vice President of Nursing
> Operations.

Does this sound far-fetched to you? It's up to you to select the type of nursing you like to do and are best suited for. The key to making the right career decision is self-understanding. Through self-evaluation, you can determine who you are and what you like. This knowledge will assist you in setting an appropriate career goal that will increase your negotiating power by focusing your job search. Setting career goals will provide criteria with which you can weigh job offers and options. See Chapter 22 for information on interviewing and a discussion of self-assessment strategies that will assist you in feeling more comfortable about how to get that first job that you really want.

"You can't consistently perform in a manner that is inconsistent with the way you see yourself" (Zig Ziglar).

WHY SET A CAREER GOAL?

Why should you set a career goal? The answer to this question is simple. Each time you succeed in meeting a career goal, you increase your self-confidence and self-esteem. A career goal defines who or what you wish to be professionally. In addition, it will help tie together the elements of your job search—the résumé writing, the research, the employer contacts, and the interview process—by giving you a direction. Remember, you cannot set a "wrong career goal"; there may be times when you will need to assess your direction then redefine and redirect your career goal. Career goals are not end results—they are the roadmap to give you direction to where you want to go.

It's helpful to set both long-term and short-term career goals. Your long-term goal of becoming a vice president of nursing may be your ultimate goal. You must also recognize in the meantime what you would like to accomplish, such as being able to assess a patient in less than 45 minutes or being able to function fully as a staff member. Whatever your goals, it helps to have a plan. Find a nurse who enjoys nursing and is currently practicing; talk with them about where you want to go in nursing. Maybe you don't know what you want. Start in the direction of an area you like—you can always change directions. Having a direction and goals is important to researching jobs, comparing offers, and choosing a satisfying career position.

When interviewing hospitals or other institutions, check their mission statement. What is it the institution is committed to achieving? Do you see evidence that they are committed to the mission statement, or is it just a statement? Does the mission statement of the institution support your career goals and your concept of nursing? Don't rush through this job-searching process. There are going to be a lot of job offers, so don't jump into something that does not fit your needs. Think about your career goals and what your needs are as a recent graduate. How can you best launch your career in nursing? (Critical Thinking Box 21-2).

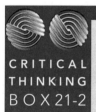

CRITICAL
THINKING
B O X 21-2

Where do you want to be in 6 months? In 5 years?

WHAT EMPLOYMENT OPPORTUNITIES ARE AVAILABLE?

You have a world of nursing to choose from; there are incredible opportunities available to begin your practice as a graduate nurse. The largest employers are hospitals or acute-care facilities. In hospitals there are a wide variety of positions, although often recent graduates are placed in staff nurse positions. If it is a general hospital, you need to choose what areas interest you most. Your first position may not be exactly what you want, but remember, it is the first step toward your career goal. As you build your competence and self-esteem, you may find just the position you want. In many hospitals, staff positions represent many different levels and areas, especially if the hospital participates in clinical or career ladders. Staff nurse positions are one of the most challenging, in addition to providing an "incubator" to begin your nursing practice. Charge positions may involve responsibility for a particular staff or a particular day or they may involve managing staff for an entire unit. There are a variety of opportunities in management as your experience level increases and you continue your education. Many institutions now refer to the person charged with the management of all of nursing as *vice president:* these persons usually have a master's or doctoral degree in nursing. Exact job titles depend on the organizational structure of the institution. It is very important in your first few years of nursing to watch the trends in nursing, realize what opportunities are available, know where your interests are, and understand what it will take (experience and education) to get you where you want to be.

Entry-level positions in the hospital are usually staff nurse positions. In the current nursing crisis the staff nurse positions are the areas of critical need. Staff nurse positions in medical-surgical nursing are one of the most demanding—and rewarding—positions. Frequently nurses begin their career here with the intention to move on to greener pastures; however, the rewards and challenges more than fulfill their needs. It is important that your first position offer you an opportunity to further develop your nursing skills. Whether it is working in the emergency department, day surgery, specialty units, or medical surgical units, staff nurse positions give you a very valuable opportunity to polish your time management, patient care organization and nursing skills (Fig. 21-1). Once you are confident with skills, procedures, and the overall practice of nursing, then you may be ready to move on to new challenges. This may be 6 months for some recent graduates; for others it may take a year or more. Take the time to reinforce your nursing competencies, it will prepare you for your future practice in nursing. Other areas in which nurses may also find employment include community health, home health care, and nursing agencies. Working in the community in such positions as occupational health, school health, and the military often requires a bachelor's degree in nursing and at least 1 year of hospital nursing, or both.

WHAT ABOUT ADVANCED DEGREES IN NURSING?

There are many advantages to advanced degrees in nursing. Review Chapter 4 for the different choices regarding an advanced degree. One of the most important aspects of obtaining an advanced degree is your experience as a nurse that helps you to determine what direction you want to go. Don't expect this to come early in your career; it may take a little time as you sample different areas of practice to determine whether you want an advanced degree and in which area to focus. If you are an associate degree graduate, you might want to consider the basic requirements for your bachelor's degree, including what schools are available and what their requirements are. This is an area you can begin to work on immediately after graduation. Remember, you can do this a little at a time without having to declare an area of special interest. Although an advanced degree is important to some nurses, others may prefer special education programs that do not lead to an advanced degree, but expertise in a specialty practice area. Keep an open mind as you begin to investigate this great world of nursing.

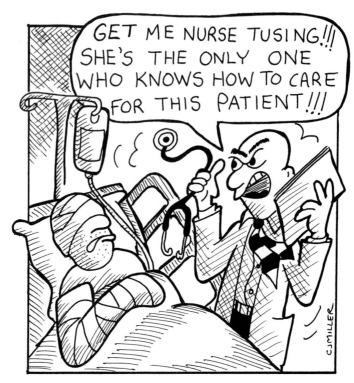

FIGURE 21-1
Being competent has its rewards.

RÉSUMÉ WRITING

HOW DO I WRITE AN EFFECTIVE RÉSUMÉ?

Design your résumé by using the KISS principle—Keep It Simple, Sincerely! (That is, use concise wording and make it easy-to-read, informational, and simple.)

Nurses are not famous for exceptional skills in putting together their own résumés! Most nurses would rather be taking care of patients and families. However, all nurses should keep a current résumé handy. It helps you keep track of where you have been and what you have done. You do not have to be a computer wizard. You can do this.

Your résumé is the first introduction a prospective employer will have to you. It will give the employer a basic idea of who you are professionally and what your objectives are for your nursing career. While defining your strengths, it is important not to overstate your skills. Most employers in this economic time are willing to train you on all or some of the components of the position you are applying for. A résumé is a concise, factual presentation of your educational and professional history (Box 21-1). Don't be surprised if a recruiter suggests other areas to you than what you have initially indicated on your résumé or in your interview. Be open to suggestions; they may have some ideas or considerations you have not even thought about.

BOX 21-1   Résumé Guidelines

❑ Catch all typos and grammatical errors, have someone proofread your resume.

❑ Present a clear objective that emphasizes your skills and strengths.

❑ A good first impression is critical—if written, it should be neat, appearing on white paper or off-white paper.

❑ Avoid using the "I" or "me" words in your résumé.

❑ Keep the information concise, preferably to one or two pages.

❑ Rule of thumb on work experience is to show most current work experience. Generally the last 10–15 years, unless there is something in your background that is critical to note.

❑ Don't try to impress anyone with big words, jargon for the profession is okay if everyone knows what it is.

❑ Don't inquire about salary or benefits in your résumé—not the right time or place for that.

❑ Don't exaggerate about what you can and cannot do—the potential employer will check it out.

❑ Do present yourself in a positive light.

❑ Your résumé should be neat and visually appealing.

❑ Don't list all of your references. Be prepared to provide them with a list when asked. You may want to have different references for different types of positions.

WHAT INFORMATION IS NECESSARY FOR A RÉSUMÉ?

Here are the components of a résumé. Be sure to proofread what you write for spelling and grammar. Don't forget that this is the first impression someone may have of you.

Demographic Data: Who Are You? Your name, address, telephone number, and e-mail address should be at the top of the page. Be sure to give correct, current information so the employer can easily contact you. If you need to give an alternate telephone number or e-mail address, please note their name and advise that person that a prospective employer may be calling for you. Keep in mind that you never put personal information such as your social security number, marital status, number of children, or your picture on a résumé.

Professional Objective: What Position Are You Applying For? There is a wide variety of ways to address this aspect. However, it is very important that you describe the position you are applying for and in what department/area of nursing you are interested. With the widespread use of the Internet, it has become increasingly easy to view job openings and be more educated and decisive about what you are looking for. You can identify several areas (if you have more than one area of preference). This ultimately is your short-term goal. You may also state a long-term goal (e.g., administration, quality assurance, case management, transplant team).

Education: Where Did You Receive Your Education, High School To Present? List your education in chronological order, beginning with high school. List the month/year of graduation and what degree was received, if any. If you have degrees other than nursing, you also want to include these in the chronological order in which you received them. This section will contain certifications or special training you have received, where you received it, and the date you completed it. If you are currently enrolled in school, be sure to include that as well.

Professional Experience: What Do You Know How To Do? "Easy to read" is the goal. It is very important to put this section in chronological order beginning with the present. You want the prospective employer to see what you have been doing most recently. List your current or previous employer, position held, dates from and to, and a brief description of your responsibilities. This is a good place to highlight special skills that you feel may be important to your prospective employer. This section will be different for a experienced nurse than for a recent graduate nurse. Nevertheless, it is important to list your employment history through the past 7 years. Include those areas of employment that may not be associated with nursing or the health care field. Whatever experience you have as an "employee" is necessary to demonstrate your ability to work with people, handle stress, be flexible, and so forth. It is not necessary to list clinical rotations you have completed during nursing school, most of those rotations are standardized. If you have not had any experience and this will be your first job, state that also. It is important for managers and staff educators to be aware of the levels of experience of the recent graduates.

Licensure: What Can You Do and Where Can You Do It? This is a very important area of information for nurses. With the implementation of the Multi-State Licensure Compact (see Chapter 17), you may only have to be licensed in one state. It is your responsibility to know which states will honor your license and which ones will require you to obtain a separate license. As a general rule, you will be required to be licensed in the state of your residence, then possibly in another state of practice, depending on the licensure compact of the states involved. List the state your license was issued and the expiration date. For security reasons, do not list your license number.

Professional Organizations: What Do You Belong To? You may list organizations in which you are a member or have held an office. It is good to list professional and community groups. This section is optional.

Honors and Awards: What Did You Receive Recognition For? If you have received recognition for special skills or volunteer work, you may want to include it here. You may also include any scholarships you have received. This is also an optional section.

References: Who Knows About You? A simple line at the bottom of the résumé "References provided on request" will suffice. Be prepared with a separate typed sheet that lists at least 3 references. Provide the names and telephone numbers of two professionals with whom you have worked and one personal reference. Always notify your references that you have listed them and that they may receive a telephone call about you. Look at the example of a résumés (Fig. 21-2) and adapt it to what works best for you. It is preferable to keep your résumé under 1 page, but this is not always possible. If you need further examples of résumés or formats, check the Internet for samples (http://resume.monster.com). Several of the popular word-processing programs also have résumé formats in the section for office forms.

WHAT ELSE SHOULD I SUBMIT WITH MY RÉSUMÉ?

Along with your résumé you should enclose a cover letter that gives a brief introduction (Box 21-2) (Fig. 21-3). Summarize your important strengths or give information regarding change of specialty but remember that this letter should be less than one page. If you have talked with a recruiter and have a specific name, then send it to them. You do not have to address it to a specific person, it will be distributed to the recruiter who handles the units where you have indicated an interest. Simply addressing it to "Nurse Recruitment" will usually get it to the right person.

WHAT ARE THE METHODS OF SUBMITTING RÉSUMÉS?

There are a variety of ways to submit résumés: hand-carry it, submit it electronically by means of e-mail or the hospital Web site, or mail it through the post office. You will probably want to send it to the nurse recruitment department of your favorite medical institution. One of the most popular methods for nurses to send résumés is through the Web site of the medical institutions they are most interested in. This is an excellent way to submit your résumé, but remember to follow-up with a telephone call if you have not heard from a recruiter within 1 week. You can also directly e-mail your résumé to a recruiter. E-mail addresses are readily available through business cards, Web sites, and word of mouth. Beware, your e-mail first page will be the cover letter when you submit your résumé by using e-mail. The same résumé writing principles apply to all electronically submitted résumés because your résumé will be printed for review. There are also many large job search Web sites available on the internet. You can post your résumé on any of these by using their specific formats but remember that businesses must pay a fee to search for applicants. It is important to remember that not all of the institutions belong to every job search Web site. Use discretion regarding where you want to post your résumé; if you are interested in a specific institution, it is best to review their Web site for positions available and guidelines for submitting résumés.

Linda Smith

123 Any Street

Dallas, TX 77777

972-555-5555

E-mail: lsmith@hotmail.com

Objective:

To obtain a staff nurse position in Hematology-Oncology.

Education:

Memorial High School, Dallas, Texas, graduated 05/1998.

El Centro College, Dallas, Texas

ADN, awarded June 2002

Experience:

10/2000 to present–Baylor Hospital, Dallas, Texas–nurse tech, part-time

02/1997 to 06/1999–Kroger's Supermarkets, cashier

Licensure:

Eligible for NCLEX May 2002 (Texas)

Certifications: CPR expires 03/2002

Professional Organizations:

Texas Nursing Students Association

References: on Request

FIGURE 21-2
Résumé.

BOX 21-2 Reminders for Cover Letters

❏ 8$\frac{1}{2}$ × 11-inch paper, white, off-white, light blue
❏ Typed with no mistakes
❏ No smudges
❏ 1$\frac{1}{2}$–2-inch margin on all sides
❏ Signed, usually with black ink
❏ No abbreviations
❏ Use business letter format

Linda Smith

111 Anyplace Blvd.

Boise, ID 30203

(712) 555-5555

Nurse Recruiter

Medical Center of Texas

222 Medical Way

Dallas, TX 77777

Dear Nurse Recruiter:

There is a Diabetic Educator position posted on your Web site. I would like to apply for the position and have attached my résumé for your review. I currently have 1 year of experience in this role in a 220-bed hospital. Before that I worked for 2 years on a medical/surgical unit with a large population of new and established diabetic patients.

   I will be relocating to the Dallas area in 2 months and will be in Dallas September 10 and 11 for interviews. Please let me know if this would be a convenient time to schedule an interview. I have voice mail on my phone, so you may leave me a message. I look forward to meeting with you. Please feel free to contact me.

Sincerely,

Linda Smith

FIGURE 21-3
Cover letter.

Now that you have your résumé ready to submit, you will need to identify prospective employers. How do you do that? One of the first things you can do is *network*. *Networking* is contacting everyone you know and even some people you don't know to get information about their specific organization or institution. Places that you can network are at your facility during clinical, at student organization programs, at career days at colleges, and at career opportunity fairs. Attend local chapter meetings of nursing organizations. Check the Sunday newspaper. Read nursing journal employment sections. When you have identified the institutions where you would like to discuss possible employment, send them your résumé. If you have not heard from them within 7 to 10 days, give them a call to make sure your résumé was received and to schedule an interview. Keep track of all this information on your record of contacts and résumés sent so that you will have easy access to the information (Fig. 21-4). It will be important to document your follow up actions and results—don't forget to keep copies of correspondence and notes on any conversations with potential employers. Remember to date all entries—briefly put

Employer Address and Phone Number	Interviewer and Title	Date Résumé Sent	Date and Time of Interview	Inquiry of Application Letter	Application Submitted	Thank You Letter Sent After Interview	Job Offer Received	Confirmation of "No Thank You" Letter Sent	Comments or Notes

FIGURE 21-4

Record of employer contacts and résumés sent.

information received, interviews requested and granted, résumés sent, and job offers received. Box 21-3 presents a summary of the steps to finding the job you want.

BOX 21-3   Your Checklist for Finding a Job

❑ Define your goals.
❑ Develop your résumé.
❑ Identify potential employers.
❑ Send your résumé and cover letter.
❑ Return a follow-up phone call.
❑ Schedule an interview.
❑ Send a follow-up letter.
❑ Keep record of employer contacts (Fig. 21–4).
❑ Make an informed decision where to work.

WHAT IS THE DIFFERENCE BETWEEN A RÉSUMÉ AND A CURRICULUM VITAE?

A curriculum vitae (CV) is a summary of your educational and academic background and is similar to a résumé. Unlike the résumé, however, your CV grows longer as you become more accomplished. You may want to include your continuing-education experiences and any publications (book chapters, journal articles.) Most CVs run 2 to 4 pages or more. As with a résumé, you may need several different CVs emphasizing different skills and experiences, depending on the positions or activity for which you are submitting the CV.

EMPLOYMENT CONSIDERATIONS: HOW DO YOU DECIDE ON AN EMPLOYER?

In 1980 the American Academy of Nursing identified criteria for what was designated as "magnet hospitals." This designation recognized hospitals for their lower turnover rates, visionary leaders, value they placed on education, and ability to maintain open lines of communication. To identify magnet hospitals in your area, check the Web site www.nursingworld.org.ancc (Valentino, 2002). In your search for a job, it is important to look for institutions/hospitals that create a work environment that supports professional nursing practice. In the current job market, locating magnet hospitals in your community would be an important consideration in your job search.

Sign-on bonuses are one of the current trends to attract nurses. Be cautious: carefully read and evaluate what is connected with the sign-on bonus. How long will you have to work to receive any of the bonus, and when will it be paid? How long do you have to work for the institution? For example, half of the sign-on bonus may be paid after 6 months of employment, but the remaining amount may not be paid until after 2 or 3 years of employment. Is the sign-on bonus in any way tied to the area in which you will be working? If you originally wanted to work in an intensive care unit but decided after 6 months that was not the area for you, can you transfer to another unit without losing your sign-on bonus?

WHAT ARE "BENEFITS"?

Salary, job responsibilities, and facility location are not the only major considerations in choosing an employer—don't forget to consider the total compensation package (that is, your benefits). Often, benefits are overlooked because their cost is less visible than the exciting new salary that you'll be receiving. Some organizations spend as much as 40% of their total employee payroll to provide this extra compensation. You should consider them your "hidden paycheck."

Most employers offer similar types of benefits in their total compensation packages. For example, most employers have some type of specific traditional plan. Some may even have a flexible plan that offers a number of options from which to choose (Box 21-4).

BOX 21-4   Benefit Package Options

❑ Health and life insurance
❑ Accidental death and dismemberment coverage
❑ Sick or short-term disability pay
❑ Vacation pay
❑ Profit sharing and retirement plan
❑ Long-term disability leave
❑ Dental and/or vision care
❑ Parking
❑ Tuition reimbursement
❑ Loan programs
❑ Dependent care programs
❑ Health and wellness programs

Regardless of the package you decide on, don't forget that there is usually a waiting period before the coverage is effective. Check with your institution—coverage with some health plans begins on one's first day of employment, but not always. Sometimes waiting periods may be as long as 3 to 6 months. Pension plans may require an even longer time before an employee is eligible to participate or at least be "vested." Vested means that the money that the institution invests in your retirement fund actually belongs to you after a specified period of time. Check with your employer to see what their retirement program offers.

Take a few minutes to look at some of the basic benefits that you'll need to decide on.

Health, Dental, and Vision Insurance. Health insurance may be contracted through companies such as Blue Cross/Blue Shield, Prudential, Metropolitan Life, and Mutual of Omaha, to name just a few. With these plans, you frequently receive health care from the physician and facility of your choice and the insurance company pays for it on a fee-for-service basis. Check to see what the co-payments are and if the insurance companies pay for well visits or physical examinations. Also check to see if there is a prescription drug plan included. All of these are subject to the conditions of each individual plan.

Other plans give you the opportunity to go to health maintenance organizations. In this situation, your family must go to a specified group of physicians or other health care professionals to get benefit coverage for the service. These services are covered on a prepaid basis. Usually your out-of-pocket expenses with health maintenance organizations are less. Table 21-1 provides a description of various health insurance terms that you need to know.

Another example of insurance coverage is through a preferred provider organization, in which your employer or insurance company arranges for fee-for-service health care with a specific provider at a predetermined rate. With a preferred provider

TABLE 21-1

Health Insurance Terms You Need to Know

Term	Definition
Coinsurance	The portion of your medical bills that you are responsible for paying after you have met the deductible. A ratio of 80/20 is standard, with you paying 20%.
Exclusions	Specific items not covered under your policy. Some policies exclude physical examinations, and health carriers can now legally exclude the treatment of AIDS.
First-dollar coverage	This policy pays all medical bills without a deductible. Almost impossible to find because coverage is so expensive.
Precertification	Some carriers require preapproval for receiving nonemergency treatments. These carriers may not cover certain treatments or will pay only partial benefits if precertification is not acquired. Your physician should be award of this when choosing treatment methods for you.
Preexisting condition	An illness or condition you have before your policy is issued. Some preexisting conditions are never covered. Most companies will not pay for the treatment of a preexisting condition for at least a year after your policy is effective.
PPO	Under a PPO system, the list of health care providers from whom you can choose is limited. Your physician may not be included on that list.
Reasonable and customary	The rates generally charged for specific treatments in your area. If a physician's fees are considerably higher than the fees charged by most physicians, your insurance company may cover only partial fees.
Waiting period	The period of time at the start of your coverage during which your carrier will not pay for certain treatments.

AIDS, Acquired immune deficiency syndrome; *PPO*, preferred provider organization.

organization, you are free to select a physician or facility for insurance coverage; however, you must go to one of the preferred providers within the organization or insurance company to obtain the lowest cost for health care.

Vision plans and dental plans may cover regular exams and provide for corrective lenses or preventive dental work. This may be at an additional rate. As with any policy there are certain out-of-pocket expenses such as deductibles that have to be met. Whatever plan you choose, be sure to determine whether or not you want to arrange coverage for your dependents or spouse. After you terminate your employment at that facility, don't forget that the institution is required by law to offer you continued coverage (COBRA) at your expense for your health insurance for a specified period of time.

Life Insurance and Death and Dismemberment. Check to see what type of basic life insurance is offered by your employer. The amount of the coverage could be fixed at an amount or it might be based on a percentage of your salary. Often this life insurance is available upon employment and may not cost you a penny. Take advantage of this. This is a smart decision. Here's a tip: It's certainly easier and often less expensive to purchase life insurance when you're just starting your career. What type of life insurance should you consider? Basically, there are two types: employer-sponsored and individually purchased life insurance.

Disability Coverage. Short-term and long-term disability coverage becomes effective if you're unable to work, either temporarily or permanently. This is helpful to you because you can collect a major percentage of your salary while disabled.

Vacation and Sick Leave. Time off, in days or hours, is accrued during pay periods. These plans often give you a certain number of days based on your length of employment. Determine at what point after employment you will begin to accrue vacation time. Some institutions may give you a percentage of pay or a dollar amount if you don't use your accrued or allocated leave.

Education Assistance. Employers often offer incentives for you to go back to school, ranging from the provision of a flexible work schedule to tuition reimbursement for continuing-education credits or degree completion.

Pensions, Tax Deferments, Annuities, and Savings Plans. You're never too young to think about retirement. Usually a percentage of your paycheck is automatically deducted and placed into your retirement fund each pay period. Some of these plans allow taxes to be deferred until you make a withdrawal from these funds. The deduction may be a contribution to Medicare or to a tax-sheltered optional retirement program.

Reimbursement Accounts ("Cafeteria Plans"). "Cafeteria plans" are reimbursement spending accounts that operate under Section 125 of the Internal Revenue Service Code. Employers may offer employees two different types of reimbursement accounts: health care and dependent day care. Each item is paid for with pretax dollars. This may translate into a big savings for you; with a cafeteria plan you have more money to spend as the amount of income that is taxed is reduced.

Dependent Care for Children and Elderly Family Members. Be sure to check with your employer to see what kind of on-site care or financial assistance that may be available to your children or elderly family members.

Health-Wellness Programs. You may wish to participate in a health-wellness program, which might include instruction in smoking cessation, weight reduction, and fitness in addition to employee assistance programs. These may be available to promote a healthy lifestyle, which reduces employee absence and increases productivity.

When doing your job search, reviewing benefits is a major part of your decision. So, as a new graduate, be sure to familiarize yourself with all the options that are available to you. The human resources department of the hospital or institution will be able to answer your questions. The decisions you make soon after graduation as well as in the early months of employment will have a far-reaching effect on your future.

WHAT IF I DON'T LIKE MY FIRST POSITION?

It is not uncommon to experience frustrations during your first work experience. Go back to Chapter 1 on reality shock, and review it for some suggestions on how to handle your situation. You also need to keep in touch with the nurse recruiter that hired you. Nurse recruiters can offer further support and assistance. Recruiters know where other recent graduates are working in the institution and may provide you with a network of individuals who can offer suggestions and support to improve your situation. In addition, recruiters also know the staffing needs of other areas in the hospital and may suggest transferring. A good way to get an idea of other areas where you may be interested in working is to "shadow" a staff nurse in that area. This means you would spend a day "shadowing" this staff nurse as they perform their job. This provides you with a good insight as to what the job requires and the working conditions of that area. When you take your first position, plan on staying there for at least a year. You want to avoid "job hopping," or changing jobs whenever you don't like what is going on with your current position. Remember, other positions have their benefits and problems, the grass may not be greener on the other side of the fence. Don't trade one set of problems for another set that may be even more difficult.

WHAT IF IT IS TIME FOR YOU TO CHANGE POSITIONS?

If you think it is time to change positions or explore other options, it is important to submit a letter of resignation (Fig. 21-5). Give at least 2 weeks notice. Check your contract to see if you agreed to give more than 2 weeks' notice and, if possible, give 4 weeks' notice. If you are leaving on less than amicable terms, do not express this in your resignation letter. You can always take grievances to the personnel or human resources department.

Finding your niche in the workplace can sometimes be overwhelming. Take the plunge and start looking. This is one of those situations that a little preparation and

November 1, 2000

Linda Smith
101 Anywhere Street
Dallas, TX 77777
214-555-8888

Ms. Joan Winter
Assistant Vice President
Children's Medical Center of Dallas
1935 Hospital Street
Dallas, TX 75235

Dear Ms. Winter

It is with regret that I must submit my resignation. I have been offered a position with Hancock Hospital. My period of employment at Children's has been very positive. I feel I have gained much experience that will be of great benefit to me in my career. My last day of employment will be November 20, 2000.

Thank you for the opportunity to work at your facility and your kind consideration.

Sincerely

Linda Smith

FIGURE 21-5
Letter of resignation.

investigation goes a long way in finding what you want. A basic understanding of the process of job hunting can go a long way to minimize the frustrations and promote a positive first job experience.

REFERENCES

Joel LA: Shifting sands, *Am J Nurs* 97(9):7, 1997.

Levenson SA: Subacute settings: making the most of a new model of care, *Geriatrics* 53(7):69-75, 1998.

Schreiber C: Thinning ranks, *Health Week* 4(19):15, 1999.

Valentino LM: Future employment trends in nursing. The nursing shortage has struck just about everywhere in the United States and there's no relief in sight—but its effects vary by region and specialty, *Am J Nurs* 102 Suppl (1):248, 2002.

ADDITIONAL READINGS

Berens M: Plan aims to head off nursing crisis, Feb 15, 2001. http://www.ChicagoTribune.com.

Bozell J: *Anatomy of a job search—a nurse's guide to finding and landing the job you want*, Philadelphia, 1999, Springhouse.

Buck JT, Matthews WR: *101 ways to power up your job search*, New York, 1997, McGraw-Hill.

Deluca MJ, Deluca, NF: *Wow!: Resumes for creative careers*, New York, 1997, McGraw-Hill.

Hansen K, Hansen R: *Dynamic cover letters: how to sell yourself to an employer by writing a letter that will get your resume read, get you an interview*, and get you the job, 1995, Ten Speed Press.

Krannich RL, Krannich CR: *101 dynamite answers to interview questions: sell your strengths!* ed 3, New York, 1997, Impact.

Krannich RL, Krannich CR: *201 dynamite job search letters*, ed 3, New York, 1997, Impact.

Mason DJ: No shortage of opportunities: evaluate your options and demand support of excellence, *Am J Nurs* 102 Suppl (1):13, 2002.

Morgan D: *10 minute guide to job interviews (10 minute guide)*, New York, 1998, Macmillan.

Newby PK: Pack up your benefits in your old kit bag. . . . *Benefits Review*, Nov/Dec, 35, 1990.

Potter R: *100 best resumes for today's hottest jobs*, New York, 1998, Macmillan.

The American Journal of Nursing: career guide, New York, 2002, Am J Nurs.

Ulrich B: Formula for the future, *NurseWeek*, 6 (14):4, 2001.

Vallano A: *Careers in nursing: manage your future in the changing world of healthcare*, New York, 1999, Kaplan.

INTERNET RESOURCES

http://www.nursingcenter.com/
http://www.nursing.net
http://www.healthleaders.com

Internet sites for writing résumés
http://www.resumenet.com
http://www.avalanche.bc.ca
http://resume.monster.com

Internet sites for posting résumés
http://www.uww.edu/StdRsces/career/jobsearc/d10a.htm
http://www.peachnet.edu/galileo/internet/jobs
http://www.careermosalc.com/cm/rwc2.html

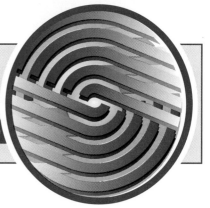

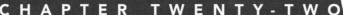

CHAPTER TWENTY-TWO

Interviewing for Employment

ALICE B. PAPPAS, PhD, RN

OK world, here I come—ready or not!
   —Unknown

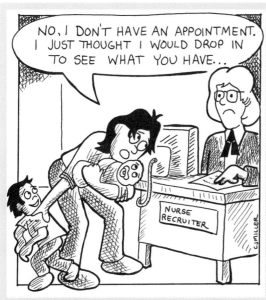

The first impression is a lasting one—make it count for you, not against you.

After completing this chapter, you should be able to:

■ Describe the essential steps involved in the interviewing process.

■ Discuss the typical questions asked by interviewers.

■ Analyze your own priorities and needs in a job. Identify short-term career goals.

The process of interviewing involves a major transitional step between school and the real world of nursing. With graduation in sight you are eager but probably a little anxious about moving into the workplace, looking for the perfect match to your hard-earned diploma or degree.

As you consider possible employment opportunities, approach the upcoming interviews as you would any graded class assignment: Do your homework! Careful preparation is the key to a successful interview. Despite claims to the contrary, few worthwhile job offers happen to someone who just walks into the personnel or nursing office. The continued expansion of the health care field has created a vast array of opportunities for recent graduates. You have developed marketable skills that are in demand, but to sell yourself successfully to prospective employers, you must be prepared.

 Plan your campaign each step of the way to enhance your chances for success!

Give yourself ample time to consider what type of position you want and need, in addition to the possibilities and limitations of the job market under consideration. You can compare the process with the selection of a marriage partner, car, home, or any other major life choice. After all, this position will help define who you are and influence your career path. Become informed and selective in the process. Too often, recent graduates accept their first positions without sufficient knowledge of their own needs or the organizations they select. Days or weeks into the job, surprise and disappointment set in as the reality of the situation becomes obvious: "I'm not happy in this position," "I can't believe I took a job like this," or "They never said anything about this during the interview." Although there is no guarantee that a job will be heaven-sent and wonderful, job dissatisfaction and turnover can be decreased if careful consideration is given to possible job selection before setting off for the actual interview.

The following steps are suggested as a guide to thorough background preparation. (See Chapter 20 for more information on job opportunities and résumé writing.) Critical Thinking Box 22-1 will help you identify your clinical interests and the possible reasons for these preferences. Hint: This will also help you answer interview questions about your choices.

CRITICAL THINKING BOX 22-1

ASSESS YOUR WANTS AND DESIRES, LIKES AND DISLIKES

Identify your interests and the possible reasons for them.

Interests	Reasons
1. I prefer to work with clients whose age is _____	_____ _____

(continued)

CRITICAL THINKING BOX 22-1

ASSESS YOUR WANTS AND DESIRES, LIKES AND DISLIKES *(Cont'd)*

Interests

2. I prefer to work in a small hospital versus a large medical center _____

3. I prefer rotating shifts versus straight shifts _____

4. I prefer an internship versus general orientation _____

5. I prefer to have a set routine or constantly changing environment _____

6. I prefer these areas (e.g., geriatrics, pediatrics, community health, medical) _____

7. Which of my religious beliefs or values might have an impact on where I work? _____

Reasons

_____
_____
_____
_____
_____
_____
_____
_____
_____
_____
_____
_____
_____
_____
_____
_____
_____
_____
_____
_____
_____
_____

SELF-ASSESSMENT

WHAT ARE MY CLINICAL INTERESTS?

Next, start writing down possible settings where you could pursue these interests. For example, if you thrive in a fast-paced environment with high-acuity patients, a critical care unit or emergency department may be for you. Within this category, however, are many specialties. Do you enjoy the medical or the surgical aspects? Cardiac or general medicine? Depending on your interests, there may be a number of possible paths to pursue (Fig. 22-1).

As you identify areas of clinical interest, try to prioritize them. This step may seem like a nonissue if you "eat, sleep, and drink" one specific specialty, but many

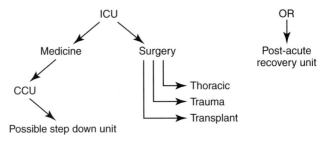

FIGURE 22-1
The environment in which I would like to work
CCU, Critical care unit; *ICU*, intensive care unit.

people have two or more strong interests and this step helps to outline some possibilities. Believe it or not, some senior students confess to liking every clinical rotation and are up in the air about which direction to take. If that description fits you, hang in there—you are not alone! There is a smorgasbord of job opportunities in nursing. You may have to sample several areas before you find the one that really fits your needs on a long-term basis. That's a major advantage of nursing as a health career choice—if you get into an area you don't like, you have the option to change! Keep in mind that all nursing experiences, both negative and positive, can contribute to your career in a productive way. The more areas you sample, the broader your knowledge base. Recruiters like flexibility in recent graduates, but let's try and narrow your interests just a bit. Perhaps you can identify what you liked about each rotation and then prioritize possible interests or identify common experiences.

> Peds—enjoyed the children and opportunity to teach families.
>
> Med/Surg—diabetic patients were challenging, staff was friendly, opportunities for teaching postoperative patients.
>
> Gerontology—enjoyed opportunities to get to know patients, liked being able to have continuity with long-term care patients.
>
> Psych—increased communication skills and self-confidence.
>
> OB—teaching opportunities, enjoyed challenge of caring for high-risk OB population.
>
> Intensive care unit (ICU)—increased technical skills and learned to prioritize, opportunity to work with complex patients, supportive environment with staff.
>
> Community—working with families, opportunity to be more autonomous.

From this example, you can see that teaching, communication skills, working with families, challenging environments, and supportive staffs are common themes. Remember these characteristics; they are important starting points for identifying your areas of interest. Depending on how you prioritize them, they can be applied in a variety of settings. The specific job market you are looking at may then narrow your interest to a more manageable list. For example, communication skills and family teaching may be your priority. As a result, community health may be a strong interest, but job inquiries reveal that staff positions prefer at least one year's experience in an acute-care setting. Knowing this fact eliminates a possible nonproductive search; it may also be useful information for later career planning. Where could you work to obtain the experience to promote your interest in community health?

WHAT ARE MY LIKES AND DISLIKES?

Another way to approach self-assessment involves identification of your likes and dislikes. This is related to interests, but on a more personal level. The job you eventually select may have some drawbacks, but it should meet many more of your likes than dislikes in order to be a good "fit."

Write out your responses to the following questions:

1. Do you enjoy an environment that provides a great deal of patient interaction, or do you thrive in a technically oriented routine?

Think back to your clinical rotations and see if you can find a pattern to what was most enjoyable or disagreeable.

- I liked opportunities for using many technical skills.
- I was uncomfortable with slower-paced routines (e.g., postpartum, nursery).
- I liked to see the results of care as soon as possible (e.g., postoperative recovery).
- I disliked the constant turnover of patients every day.

2. Do you enjoy working closely with other staff or prefer a more autonomous role in patient care?

This question may influence a setting with primary care or team nursing. Why did you like or dislike one type or the other? Talk over your responses with some friends who may have had other experiences and get their opinions as well. Remember that the trend toward interdisciplinary care approaches is decreasing options for "autonomous" practice.

3. Do you learn best in a highly structured environment or in more informal on-the-job training?

Knowing your learning style can guide your interest in and selection of an internship or orientation program. For example, internships range from formal classes with lengthy preceptorships to more informal orientations of fairly short duration. Remember that a program that meets your needs may not be the answer for your best friend. Write down what you would like from an orientation or internship program. Look over your list and prioritize what you need and want.

4. Do you really like making autonomous decisions, or do you want and need more direction and supervision at this point in your professional development?

You will shortly have completed nursing school, backed up by employment in an ICU throughout your senior year. Are you ready to be a 3 to 11 PM charge nurse in a small rural hospital, or do you want a slower transition to such responsibility? If this situation were offered, would you be flattered, frightened, or flabbergast? Write down your reaction and consider how you would respond to the recruiter who offers you such a position.

5. How much physical energy are you able and willing to expend at work?

Running 8 to 12 hours a day may or may not act as a tonic. Think back to the pace of your clinical rotations, and consider how your body reacted (minus the anxiety associated with instructor supervision, if you can!). Would you prefer a unit that has some predictable periods of frenzy and pause, or do you thrive on the unpredictable?

6. Are you a day, evening, or night person?

In other words, are there certain times of the day when you are at your best? How about your worst? Be honest and realistic with your answers. Very few people are equally efficient and effective 24 hours a day. If your body shuts down at 10 PM, or you resist all efforts to wake up before 9 AM, certain shifts may need to be eliminated. However, if the job market is tight in your area of interest, the available positions may be on less-desirable shifts and you may need to make adjustments in other areas of your life to temporarily acclimate better to a position.

7. Do you like rotating shifts, or, perhaps more realistically, can you work rotating shifts?

One aspect of reality shock for some recent graduates is the realization that straight days ended with the last clinical rotation in school. Hospital and long-term care staffing is 24 hours a day, 7 days a week. In other words its a "24-7 profession"—a possibly unpleasant aspect of nursing, but a real one nonetheless. Assess your ability to work certain shifts, and try to strike a flexible approach. Identify a possible rotation pattern (e.g., days/evenings or evenings/nights) or your willingness to work a straight evening or night position. The increased trend of 12-hour shifts (7 AM-7 PM or 7 PM-7 AM) can be very demanding for days assigned but is very popular with many nurses because of the increased days off.

Consider the impact of these choices on your family, social, and recreational needs. If there are certain shifts you must rule out, recognize that this may limit your job choices and plan accordingly. Giving some thought to your flexibility ahead of time will help you avoid committing to any and all shifts during an interview and will facilitate your job hunt.

8. Can you work long hours (e.g., 12-hour shifts) without too much tension and fatigue?

The 12-hour staffing option offers flexibility (e.g., 3 days on, 4 days off) but leaves some people exhausted and irritable. Consider your personal needs outside of work when you respond to this item. Can you climb into bed or put your feet up after a nonstop 12-hour shift, or do you need to pick up family responsibilities when you walk in the door? The four days off may well compensate for three days of fatigue, but map out your needs before you interview.

9. Do you like making decisions quickly or generally favor a more relaxed approach to clinical problems?

In general, ICU and telemetry require more immediate reactions than adolescent psych and orthopedics. Does the ICU environment excite or bewilder you? Would you prefer a slower pace? Don't criticize yourself for your likes or dislikes. Slower-paced units require different strengths, not less knowledge. You have nothing to gain by working in an ICU if you dislike the setting. Meet your own needs, not someone else's.

10. What do you need in a job to be happy?

This does not mean money or benefits, but rather the sense that the job is worth getting excited about. Think about past employment you've had, whether health care–related or not. What did you like or dislike about the job? What made you stay? Possible answers include opportunities for growth, advancement, working with people you respect, or collegiality. Remember, your answers should include things that are important to you. You may want to compare your answers with those of others whose opinions you value to gain a broader perspective.

WHAT ARE MY PERSONAL NEEDS AND INTERESTS?

A third aspect of self-assessment focuses on personal needs and interests. How much time and effort are you willing and able to give to your career at this point in time? Will work be a number one priority in your life, or does family or continued education take precedence?

Is relocation a possibility? If you are considering relocation, decide how you will gather information on possible job opportunities in the area or areas under consideration. Include newspapers, Internet Web sites, professional journals, and possible family or other personal contacts as sources of information. If this is a voluntary move, develop a list of pros and cons for each location under consideration. Include your personal interests in the decision (e.g., cost of living, possible relocation allowance, access to recreational activities, opportunities for advanced education, and clinical opportunities).

How much are you willing to commute? The job opportunity may be terrific, but can you live with a 1-hour commute each way? Find out the probable commuting time for the hours and days you want to work and add this piece of information to your collection of facts about various institutions. If you are remaining in the same locale, this may be common knowledge, but if you are relocating, this will determine the need for housing arrangements.

What salary range are you willing to consider? Although starting salary for recent graduates is generally nonnegotiable, differentials for evenings, nights, and weekends create a range of salary possibilities. If you want an extended internship, a lower starting salary may be offered. Are you willing and able to trade this off for the benefits of an extended internship? Some areas of the country offer considerably higher salaries than others, but factor in the cost of living before you move out of town. You may be unpleasantly surprised by a monthly rent that swallows up your salary.

Is overtime desirable in your life? Can it be reasonably juggled with other interests and time demands? The extra money may sound great and look impressive on your paycheck, but do not put unreasonable demands on your physical and emotional well-being. Staffing needs create overtime in many settings, but give some thought to what kind of overtime you can and cannot do when the question is asked.

As the nursing shortage worsens, there has been concern regarding mandatory overtime. Mandatory overtime has been such a hot issue that states are now passing laws prohibiting it. The Safe Nursing and Patient Care Act of 2001 was introduced at the federal level to address this issue (Carr, 2002). When it will be passed and the implications are still unclear. Make sure you have a clear understanding of the overtime policy before you agree to a position.

WHAT ARE MY CAREER GOALS?

The final step of your self-assessment is the development of career goals. Yes, you really do need to have some goals. You are the architect of your professional future, so take pen to paper and start designing. Consider your answers to the following questions.

What do you want from your first nursing position? Possible answers might include developing confidence in decision-making, more proficiency with technical skills, and increased organizational abilities.

What are your professional goals for the first year? Third year? Fifth year? If you cannot imagine your life, let alone your career, beyond 1 to 2 years, relax. Many people feel uncertain planning beyond their initial position. Close your eyes and try to imagine yourself one year out of school. Compare yourself with recent graduates you have seen during your rotations, and try to imagine the roles they are developing. The following are possible answers:

- First-year goal
  - Becoming a competent staff nurse in pediatrics or ICU.
- Third-year goal
  - Achieving certification in your specialty area.
  - Involvement in a professional organization.
  - Possibly moving into a charge position on your unit.
  - Returning to school for advanced education.
- Fifth-year goal
  - Completing an advanced degree or moving into a management position.

If you honestly do not think you will return to school at this point in your life, don't feel as though you should fake your answer. Develop a comfortable response to a question regarding your goals for the first year, and consider what you might want to be doing after that time. Remember, it is far easier to gauge how your career is progressing if you have established goals to which you can refer. This is also a favorite question posed during interviews, so spend some time thinking about it! Recruiters are interested in nurses with a plan. They are encouraged to "hire for attitude and provide training for skills." Prepare to have an enthusiastic attitude toward your future as a professional.

RESEARCHING PROSPECTIVE EMPLOYERS

HOW DO I GO ABOUT RESEARCHING PROSPECTIVE EMPLOYERS?

Media Information.

Newspapers. It's time to start reading the Sunday employment section to get specific information about current openings in your area. Scan the advertisements to see whether any are targeted specifically to graduating seniors. Focus on these initially because they will include information on possible internships or specialized orientations, in addition to specific openings for graduate nurses. The advertisements will also give you a name and number to contact for further information. Clip the advertisements that interest you, and start a file for each potential employer.

Online Searches. Electronic job searches are growing in popularity and are increasingly useful for accessing information for both local and distant nursing opportunities. Some recruiters believe that use of the Net is far more cost-effective than advertising in newspapers. Online/electronic searches may reveal Web sites for specific hospitals/institutions. You may then review the positions available within that one institution. If you intend to use this method to follow-up on a job posting, be prepared to submit your flawless résumé electronically and spell-check all of your correspondence before you click the send button.

Job Fairs/Open Houses. You may have the opportunity to attend a nursing job fair or hospital open house as a soon-to-be graduate nurse. Take advantage of this opportunity to collect information about specific employers and possibly make initial contacts for later interviews. Leave your jeans and tennis shoes at home on these occasions, though. Take some time with your appearance because first impressions are important! (See Box 22-1 for specifics regarding physical appearance and grooming.)

BOX 22-1 The Dos and Don'ts of Dressing for Interviews

DO

❑ Look over your wardrobe and select a conservative outfit. Ladies, if you own a suit, consider wearing it, but don't blow your budget buying an outfit you will never wear again. Other acceptable outfits include a business-type dress or skirt with coordinated top. The two tried-and-true rules for job interview attire are dress conservatively and professionally. Although a nursing shortage may loosen the rules a bit, the impression you convey by your outfit is likely to be remembered.

❑ Be conservative with makeup and hairdo.

❑ Wear minimal jewelry—you don't want to jingle and rattle with every move.

(continued)

> **BOX 22-1   The Dos and Don'ts of Dressing for Interviews *(Cont'd)***
>
> ❑ Wear hose with a skirt or a dress—bare legs may be fashionable, but not for a professional interview.
> ❑ Consider a suit or jacket with coordinated slacks, shirt, and tie for men.
> ❑ Take a few minutes to look yourself over in the mirror.
>
> **DON'T**
> ❑ Wear casual clothes such as tee shirts, jeans, tennis shoes, or sandals. They may reflect the "real" you, but this is not the place to show that aspect of your personality.
> ❑ Be guilty of poor grooming or hygiene.
> ❑ Wear brand-new shoes, which may turn your day into a "painful" experience.
> ❑ Bring your children with you. You should leave them at home. Do not expect the staff to act as baby sitters.

If you plan to formally interview at the institution in the future, take home their brochure and become familiar with the information it contains. Recruiters appreciate applicants who know some basic facts about their institution. It will also help you respond to one of their favorite lines of questioning: "Why do you want to work for our institution?" or "In what ways do you feel you can contribute to our organization?"

Employee Contacts. If you have a friend or family member—or simply know someone—who works at an institution you are considering for employment, make an effort to speak with him or her about the job environment. As insiders they may be able to provide you a perspective about the employer that the advertisement, recruiter, or interview cannot. Possible questions you may want to ask them include "Why do they enjoy working there?" "What was orientation like?" and "How is employee morale?"

Personnel/Recruitment Contacts.

Letter-Writing Campaign. Plan to send your résumé with a cover letter, and triple-check both for grammatical errors. Your résumé and cover letter are the first impression you will make with a prospective employer. Careless grammar and poor presentation can make the difference in ever getting an invitation to interview. You can obtain addresses through advertisements or telephone contact. Make sure you include your telephone number in the mailing so that you can be contacted if necessary and the probable date you would like to begin employment. (See Chapter 21 for résumé tips.)

Telephone Contact. Before you pick up the telephone, get out your calendar and start planning likely dates for possible interviews, in addition to the approximate date you want to begin working. Armed with this information, you can comfortably answer questions beyond the fact that you would like them to send you a brochure and an application. Depending on the institution you contact, human resources or nurse recruitment may want you to send a résumé or may press you to set up an appointment for an interview.

Personal Contact. If you plan to just stop by personnel or nurse recruitment for a brochure and an application, make sure you give some thought to your appearance. Tee shirts, shorts, and jeans are not appropriate and have caused otherwise well-qualified applicants to be passed over for further consideration. Again—remember that first impression!

WHAT DO I NEED TO KNOW TO ASSESS THE ORGANIZATION?

Now that you have described yourself and have thought about the kind of setting in which you work best, continue these exercises on a consistent basis. This ongoing analysis will help you make decisions about the kind of organization that is best for you and put you in a position to determine what kind of organization fits you.

HOW DO YOU GO ABOUT ASSESSING AN ORGANIZATION TO FIND WHAT YOU WANT?

Talk to People in the Organization. One obvious answer is to ask the people who work in that organization. When you interview for a position, you can meet people who work in the specific setting in which you are interested. Ask questions that will help you learn about certain situations. Think of scenarios to present to staff to determine their reactions to situations. How people handle these questions will give you great insight into the way the organization works. If they feel uncomfortable with your approach, you will know that this kind of approach is not usual for them. If they rise to the occasion and very openly and candidly discuss their reactions, this will give you a different perspective on their viewpoints. Take some time to think about questions and situations you would like to present when you talk to people in various facilities.

Read and Analyze the Recruitment Materials. Organizations also present themselves to you through their documents. When organizations send recruitment materials to you or advertise online, they are telling you the things they want you to know about them. Organizations spend a great amount of time and money on material that they believe presents their philosophy and attitude toward patients and employees. What an organization chooses to tell you tells you about the organization. Carefully analyze the materials presented to you. This is another way of determining the values the organization lives by and deems important. All of these materials are intended to make a statement to you about who they are.

Is There a Mission or Philosophy Statement? There are other written documents to examine. For example, a specific nursing unit may have a mission statement that tells you who they are and what they are about. The department of nursing will have a philosophy statement that should be the organizing framework around which the members structure themselves in delivering nursing care. In some organizations, staff know what this mission statement says and how it provides direction to them. In other organizations, staff will be unfamiliar with the statement of philosophy. All of these written materials should send a message to you about the organization. Do your observations during the interview process support the organizations mission/philosophy statements? (Critical Thinking Box 22-2)

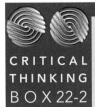

CRITICAL THINKING BOX 22-2

What are some observations that you may have during your interview process that would cause you to have second thoughts about accepting a position at the institution?

Evaluate the Reputation of the Leadership. Organizations are guided by people at the top and take on the characteristics these people support. What do you know about the chief executive officer? This person sets the stage and the direction for the organization. You can gather information about the chief executive officer by asking people during the interview what this person is like. People in the community will also be familiar with this person and will give you insight into the values and characteristics that this person represents. If there has been stability in the top-level executive team over a period of years, that tells you one thing. If there has been constant change, with people continually leaving, that tells you another thing about the organization.

The same can be said for the chief nursing officer. This person sets the direction for the nursing organization, either by active design or benign neglect, and sets into motion an organization that structures the beliefs about patients, staff, and nursing. It is very important to talk with nurses who are working with this person and determine how they feel about the management in their organization. Has he or she had a successful tenure? Is this person well respected? Can people point to a strategic direction and philosophy this person has given to the organization?

Is a Nursing Theory or Philosophy Used? Some nursing divisions organize themselves around a nursing theorist or a philosophy of care. Orem's self-care theory, Neuman's systems model, and King's theory of goal attainment are examples of organizing frameworks that nursing organizations have adopted. If an organization does not have a nursing theorist, it often adopts a philosophy or model according to which it operates. The organizing framework that is adopted will determine how the organization is developed. From the organizing framework will come the goals and objectives of the department of nursing. These goals and objectives will provide you with a long-range view of the direction of this organization. Individual nursing units also occasionally have such an organizing framework on which to base their direction of care. It is appropriate to find out information like this so you know if you can agree with the organization's direction or philosophy. The more you know about an organization upfront, the more likely you are to select the "best fit" for your talents and goals.

THE INTERVIEW PROCESS

HOW DO I PLAN MY INTERVIEW CAMPAIGN?

Set Up Your Schedule. Keep the following points in mind:

- Agencies usually have specific dates for orientations, internships, and preceptorships.
- Identify when you want to begin employment, and mark your calendar.
- Work backward from this date to plan dates and times for interviews.
- Plan no more than two interviews in one day. If you do, beware of information overload and the risk of being late for at least one interview. Have two or three possible dates available on your calendar before you call the human resources office or nurse recruitment. Advance planning will keep you from fumbling on the telephone when they tell you that your first choice is unavailable!

While you are on the telephone, ask some questions about their interview process. How much time should you plan for the interview? It may range from under 1 hour to a half day. Ask about the job description on the telephone if you have not seen it in the newspaper or online. Becoming familiar with both the job description and the prospective employer is a critical key to interview success.

What does the interview process involve? It may involve tours and multiple interviews including human resources, nurse recruitment, one or more clinical managers, and possibly staff. If you are applying for an internship, it is not unusual to be interviewed by a panel of three or four people. Knowing this ahead of time may increase your anxiety, but it is less stressful than being surprised by this fact at the door.

Will more than one interview be required? Some institutions will use the first interview as a screening mechanism. You may be asked to come back for a follow-up interview.

How do you get to the human resources or nurse recruitment office? Ask for directions ahead of time if you are unfamiliar with the area. Have a good idea of the time involved for travel. Arriving late for an interview may create a very poor initial impression.

Will you be able to meet with clinical managers from different areas on the same day? Are there new graduates in the area with whom you can talk? This is important if you are interested in more than one clinical area.

Will a tour of the unit be included? If this is not a standard part of the interview process, express interest in having one so you can get a more realistic idea of the setting and possibly meet some of the staff.

Prepare to Show Your Best Side. Develop your responses to probable interview questions (Box 22-2). If you don't plan possible responses, you run the risk of looking wide-eyed as you fumble for an answer or ramble on around the subject.

> **BOX 22-2 Key Points to Remember About Your Responses During an Interview**
>
> ❑ Answer honestly.
> ❑ Do not brag or gloat about your achievements, but do show yourself in a positive light.
> ❑ Remember that you are your best salesperson!
> ❑ Do not criticize past employers or instructors. It is more likely to reflect unfavorably on you than on them.
> ❑ Do not dwell on your shortcomings. Turn them into areas for future development: "I need to improve my organization skills. Managing a group of patients will be a challenge, but I am looking forward to it."
> ❑ Demonstrate flexibility and a willingness to begin work in an area of second or third choice if the job market is limited.

In Critical Thinking Box 22-3 are examples of interview questions with which you should be familiar with. How would you answer these questions?

CRITICAL THINKING BOX 22-3

SAMPLE OF INTERVIEW QUESTIONS

The following is a sampling of interview questions you should be familiar with. Prepare your responses.

1. What area or areas of nursing are you interested in and why?

_____

_____

2. Tell me about your clinical experiences. Which rotations did you enjoy the most? Why?

_____

_____

_____

3. Which one did you enjoy the least? Why?

_____

_____

4. What do you feel are your strengths? Why?

_____

_____

(continued)

SAMPLE OF INTERVIEW QUESTIONS *(Cont'd)*

5. How about your weaknesses? Why?

_____

_____

_____

6. Why do you want to work for our organization?

_____

_____

_____

7. What qualifications do you have that make you believe that you will be successful in this staff position?

_____

_____

8. What skills do you feel you have gained from your past work experiences that may help you in this position?

_____

_____

9. Tell me a little about yourself. How would others describe you?

_____

_____

_____

10. What are your future career plans? Where do you expect to be in two or three years? Five years?

_____

_____

_____

11. We do not have any openings at the present time in the areas in which you have indicated an interest. Would you be willing to accept a position in another area?

_____

_____

_____

(continued)

CRITICAL THINKING BOX 22-3

SAMPLE OF INTERVIEW QUESTIONS (Cont'd)

12. How do you handle stress in the work setting?

_____

_____

_____

_____

Spend some time looking over your answers. Do they describe you accurately? Rework your answers until you feel comfortable with them, but don't try to memorize the words. They should serve as a guide for the upcoming interiew.

Rehearse the Interview. If you role-play a possible interview, it will probably increase your comfort level for the real thing. Following are some suggestions for a rehearsal:

- Dress for the part. It will add some authenticity to the situation.
- Choose a supportive friend or family member to role-play the interviewer.
- Practice your verbal responses to sample questions.
- Ask for constructive feedback regarding your appearance, body language, and responses.

Many applicants say they have no questions at the end of the interview. This may be true, or it may reflect the urge to end the interview and relax! Some words of advice: Prepare a few questions! This will be your opportunity to gather important details and possibly impress the interviewer with your interest. The following is a sampling of possible questions:

- What are your expectations of recent graduates?
- What is your evaluation process like?
- Who will evaluate me, and how can I get feedback about my performance?
- I'd like some more information about your preceptorship program. How long will I have a preceptor, and what can I expect from the preceptor?
- What is the nurse-to-patient ratio on each of the shifts I may be working?
- What is your policy regarding weekend coverage?
- What opportunities are there for professional development?

Look over the recruitment brochures for additional ideas on questions. This shows that you are interested in the institution and have done your homework.

STRATEGIES FOR INTERVIEW SUCCESS

One of the most important strategies for successful interviewing is to dress for success (see Box 22-1).

Watch your interviewing etiquette. Your parents taught you to mind your manners, and this is an opportunity to put that education to good use.

Make sure you know the name and title of the individual who is scheduled to meet with you.

CRITICAL FIRST 5 MINUTES!

The initial 5 minutes of an interview are critical. Research shows that the decision to continue interest or possibly hire is made during this time.

Arriving early may give you a chance to look over additional information about the institution or possibly give you more time for your interview. If you are delayed or cannot keep the appointment, call the interviewer to reschedule.

Be aware of your body language; that is, establish eye contact with the interviewer and maintain reasonable eye contact during the interview. Try to avoid or minimize distracting nervous mannerisms. Keep your hands poised in your lap or in some other comfortable position. If you "talk with your hands," try not to do this continually. If you cross your legs, don't shake your foot. If offered coffee or another drink, decide whether this will relax you or complicate your body language. Show enthusiasm in your voice and body language. Do not smoke or chew gum. Give a winning smile when you are introduced and offer to shake hands. Women sometimes have a problem with shaking hands. Practice it at home to become more comfortable. Demonstrate interest in what the interviewer has to say. Do not argue with or contradict the interviewer! Wait to ask about salary and benefits until all other aspects of the interview have been completed, including your other questions! Salary and benefits are important aspects, but they should not dominate your conversation. If you want to take some notes during the interview, ask the interviewer if he or she minds. This is generally quite acceptable. Bring along your list of questions, and if you can't recall them when given the chance, ask to take out your list. Do not check off information during the interview as if you were grocery shopping!

PHASES OF THE INTERVIEW

The interview is generally divided into three areas, each of which serves a particular purpose. The first is the *introduction.* This is a lightweight section that should help to put you somewhat at ease. Some effort to break the ice will be made, and the communication may focus on the traffic, the weather, or the excitement you probably feel about your upcoming graduation. Take some slow, deep breaths and make a conscious effort to relax. Remember that you are making an initial impression with your verbal and nonverbal behavior.

The second phase involves *fact-finding.* Depending on the skill and style of the interviewer, you may be unaware of the subtle change in conversation, but questions about you will most likely now be asked. Remember the answers you rehearsed, and make an effort to use that information. Your résumé may be used as a source of questions, so make sure you can speak about its contents and that every item on the résumé can be verified. Studies have shown that up to 35% of all job applicants have some inaccurate or misleading information on their résumés. The information that you provide on the résumé will be verified, and deliberate and "accidental" inaccuracies could cost you the job. Be prepared to offer your references and possibly explain why you have selected these particular individuals. If you have a tendency to give short responses or avoid answering questions, a skilled interviewer will reword the question or possibly note that you do not answer questions well. Interviewers strive to have the applicant talk about 90% of the time, so consider this your audition. They are really interested in getting to know you as a prospective "fit" with their institution, so be both enthusiastic and honest.

Some institutions are asking students or recent graduates to bring in a portfolio reflecting their school experiences. Included in this portfolio might be your skills checkoff sheets. This is particularly beneficial if it is signed by the faculty with occasional positive comments. Include in the portfolio some of your best nursing care plans. If you have been in a variety of clinical agencies, it is appropriate to include a list that also indicates the type of experience (e.g., Memorial Hospital—obstetrics). The portfolio should reflect your best schoolwork and present you in a positive light. If the interviewer does not ask for a portfolio, then you may offer it for their review.

The *closing* is the last phase of the interview process. The interviewer may summarize what has been discussed and give you some ideas about the next step in the process (e.g., a tour, a meeting with clinical managers, or a follow-up interview). This is your time to ask questions. However, if you feel full of facts and unable to ask any questions at this time, leave the door open to future contacts by saying "I believe you answered all my questions at this time, but may I contact you if I have some questions later on?"

After the initial interview, you may tour the area in which you will work. Show interest when this tour is offered, and use it as an opportunity to observe the surroundings for such things as professional behaviors and organizational and environmental factors. If you have the chance, interact with the staff, especially with recent graduates. Ask what they enjoy about their unit and job position. Before leaving, make sure you thank the interviewer for his or her time and interest.

HOW DO I HANDLE UNEXPECTED QUESTIONS OR SITUATIONS?

OK, you did your homework and you're prepared for anything, but out of the blue you are asked a question you never expected. What should you do? Saying "No fair" is not a good answer! Take a deep breath, pause, and consider saying something like this: "That's an interesting question. I'd like to think about my answer for a minute if you don't mind. Can we come back to that subject later in the interview?" Given a temporary break, you will have time to develop your thoughts on the subject. Don't ignore the question, however, because the interviewer will most likely bring it up again. Suppose you answer the question but feel your response was incomplete or off the mark. Look for an opportunity at the end of the interview to bring up the subject again, saying something like "I've had some time to think about an earlier question and want to add some additional information, if you don't mind."

JOB OFFERS AND POSSIBLE REJECTION

Let's consider a positive outcome first. If you are offered a position during or at the end of the interview, three possible reactions are likely:

- You are not ready to say yes or no. This is your first interview, and you have two more interviews scheduled.
- You would like very much to work here. The job offer is just what you're looking for.
- You don't want the position. It is not what you thought it would be, or something about the institution turns you off.

Whichever decision you make about the job offer, the following are helpful tips for your response:

1. Be honest. If you have other interviews to complete, say so. Be prepared to tell the interviewer when you will make your decision about the job offer
2. Avoid being pressured to say "yes" if you are not ready to commit to the job or feel that the position does not meet your needs.
3. Be polite. Ask for some time to consider the offer if you are unsure of what you want to do at present.
4. If you know the offer does not interest you, decline the offer graciously and express appreciation for their interest in you.
5. Accept the offer and smile!

Suppose you receive a rejection or no job offer for the position, despite your interest and preparation. Before you leave in a state of dejection, find the courage to ask for a possible explanation if it hasn't been made clear at this point. If you do not find out about the rejection until later, consider calling the interviewer for this information. Common reasons for rejection include the following. See if any of these factors might apply to you.

Lack of opening for your interests and skills. They liked you but couldn't find a spot right now, or a more qualified candidate was selected for the position.

Poor personal appearance, including inappropriate clothes. You stopped by for the interview on your way to work out.

Lack of preparation for the interview. You were unable to answer questions intelligently or showed lack of knowledge of, or interest in, the employer.

Your answers were superficial or filled with "I don't know."

Poor attitude, dominated by "What's in this for me?" instead of "How can I contribute to the organization?" Your first question focused on salary and perks.

Answers and behavior reflected conceit, arrogance, poor self-confidence, or lack of manners or poise. They should hire you just because you showed up! Or a résumé and responses that did not reflect initiative, achievements, or reliable work history.

You have no goals or future orientation. After all, you just want a job.

Perceived lack of leadership potential. You like being a follower in all situations and do not want to make decisions.

Poor academic record without a reasonable explanation. You worked as hard as you could in school, but the teachers didn't like you; you lacked appropriate references; or your references were not available or did not reflect favorably on you.

Lack of flexibility. Unwilling to begin work in an area that is not your first or second choice. Consider how rigid you can afford to be at this particular point in time or at this institution.

 If at first you don't succeed, try, try again.

POSTINTERVIEW PROCESS

Now that the interview is over, you may want to relax, celebrate, or jump in your car to make your next interview appointment. Stop for a few minutes, and jot down some notes about the interview. This is particularly important if you have another interview the same day. Critique the interview. Consider the following questions:

1. What do you think were your strengths and weaknesses?
2. Is there anything you wish you had or had not said? Why?
3. Were there any surprises?
4. How do you feel you handled the situation?
5. What can you do differently the next time?

Be sure to write down details about the job, which will help you decide on its relative merits and drawbacks. If you do not do this, you may not be able to distinguish job A from job B by the time the interviews are finished. You may experience information overload after a number of interviews, but if you have taken notes about each, the sorting out process will be easier. (Chapter 21 includes an employer contact record-keeping chart for this process.)

After the interviews are over, rank your job offers against your personal list of priorities to make an informed choice. This may be an unnecessary step for you if you were sold on a particular interview. However, it is a good idea to consider interviewing at least two institutions, if only to strengthen your decision about the first interview. It will help eliminate possible doubts about your choice later on. If there is a job you think you are really interested in, do a couple of other interviews first. This will give you some experience in interviewing. You may then be able to conduct a more positive interview for the position in which you are really interested. More interviews may also open your eyes to other possibilities.

FOLLOW-UP COMMUNICATION

Remember how nice it is to get a thank-you note in the mail or a telephone call of appreciation? Well, the same idea carries over to the work world: Write those letters!

Follow-up Letter. Take a few minutes to write a note of thanks to the interviewer for the time and interest spent on your behalf. You may want to include additional information in the note: your continuing interest in the position if you hope an offer will be made, the date you will be making your job decision, additional thanks for any special efforts extended to you (lunch, individualized tour), and any change in telephone numbers and appropriate times when they may be able to contact you. Use plain thank-you note cards, not frilly or cute. This is a situation where a handwritten note is certainly acceptable, just make sure it is legible and neat. Recruiters frequently comment on the positive aspect of a follow-up letter, and it may serve to keep your name at the top of the list because of your attention to interpersonal communication. It also helps to "separate you from the pack of applicants."

Letters of Rejection. As soon as you make up your mind regarding job offers, notify other prospective employers of your decision. Decline their job offer graciously and include an expression of appreciation for their interest in you. The format for this letter should follow the standard rules of business letters that were discussed in Chapter 21. Remember, you have accepted a position elsewhere, but your career could take a turn in the future that may bring you back to the institution you are now declining. Leave a positive impression with human resources and recruitment.

Telephone Follow-up. On the basis of the interview, you should have a pretty clear idea of the "how" and "when" of further contact. A telephone call may be appropriate when you haven't heard from a recruiter by an agreed-upon date. You can contact a recruiter or interviewer by telephone to decline a job offer, but a personal letter is preferable to leaving a telephone message. Remember to be unfailingly polite to everyone you speak to on the telephone. Secretaries and other support personnel will remember and pass on unfavorable impressions to their superiors. Recruiters do not want to hire staff who are rude or impatient. They know that this behavior is likely to be shown toward patients and families as well.

 Good luck with your interviews! Just remember . . . Success lies not in achieving what you aim at, but in aiming at what you ought to achieve.

ADDITIONAL READINGS

Aisenstein TJ: Taking charge—how to land the job you want, RN, 53(2):15-18, 1990.

Cool reception, *Nursing* 29(12):12-14, 1999.

Farber GM: Job hunting in the world of nursing, *Imprint* 42(1):21-22, 1995.

Flanagan L: *Entering and moving in the professional job market: a nurse's resource kit* (ANA Pub. #ECO-146), Kansas City, Mo, 1988, ANA

Get Wired, Get Hired? (July, 1998). *PC World.* http://web5.searchbank.com/infotrac/session/173/52/ 5103287w5/11!xrn2

Hugg A: Universal language, *NurseWeek,* 7(2):30-32, 2002.

Hayden H, Kumpf P: Marketing yourself part 3: the interview, *Health Promot Pract* 1(4):314-318, 2000.

Glasser G: Your mama taught you better, *RN* 53(6):120, 1990.

Make a good first impression, *Crit Care Nurse Suppl* 7-8, 2000.

Make a good first impression. (September 4, 2001). http://www.critical-care-nurse.org/CC...9ca7 fe3e7732222d88256a070081991c?OpenDocumen

Navarra T: Interviewing mistakes: an ounce of prevention is worth a pound of cure, *Nurs Spec Career Fitness Online* 2000, at http://community. nursingspectrum.com/MagazineArticles/srticle.cfm?AID=1013

Russo C: How to interview on your own terms: the rising demand for nurses increases your negotiating power, *Am J Nurs Career Guide* :16-18, 2001

Schmalz KJ: Marketing yourself, part 2: the unwritten dress code: how to dress for the job interview, *Health Promot Pract* 1(3):229-233, 2000.

Tyler L: Watch out for "red flags" on a job interview, *Hospitals* 64(14):46, 1990.

Washington R: A practical guide to interviewing, *Imprint* 37(5):38-39, 1990-1991.

INTERNET RESOURCES

http://www.tbrnet.com/interviewing/index.html
http://www.quintcareers.com/intvres.html
http://www.careercity.com/content/interview/
http://www.carnegieresources.com/interview.htm
http://www.resumesystems.com/career/interview.htm
http://www.quintcareers.com/interview_questions.html

Here are some great sites for "virtual interview" practice!
http://content.monster.com/jobinfo/interview/virtual/
http://www.interviewcoach.com/virtual.html
http://www.western.edu/career/Interview_virtual/Virtual_interview.htm

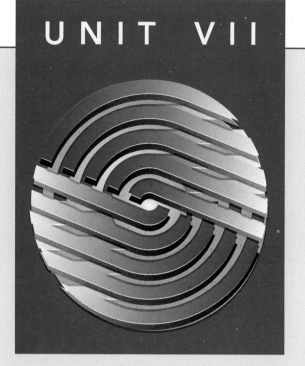

UNIT VII

THRIVING . . . NOT JUST SURVIVING

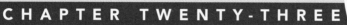
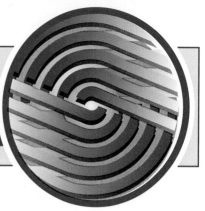
Self-Care Strategies

BARBARA J. MICHAELS, EdD, LMFT, RN

I will use words which emanate power, strong words to guide me. My words today will be strong and powerful. I will choose words that convey a sense of mastery, competence, and ability: I can. I will. I am. I do. . . .

—*Rochelle Lerner, 1985*

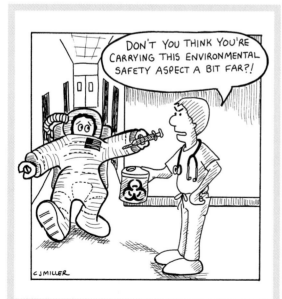

Nurses must be aware of potential threats to their health.

After completing this chapter, you should be able to:

▨ Identify potential threats to your health and well-being.

▨ Describe how impediments to your health and well-being affect you personally and professionally.

▨ Discuss the implications of caring for the self.

▨ Identify strategies for self-care.

▨ Formulate a plan of care for yourself that is based on identified deficits in self-care.

F or nurses to effectively take care of their patients, they must first take care of themselves. As a new graduate in your first year of practice, you need to make "taking care of yourself" a top priority. The work environment will be demanding; you will be exposed to learning opportunities and be introduced to a whole new area of professional responsibilities. How you perceive yourself often determines how effective you are as a nurse. The way you feel about yourself will be influenced by your values, actions, successes, and failures during your first year after graduation. Self-care is the foundation that will assist you in thriving in nursing instead of just surviving.

POTENTIAL OCCUPATIONAL THREATS TO HEALTH AND WELL-BEING

There are many potential threats to health and well-being that nurses encounter on a daily basis. Some of these potential threats, such as mental and physical fatigue associated with rotating work schedules and work-related injuries, have been a part of nursing practice for many years. Others, such as exposure to human immunodeficiency virus (HIV) infection, are relatively new. In either case, nurses must learn to deal with these threats—or deal with the consequences of chronic back pain, sleep deprivation, or communicable diseases, such as acquired immunodeficiency syndrome (AIDS) and tuberculosis. See Box 23-1 for five major categories of workplace hazards and examples in each category, and see Critical Thinking Box 23-1.

WHAT ROLE DOES THE FEDERAL GOVERNMENT PLAY IN MAINTAINING ENVIRONMENTAL SAFETY?

In 1971 the federal government created the Occupational Safety and Health Administration (OSHA). The purpose of this agency is to establish safety and health

---

 BOX 23-1 Categories and Examples of Occupational Health Hazards for Nurses

Biologic/infectious HIV or HBV: exposure, needlestick injuries.

Chemical: exposure to sterilizing agents, chemotherapy drugs, and latex.

Environmental/mechanical: back injuries, shift work, and violent behavior toward health care workers.

Physical: radiation exposure and eye and skin injuries from lasers emitting nonionizing radiation.

Psychological: work overload, shift work, lack of staffing and resources, dealing with family members, and dealing with dying patients, especially children.

(Modified from Rogers B: Is health care a risky business? As I see it [Opinion column], *Am Nurse* 1997.)

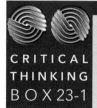

CRITICAL THINKING BOX 23-1

During your most recent clinical experience, what can you identify as a potential hazard to your safety?

standards in the work environment. OSHA requires employers to provide a safe work environment for employees to comply with the OSHA safety and health standards. Specific employee training regarding occupational health and environmental conditions includes environmental safety, fire, hazardous materials, medical and first aid, material handling and storage, and machine handling. Examples of OSHA requirements are safety glasses, sharps containers, handling and control of radioactive materials, and protective outer clothing. Several important employee rights are listed in Critical Thinking Boxes 23-2 and 23-3.

AM I REALLY IN DANGER OF CONTRACTING AIDS?

AIDS is a very real threat to health professionals. Before the late 1970s, a mention of AIDS was not to be found in the professional literature. Today articles about AIDS

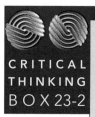

CRITICAL THINKING BOX 23-2

THINK ABOUT . . .

Think How These Employee Rights Apply To Client Care

❑ Request an inspection if they believe an imminent danger exists or a violation of a standard exists that threatens physical harm.

❑ Have a representative (such as a union steward) accompany an OSHA compliance officer during the inspection of a workplace.

❑ Advise an OSHA compliance officer of any violation of the act that they believe exists in the workplace, and question, and be questioned privately by, the compliance officer.

❑ Have regulations posted to inform them of protection afforded by the act.

❑ Have locations monitored in order to measure exposure to toxic or radioactive materials, have access to the records of such monitoring or measuring, and have a record of their own personal exposure.

❑ Have medical examinations or other tests to determine whether their health is being affected by an exposure, and have the results of such tests furnished to their physicians.

❑ Have posted on the premises any citations made to the employer by OSHA.

From Bittel LR, and Newstrom JW (1990). *What every supervisor should know* (6th ed.). New York: McGraw-Hill, with permission.

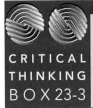

What do you see in the hospital as a result of the requirements of OSHA?

not only are found in nursing literature but appear almost on a regular basis in the daily newspapers. Of particular concern has been the number of cases in which patients have contracted AIDS from a health professional who was careless in the use of standard precautions. To prevent transmission of HIV, nurses and health care workers must adhere to standard precautions. In an editorial in the *American Nurse*, Barbara Fassbinder (1992), who is one of the first three health care workers known to have contracted HIV through a non-needlestick injury in 1986, shared the following message with all health care workers:

"Listen to the experts and take universal precautions seriously. Your life depends on it. That is my message. It is a simple message, and yet one that is too often ignored in the workplace for a variety of reasons, including inconvenience and denial that anything bad can ever happen. A few moments of inconvenience may save your life. And if you think nothing bad can ever happen to you, I'm living proof that can be a fatal attitude."

When standard precautions are correctly implemented, contracting AIDS from a patient is highly unlikely. Nurses who work in emergency departments and surgery are in areas of high risk of exposure to HIV. Another area of increasing concern about exposure to blood and body fluid contamination is in labor and delivery. The American Nurses Association does not promote mandatory testing of patients, nor does the Centers for Disease Control. Both organizations believe that the transmission of AIDS is halted by strict adherence to standard precautions, in addition to the education of both consumers and health care professionals. Mandatory testing for HIV status of employees may be required by some institutions; however, written, valid consent must be obtained for the test to be performed. The results of the test cannot be used to determine employment. If an employer discriminates on the basis of HIV status, two federal laws are violated, the Rehabilitation Act and the Americans With Disabilities Act. It is recommended that employers not require testing but encourage employees to determine their HIV status. To obtain more information regarding employment rights of HIV-positive health care workers, contact the National AIDS Clearinghouse at the Centers for Disease Control in Atlanta for their catalog. Additional material can be found on the AIDS Line database. Another source of information is the American Nurses Association's *Compendium of HIV/AIDS position policies and documents* (1994).

IS SUBSTANCE ABUSE REALLY A PROBLEM FOR NURSES?

The incidence of substance abuse among nurses is high. Approximately 10% of nurses are chemically dependent, and for many, substance abuse begins while attending nursing school (Coleman et al, 1997). Researchers have found that nurses in recovery from chemical dependency were likely to have been in the upper one-third of their graduating class and were considered very competent by their nursing colleagues.

There is considerable stigma associated with the diagnosis of chemical dependency or alcoholism. The nursing profession has chosen to use the term impaired professional for the nurse who is impaired because of the use of alcohol or other drugs or because of psychological dysfunction. If you suspect a nurse of chemical dependency or another major psychological problem such as major depression or bipolar disorder, do not ignore it. Programs to help impaired nurses have been in place since 1982. There are many state-run programs that provide intervention and subsequent support and monitoring during the recovery of an impaired nurse. In this way a practicing nurse does not need to lose his or her license. When the program is successfully completed, usually after approximately 2 years, the nurse is deemed successfully treated. Programs for identifying and monitoring the impaired nurse vary from state to state (Critical Thinking Box 23-4).

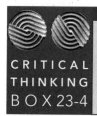

CRITICAL THINKING BOX 23-4

What type of program does your state offer for impaired nurses?

IS BURNOUT INEVITABLE FOR NURSES?

Much has been written about the concept of burnout in nurses. In early research, burnout was thought to be a problem within a nurse or a problem inherent in the nursing profession. However, the stressors in the current workplace caused by restructuring, increased use of unlicensed personnel, and staffing shortages have increased the potential for burnout among nurses employed in hospitals or in other types of health care delivery systems. Over the years, nurses have learned to recognize and manage burnout related to caring too much for their patients. What nurses are currently struggling with is that they are working in toxic environments that are not congruent with their personal philosophies of nursing care.

Burnout associated with job stress can leave nurses vulnerable to depression, physical illness, and alcohol and drug abuse. Symptoms include a loss of energy, weariness, gloominess, dissatisfaction, increased illness, decreased efficiency, absenteeism, and self-doubt. Burnout typically progresses through five stages that are particularly notable within the work setting: initially a feeling of enthusiasm for the job, followed by a loss of enthusiasm, continuous deterioration, crisis, and finally devastation and the inability to work effectively. The perfectionist, overly unselfish, and passive personality types are the most prone to burnout (Hudson, 1995) (Critical Thinking Box 23-5).

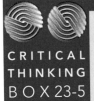

What are the characteristics you have observed in a nurse experiencing "burnout"?

The concepts of managed care, capitation, cost containment, and shortened hospital stays are often not compatible with the emphasis on quality care and customer service. These opposing philosophies create conflict for nurses and lead to burnout that is not as easily remedied as burnout caused by internal factors. Hospital restructuring can be very stressful for those involved in the changed institutional philosophy. Cross training and changes in job description and staffing structure contribute to burnout.

It is important to recognize clearly the mission of the hospital or corporation when you apply for your first job. Is their mission similar to yours? Will you be able to give the quality care that you want to deliver, or will you be required to compromise your values to fit into the system?

There are many strategies designed to combat burnout, and many of them are detailed in this chapter on self-care. However, nurses today will need to determine whether their burnout is caused by internal or external factors. In some cases it may be necessary for the nurse to change to a place of employment that is more in line with her or his belief system.

EMPOWERMENT AND SELF-CARE

Learning about self-care is really about empowerment. The word *power* comes from the French word *pouvoir*, which means "to be able." To empower means to enable—enable self and others to reach their greatest potential for health and well-being. However, the concept of enabling is seen in a negative light because it refers to doing things for others that they can do for themselves. Actually, preventing friends and loved ones from dealing with consequences for their behavior is very disempowering.

With empowerment comes a feeling of well-being and effectiveness. There are times and situations in our lives when we feel more or less powerful. Examples of occasions when one feels powerful or powerless are given in Box 23-2. You may find as you read through the list that there are some situations in your life in which you do feel powerful and some in which you don't. Self-assessment of our sense of well-being and self-esteem helps us to know where to begin. Because change is a constant and all of us are in varying states of emotional, physical, and mental change at any given time, it is important to assess ourselves on a regular basis. As a matter of fact, knowing one's self is the very first step in learning to care for one's self. Empowerment in all spheres of our being is very important. Examine the Holistic Self-Assessment Tool (Critical Thinking Box 23-6), which includes measures of our emotional, mental, physical, social, spiritual, and choice potentials.

Emotional wholeness is about our ability to feel. The ability to express a wide range of emotions is indicative of good mental health. Nurses are often very good at helping their patients "feel" their feelings but often have a difficult time feeling and expressing their own.

Experiencing mental wholeness implies that we maintain our childlike ability to dream and fantasize about the future. Nurses frequently have an overabundance of

---

BOX 23-2 Examples of Times When One Feels Powerless or Powerful

I Feel Powerless When
- ❏ I'm ignored
- ❏ I get assigned to a new hospital unit
- ❏ I can't make a decision
- ❏ I'm exhausted
- ❏ I'm being evaluated by my instructor
- ❏ I have no choices
- ❏ I'm being controlled or manipulated
- ❏ I have pent-up anger
- ❏ I don't think or react quickly
- ❏ I don't speak loudly enough
- ❏ I don't have control over my time

I Feel Powerful When
- ❏ I'm energetic
- ❏ I get positive feedback
- ❏ I know I look good
- ❏ I tell people I'm a nurse
- ❏ I have clear goals for my career
- ❏ I stick to decisions
- ❏ I speak out against injustice
- ❏ I allow myself to be selfish without feeling guilty
- ❏ I tell a good joke
- ❏ I work with supportive people
- ❏ I'm told by a patient or family that I did a good job

Adapted from Josefowitz N (1980). *Paths to power.* Menlo Park, CA: Addison-Wesley, p. 7, with permission.

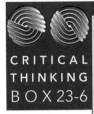

HOLISTIC SELF-ASSESSMENT TOOL

EMOTIONAL POTENTIAL

_____ I push my thoughts and feelings out of conscious awareness (denial).

_____ I feel I have to be in control.

_____ I am unable to express basic feelings of sadness, joy, anger, and fear.

_____ I see myself as a victim.

_____ I feel guilty and ashamed a lot of the time.

_____ I frequently take things personally.

SOCIAL POTENTIAL

_____ I am overcommitted to the point of having no time for recreation.

_____ I am unable to be honest and open with others.

_____ I am unable to admit vulnerability to others.

_____ I am attracted to needy people.

_____ I feel overwhelmingly responsible for others' happiness.

_____ My only friends are nurses.

PHYSICAL POTENTIAL

_____ I neglect myself physically—overweight/underweight, lack of adequate rest and exercise.

_____ I feel tired and lack energy.

_____ I am not interested in sex.

_____ I do not engage in regular physical and dental check-ups.

_____ I have seen a doctor in the past six months for any of the following conditions: migraine headaches, backaches, gastrointestinal problems, hypertension, or cancer.

_____ I am a workaholic—work is all-important to me.

SPIRITUAL POTENTIAL

_____ I see that events that occur in my life are controlled by external choices.

_____ I find the world a basically hostile place.

_____ I lack a spiritual base for working through daily problems.

_____ I live in the past or the future.

_____ I have no sense of power greater than myself.

MENTAL POTENTIAL

_____ I read mostly professional literature.

_____ I spend most waking hours obsessing over people, places, or things.

(continued)

CRITICAL
THINKING
BOX 23-6

HOLISTIC SELF-ASSESSMENT TOOL *(Cont'd)*

_____ I am no longer able to dream or fantasize about my future.

_____ I can't remember much of my childhood.

_____ I can't see much change happening for myself, either personally or professionally.

CHOICE POTENTIAL

_____ I have difficulty making decisions, I am prone to procrastination and am frequently late for personal and professional appointments.

_____ I find it difficult to say no.

_____ I find myself unwilling to take reasonable risks.

_____ I find it difficult to take responsibility for myself.

concrete knowledge of the practice of nursing. We appreciate the challenge of a difficult patient. However, because of the mental and physical demands of the nursing profession, we often don't take time out to learn other disciplines.

Nurses frequently neglect their physical health. We make certain that our patients receive excellent health education and discharge instructions and worry when they are noncompliant. As nurses, however, we do not always follow through when it comes to such things as physical exams, mammograms, and dental health for ourselves. We work long hours and don't plan adequate time for physical recuperation.

Because our profession is such a demanding one, we often don't take the time to cultivate our social potential. When we do spend time with friends, it is because they "need" us. When we get together with friends who are nurses, we spend the time together talking about work.

Spiritual potential simply means that we have a daily awareness that there is something more to living than mere human existence. The lives of nurses with spiritual potential have meaning and direction.

The ability to know that we have choices in life is the final area of the assessment tool. Nurses without "choice power" see life as black and white, with little gray in the middle. Awareness of our choices eliminates the black and white extremes and enables us to act rather than react in situations. Nurses with choice power are able to make decisions and take risks and feel good about it.

Remember to use this tool not only to assess the negatives in your life, but also to assess areas in which you are experiencing growth. You can't survive nursing school, for example, and not experience growth in all areas.

SUGGESTED STRATEGIES FOR SELF-CARE THAT ARE BASED ON THE HOLISTIC SELF-ASSESSMENT TOOL

Not having our life in a state of balance and not having a vision for the future often reflect a state of poor self-esteem. Nathaniel Branden (1992), often referred to as the father of the self-esteem movement, has identified several factors found in individuals with healthy self-esteem. These include the following:

- A face, manner, and way of talking and moving that project the pleasure one takes in being alive.
- Ease in talking of accomplishments or shortcomings with directness and honesty.
- An attitude of openness to and curiosity about new ideas, new experiences, and new possibilities of life.
- Openness to criticism and comfortable about acknowledging mistakes because one's self-esteem is not tied to an image of perfection.
- An ability to enjoy the humorous aspects of life in one's self and others (Branden, p. 43).

The key to developing healthy self-esteem is to become aware of the areas that need the most repair and work on them. However, it is essential to maintain a sense of balance; going overboard in one or two areas is counterproductive. For example, a nurse who exercises five times a week, follows a healthy diet, and sleeps well but is emotionally numb and does not have a clear vision for her future is out of balance. It is a good idea to use this tool (Critical Thinking Box 23-6) every 6 months to a year—similar to taking an inventory at home or in a business.

AM I EMOTIONALLY HEALTHY/EMOTIONALLY INTELLIGENT?

Being emotionally healthy means that you are aware of your feelings and are able to acknowledge them in a healthy way. In the best-selling book *Emotional intelligence*, Goleman (1995) states that emotional intelligence consists of the following five domains: knowing one's emotions, managing emotions, motivating one's self, recognizing emotions in others, and handling relationships. It is certainly best when the basics of emotional intelligence are taught by parents who are good emotional coaches. However, it is never too late to learn.

Nurses who have good emotional health know when they are feeling fearful, angry, sad, ashamed, happy, guilty, or lonely, and they are able to distinguish these feelings. They have found appropriate ways to express their feelings without offending others. When feelings are not expressed or at least acknowledged, they frequently build up, which results in emotional binging. Sometimes our bodies take the brunt of unacknowledged feelings in the form of headaches, gastrointestinal problems, anxiety attacks, and so on.

Feelings or emotions are neither good nor bad. They are indications of some of our self-truths, our desires, and our needs. Critical Thinking Box 23-7 is an exercise to help access and acknowledge feelings.

WHAT ABOUT FRIENDS AND FUN? HOW DO I FIND THE TIME?

An occupational hazard of nurses is overcommitting, both personally and professionally. As a result, they frequently have difficulty in meeting their social potential. Michaels (1990) found that student nurses were very remiss in engaging in recreational activities. However, the findings indicated that students who did engage

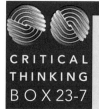

EXERCISE TO HELP ACCESS AND ACKNOWLEDGE FEELINGS

1. Turn your attention to how you are feeling. What part of your body feels what?
2. Recognize to yourself that this is how you are feeling, and give it a name. If you hear an inner criticism for feeling this way, just set it aside. Any feeling is acceptable.
3. Let yourself experience the sensations you are having. Separate these feelings from having to do anything about them.
4. Ask yourself whether you want to express your feelings now or some other time. Do you want to take some other action now or later? Remind yourself that you have choices.

BOX 23-3   Some Pleasurable Activities

Go on a picnic with friends.

Invite friends over for a potluck dinner.

Go to a movie.

Plan celebrations after exams or completing a project.

Introduce yourself to three new people.

Visit a museum.

Call an old friend.

Play with your children.

Borrow someone else's children for play.

Volunteer for a worthwhile project.

Get involved in religious or spiritual activities.

Spend some time people-watching.

Take up a new hobby.

Invite humor into your life.

in recreational activities on a regular basis were less depressed and scored lower on tools used to measure depression, burnout, and co-dependency.

Student nurses often say they do not engage in recreational activities because they cost money and that all their money goes into living expenses. First of all, it is important to include some money in your monthly budget for fun. Depriving yourself of time for recreation on a regular basis may lead to impulsive recreational spending such as a shopping binge with credit cards or money allotted for something else. Second, there are many things to do and places to go that are pleasurable and do not cost a lot of money. Several examples are found in Box 23-3.

Another area in the social arena in which many nurses have difficulty is forming relationships outside of nursing. If you spend all your free time with nurses, chances are that you will "talk shop." Nursing curricula are very science-intensive because there is so much to learn in such a short period of time. Cultivate some friends who have a liberal arts or fine arts background. Choose friends who have different political opinions or come from a different part of town, a different culture, or a different socioeconomic class.

SELF-CARE

HOW DO I TAKE CARE OF MY PHYSICAL SELF?

Nurses are great when it comes to patient education. As a matter of fact it is one of nursing's strengths as a profession. Sometimes we have difficulty applying this information to ourselves. Taking care of ourselves physically is very important (Fig. 23-1). Our

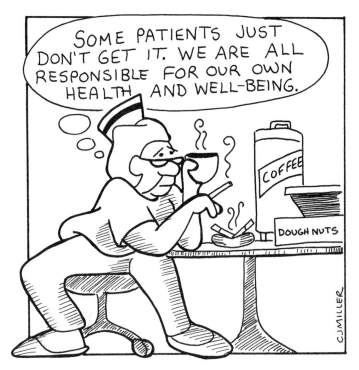

FIGURE 23-1
How do I take care of my physical self?

profession is both mentally and physically challenging. Taking care of ourselves physically entails getting proper nutrition and adequate sleep and exercising on a regular basis.

The *Clinician's handbook of preventive services: put prevention into practice* (1998) from the U.S. Department of Health and Human Services recommends the following:

- **Fats and cholesterol:** Select low-fat/low-cholesterol foods such as lean meat, fish, poultry, and low-fat products. Avoid butter, deep-fried foods, marbled meats, and processed cheeses.
- **Complex carbohydrates and fiber:** Choose whole-grain bread and cereal products, pastas, vegetables, and fruits naturally high in complex carbohydrates. Avoid desserts and canned fruits that contain refined sugars.
- **Sodium:** Select food naturally low in salt and cut down the amount of salt added during food preparation and at the table. Reduce intake of foods such as ham, bacon, salted snacks, and other highly processed foods.
- **Alcohol:** Consume no more than two drinks a day: alcohol contains only empty calories.
- **Exercise:** Incorporate 30 minutes or more of moderate-intensity physical activity, such as walking, into your schedule (preferably daily).

A good exercise program is one that includes activities that foster aerobic activity, flexibility, and strength. A very important part of an exercise program is that it be a regular habit. To be effective, the program should take 3 to 6 hours a week. And it doesn't have to cost money. You don't have to belong to a gym or invest in exercise equipment. Aerobic activities include walking, jogging, swimming, bicycling, and dancing. Minimal fitness consists of raising your heart rate to 100 beats/min and keeping it there for 30 minutes (Fig. 23-2).

STRATEGIES TO FOSTER MY SPIRITUAL SELF—DOES MY LIFE HAVE MEANING?

People who have a sense of spiritual well-being find their lives to be positive experiences, have relationships with a power greater than themselves, feel good about the future, and believe there is some real purpose in life. If we find that our lives lack meaning and our spiritual health is lacking, how do we go about finding spiritual well-being?

Daily prayer and meditation are very important in maintaining a spiritual self. M. Scott Peck (1978) states that the process of spiritual growth is an effortful and difficult one because it is conducted against a natural resistance, a natural inclination to keep things the way they were, to cling to the old maps and old ways of doing things, to take the easy path. Reading religious or philosophical material and studying the great religions are two examples of ways to foster spiritual growth. There are also many spiritual books, enough reading for a lifetime.

In addition to reading what others have written about the subject, many people access their spiritual selves with the practice of meditation. Meditating allows us time to become quiet, heal our thoughts and bodies, and be grateful. A sample meditation on gratitude and healing is included in Box 23-4.

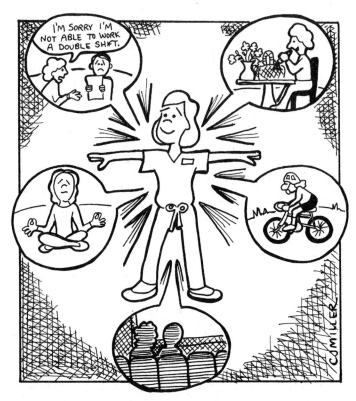

FIGURE 23-2
Learn to take care of yourself.

 BOX 23-4 A Meditation on Gratitude and Healing

Take a deep breath and gently close your eyes. Give a few big sighs . . . sighs
of relief . . . and see if your body wants to stretch a little . . . or yawn . . .
(pause).

Now pay attention to the rhythm of your breathing . . . Feel your body rise gently
as you breathe in, and relax as you breathe out . . . (pause for several breaths)
. . . every outbreath is an opportunity to let go . . . to feel the pleasant warmth
and heaviness of your body . . . a little more on each outbreath . . . (pause).

Now, as you breathe in, imagine your breath as a stream of warm, loving light
entering through the top of your head. Let it fill your forehead and eyes . . .
your brain . . . your ears . . . and nose . . . feel the light warm and relax
your tongue, your jaws, and your throat. Let your whole head float in an
ocean of warm light . . . growing brighter and brighter with each breath . . .
(pause) . . . Thank your eyes for the miracle of sight . . . your nose for the
fragrance of roses and hot coffee on cold mornings (or whatever you like)
. . . your ears for the richness that sound is . . . your tongue for the pleasure
of taste . . . and let the light fill and heal every cell of your senses. . . .

(continued)

BOX 23-4   A Meditation on Gratitude and Healing *(Cont'd)*

Breathe the light into your neck . . . let it expand gently into your shoulders . . . and breathe it down your arms . . . and into your hands . . . right to the tips of your fingers . . . Thank you arms and hands for all you have created and touched with your life. . . . All the people you have hugged and held to your heart . . . Rest in the warmth and love of the light . . . light that grows brighter with every breath. . . .

And breathe the warm light into your lungs and your heart . . . feeling it penetrate your entire chest, filling every organ, every cell with love. As you breathe, send gratitude to your lungs for bringing in the energy of life— and to your heart for sending life to all the cells of your body, for serving you so well for all these years . . . rest in the gratitude and love . . . in the light that continues to grow brighter with each breath . . . (pause).

And breathe the light into your belly, feeling it penetrate deeply into your center, into the organs of digestion and reproduction . . . and sense the miracle of your body . . . the mystery of procreation and of the ability to beget life . . . let the light expand through your torso and down into your buttocks . . . growing warmest and brighter . . . balancing and healing all the cells of your body. . . .

Breathe the light into your thighs . . . into bone and muscle, nerve and skin, alive with the energy of light . . . comforted in your caring and your love . . . and let the light expand into your calves . . . and your feet . . . right to the soles of your feet . . . feeling gratitude for the gift of walking . . . letting the lovelight grow brighter and brighter. . . .

Rest in the fullness of the light . . . enjoying the lifeforce . . . and, if there is any place in your body that needs to relax or to heal, direct the light there and hold that part of yourself with the same love you would give to a hurt child . . . (pause).

Now, as you breathe, sense how the light radiates out from your body . . . just as a light shines in the darkness, surrounding you in a cocoon of love . . . and you can sense that cocoon extending all around your body, above and below you, and to all sides, for about three feet . . . like a giant cocoon . . . a place of complete safety where you can recharge your body and your mind . . . (pause).

And you can imagine the light around other people . . . surrounding them with the same radiance of love, gratitude, and healing . . . see your loved ones in the light . . . see those whom you think of as your enemies in the light . . . then let the light expand until you can imagine the entire world as an orb of light . . . (pause) . . . amidst a universe of light (pause) all connected . . . all at peace . . . and feel the wonder and majesty of creation . . . (pause).

Now for a minute or two just rest . . . just breathe . . . returning to the warm, comfortable feelings within you . . . (long pause).

Begin fading out the music now, and then read the instructions for reorientation.

And now, begin to reorient yourself to the room . . . slowly and at your own pace . . . bringing the peace and gratitude back with you.

From Borysenko J (1987). *Minding the body, mending the mind.* Menlo Park, CA: Addison-Wesley, with permission.

HOW DO I INCREASE MY MENTAL POTENTIAL? IT'S OK TO DAYDREAM. . . .

Nursing students get considerable opportunity to exercise their mental potential while they are in nursing school. This activity, however, is primarily in the form of formal education. There are many other ways to exercise this potential. One of the first ways is to concentrate on removing negative thoughts or self-defeating beliefs from our minds. Examples of statements that nursing students frequently make are:

- "I must make A's in nursing school."
- "I must have approval from everyone, and if I don't, I feel horrible and depressed."
- "If I fail at something, the results will be catastrophic."
- "Others must always treat me fairly."
- "If I'm not liked by everyone, I am a failure."
- "Because all my miseries are caused by others, I will have no control over my life until they change."

If you relate to any of these statements, you have some work to do on your belief system. You are setting yourself up for failure by having extremely high expectations of yourself. You are also giving other people power over your own destiny. Remember, you can't change others. The only person you can change is yourself.

One way that we can change these internal beliefs is to learn how to give ourselves daily affirmations (Fig. 23-3). Simply put, affirmations are powerful, positive statements concerning the ways in which we would like to think, feel, and behave. Some examples are "I am a worthwhile person"; "I am human and capable of making mistakes"; and "I am able to freely express my emotions." Always begin affirmative statements with "I" rather than "you." This practice keeps the focus on self rather than others and encourages the development of inner self-worth.

The power of affirmation exercises lies in consistency—repetition encourages ultimate belief in what is being said.

Begin each day with some affirmations. Try some of the examples in Box 23-5. These enable us to feel better about ourselves and consequently raise our self-esteem. Stand in front of a mirror and tell yourself that you are a special person and worthy of self-love and the love of others. Another suggestion is to record some positive affirmations on your telephone answering machine and call your telephone number in the middle of the day or when you are having a slump or attack of self-pity; hearing you own voice say you are okay can have a very positive effect. For example, "Hello—Glad you're having a great day, please leave a message." Also consider signing up to receive a daily affirmation from a Web site listed at the end of this chapter: http://www.rutts.com. When you sign up for this free service, you receive a daily affirmation in an e-mail message (Critical Thinking Box 23-8).

WHAT ARE MY CHOICES, AND HOW DO I EXERCISE THEM?

Many of us negotiate our way through life never realizing that we have many choices. We remain victims, waiting for life to happen, rather than taking a proactive stance. In his best-selling book *Seven habits of highly effective people*, Stephen Covey (1989)

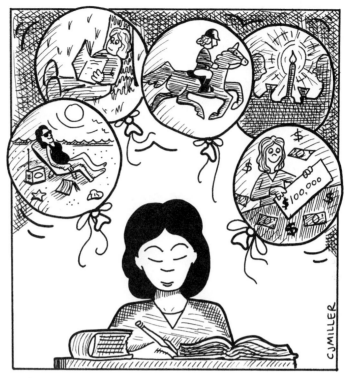

FIGURE 23-3
Daydream: Send up your brain balloons!

BOX 23-5   Affirmations

❏ I am a worthwhile person.
❏ I am a child of God.
❏ I am willing to accept love.
❏ I am willing to give love.
❏ I can openly express my feelings.
❏ I deserve love, peace, and serenity.
❏ I am capable of changing.
❏ I can take care of myself without feeling guilty.
❏ I can say no and not feel guilty.
❏ I am beautiful inside and out.
❏ I can be spontaneous and whimsical.
❏ I am human and capable of making mistakes.
❏ I can recognize shame and work through it.
❏ I forgive myself for hurting myself and others.

(continued)

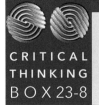

BOX 23-5   Affirmations (Cont'd)

❑ I freely accept nurturing from others.
❑ I can be vulnerable with trusted others.
❑ I am peaceful with life.
❑ I trust the process with life.
❑ I am free to be the best me I can.
❑ I love and comfort myself in ways that are pleasing to me.
❑ I am automatically and joyfully focusing on the positive.
❑ I am giving myself permission to live, love, and laugh.
❑ I am creating and singing affirmations to create a joyful, abundant, fulfilling life.

CRITICAL THINKING BOX 23-8

What are some positive affirmations that work for you, and how can you increase the effectiveness of these affirmations?

states that the very first habit we must develop is to be proactive. We stop thinking in black and white and come to realize that in every arena of our lives, we have choices about how to respond and react. Covey differentiates between people who are proactive and people who are reactive. Examples of proactive versus reactive language are included in Box 23-6. Pay attention to your own language patterns for the next few weeks. Are there times when you could say "I choose?" You can choose to respond to people and situations rather than react. Exercising our choice potential also entails that we act responsibly toward others. We recognize that other people have the right to choose for themselves and to be accountable for their own behavior.

BOX 23-6   Examples of Proactive and Reactive

There's nothing I can do.	Let's look at our alternatives.
That's just the way I am.	I can choose a different approach.
He makes me so mad.	I control my own feelings.
They won't allow that.	I can create an effective presentation.
I have to do that.	I will choose an appropriate response.
I can't.	I choose.
I must.	I prefer.
If only.	I will.

Before we can act responsibly toward others, we must first act responsibly toward ourselves. This involves self-acceptance and self-love. In his book *Born for love: reflections on loving*, Leo Buscaglia (1992) states this very eloquently:

> Being who we are people who feel good about themselves are not easily threatened by the future. They enthusiastically maintain a secure image whether everything is falling apart or going their way. They hold a firm base of personal assuredness and self-respect that remains constant. Though they are concerned about what others think of them, it is a healthy concern. They find external forces more challenging than threatening.
>
> Perhaps the greatest sign of maturity is to reach the point in life when we embrace ourselves—strengths and weaknesses alike—and acknowledge that we are all that we have; that we have a right to a happy and productive life and the power to change ourselves and our environment within realistic limitations. In short, we are, each of us, entitled to be who we are and become what we choose (p. 177).

REFERENCES

American Nurses Association: *Compendium of HIV/AIDS position policies and documents*, Pub. No. PR8, Kansas City, Mo, 1994, ANA.

Buscaglia L: *Born for love: reflections on loving*, Thorofare, NJ, 1992, Random House.

Coleman EA, Honeycutt G, Ogden B, McMillan DE, et al: Assessing substance abuse among health care students and the efficacy of educational interventions. *J ProfNurs* 13(1): 28-37, 1997.

Covey S: *Seven habits of highly effective people*, New York, 1989, Simon & Schuster.

Fassbinder B: It's time to face the enemy—together, *Crit Care Nurse* 12(7):112, 1992.

Goleman D: *Emotional intelligence*, New York, 1995, Bantam Books.

Hudson S: Job-related burnout said to be increasing, *NurseWeek* 8(17):1, 1995.

Michaels B: *Antecedents to professional impairment: burnout, depression, codependency and alcohol use in community college nursing students*, Nova University, Ft Lauderdale, Fla.

Peck MS: *The road less traveled*, New York, 1978, Simon & Schuster.

Rogers, B: Is health care a risky business? As I see it (opinion column) *American Nurse*, 1997.

US Department of Health and Human Services, Office of Disease Prevention and Health Promotion: *Clinician's handbook of preventive services: put prevention into practice*, Washington, DC, 1998, Public Health Service.

ADDITIONAL READINGS

American Nurses Association: *Addictions and psychological dysfunction in nursing: the profession's response to the problem*, Kansas City, Mo, 1984, ANA.

Beattie M: *Beyond co-dependency*, New York, 1989, Harper & Row.

Bissell L, Haberman PW: *Alcoholism in the professions*, New York, 1984, Oxford University Press.

Borysenko J: *Minding the body, mending the mind,* Menlo Park, Calif, 1987, Addison-Wesley.

Carson W: AIDS and the nurse—a legal update, *Am Nurse* 25(3):18, 1993.

Cullen A: Burnout: Why do we blame the nurse? *Am J Nurs* 95(11):23-27, 1995.

Duquette A, et al: Factors related to nursing burnout: a review of empirical knowledge, *Issues Ment Health Nurs* 15(4):337-358, 1994.

Ellison CW: Spiritual well-being: conceptualization and measurement, *J Psychol Theol* 11: 330-340.

Hall SF, Wray LM: Co-dependency: nurses who give too much, *Am J Nurs* 89(11):1456-1460, 1989.

Josefowitz N: *Paths to power,* Menlo Park, Calif, 1980, Addison-Wesley.

Legal Questions. HIV testing: condition of employment, *Nursing* 23(2):67, 1993.

Lerner R: *Daily affirmations,* Pompano Beach, Fla, 1985,: Health Communications.

Meisenhelder JB: Contributing factors to fear of HIV contagion in registered nurses, *Image J Nurse Sch* 26(1):65-69, 1994.

Perry BL: Chemical dependency among nurses: are policies adequate? *Nurs Manage* 26(5), 52-56, 1995.

Robbins CE: A monitored treatment program for impaired health care professionals, *J Nurs Adm* 17(2):17-21, 1987.

Skinner K, Scott RD: Depression among female registered nurses, *Nurs Manage* 24(8):42-45, 1993.

Zerwekh J, Michaels B: Co-dependency: assessment and recovery, *Nurs Clin North Am* 24(1):109-120, 1989.

INTERNET RESOURCES

Occupational Safety and Health Administration
http://www.osha.gov

National Institute on Drug Abuse
http://www.nida.nih.gov

Join Together Online
http://www.jointogether.org/sa

Web of Addictions
http://www.well.com/user/woa

HIV/AIDS Resources Sampler
http://www.nnlm.nlm.nih.gov/pnr/samplers/aidspath.html

CDC National AIDS Clearinghouse
http://www.cdcnac.org

MedWeb at Emory University
http://www.medweb.emory.edu/MedWeb

Daily Affirmations
http://www.rutts.com/AffirmationsADay.htm

The Daily Motivator
http://greatday.com

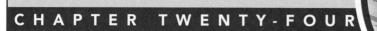

CHAPTER TWENTY-FOUR

NCLEX-RN and the New Graduate

JO CAROL CLABORN, MS, RN, CNS

The way I see it, if you want the rainbow, you gotta put up with the rain.
    —Dolly Parton

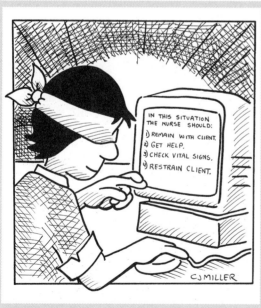

Don't take unnecessary chances. . . .
understand the NCLEX process.

After completing this chapter, you should be able to:

■ Discuss the role of the National Council of State Boards of Nursing.

■ Discuss the implications of computer adaptive testing.

■ Identify the process and steps for preparing to take the National Council Licensure Examination for Registered Nurses.

■ Identify criteria for selecting a review book and a review course.

Planning and preparing for the National Council Licensure Examination for Registered Nurses (NCLEX-RN) are essential components of the transition process. As with other aspects of transition, planning begins before you graduate. Planning ahead will assist you with more comprehensive preparation, in addition to decreasing your anxiety about the examination. Being prepared and knowing what to expect will help you to maintain a positive attitude.

THE NCLEX-RN

WHO PREPARES IT, AND WHY DO WE HAVE TO HAVE IT?

The National Council of State Boards of Nursing (NCSBN) is the governing body for the committee that prepares the licensure examination. Each member board or state determines the application process and deadlines in their state, in addition to the mechanics of administering the examination. The NCLEX represents a national examination with standardized scoring. All candidates in every state are presented with questions based on the same test plan. Every state requires the same passing level or standard. There is no discrepancy in passing scores from one state to another.

The NCLEX is **not** designed to determine everything you know or to determine whether you are a capable clinical specialist. Your performance on the NCLEX will not influence entry into baccalaureate or graduate programs. The NCLEX is used to regulate entry into nursing practice in the United States. The purpose of the examination is to determine whether the candidate is competent to perform safe, effective entry-level nursing care (NCSBN, 2001). Upon successful completion of the examination, you will be granted a license to practice nursing in the state in which you applied for licensure. Licensure is currently in a significant change process. There are many nurses who maintain a current license in multiple states. The increase in nursing practice across state lines, the growth of managed care, and the advances in telehealth medicine prompted an in-depth research project that was conducted by the NCSBN in the late 1990s. As a result of that research the Mutual Recognition Model for Multistate Regulation has been implemented. This is frequently referred to as the Nurse Licensure Compact. As of May 2002, the compact has been enacted through the state legislatures of 18 states (WCSBN, 2002, news release).

HOW WILL THE NURSE LICENSURE COMPACT AFFECT YOUR LICENSE?

The nursing license in the compact states will function much like a driver's license. The individual will hold one license issued in the state of residence but is responsible for the laws of the state in which they are driving. The individual nurse may practice in another state; however, the nurse must comply with the Nurse Practice Act of the state in which he or she practices. The transition process has begun; how fast it is implemented will depend on individual states. The Nurse Licensure Compact must be passed by the state legislature in each participating state. For more information on this process, please refer to Chapters 18 and 20. Watch your state nursing organization and Board of Nursing newsletters to see where your state is in the process of joining the Interstate Compact on Nurse Licensure.

Before the Nurse Licensure Compact is implemented, the respective states will continue to require the nurse to be licensed in the individual state of practice. Transfer of nursing licenses between states is a process called "licensure by endorsement." If you wish to practice in a state in which you are not currently licensed, you must contact the State Board of Nursing in the state in which you wish to practice. The State Board of Nursing will advise you of the process to become licensed in that state. This process does not change your successful completion of the NCLEX, nor do you have to take the examination again. All states recognize the successful completion of the NCLEX, regardless of the state in which you took the examination or where your license was issued (Critical Thinking Box 24-1).

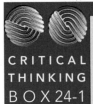

CRITICAL THINKING BOX 24-1

What is the status of the Nurse Licensure Compact in your state?

The content of the NCLEX is based on a test blueprint that is determined by the National Council. The blueprint reflects entry-level nursing practice as identified by research and the Job Analysis Study of Newly Licensed Registered Nurses. This research study is conducted by the National Council every 3 years. The job analysis research in 1999 indicated that the majority of new graduates were continuing to work in a general medical–surgical environment. The majority of entry-level nurses indicated they cared for acutely ill patients. Patients with stable and unstable chronic conditions and terminal patients were the next largest group. The majority of entry-level nurses indicated they cared for adult and geriatric patients with stable chronic conditions, those who were acutely ill, or those who had unstable chronic conditions. The majority of the new graduates surveyed also indicated their primary responsibility was in the delivery of direct patient care. The hospital and long-term care facilities were the primary employers of the new graduate. A significant number of new graduates indicated that they have administrative responsibilities. The test plan in this chapter was implemented in April 2001 and will be used until April 2003. A new test plan is implemented every 3 years. This represents the time required to conduct the research, analyze the data, and implement a new test plan on NCLEX (Hertz, 2000).

WHAT IS THE NCLEX-RN TEST PLAN?

The examination is made up of questions that are designed to test the candidate's ability to apply the nursing process and to determine appropriate nursing responses and interventions to provide safe nursing care. The test plan is based on the nursing process and areas of patient needs.

Nursing Process. Each of the five phases of the nursing process has equal importance and are equally represented in the test bank. All questions in the test bank are categorized according to the appropriate level of the nursing process.

Patient Needs. There continues to be four levels of patient needs identified in the Job Analysis Study (Hertz, 2000). Each level of patient need is assigned a percentage that reflects the weight of that category of patient need on the NCLEX-RN. The approximate percentages of each area are as follows:

> Safe, effective care environment: 23%
> Health promotion and maintenance: 10%
> Psychosocial integrity: 15%
> Physiological integrity: 52% (Hertz, 2000)

In April 1994, the NCSBN implemented computer adaptive testing (CAT) for the NCLEX for both practical/vocational nurses (NCLEX-PN/VN) and registered nurses (NCLEX-RN). This represented a major advance in the implementation and administration of the examination. The information presented here is a brief introduction to the NCLEX-RN CAT. It is important that you carefully follow the information and instructions you receive in your NCLEX Candidate Bulletin, in addition to information from your state board of nurse examiners.

WHAT DOES CAT MEAN?

With CAT, each candidate receives a different set of questions via the computer. The questions are assembled interactively as the candidate progresses through the examination. The computer develops an examination based on the test plan and selects questions to be presented on the basis of the candidates' responses to the previous question. The number of questions each candidate receives and the testing time for each candidate will vary (Collected Works, 2002). As candidates answer questions correctly, the questions will get progressively more difficult. When candidates miss questions, the computer will select an easier question to present (NCSBN, 2001). The questions presented will reflect the NCLEX test plan based on the nursing process, patient needs, and the Job Analysis Study.

"Tryout" questions will continue to be integrated into the examination. The NCSBN Examination Committee evaluates the statistical information from each of these questions to determine if the question is valid and to identify the level of difficulty of the test item (NCSBN, 2002, candidate bulletin). Don't get alarmed—these questions are not counted in the grading of the examination, and time has been allocated for the candidate to answer these questions.

What Is the Application Process for NCLEX CAT? About 2 to 3 months before graduation, the school of nursing will have each candidate complete an application form and send it to the state board of nurse examiners. Upon completion of the nursing program, the school will verify the graduate's status with the board of nursing. After the forms have been processed, each candidate will then receive an Authorization to Test with instructions and the telephone numbers and addresses of the centers that will be administering the examination. Read your instruction packet carefully. An Authorization to Test will be required for scheduling your testing date and for admission into the testing center. Application forms for the examination may be obtained by contacting the respective board of nurse examiners. All candidates will be thumb-printed and photographed at the testing location.

Where Do I Take the Test? There are testing sites in every state. Each candidate will receive information regarding the location of the centers and may select the center that is most convenient. There will be several testing stations at each center. A candidate may take the test at any of the testing sites in the United States; however, license to practice will be issued only in the state where the candidate's application was submitted.

When Do I Take the Test? After receiving the Authorization to Test (ATT), a candidate may contact the desired center to schedule the examination. The location and telephone numbers of the testing centers will be included in the information. Plan on receiving your ATT about 2 to 3 weeks after you finish school. You may schedule your examination as soon as you receive the ATT; that means you may receive the ATT on Wednesday, call the location of your choice and if you want to take the examination the next day and there is space available, you may do so. The testing center staff will schedule the examination appointment. They will also advise you of the testing center hours.

During the last two months of school, begin to plan when you would like to take the examination. The examination should be taken within about 6 weeks of graduation. Take into consideration some study time and whether a formal review course is available. It is important that you take the examination soon after graduation, if you wait too long your level of comprehension of critical information is decreased. Finish school, take a review course if you want, get your ATT, and go take the examination. This is not a good time to plan a vacation, bring your mother to live with you, get married, or engage in other activities that cause a crisis in your life (Critical Thinking Box 24-2).

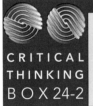

CRITICAL THINKING BOX 24-2

When do you want to take your NCLEX? Review Boxes 24-1 through 24-3 to help you get started on thinking about this process.

How Much Time Do I Have and How Many Questions Are There? Each candidate is scheduled for a five-hour time slot. The average time for testing has been around two hours, and the average number of questions answered has been in the range of 110 to 145 (NCSBN, 1998). Each candidate must answer at least 75 questions. Remember, these numbers are averages. If you answer 76 or 150 questions, or if you take the test for 1 hour or 2 hours, it is no indication of a pass or fail score. It just means you have "turned your test in" and the test has been completed. The examination will end when the student:

- Measures at a level of competence above or below the standard and at least 75 questions have been answered.
- Completes a maximum of 265 questions.
- Has been testing for the maximum time of 5 hours (NCSBN, 2002, candidate bulletin).

Do I Have to Be Computer-Literate? It is not necessary to study from a computer, nor is it necessary that you be "computer literate." Research has demonstrated that candidates who were not accustomed to working on a computer did as well as those who were very comfortable with the computer. So, prior computer experience is not a prerequisite to passing the NCLEX!

How Will I Keep the Computer Keys Straight and Deal With a Mouse? The only time you will use the keys and keyboard is to enter your name and identification code. After that information has been entered all the keys become inactive and you will use the mouse to select your answers and progress through the examination. When a candidate confirms an answer, the computer screen automatically progresses to the next question. At the testing site, each candidate is given an orientation to the computer and will go through a practice/orientation process. Every effort is made to make sure that the candidate understands and is comfortable with the testing procedure and equipment.

What Is the Passing Score? Every state has the same passing criteria. Specific individual scores will not be available to you, your school, or your place of employment. You cannot obtain your results from the testing center. Your score will be reported directly to you as pass or fail. A composite of student results will be mailed to the respective schools of nursing. There is no specific published score or

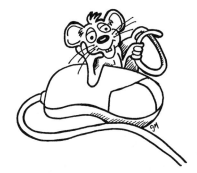

As of 2002, the use of the computer mouse makes navigating the CAT easier.

number that represents passing. If a candidate is not successful, some states offer an opportunity for the them to review their examination. This is usually a rather costly activity, and does not benefit the student because when they take the examination again they will get a totally different set of questions.

How Will I Know I Have Passed? The examination scores are compiled at a national testing center and sent directly to state boards of nursing. The majority of state boards of nursing are able to advise the candidates in writing of their results within three to four weeks of taking the examination. Check your candidate bulletin as well for the information from your state regarding the availability of results online or from an automated telephone verification system. Do not call the state board of nursing to inquire about your pass or fail status; they cannot release information on the telephone.

WHAT ARE THE TECHNICAL ASPECTS OF THE NCLEX?

The majority of the questions are multiple choice, with four options (Fig. 24-1). Each question will stand alone and will not require information from previous questions to determine the correct answer. All of the information for the question will be available on the computer screen. If you need scratch paper, it will be provided and you will be required to turn it in. You may not take calculators into the examination; however, a "drop down" calculator will be available on the screen for math calculations. Everyone will be tested according to the same test plan, but candidates will receive different questions. There is only one answer to each question; you do not get any partial credit for another answer—it is either right or wrong. All questions must be answered, even if you have to make a wild guess. The computer selects the next question on the basis of the response to the previous question. (You don't get another question until the one on the screen is answered.) You will not be able to go back to a previous question once that question is removed from the screen. (You can't go back and change your answer to the wrong one!) There will be a mandatory ten-minute rest period after two hours of testing. If you need to take a break before the 2 hours, notify one of the testing center representatives (NCSBN, 2002, candidate bulletin).

There is not a lot of storage area at the testing sites. There are some small lockers for your personal items. So do not take your textbooks, all your notes from school, your lucky stuffed bear, or any other materials you have been carrying around in that pack for the past 2 years!

What If I Need to Change the Time or Date I Have Already Scheduled? You can change your testing date and time if you advise the testing center before noon, two business days before your scheduled appointment. You can then reschedule the test at no additional cost. If a candidate does not reschedule within this time frame or does not come at the scheduled testing time, then an additional registration form and fee will be required (NCSBN, 2002).

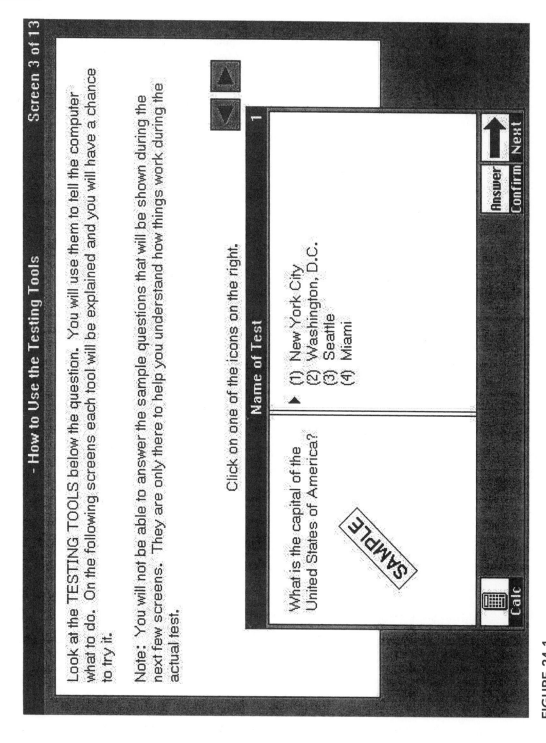

FIGURE 24-1
Sample Page of Testing Tutorial from NCSBN.

What Are the Advantages of CAT for the Candidate? The environment is quiet and conducive to testing. The work surface is large enough to accommodate both right- and left-handed people with adequate room for the computer and scratch paper. The time frame is much more relaxed—there is a total of five hours. Each candidate can work at his or her own pace. Each person has her own testing station or cubicle. There should be a minimal amount of distraction, if any, by the other candidates who are testing at the same time. If a graduate has to retake the examination, the parameters for retesting are established by the respective state board of nursing. The National Council requires the candidate to wait at least 91 days after the first examination before scheduling a second time. Candidates who take the examination again will not be given the same questions.

PREPARING FOR THE NCLEX-RN

WHERE AND WHEN SHOULD I START?

Six Months Before the NCLEX

Make sure you know the deadlines and application process for your state. Your school will advise you of the specific dates the forms are due to the state office. Make sure you follow the directions exactly. State boards of nursing do not respond favorably to applications that are not submitted on time or are submitted in an incorrect format. A listing of the state boards of nursing can be found in Appendix A. If you plan on applying for licensure in another state, it is your responsibility to contact the board of nursing in that state to obtain your papers for application. Plan early to investigate the feasibility of taking the examination in another state.

Investigate review courses. Review courses can assist you in organizing your study materials and identifying areas in which you need to focus your study time. The percentage of graduates passing the examination is higher for those who participated in a formal review course (Zerwekh, 1986)

Plan an expense account for the end of school and for the NCLEX. Frequently students are caught at the end of school with unexpected expenses, one of which may be the fees for the NCLEX. Start a small savings plan—maybe $5 a week—to help defray these expenses. For family and friends who want to "give you something for graduation," you might tell them of your "wish list," including those expenses incurred at graduation (Box 24-1).

Two Months Before the NCLEX: What Do I Need to Do Now?

If you have a job, discuss with your supervisor your anticipated NCLEX-RN test date. Submit your request for days off *in writing* as soon as your test date is confirmed. This is something you want to make sure they understand. Supervisors may not be aware that each candidate can schedule their own testing date.

BOX 24-1   Budget for the End of School and the NCLEX

HOW MUCH IS IT GOING TO COST ME TO GET OUT OF SCHOOL?

❏ *Required Expenses*

Graduating fees from college or university   _____

Application fees for NCLEX-RN   _____

Passport-type picture (may be required for state   _____
    application)

❏ *Expenses to take NCLEX-RN*

Travel—car, bus, airfare   _____

Hotel accommodations at NCLEX testing site   _____

Miscellaneous (food, transportation to site, etc.)   _____

❏ *Optional Expenses*

School pin   _____

Uniform or cap and gown for graduation   _____

Graduation expenses passed on to graduate   _____

Graduation pictures (class or individual)   _____

Graduation invitations   _____

Commercial pretesting   _____

NCLEX-RN review course (need to plan this   _____
    before school is out)

NCLEX-RN review book(s) (get these early—   _____
    really helps with the last year of nursing
    school!)

❏ *Expenses After Graduation (It's Not Over Yet!)*

Professional organizations (most organizations   _____
    will give a discount on new membership to the
    graduate nurse)

Professional journals   _____

Uniform, scrub suits, shoes to begin new job   _____

Professional liability insurance (check with the   _____
    school regarding transfer from school policy to
    individual policy)

_____

NCLEX-RN, National Council Licensure Examination for Registered Nurses.

Plan on taking off the day before the examination and, if possible, the day after also. This will allow you time to relax and, if necessary, travel to and from the testing site.

Decide how you are going to get to the test site and will it be necessary for you to stay overnight. If the closest testing site is not easily accessible, is more than a one-hour drive away, or involves driving through a heavily congested traffic area, you may want to consider staying overnight in a hotel room close to the site. For some graduates this will prevent unnecessary hassle and increased anxiety on the day of the examination.

Are you going with a group or by yourself? How will you feel if the group is finished and you are still working on your examination? Will you feel rushed because everyone is waiting for you? Don't create a situation to increase your anxiety at one of the most important times of your nursing career. If you are okay with the group waiting for you, and everyone understands the situation, then it may be a source of support for you. If a group of graduates are traveling together and are able to schedule the examination on the same day, consideration should be given to planning the hotel accommodations. *Don't have a crowd in your room.* Plan on having your own bed. Five people in a room designed for two or four will not be conducive to sleep the night before the examination. If you are rooming with another person, select someone you like and can tolerate in close quarters for a short period of time. Surround yourself with people who have a positive attitude; you don't need complainers and negative thinkers.

Develop a plan for studying. Do you need to study alone, or do you benefit from group study time? Set yourself a study schedule that you can realistically achieve. Two to three hours a day for two or three days a week is realistic; eight hours a day on your days off doesn't work. If you take a formal review course, plan your study time to gain the most from the course. A review course is not meant to be your only study time. When you finish a review course, you should have a much better idea regarding what is going to be tested, how it will be tested, and where you need to focus some study time. Priority areas to study are those you are the weakest in; focus on those first.

The Day Before the BIG DAY.

Make sure you have all of the papers required for admission. Read your information packet again. The Authorization to Test that you received from the testing service will be required at the testing site. The information packet that you receive should have all of the necessary information and directions needed for the test site. Check to see if there is anything else you will need to take with you to the site.

Make a "test run" the evening before the test. Find the parking areas. If your hotel is within four to six blocks of the test site, the walk will be a terrific way to help reduce anxiety and get the blood circulating to your brain! Whether you drive or walk to the site, go the day before to make sure you know where you are going.

Go to bed early, don't study, cram or party! Plan on eating a light dinner, something that will not upset your stomach—you don't need to be up half of the night with heartburn and/or diarrhea!

The BIG DAY Is Here.

Eat a well-balanced breakfast, not sweet rolls and coffee. Protein and complex carbohydrates will help sustain you during the examination. Eat light, something that is nourishing, but not heavy. Don't drink a lot of coffee—you don't need to be distracted by frequent bathroom trips.

Dress comfortably. Anticipate that the temperature at the testing sites will be a little cool rather than too warm. Don't wear tight clothes that restrict your breathing when you sit down! Dress casually and comfortably and be prepared with a sweater or light jacket just in case you need it.

Arrive at the test site a little early. This will allow you time to get checked in and prevent anxiety about being late.

HOW DO I SELECT AN NCLEX REVIEW COURSE?

There are many review courses available to assist the graduate nurse in preparing for the NCLEX. Before you sign up, evaluate which course will be most beneficial to you. In considering a review course, remember the objective is review, not primary learning (Box 24-2).

BOX 24-2   Selecting an NCLEX Review Course

Here are some questions to consider:

Where Am I Going to Work?
Will the institution pay for the review? _____
Will the institution pay the initial fee or do I need to plan for
    reimbursement? _____
Does the Institution Provide an On-Site Review?
Who teaches it? _____
Is it an independent company or hospital employees? _____
Review Course Instructors
Who will teach the class? Your faculty from school? Or, review course faculty
    trained by the review company? _____

(continued)

BOX 24-2   Selecting an NCLEX Review Course (Cont'd)

What Type of Instructional Material Is Used?

Does it cost extra outside the registration fee? _____

If it is additional to registration fee, where do I get it? _____

Can I keep all of the instructional materials? (books, testing booklets, audio tapes, and so forth) _____

Does the instructional material include practice test questions in the NCLEX format? _____

Can I get any of the course materials ahead of time to begin studying? _____

How Are the Classes Conducted?

How many days? _____

Are days consecutive or spread over several weeks? _____

What are the hours each day? _____

What type of audio-visual aids are used? _____

What is the teaching style (group work, lecture, home study, group participation, testing practice, and so forth)? _____

What is the average size class for the area? _____

How Much Does It Cost?

What is the total price? _____

Does this include all of the class materials? _____

What is the per-hour or per-day cost? (This will help to evaluate cost effectiveness of various types of programs.) _____

Are there group rates, and what are they? _____

Are there early registration discounts? _____

When does the money have to be in? _____

Are there any "extra incentives?" _____

How Do I Pay for It?

Is there a payment plan? _____

Can I make an early deposit to hold my space? _____

When is the deposit due? When is the final amount due? _____

If I change my mind after I make the deposit, can I get the deposit back? _____

Is There a Guarantee?

What is the guarantee? _____

Can I take the review over again? _____

Does it have to be in the same location as the first time? _____

(continued)

BOX 24-2   Selecting an NCLEX Review Course (Cont'd)

What do I have to do to qualify for the guarantee? _____

Do I get further assistance in identifying areas of need and studying for next time? _____

What Is the Pass Rate and How Is It Determined?

Is it based on all new graduates who took the review? _____

Is it a company survey of participants after NCLEX? _____

Is it based on all participants or only the first-time takers? _____

Is it based on the company projected success rate? _____

Did the review company answer all of my questions in a courteous manner and seem interested in my business? _____

Do you know anyone who has taken a review? _____

What are their recommendations? _____

What Type of Review Courses Are Available? Evaluate your geographic location. Which review courses are easily accessible? Are you considering traveling to another city to attend a review course? Collect data on all of the courses, then compare them to see which one best meets your needs and budget. Check with your prospective employer regarding time off and scheduling. Plan ahead and make an intelligent decision regarding review courses. Do not feel that you must sign up with the first review company that contacts you!

Carefully evaluate your need for a review course. Are you the type of student who can plan study time, establish a study review schedule, and stick to it? Were you in the top 25% of your graduating class? Have you had experience working in a hospital with adult medical–surgical patients, other than while you were in school? As a new graduate do you feel prepared for this examination? If you can answer yes to all of these questions, you may not want to consider a review course in your preparation for the NCLEX-RN. The majority of graduates are able to say yes to one or two of these questions, but not to all of them.

What Are the Qualifications of the Review Course Instructors? To teach a review course effectively, the instructor needs to be familiar with the NCLEX. That ability is most often found in instructors who have teaching experience in a school of nursing. Some hospitals provide in-house review courses taught by excellent educators and clinical specialists. Determine if these instructors are familiar with the NCLEX plan. Information that is not a focus of the NCLEX plan does not need to be included in a review course. It is also important to find out if the review course faculty are from a school of nursing in your immediate area. It is possible that you will be paying for a review course to be taught by someone from your nursing school faculty. A review course will be more effective if it is taught by someone with a different perspective. This helps to anchor information and reinforce previous learning. Look for a course that brings faculty in from areas outside your school.

What Type of Instructional Materials Are Used in the Course? Are the materials an additional course expense? Do you get to keep the materials after the course is over? Are handouts, workbooks, audiotapes, books, and other materials used to enhance learning? Be concerned if there are no course outlines, workbooks, handouts, or books; you might spend all of your time writing and miss listening to the necessary information. Do the course materials include practice test questions that are similar in format to the NCLEX? Ask about the format used to organize the material (e.g., integrated, blocked, systems). How does the format compare to the NCLEX plan of patient needs and nursing process that is described in your Candidate Bulletin from the National Council? These are all important questions to ask.

How Is the Course Taught? Are visuals used to enhance learning? Is the presentation given by a "live person"? Some courses may be given using videos and audiotapes rather than a person who will speak to you and answer your questions.

Does the Course Include Instruction in Test-Taking Skills and Practice? Test-taking skills and practice are a very important aspect of a review course. The graduate needs to begin to practice testing strategies and use them in answering questions written by someone other than their nursing school faculty.

How Much Does the Course Cost? Most review courses cost about $200 to $300. Frequently there is a discount for early registration, and there may also be a discount for group registration. Make sure you understand the review company policy regarding deposit and registration fees. Make sure you understand the cancellation policy. Some companies will let you pay a deposit, with the total amount due by a certain date. Check out the possibility of organizing a group; some courses give a free review or a discount to the group organizer.

How Long Does It Last? Is the course three, four, or five consecutive days? Is it given only in the evenings? Is it taught only on the weekend for six weeks? This is very important to determine early in your evaluation of review courses. Compare the price with the length of the course; are you getting your money's worth? Notify your employer as soon as possible if you need to fit the review into your work schedule. Most hospitals will arrange the new graduate's schedule to allow attendance at a review course. Some hospitals even provide a review course as a benefit to the new graduate nurse employee! Once you have determined which review course you wish to take, discuss it with your prospective employers or notify your current employer as soon as possible. It is important to provide adequate advance notice to your employer so that staffing schedules may be planned.

Where Is the Course Held? Are you going to have to drive for an hour every day? Will you need to obtain a hotel room? Ask about parking. What is the availability of inexpensive restaurants in the area? Is food going to be a major expense?

What Are the Statistics Regarding the Pass Rate for the Company? It is very appropriate to inquire about how the pass rate statistics are determined by the review company. Check the Web page for the NCSBN (http://www.ncsbn.org) to determine the most current statistics for passing the NCLEX. Appendix A has a listing of the Web addresses for the State Boards of Nursing. The review company must obtain the results directly from course participants or from schools of nursing. The National Council does not make this information available to the review companies. Find out whether the advertised pass rate is based on actual responses from participants or from projected figures from the company.

Does the Review Company Offer Any Type of Guarantee? Some review companies will offer you a free review course, further assistance, or a home study guide if you are not successful on the examination. Find out what the guarantee means and who is eligible for it. Make sure you get in writing what you must do to be eligible and to file for the benefit.

What Is the Size of the Class? Some review course classes will have several hundred participants. One problem resulting from a large class is that if you don't get there an hour early, you don't get a seat where you can see or hear. There are some review companies that limit the enrollment depending on the classroom environment. Ask about the size of the class and the classroom environment.

When Is the Course Offered? Some graduates prefer to take a review course just before the examination so that the information is still fresh in their minds. Most graduates prefer to take the review within 1 to 2 weeks before the examination. This time frame generally works very well; the review course is scheduled during the time you are waiting for your Authorization to Test. When you receive your authorization, you are ready to schedule the examination. This schedule allows time to organize and study those areas that are your weakest. If you have only one review course available, how does it fit with your plans for scheduling the examination? Another aspect to consider is your employment schedule. Can you get time off from work? If your employer will not give you the time off, you may need to take a review course as early in the day as possible so you can go to work. Try to arrange your review course time so you can focus on reviewing the information. If you have to work nights or evenings during the course, you will not benefit as much from the review.

Call the review company to get your questions answered. Do they spend time on the telephone with you, or are they in a rush to get you off the telephone? Ask what makes their course better than another course. Is the company representative friendly and knowledgeable, and does that person demonstrate concern for answering all of your questions?

Ultimately each graduate must decide whether to take a review course and which review course is right. The more informed you are regarding a review course, the more intelligent a decision you can make.

NCLEX-RN REVIEW BOOKS

Which One Is Right for You? It is important to select a review book that meets your study needs. The first step is to check out your choices. Nursing faculty, friends with review books, the school library, and the local nursing textbook stores are all sources of information regarding review books. There are two main kinds of nursing review books: those with content review and those that consist totally of review questions. Evaluate how the book will be used: is it for study during school or is it specifically for review for the NCLEX? For example, if you bought the review book to study pediatric nursing, you may be disappointed. The focus of the NCLEX is not on pediatrics; therefore, it is not often a strong component in review books. If you wish to use a review book to identify priority aspects of care in the medical-surgical patient, a review book can be of great benefit. The following discussion of review book selection is directed primarily toward review books that contain content review. Take notes as you read the different selections; it is hard to remember all the positive and negative points of each book (Box 24-3). Frequently students find the review books to be of great benefit during school in assisting them to organize and understand a large amount of information. Plan on purchasing a review book while you are still in nursing school. Review books are revised about every three years.

Do an Overview. Is the type style and size comfortable to read? Does the page layout enhance reading and finding information? Are there graphics, charts, or diagrams? Is the information outlined or is it narrative in style? Is it difficult to read a constant narrative text?

Scan the Table of Contents. Is the information presented in a logical sequence? How is the information organized? It is important that the information be organized in a manner that is logical to you. The NCLEX is based on an integrated format that uses the nursing process and patient needs. Read the introduction to see how these areas were considered in the organization of the text. Quickly scan the table of contents, and check the number of pages in various areas of subject material. What is the focus of the material?

Evaluate Chapter Layout. How well is the material organized within the chapter? Are there major headings and subheadings to assist you in finding information quickly? Some texts use two-toned shading, boxes, or a second color to highlight divisions of content or priority information. These may not be points you have identified in previous textbooks; however, these devices help to decrease the monotony of constant reading and to increase interest in the material presented.

Evaluate Content. Select a topic or topics you would like to read about in each of the review books you are considering. Select the priority nursing concepts and interventions you want to identify (e.g., nursing care of a patient with diabetes). Evaluate the information regarding the adult, pediatric, and obstetric patient. How does the information compare in the review books you are considering? Is the material logically organized? Does it contain the major concepts of care for that

---

BOX 24-3 Selecting a Review Book: Where Do I Start?

Here are some questions to consider:

Does the review course I am considering provide a review book? _____

What does the review book look like? _____

❑ Type style: is it easy to read? _____

❑ Outline or narrative format? _____

❑ Quality of the paper: does it bleed through when highlighted? _____

Is the table of contents helpful? _____

What is the organization pattern of the book? _____

Is the information blocked or integrated? _____

Is the primary focus on nursing care? _____

Are the high-priority areas easily identified and adequately covered? _____

Is there a comprehensive index? _____

How easy is the information to find and to understand? _____

Does it cover the priorities of nursing care? _____

Where are the medications, treatments, and diagnostics for each of these
  topics? _____

Are there test questions included in the content review book? _____

Are the questions at the end of each chapter? _____

Are the questions in a study guide format? _____

Are there sample tests to practice test-taking skills? _____

Are the sample tests integrated, blocked (pediatrics, obstetrics, medical), or
  reflective of previous chapter material? _____

Does the book include the correct answers and rationale for all of the test
  questions? _____

Is information repeated in different areas? _____

What is the focus of the content? _____

Test-taking strategies—are they included in the book and easy to understand?
  _____

---

particular example? The focus of the book should be toward nursing care, not medical diagnosis, pharmacology, or pathophysiology. In evaluating the currency of content, keep in mind that you can't expect information that came out last month to be reflected in any textbook. The focus of NCLEX is to evaluate entry-level nursing care that is common practice across the country. Remember, the NCLEX is more heavily weighted toward the medical-surgical patient.

Evaluate the Index. Take several common topics and look them up in the index. A good index is critical to finding information in a timely manner.

Test Questions. Are test questions included in the text? Questions may be found after each of the main chapters or grouped together at the end of the book. Check to see if a rationale for the correct answer is included for each question. Does a computer disk of questions come with the book? How many questions are on the disk? Are the computer questions different from the questions in the book? You may be expecting the disk to have new practice questions and it only has the questions that are in the book. If a computer disk of questions comes with the book, can the disk be used indefinitely, or does it disintegrate after so many uses?

Test-Taking Strategies. Does the book include information on test-taking strategies for multiple-choice questions? Test-taking strategies help you to be more "test wise." These strategies can be of great benefit while you are still in school, in addition to while you prepare for the NCLEX.

WHAT DIFFERENCE DO TEST-TAKING STRATEGIES MAKE?

Information on test-taking strategies can be of benefit to you now and later. Start putting into practice some of these tips, and they will be second nature when you take the NCLEX.

Knowing how to take an examination is a skill that is developed through practice. Look back at the beginning of nursing school and your first nursing examination—have you come a long way from there! How many times during school have you reviewed a test and discovered you knew the right answer, but marked the wrong one? Nursing faculty and those responsible for the NCLEX are not sympathetic to your claim that you "really meant this answer and not the one I marked." How many times did you go back and change an answer from the correct response to the wrong one? If these are common errors you experienced during nursing school, you need to incorporate testing strategies into your testing skills. Some of the testing practices you have developed over the years may be positive, some may be negative. Take the time to implement good testing practices—get the question right the first time! Analyze where you are with testing skills, get rid of the negative, and retain the positive.

NCLEX Testing Tips

NCLEX Hospital. For this examination to be appropriate to all candidates nationwide, it is important that there be a base for the vast knowledge that is to be tested. Therefore, when you are taking the NCLEX, consider yourself working in the NCLEX Hospital. It is a great place to work—everything works like it is supposed to, great equipment, plenty of staff and the best nursing care possible. The patients all have conditions that respond just like the book says they are supposed to respond. Study according to your textbooks. Your clinical experience is complementary to your academic study. Do not focus on the unusual, unexpected, or strange things that happened to you during clinical rotations.

NCLEX Patients. Focus on the patient in the question you are working on. As far as the NCLEX Hospital is concerned, that is the only patient you are to be concerned about. Do not worry about the 5 or 6 other patients you may have assigned to your care, in the NCLEX Hospital you are taking care of one patient at a time. Your priority concern is the patient in the current question you are trying to answer.

Medication Administration. Know the five rights and the common nursing implications of medications. Most of the time both the trade name and generic name are provided in the question. A good strategy is to study the medications according to the classification. What are the nursing implications regarding administration of corticosteroid medications?

Calling for Assistance. Be careful in questions that the right answer appears to be to call someone else to take care of the problem. This is a nursing examination; therefore, identify the best nursing management. This includes questions that include calling the doctor, respiratory therapist, housekeeping, chaplain, social worker, etc. Make sure there is not something you need to do for the patient before notifying someone else regarding the problem. If the patient is experiencing difficulty, his condition is changing and there is nothing you can do, then call the doctor. This is particularly true in situations in which the patient is experiencing a problem with impaired circulation.

Positioning. Watch questions that have particular positions in the stem of the question, or include positions in the options. Is the patient's position necessary to prevent complications, treat a current problem, or is it primarily for comfort? As you are reviewing, watch the questions that include conditions that require a specific position in the care of that patient.

Delegation and Supervision. The NCLEX will contain questions in these areas. Some common considerations to make when evaluating these questions:

- Do not delegate the steps of the nursing process.
- Delegate to someone else the most stable patient with the most predictable response to care.
- Do not delegate teaching or evaluating responsibilities.
- Delegate those tasks that have the most specific guidelines—collecting a urine sample, feeding, providing hygiene, ambulating, etc.

Setting Priorities. Determine the most unstable patient who requires nursing care to prevent immediate complications—take care of this patient first. Keep in mind the steps of the nursing process (assessment is first), and Maslow's hierarchy of needs (breathing is first).

Doctor's orders. Most often when an option is presented that requires a doctor's order; there is already a doctor's order for the action. If the question states "a dependent nursing action . . . " or "the nurse would initiate what action . . . ," then consider the possibility of whether or not you need a physician's order for the activity.

Be aware—the expected answer you are looking for may not be included in the options! This is not uncommon on NCLEX questions. Consider the principles and concepts of care for a patient with the problem presented.

TEST ANXIETY—WHAT IS THE DISEASE? HOW DO YOU GET RID OF IT?

Frequently students and graduates focus on their "test anxiety" as the reason for not doing well on examinations. Test anxiety is something that only you can change. You are the one allowing the anxiety to affect you in a negative way. The only person responsible for your test anxiety is you, and the only one who can do anything about it is you. Look at some simple steps to decrease your anxiety regarding testing.

- Plan ahead. Don't wait till the last minute to read the 150 pages in your textbook, review all your classroom notes, and read the 10 articles assigned for the test. Plan study time and stick to it!
- Set aside study time for when you are at your best. Frequently, study time is scheduled at a time when everything else (laundry, meals, housecleaning, yard work, and so on) is completed. You are defeating your purpose and increasing your anxiety when you try to study at a time when you are tired and not receptive to learning.
- Give yourself a break! Plan your study time to include a break about every hour. Your retention of information begins to decrease after about 30 minutes and is significantly decreased after an hour.
- Think Positively! If your friends are "negative thinkers," don't plan on studying with them. Go to the movies or play sports with them, but don't study with them. Anxiety and negative thinking are contagious—don't expose yourself to the disease!
- Don't cram. The NCLEX is not written to evaluate memory-based information. Test questions focus on the application of principles and the analysis of information to determine an appropriate nursing response or action (Hertz et al, 2000). Don't jeopardize your critical-thinking skills by staying up late and cramming.

Just thinking about an examination can cause some students an increase in anxiety. It seems as though during the last year of school, particularly the last semester, tests become a major source of anxiety. Everyone knows fellow students who become obsessed with the idea that they are going to fail an important examination. It is essential that examinations be viewed in a positive manner—get rid of those negative thought "tapes"! Put yourself in charge of your feelings. Replace those negative thoughts and ideas with positive ones: "I will pass this test." Write down positive affirmations and put them on your bathroom mirror, on your refrigerator, anywhere you will see them often. Potential employers, state boards of nursing, your spiritual advisers, and your neighbors are not going to think less of you if you are not at the top of the class. Keep in mind that your employers and the state boards do not care what your grades were in school or on the NCLEX—they just want to know that you can pass the NCLEX and practice nursing safely. Give yourself permission to be in the middle—an average student on grades, but one who is concerned about professional, safe nursing practice.

WHAT ARE STRATEGIES FOR ANSWERING MULTIPLE-CHOICE QUESTIONS?

On the NCLEX, multiple-choice test questions have a stem in which the question is presented and four options from which to choose an answer. Of these four options, three are meant to distract you from the correct answer. There is only one correct answer. The majority of NCLEX questions will be multiple-choice questions in which the options give you the choice of four answers, not a combination of the four options (e.g., 1. A, B, C).

Read the Question (Stem) Carefully. Do *not* read extra meaning into the question. Make sure you read the stem correctly and understand exactly what information is being requested (do you tend to make the patient sicker than he really is by the time you finish the question?).

Create a Pool of Information. What do you anticipate the answer to include? What are the concepts of care regarding a patient with the condition or problem presented? Get a general idea before you read the options.

Evaluate All the Options in a Systematic Manner. Focus on what information is being requested, then carefully go through each option. Do not stop with the first correct answer; the last option may be more correct or more inclusive of information.

Eliminate Options You Know Are Not Correct. And leave them alone! Once you have eliminated an option, don't go back to it unless you have gained more insight into the question. Frequently your initial response to a question is correct.

Identify Similarities in the Options. Find the one that is different. The option that is different may be the correct answer. For example, in a question dealing with a low-residue diet, three of the options might contain a vegetable with a peeling, but one might not—that one is probably the correct answer. Evaluate options that contain several suggested patient activities; are the activities similar, but with one that is different?

Evaluate Priority Questions Very Carefully. Keep in mind the nursing process and Maslow's hierarchy of needs. You must obtain adequate assessment information before proceeding with the nursing process. According to Maslow, physical needs must be met before psychosocial needs—your mental health patient must have basic physical needs met before you can focus on the mental health needs. When considering the physical needs, respiratory needs are a priority. (You've got to breathe first!)

Select Answers that Focus on the Patient. Choices that focus on hospital rules and policies are most often not correct.

Analyze your testing skills so that you will know where to start to improve them. Once you have identified your testing weaknesses, organize a plan to correct the problem areas. One of the most difficult things to do is to change the way you are used to doing something, even when it makes life easier. Get an early start on evaluating testing skills; it can make a significant difference in the remaining examinations in nursing school.

Wow! NCLEX deadlines, review courses, testing skills, review books, money, license . . . and all you thought you needed to do was graduate from nursing school! There are a lot of steps in between graduating from nursing school and being successful on the NCLEX. The key to surviving it all with a smile is careful planning and implementing those plans during your role transition. (That sounds a lot like the nursing process, doesn't it?) The NCLEX-RN is one of the most incredible opportunities of your life. This examination will open the doors for you as you begin one of the most fantastic experiences of a lifetime: a career in nursing.

 Just say to yourself "I can do it . . . I can pass NCLEX!

REFERENCES

Hertz JE et al: *1999 practice analysis of newly licensed registered nurses in the United States*, Chicago, 2000, NCSBN.

National Council of State Boards of Nursing, Inc: *NCLEX Candidate Bulletin*, Chicago, 2002, NCSBN.

National Council of State Boards of Nursing, Inc: *Issues* 20(4), 1999.

National Council of State Boards of Nursing, Inc: *Collected Works, 2002.* Accessed Sept. 10, 2002. Available at http://www. ncsbn.org.

National Council of State Boards of Nursing, Inc: *Recent News Releases: NCSBN Welcomes Two More States to the Nurse Licensure Compact.* Available at http://www.ncsbn.org.

Zerwekh J: *A Delphi study of factors influencing nursing students to enroll in review courses* (dissertation), East Texas State University, 1986.

ADDITIONAL READINGS

National Council of State Boards of Nursing, Inc: *Introduction to computerized adaptive testing (CAT) for NCLEX* (video), Chicago, 1992, NCSBN.

Rayfield S: *NCLEX-RN 101: how to pass*, ed 3, Shreveport, La, 1998, ICAN.

Zerwekh J: Evaluating multiple choice questions, *Healthc Trends Transit* 16-17, 1994.

Zerwekh J: Which NCLEX book is best? *Graduating Nurse*, Spring, 22-24.

Zerwekh J: Selecting a review course, *Health Trends Transit* 18-21, 1994.

Zerwekh J, Claborn JC: *NCLEX-RN: a comprehensive study guide*, ed 5, Dallas, 2002, Nursing Education Consultants.

INTERNET RESOURCES

Nursing Education Consultants, Inc.
http://www.nursinged.com

NCSBN student Web area
http://www.nclex.com

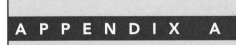
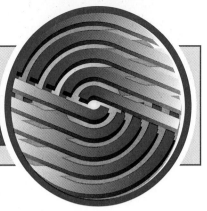

Contact Information and Web Sites

Alabama Board of Nursing
770 Washington Avenue
RSA Plaza, Suite 250
Montgomery, AL 36130-3900
Phone: 334-242-4060
Fax: 334-242-4360
Contact Person: N. Genell Lee, MSN, JD, RN, Executive Officer
Web Site: http://www.abn.state.al.us

Alaska Board of Nursing
Department of Community & Economic Development
Division of Occupational Licensing
3601 C Street, Suite 722
Anchorage, AK 99503
Phone: 907-269-8161
Fax: 907-269-8196
Contact Person: Dorothy Fulton, MA, RN, Executive Director
Web Site: http://www.dced.state.ak.us/occpnur.htm

American Samoa Health Services
Regulatory Board
LBJ Tropical Medical Center
Pago Pago, AUSTRALIA 96799
Phone: 684-633-1222
Fax: 684-633-1869
Contact Person: Etenauga Lutu, RN, Executive Secretary

Arizona State Board of Nursing
1651 E. Morten Avenue, Suite 210
Phoenix, AZ 85020-4313
Phone: 602-331-8111
Fax: 602-906-9365
Contact Person: Joey Ridenour, MN, RN, Executive Director
Web Site: http://www.azboardofnursing.org

Information retreived from National Council State Board of Nursing's Web site: http://www.ncsbn.org/public/regulation/boards_of_nursing_board.htm. Accessed Sept. 5, 2002.

Arkansas State Board of Nursing
University Tower Building
1123 S. University, Suite 800
Little Rock, AR 72204-1619
Phone: 501-686-2700
Fax: 501-686-2714
Contact Person: Faith Fields, MSN, RN, Executive Director
Web Site: http://www.arsbn.org

California Board of Registered Nursing
400 R Street, Suite 4030
P.O. Box 944210
Sacramento, CA 94244-2100
Phone: 916-322-3350
Fax: 916-327-4402
Contact Person: Ruth Ann Terry, MPH, RN, Executive Officer
Web Site: http://www.rn.ca.gov

California Board of Vocational Nurse and Psychiatric Technician Examiners
2535 Capitol Oaks Drive, Suite 205
Sacramento, CA 95833
Phone: 916-263-7800
Fax: 916-263-7859
Contact Person: Teresa Bello-Jones, JD, MSN, RN, Executive Officer
Web Site: http://www.bvnpt.ca.gov

Colorado Board of Nursing
1560 Broadway, Suite 880
Denver, CO 80202
Phone: 303-894-2430
Fax: 303-894-2821
Contact Person: Patricia Uris, PhD, RN, Program Administrator
Web Site: http://www.dora.state.co.us/nursing

Connecticut Board of Examiners for Nursing
Dept. of Public Health
410 Capitol Avenue, MS# 13PHO
P.O. Box 340308
Hartford, CT 06134-0328
Phone: 860-509-7624
Fax: 860-509-7553
Contact Person: Jan Wojick, Board Liaison
Web Site: http://www.state.ct.us/dph

Delaware Board of Nursing
861 Silver Lake Blvd
Cannon Building, Suite 203
Dover, DE 19904
Phone: 302-739-4522
Fax: 302-739-2711
Contact Person: Iva Boardman, MSN, RN, Executive Director

District of Columbia Board of Nursing
Department of Health
825 N. Capitol Street NE, 2nd Floor
Room 2224
Washington, DC 20002
Phone: 202-442-4778
Fax: 202-442-9431
Contact Person: Bonnie Rampersaud, Acting Program Manager for Program Licensing

Florida Board of Nursing
Capital Circle Officer Center
4052 Bald Cypress Way, Room 120
Tallahassee, FL 32399-3252
Phone: 850-488-0595
Contact Person: Dan Coble, RN, PhD, Executive Director
Web Site: http://www.doh.state.fl.us/mqa

Georgia State Board of Licensed Practical Nurses
237 Coliseum Drive
Macon, GA 31217-3858
Phone: 478-207-1300
Fax: 478-207-1633
Contact Person: Jacqueline Hightower, JD, Executive Director
Web Site: http://www.sos.state.ga.us/ebd-lpn

Georgia Board of Nursing
237 Coliseum Drive
Macon, GA 31217-3858
Phone: 478-207-1640
Fax: 478-207-1660
Contact Person: Shirley Camp, BSN, JD, RN, Executive Director
Web Site: http://www.sos.state.ga.us/ebd-rn

Guam Board of Nurse Examiners
P.O. Box 2816
1304 East Sunset Boulevard
Barrgada, GU 96913
Phone: 671-475-0251
Fax: 671-477-4733

Hawaii Board of Nursing
Professional & Vocational Licensing Division
P.O. Box 3469
Honolulu, HI 96801
Phone: 808-586-3000
Fax: 808-586-2689
Contact Person: Kathleen Yokouchi-Tokumoto, MBA, BBA, BA, Executive Officer
Web Site: http://www.state.hi.us/dcca/pvl/areas_nurse.html

Idaho Board of Nursing
280 N. 8th Street, Suite 210
P.O. Box 83720
Boise, ID 83720
Phone: 208-334-3110
Fax: 208-334-3262
Contact Person: Sandra Evans, MA, EdD, RN, Executive Director
Web Site: http://www.state.id.us/ibn/ibnhome.htm

Illinois Department of Professional Regulation
James R. Thompson Center
100 West Randolph, Suite 9-300
Chicago, IL 60601
Phone: 312-814-2715
Fax: 312-814-3145
Contact Person: Deborah Taylor, RN, Ed.D Nursing Act Assistant Coordinator
Web Site: http://www.dpr.state.il.us

Illinois Department of Professional Regulation
320 W. Washington St.
3rd Floor
Springfield, IL 62786
Phone: 217-782-8556
Fax: 217-782-7645

Indiana State Board of Nursing
Health Professions Bureau
402 W. Washington Street, Room W041
Indianapolis, IN 46204
Phone: 317-234-2043
Fax: 317-233-4236
Contact Person: Kristen Kelley, Director of Nursing of IN BON
Web Site: http://www.state.in.us/hpb/boards/isbn

Iowa Board of Nursing
RiverPoint Business Park
400 SW 8th Street, Suite B
Des Moines, IA 50309-4685
Phone: 515-281-3255
Fax: 515-281-4825
Contact Person: Lorinda Inman, MSN, RN, Executive Director
Web Site: http://www.state.ia.us/government/nursing

Kansas State Board of Nursing
Landon State Office Building
900 SW Jackson, Suite 551-S
Topeka, KS 66612
Phone: 785-296-4929
Fax: 785-296-3929
Contact Person: Mary Blubaugh, MSN, RN, Executive Administrator
Web Site: http://www.ksbn.org

Kentucky Board of Nursing
312 Whittington Parkway, Suite 300
Louisville, KY 40222
Phone: 502-329-7000
Fax: 502-329-7011
Contact Person: Sharon Weisenbeck, MS, RN, Executive Director
Web Site: http://www.kbn.state.ky.us

Louisiana State Board of Practical Nurse Examiners
3421 N. Causeway Boulevard, Suite 203
Metairie, LA 70002
Phone: 504-838-5791
Fax: 504-838-5279
Contact Person: Claire Glaviano, BSN, MN, RN, Executive Director
Web Site: http://www.lsbpne.com

Louisiana State Board of Nursing
3510 N. Causeway Boulevard, Suite 501
Metairie, LA 70002
Phone: 504-838-5332
Fax: 504-838-5349
Contact Person: Barbara Morvant, MN, RN, Executive Director
Web Site: http://www.lsbn.state.la.us

Maine State Board of Nursing
158 State House Station
Augusta, ME 04333
Phone: 207-287-1133
Fax: 207-287-1149
Contact Person: Myra Broadway, JD, MS, RN, Executive Director
Web Site: http://www.state.me.us/boardofnursing

Maryland Board of Nursing
4140 Patterson Avenue
Baltimore, MD 21215
Phone: 410-585-1900
Fax: 410-358-3530
Contact Person: Donna Dorsey, MS, RN, Executive Director
Web Site: http://www.mbon.org

Massachusetts Board of Registration in Nursing
Commonwealth of Massachusetts
239 Causeway Street
Boston, MA 02114
Phone: 617-727-9961
Fax: 617-727-1630
Contact Person: Theresa Bonanno, MSN, RN, Executive Director
Web Site: http://www.state.ma.us/reg/boards/rn

Michigan CIS/Office of Health Services
Ottawa Towers North
611 W. Ottawa, 4th Floor
Lansing, MI 48933
Phone: 517-373-9102
Fax: 517-373-2179
Contact Person: Diane Lewis, Policy Manager for Licensing Division
Web Site: http://www.cis.state.mi.us/bhser/genover.htm

Minnesota Board of Nursing
2829 University Avenue SE
Suite 500
Minneapolis, MN 55414
Phone: 612-617-2270
Fax: 612-617-2190
Contact Person: Shirley Brekken, MS, RN,
    Executive Director
Web Site: http://www.nursingboard.state.
    mn.us

Mississippi Board of Nursing
1935 Lakeland Drive, Suite B
Jackson, MS 39216-5014
Phone: 601-987-4188
Fax: 601-364-2352
Contact Person: Marcia Rachel, PhD, RN,
    Executive Director
Web Site: http://www.msbn.state.ms.us

Missouri State Board of Nursing
3605 Missouri Blvd.
P.O. Box 656
Jefferson City, MO 65102-0656
Phone: 573-751-0681
Fax: 573-751-0075
Contact Person: Lori Scheidt, BS, Acting
    Executive Director
Web Site: http://www.ecodev.state.mo.us/
    pr/nursing

Montana State Board of Nursing
301 South Park
P.O. Box 200513
Helena, MT 59620-0513
Phone: 406-841-2340
Fax: 406-841-2343
Contact Person: Barbara Swehla, MN, RN,
    Executive Director
Web Site: http://www.discoveringmontana.
    com/dli/bsd/license/bsd_boards/nur_boar
    d/board_page.htm

Commonwealth Board of Nurse Examiners
P.O. Box 501458
Saipan, MP 96950
Phone: 670-664-4810
Fax: 670-664-4813
Contact Person: Elizabeth Torres-Untalan,
    RN, Chairperson

Nebraska Health and Human Services System
Dept. of Regulation & Licensure, Nursing
    Section
301 Centennial Mall South
Lincoln, NE 68509-4986
Phone: 402-471-4376
Fax: 402-471-3577
Contact Person: Charlene Kelly, PhD, RN,
    Executive Director
Nursing and Nursing Support Web Site:
    http://www.hhs.state.ne.us/crl/
    nursingindex.htm
Nebraska Center for Nursing: http://www.
    center4nursing.org

Nevada State Board of Nursing
Administration, Discipline & Investigations
1755 East Plumb Lane
Suite 260
Reno, NV 89502
Phone: 775-688-2620
Fax: 775-688-2628
Contact Person: Debra Scott, MS, RN,
    Executive Director
Web Site: http://www.nursingboard.state.nv.us

Nevada State Board of Nursing
License Certification and Education
4330 S. Valley View Blvd.
Suite 106
Las Vegas, NV 89103
Phone: 702-486-5800
Fax: 702)-486-5803
Contact Person: Don Rennie MS, RN,
    Associate Executive Director for Licensure
    & Certification
Web Site: http://www.nursingboard.state.nv.us

New Hampshire Board of Nursing
P.O. Box 3898
78 Regional Drive, BLDG B
Concord, NH 03302
Phone: 603-271-2323
Fax: 603-271-6605
Contact Person: Cynthia Gray, MBA, BS, RN, CPN, Executive Director
Web Site: http://www.state.nh.us/nursing

New Jersey Board of Nursing
P.O. Box 45010
124 Halsey Street, 6th Floor
Newark, NJ 07101
Phone: 973-504-6586
Fax: 973-648-3481
Contact Person: Patricia Lynch Polansky, MS, RN, Executive Director
Web Site: http://www.state.nj.us/lps/ca/medical.htm

New Mexico Board of Nursing
4206 Louisiana Boulevard, NE
Suite A
Albuquerque, NM 87109
Phone: 505-841-8340
Fax: 505-841-8347
Contact Person: Debra Brady, PhD, RN, Executive Director
Web Site: http://www.state.nm.us/clients/nursing

New York State Board of Nursing
Education Bldg.
89 Washington Avenue
2nd Floor West Wing
Albany, NY 12234
Phone: 518-474-3817, ext. 120
Fax: 518-474-3706
Contact Person: Barbara Zittel, PhD, RN, Executive Secretary
Web Site: http://www.nysed.gov/prof/nurse.htm

North Carolina Board of Nursing
3724 National Drive, Suite 201
Raleigh, NC 27612
Phone: 919-782-3211
Fax: 919-781-9461
Contact Person: Polly Johnson, MSN, RN, Executive Director
Web Site: http://www.ncbon.com

North Dakota Board of Nursing
919 South 7th Street, Suite 504
Bismarck, ND 58504
Phone: 701-328-9777
Fax: 701-328-9785
Contact Person: Constance Kalanek, PhD, RN, Executive Director
Web Site: http://www.ndbon.org

Ohio Board of Nursing
17 South High Street, Suite 400
Columbus, OH 43215-3413
Phone: 614-466-3947
Fax: 614-466-0388
Contact Person: Janice Lanier, RN, JD, Interim Executive Director
Web Site: http://www.state.oh.us/nur

Oklahoma Board of Nursing
2915 N. Classen Boulevard, Suite 524
Oklahoma City, OK 73106
Phone: 405-962-1800
Fax: 405-962-1821
Contact Person: Kimberly Glazier, M.Ed., RN, Executive Director
Web Site: http://www.youroklahoma.com/nursing

Oregon State Board of Nursing
800 NE Oregon Street, Box 25
Suite 465
Portland, OR 97232
Phone: 503-731-4745
Fax: 503-731-4755
Contact Person: Joan Bouchard, MN, RN, Executive Director
Web Site: http://www.osbn.state.or.us

Pennsylvania State Board of Nursing
124 Pine Street
Harrisburg, PA 17101
Phone: 717-783-7142
Fax: 717-783-0822
Contact Person: Miriam Limo, MS, MSN, RN, Executive Secretary
Web Site: http://www.dos.state.pa.us/bpoa/nurbd/mainpage.htm

Commonwealth of Puerto Rico Board of Nurse Examiners
800 Roberto H. Todd Avenue
Room 202, Stop 18
Santurce, PR 00908
Phone: 787-725-7506
Fax: 787-725-7903
Contact Person: Magda Bouet, Executive Director of the Office of Regulations and Certifications of Health Care Professions

Rhode Island Board of Nurse Registration and Nursing Education
105 Cannon Building
Three Capitol Hill
Providence, RI 02908
Phone: 401-222-5700
Fax: 401-222-3352
Contact Person: Charles Alexandre, MSN, RN, Executive Officer
Web Site: http://www.health.state.ri.us

South Carolina State Board of Nursing
110 Centerview Drive
Suite 202
Columbia, SC 29210
Phone: 803-896-4550
Fax: 803-896-4525
Contact Person: Martha Bursinger, RN, MSN, Executive Director
Web Site: http://www.llr.state.sc.us/pol/nursing

South Dakota Board of Nursing
4300 South Louise Ave., Suite C-1
Sioux Falls, SD 57106-3124
Phone: 605-362-2760
Fax: 605-362-2768
Contact Person: Diana Vander Woude, MS, RN, Executive Secretary
Web Site: http://www.state.sd.us/dcr/nursing

Tennessee State Board of Nursing
426 Fifth Avenue North
1st Floor, Cordell Hull Building
Nashville, TN 37247
Phone: 615-532-5166
Fax: 615-741-7899
Contact Person: Elizabeth Lund, MSN, RN, Executive Director
Web Site: http://170.142.76.180/bmf-bin/BMFproflist.pl

Texas Board of Nurse Examiners
333 Guadalupe, Suite 3-460
Austin, TX 78701
Phone: 512-305-7400
Fax: 512-305-7401
Contact Person: Katherine Thomas, MN, RN, Executive Director
Web Site: http://www.bne.state.tx.us

Texas Board of Vocational Nurse Examiners
William P. Hobby Building, Tower 3
333 Guadalupe Street, Suite 3-400
Austin, TX 78701
Phone: 512-305-8100
Fax: 512-305-8101
Contact Person: Terrie Hairston, RN, CHE, Executive Director
Web Site: http://www.bvne.state.tx.us

Utah State Board of Nursing
Heber M. Wells Bldg., 4th Floor
160 East 300 South
Salt Lake City, UT 84111
Phone: 801-530-6628
Fax: 801-530-6511
Contact Person: Laura Poe, MS, RN,
Executive Administrator
Web Site: http://www.commerce.state.ut.us

Vermont State Board of Nursing
109 State Street
Montpelier, VT 05609-1106
Phone: 802-828-2396
Fax: 802-828-2484
Contact Person: Anita Ristau, MS, RN,
Executive Director
Web Site: http://vtprofessionals.org/nurses

Virgin Islands Board of Nurse Licensure
Veterans Drive Station
St. Thomas, VI 00803
Phone: 340-776-7397
Fax: 340-777-4003
Contact Person: Winifred Garfield, CRNA,
RN, Executive Secretary

Virginia Board of Nursing
6606 W. Broad Street, 4th Floor
Richmond, VA 23230
Phone: 804-662-9909
Fax: 804-662-9512
Contact Person: Nancy Durrett, MSN, RN,
Executive Director
Web Site: http://www.dhp.state.va.us

Washington State Nursing Care Quality Assurance Commission
Department of Health
1300 Quince Street SE
Olympia, WA 98504-7864
Phone: 360-236-4700
Fax: 360-236-4738
Contact Person: Paula Meyer, MSN, RN,
Executive Director
Web Site: http://www.doh.wa.gov/nursing

West Virginia Board of Examiners for Licensed Practical Nurses
101 Dee Drive
Charleston, WV 25311
Phone: 304-558-3572
Fax: 304-558-4367
Contact Person: Lanette Anderson, RN,
BSN, JD, Executive Secretary
Web Site: http://www.lpnboard.state.wv.us/

West Virginia Board of Examiners for Registered Professional Nurses
101 Dee Drive
Charleston, WV 25311
Phone: 304-558-3596
Fax: 304-558-3666
Contact Person: Laura Rhodes, MSN, RN,
Executive Director
Web Site: http://www.state.wv.us/nurses/rn

Wisconsin Department of Regulation and Licensing
1400 E. Washington Avenue
P.O. Box 8935
Madison, WI 53708
Phone: 608-266-0145
Fax: 608-261-7083
Contact Person: Kimberly Nania, Director,
Bureau of Health Service Professions
Web Site: http://www.drl.state.wi.us

Wyoming State Board of Nursing
2020 Carey Avenue, Suite 110
Cheyenne, WY 82002
Phone: 307-777-7601
Fax: 307-777-3519
Contact Person: Cheryl Lynn Koski, MS,
RN, CS, Executive Director
Web Site: http://nursing.state.wy.us

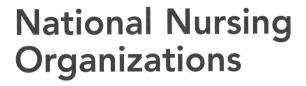

National Nursing Organizations

Academy of Medical-Surgical Nurses
E. Holly Avenue, Box 56
Pitman, NJ 08071-0056
Phone: 856-256-2323
Fax: 856-589-7463
E-mail: amsn@ajj.com
Web Site: http://amsn.inurse.com

Air & Surface Transport Nurses Association
915 Lee Street
Des Plaines, IL 60016-6569
Phone: 847-460-1170
Fax: 847-460-4001
E-mail: executive-director@astna.org
Web Site: http://www.astna.org

American Academy of Ambulatory Care Nursing
E. Holly Avenue, Box 56
Pitman, NJ 08071-0056
Phone: 800-262-6877
Fax: 856-589-7463
E-mail: aaacn@ajj.com
Web Site: http://aacn.inurse.com

American Academy of Nurse Practitioners
P.O. Box 12846
Austin, TX 78711
Phone: 512-442-4262
Fax: 512-442-6469
E-mail: admin@aanp.org
Web Site: http://www.aanp.org

American Academy of Nursing
600 Maryland Avenue, SW
Suite 100 West
Washington, DC 20024-2571
Phone: 202-651-7238
Fax: 202-554-2641
E-mail: tgaffney@ana.org
Web Site: http://www.nursingworld.org/aan

American Assembly for Men in Nursing
c/o NYSNA, 11 Cornell Road
Latham, NY 12110-1499
Phone: 518-782-9400, ext. 346
E-mail: aamn@aamn.org
Web Site: http://www.aamn.org

American Association for the History of Nursing, Inc.
P.O. Box 175
Lanoka Harbor, NJ 08734
Phone: 609-693-7250
Fax: 609-693-1037
E-mail: aahn@aahn.org
Web Site: http://www.aahn.org

American Association of Colleges of Nursing
1 Dupont Circle, NW, Suite 530
Washington, DC 20036
Phone: 202-463-6930
Fax: 202-785-8320
E-mail: webmaster@aacn.nche.edu
Web Site: http://www.aacn.nche.edu

American Association of Critical Care Nurses
101 Columbia
Aliso Viejo, CA 92656-1491
Phone: 800-899-2226
Fax: 949-362-2020
E-mail: info@aacn.org
Web Site: http://www.aacn.org

American Association of Diabetes Educators
100 W. Monroe Street, 4th Floor
Chicago, IL 60603-1901
Phone: 312-424-2426
Fax: 312-424-2427
E-mail: aade@aadenet.org
Web Site: http://www.aadenet.org

American Association of Legal Nurse Consultants
4700 W. Lake Avenue
Glenview, IL 60025
Phone: 877-402-2562
Fax: 847-375-6313
E-mail: info@aalnc.org
Web Site: http://www.aalnc.org

The American Association of Managed Care Nurses, Inc.
P.O. Box 4975
Glen Allen, VA 23058-4975
Phone: 804-747-9698
Fax: 804-747-5316
E-mail: sreed@aamcn.org
Web Site: http://www.aacmcn.org

American Association of Neuroscience Nurses
4700 W. Lake Avenue
Glenview, IL 60025-1485
Phone: 847-375-4733
Fax: 847-375-6333
E-mail: aann@aann.org
Web Site: http://www.aann.org

American Association of Nurse Anesthetists
222 S. Prospect Avenue
Park Ridge, IL 60068-4001
Phone: 847-692-7050
Fax: 847-692-6968
E-mail: info@aana.com
Web Site: http://www.aana.com

The American Association of Nurse Attorneys
7794 Grow Drive
Pensacola, FL 32514
Phone: 850-474-3646
Fax: 850-484-8762
Web Site: http://www.taana.org

American Association of Occupational Health Nurses, Inc.
2920 Brandywine Road, Suite 100
Atlanta, GA 30341
Phone: 770-455-7757
Fax: 770-455-7271
E-mail: aaohn@aaohn.org
Web Site: http://www.aaohn.org

American Association of Office Nurses
109 Kinderkamack Road
Montvale, NJ 07645
Phone: 800-457-7504
Fax: 201-573-8543
E-mail: aaonmail@aaon.org
Web Site: http://www.aaon.org

American Association of Spinal Cord Injury Nurses
75-20 Astoria Boulevard
Jackson Heights, NY 11370
Phone: 718-803-3782
Fax: 718-803-0414
E-mail: info@epva.org
Web Site: http://www.aascin.org

American Board of Nursing Specialties
4035 Running Springs
San Antonio, TX 78261
Phone/Fax: 830-438-4897
E-mail: abns@h-r-s.org
Web Site: http://www.nursingcertification.org

American College of Nurse Practitioners
503 Capitol Court, NE, #300
Washington, DC 20002
Phone: 202-546-4825
Fax: 202-546-4797
E-mail: acnp@nurse.org
Web Site: http://www.nurse.org/acnp

American Holistic Nurses Association
P.O. Box 2130
Flagstaff, AZ 86003-2130
Phone: 800-278-2462
Fax: 520-526-2752
E-mail: ahna-flag@flaglink.com
Web Site: http://www.ahna.org

American Long Term & Sub Acute Nurses Association
P.O. Box 1304
Toms River, NJ 08753
Phone: 732-573-0839
E-mail: ALSNA@aol.com
Web Site: http://www.alsna.com

American Nephrology Nurses' Association
E. Holly Avenue, Box 56
Pitman, NJ 08071-0056
Phone: 888-600-2662
Fax: 856-589-7463
E-mail: anna@ajj.com
Web Site: http://www.annanurse.org

American Nurses Association
600 Maryland Avenue, SW, Suite 100 West
Washington, DC 20024
Phone: 800-274-4262
Fax: 202-651-7001
Web Site: http://www.nusringworld.org

American Organization of Nurse Executives
1 N. Franklin
Chicago, IL 60606
Phone: 312-422-2800
Fax: 312-422-4503
E-mail: aone@aha.org
Web Site: http://www.aone.org

American Psychiatric Nurses Association
1200 19th Street, NW, Suite 300
Washington, DC 20036-2401
Phone: 202-857-1133
Fax: 202-857-1102
E-mail: info@apna.org
Web Site: http://www.apna.org

American Radiological Nurses Association
7794 Grow Drive
Pensacola, FL 32514
Phone: 866-486-ARNA (2762); 850-474-7292
Fax: 850-484-8762
E-mail: arna@puetzamc.com
Web Site: http://www.arna.net

American Society for Long-Term Care Nurses
660 Lonely Cottage Drive
Upper Black Eddy, PA 18972-9313
Phone: 610-847-5396
Fax: 610-847-5063

American Society of Pain Management Nurses
7794 Grow Drive
Pensacola, FL 32514
Phone: 888-342-7766
Fax: 850-484-8762
E-mail: aspmn@puetzamc.com
Web Site: http://www.aspmn.org

American Society of PeriAnesthesia Nurses
10 Melrose Avenue, Suite 110
Cherry Hill, NJ 08003-3696
Phone: 877-737-9696
Fax: 856-616-9601
E-mail: aspan@aspan.org
Web Site: http://www.aspan.org

American Society of Plastic and Reconstructive Surgical Nurses
E. Holly Avenue, Box 56
Pitman, NJ 08071-0056
Phone: 856-256-2340
Fax: 856-589-7463
E-mail: asprsn@mail.ajj.com
Web Site: http://www.asprsn.org

Association for Professionals in Infection Control and Epidemiology, Inc.
1275 K Street, NW, Suite 1000
Washington, DC 20005-4006
Phone: 202-789-1890
Fax: 202-789-1899
E-mail: apicinfo@apic.org
Web Site: http://www.apic.org

Association of Nurses in AIDS Care
11250 Roger Bacon Drive, Suite 8
Reston, VA 20190-5202
Phone: 800-260-6780
Fax: 703-435-4390
E-mail: aidsnurses@aol.com
Web Site: http://www.anacnet.org

Association of Pediatric Oncology Nurses
4700 W. Lake Avenue
Glenview, IL 60025
Phone: 847-375-4724
Fax: 847-375-6324
E-mail: info@apon.org
Web Site: http://www.apon.org

Association of Perioperative Registered Nurses
2170 S. Parker Road, Suite 300
Denver, CO 80231-5711
Phone: 800-755-2676 or 303-755-6300
Web Site: http://www.aorn.org

Association of Rehabilitation Nurses
4700 W. Lake Avenue
Glenview, IL 60025-1485
Phone: 800-229-7530
Fax: 847-375-4777
E-mail: info@rehabnurse.org
Web Site: http://www.rehabnurse.org

Association of Women's Health, Obstetric and Neonatal Nurses
2000 L Street, NW, Suite 740
Washington, DC 20036
Phone: 800-673-8499
Fax: 202-728-0575
Web Site: http://www.awhonn.org

Case Management Society of America
8201 Cantrell, Suite 230
Little Rock, AR 72227
Phone: 501-225-2229
Fax: 501-221-9068
E-mail: cmsa@cmsa.org
Web Site: http://www.cmsa.org

Emergency Nurses Association
915 Lee Street
Des Plaines, IL 60016-6569
Phone: 800-243-8362
E-mail: enainfo@ena.org
Web Site: http://www.ena.org

Endocrine Nurses Society
4350 E. West Hwy., Suite 500
Bethesda, MD 20814-4410
Phone: 301-941-0249
Fax: 301-941-0259
E-mail: staff@endo-nurses.org
Web Site: http://www.endo-nurses.org

Home Healthcare Nurses Association
228 Seventh Street, SE
Washington, DC 20003
Phone: 800-558-4462
Fax: 202-547-3540
E-mail: hhna_info@nahc.org
Web Site: http://www.nahc.org/hhna

Hospice and Palliative Nurses Association
Medical Center East, Suite 375
211 N. Whitfield Street
Pittsburgh, PA 15206-3031
Phone: 412-361-2470
Fax: 412-361-2425
Web Site: http://www.hpna.org

Infusion Nurses Society
220 Norwood Park South
Norwood, MA 02062
Phone: 781-440-9408
Fax: 781-440-9409
Web Site: http://www.ins1.org

International Nurses Society on Addictions
P.O. Box 10752
Raleigh, MC 27605
Phone: 919-821-1292
Fax: 919-833-5743
Web Site: http://www.intnsa.org

International Transplant Nurses Society
1739 E. Carson Street, Box 351
Pittsburgh, PA 15203-1700
Phone: 412-488-0249
Fax: 412-431-5911
E-mail: itns@msn.com
Web Site: http://www.itns.org

National Association of Clinical Nurse Specialists
3969 Green Street
Harrisburg, PA 17110
Phone: 717-234-8799
Fax: 717-234-6798
E-mail: info@nacns.org
Web Site: http://www.nacns.org

National Association of Hispanic Nurses
1501 16th Street, NW
Washington, DC 20036
Phone: 202-387-2477
Fax: 202-483-7183
E-mail: info@nahnhq.org
Web Site: http://www.nahnhq.org

National Association of Neonatal Nurses
701 Lee Street, Suite 450
Des Plaines, IL 60016
Phone: 800-451-3795
Fax: 847-297-6768
E-mail: info@nann.org
Web Site: http://www.nann.org

National Association of Orthopaedic Nurses
E. Holly Avenue, Box 56
Pitman, NJ 08071-0056
Phone: 856-256-2310
Fax: 856-589-7463
E-mail: naon@mail.ajj.com
Web Site: http://naon.inurse.com

National Association of Pediatric Nurse Associates & Practitioners, Inc.
1101 Kings Hwy. North, Suite 206
Cherry Hill, NJ 08034-1912
Phone: 877-662-7627
Fax: 856-667-7187
E-mail: info@napnap.org
Web Site: http://www.napnap.org

National Association of School Nurses
P.O. Box 1300
Scarborough, ME 04070-1300
Phone: 207-883-2117
Fax: 207-883-2683
E-mail: nasn@nasn.org
Web Site: http://www.nasn.org

National Association of Vascular Access Networks
11417 S. 700 East, PMB 205
Draper, UT 84020
Phone: 888-576-2826
Fax: 801-576-1824
E-mail: info@navannet.org
Web Site: http://www.navannet.org

National Black Nurses Association, Inc.
8630 Fenton Street, Suite 330
Silver Spring, MD 20910-3803
Phone: 301-589-3200
Fax: 301-589-3223
E-mail: NBNA@erols.com
Web Site: http://www.nbna.org

National Council of State Boards of Nursing, Inc.
676 N. Street Clair Street, Suite 550
Chicago, IL 60611-2921
Phone: 312-787-6555
E-mail: info@ncsbn.org
Web Site: http://www.ncsbn.org

The National Federation for Specialty Nursing Organizations
E. Holly Avenue, Box 56
Pitman, NJ 08071
Phone: 856-256-2333
Fax: 856-589-7463
E-mail: nfsno@ajj.com
Web Site: http://www.nfsno.org

National Federation of Licensed Practical Nurses, Inc.
893 U.S. Hwy. 70 West, Suite 202
Garner, NC 27529
Phone: 800-948-2511
Fax: 919-779-5642
E-mail: cbarbour@mgmt4u.com
Web Site: http://www.nflpn.org

National Gerontological Nursing Association
7794 Grow Drive
Pensacola, FL 32514
Phone: 850-473-1174
Fax: 850-484-8762
E-mail: ngna@puetzamc.com
Web Site: http://www.ngna.org

National League for Nursing
61 Broadway, 33rd Floor
New York, NY 10006
Phone: 800-669-1656
Fax: 212-812-0393
E-mail: nlnweb@nln.org
Web Site: http://www.nln.org

National Nursing Staff Development Organization
7794 Grow Drive
Pensacola, FL 32514
Phone: 800-489-1995
Fax: 850-484-8762
E-mail: e-mail@nnsdo.org
Web Site: http://www.nnsdo.org

National Organization for Associate Degree Nursing
11250 Roger Bacon Drive, Suite 8
Reston, VA 20190-5202
Phone: 703-437-4377
Fax: 703-435-4390
E-mail: noadn@noadn.org
Web Site: http://www.noadn.org

National Student Nurses' Association
45 Main St., Suite 606
New York, NY 11201
Phone: 718-210-0705
Fax: 718-210-0710
E-mail: nsna@nsna.org
Web Site: http://www.nsna.org

Nurses Christian Fellowship
Box 7895
Madison, WI 53707-7895
Phone: 608-274-4823, ext. 402
E-mail: ncf@ivcf.org
Web Site: http://www.ncf-jcn.org

Oncology Nursing Society
501 Holiday Drive
Pittsburgh, PA 15220
Phone: 412-921-7373
Fax: 412-921-6565
E-mail: customer.service@ons.org
Web Site: http://www.ons.org

Respiratory Nursing Society
7794 Grow Drive
Pensacola, FL 32514-7072
Phone: 850-474-8869
Fax: 850-484-8762
E-mail: rns@puetzamc.com

Sigma Theta Tau International Honor Society of Nursing
550 W. North Street
Indianapolis, IN 46202
Phone: 317-634-8171
Fax: 317-634-8188
E-mail: stti@stti.iupui.edu
Web Site: http://www.nursingsociety.org

Society of Otorhinolaryngology and Head-Neck Nurses, Inc.
116 Canal Street
New Smyrna Beach, FL 32168
Phone: 904-428-1695
Fax: 904-423-7566
E-mail: sohnnet@aol.com
Web Site: http://www.sohnnurse.com

Society for Vascular Nursing
7794 Grow Drive
Pensacola, FL 32414
Phone: 888-536-4786
Fax: 850-484-8762
E-mail: svn@puetzamc.com
Web Site: http://www.svnnet.org

Society of Gastroenterology Nurses and Associates, Inc.
401 N. Michigan Avenue
Chicago, IL 60611-4267
Phone: 800-245-7462
Fax: 312-527-6658
E-mail: sgna@sba.com
Web Site: http://www.sgna.org

Society of Urologic Nurses and Associates
E. Holly Avenue, Box 56
Pitman, NJ 08071-0056
Phone: 888-827-7862
Fax: 856-589-7463
E-mail: suna@ajj.com
Web Site: http://www.suna.org

Transcultural Nursing Society
36600 Schoolcraft Road
Livonia, MI 48150-1173
Phone: 888-432-5470
Fax: 732-432-5463
E-mail: barnes@smtp.munet.edu
Web Site: http://www.tcns.org

Wound, Ostomy and Continence Nurses Society
1550 S. Coast Hwy., #201
Laguna Beach, CA 92651
Phone: 888-224-9626
Fax: 949-376-3456
E-mail: maria@wocn.org
Web Site: http://www.wocn.org

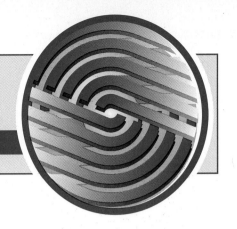

State Nurse Associations

Alabama State Nurses' Association
Karen L. Pakkala, MSN, RN, CAE, Executive
 Director
360 North Hull Street
Montgomery, AL 36104-3658
Phone: 334-262-8321
Fax: 334-262-8578
E-mail: alabamasna@mindspring.com or
 karenp.asna@mindspring.com
Web Site: http://www.nursingworld.org/snas/al
Office Hours: 8:00 AM-4:00 PM central time

Alaska Nurses Association
Camille Soleil, Executive Director
2207 East Tudor Road, Suite 34
Anchorage, AK 99507-1069
Phone: 907-274-0827
Fax: 907-272-0292
E-mail: aknurse@aknurse.org or csoleil@
 aknurse.org
Web Site: http://www.aknurse.org
Office Hours: 8:00 AM-4:30 PM Alaska time

Arizona Nurses Association
Marla Weston, RN, MS, Executive Director
1850 E. Southern Ave, Suite #1
Tempe, AZ 85282
Phone: 480-831-0404
Fax: 480-839-4780
E-mail: info@aznurse.org or marla@aznurse.
 org
Web Site: http://www.aznurse.org
Office Hours: 8:30 AM-4:30 PM mountain time

Arkansas Nurses Association
David Eubanks, MSN, RN, Chief Staff
 Officer
804 N. University
Little Rock, AR 72205
Phone: 501-664-5853
Fax: 501-664-5859
E-mail: arna@prodigy.net or deubanks@arna.
 org
Web Site: http://www.arna.org
Office Hours: 8:00 AM-4:30 PM central time

Association information retreived from constituent member organizations of the American Nurses Association, Web Site: http://www.nursingworld.org/snaaddr.htm. Accessed Sept. 5, 2002.

ANA\California

Tricia Hunter, RN, Executive Administrator
1121 L Street, Suite 409
Sacramento, CA 95814
Phone: 916-447-0225
Fax: 916-447-5568
E-mail: anacalif@pacbell.net
Web Site: http://www.anacalifornia.org
Office Hours: 9:00 AM-5:00 PM pacific time

Colorado Nurses Association

Linda Metzner, RN, MS, JD, Executive
  Director
950 S. Cherry, Suite 508
Denver, CO 80246
Association Management Alliance, Inc.
Phone: 303-757-7483
Fax: 303-758-0190
E-mail:cna@nurses-co.org or lwmetzner@
  aol.com
Web Site: http://www.nurses-co.org
Office Hours: 8:30 AM-4:30 PM mountain time

Connecticut Nurses' Association

Polly T. Barey, MS, RN, Executive Director
Meritech Business Park
377 Research Parkway, Suite 2D
Meriden, CT 06450
Phone: 203-238-1207
Fax: 203-238-3437
E-mail: polly@ctnurses.org
Web Site: http://www.ctnurses.org
Office Hours: 9:00 AM-5:00 PM eastern time

Delaware Nurses Association

Ruth Bashford, MN, RN, Executive Director
2644 Capitol Trail, Suite 330
Newark, DE 19711
Phone: 302-368-2333
Fax: 302-366-1775
E-mail: delnurse@erols.com
Web Site: http://www.nursingworld.org/
  snas/de
Office Hours: 9:00 AM-4:00 PM eastern time

District of Columbia Nurses Association, Inc.

Tom Wachter, Acting Executive Director
5100 Wisconsin Ave, N.W., Suite 306
Washington, DC 20016
Phone: 202-244-2705
Fax: 202-362-8285
E-mail: dcnurses1@aol.com
Web Site: http://dcnaonline.com
Office Hours: 9:00 AM-5:00 PM eastern time

Federal Nurses Association (FedNA)

Pamela C. Hagan, MSN, RN, Chief Programs
  Officer
600 Maryland Avenue, SW, Suite 100W
Washington, DC 20024
Phone: 202-651-7333
Fax: 202-651-7355
E-mail: FedNA@ana.org
Web Site: http://www.nusingworld.org/FedNA
Office Hours: 9:00 AM-4:30 PM eastern time

Florida Nurses Association

Paula Massey, MN, RN, Executive Director
P.O. Box 536985
Orlando, FL 32853-6985
Phone: 407-896-3261
Fax: 407-896-9042
E-mail: info@floridanurse.org or pmassey@
  floridanurse.org
Web Site: http://www.floridanurse.org
Office Hours: 8:30 AM-4:30 PM eastern time

Georgia Nurses Association

Deborah Hackman, Chief Executive Officer
3032 Briarcliff Road, NE
Atlanta, GA 30329-2655
Phone: 404-325-5536
Fax: 404-325-0407
E-mail: gna-ceo@mindspring.com
Web Site: http://www.georgianurses.org
Office Hours: 8:00 AM-4:30 PM eastern time

Guam Nurses Association
Glynis S. Almonte, BSN, RN, Executive
   Director
P.O. Box CG
Hagatna, GU 96932
Tel/Fax: 671-477-6877
E-mail: guamnurse@ite.net
Office Hours: 11:00 AM-1:00 PM pacific time

Hawaii Nurses Association
Nancy McGukin, Executive Director
677 Ala Moana Boulevard, Suite 301
Honolulu, HI 96813
Phone: 808-531-1628
Fax: 808-524-2760
E-mail: nancy@hawaiinurses.org
Web Site: http://www.hawaiinurses.org
Office Hours: 8:00 AM-4:30 PM Hawaiian time

Idaho Nurses Association
Judy Murray, PhD, RN, Executive Director
200 North 4th Street, Suite 20
Boise, ID 83702-6001
Phone: 208-345-0500
Fax: 208-385-0166
E-mail: idahonursesassn@hotmail.com or
   jmurray@boisestate.edu
Web Site: http://www.nursingworld.org/
   snas/id
Office Hours: 9:00 AM-5:30 PM mountain
   time

Illinois Nurses Association
Cathy Holmgren, RN, MBA, Executive
   Director
105 West Adams Street, Suite 2101
Chicago, IL 60603
Phone: 312-419-2900, ext. 226
Fax: 312-419-2920
E-mail: cholmgren@illinoisnurses.com
Web Site: http://www.illinoisnurses.com
Office Hours: 9:00 AM-5:00 PM central time

Indiana State Nurses Association
Ernest C. Klein, Jr, RN, CAE, Executive
   Director
2915 North High School Road
Indianapolis, INa 46224
Phone: 317-299-4575
Fax: 317-297-3525
E-mail: isnarn@prodigy.net
Web Site: http://www.indiananurses.org
Office Hours: 8:30 AM-4:30 PM eastern time

Iowa Nurses Association
Linda Goeldner, MA, MA, CHE, CAE,
   Executive Director
1501 42nd Street, Suite 471
West Des Moines, IA 50266
Phone: 515-225-0495
Fax: 515-225-2201
E-mail: iowanurses@aol.com or lkgoeld@
   aol.com
Web Site: http://www.iowanurses.org
Office Hours: 8:30 AM-4:00 PM central time

Kansas State Nurses Association
Terri R. Roberts, JD, RN, Executive Director
1208 S.W. Tyler
Topeka, KS 66612-1735
Phone: 785-233-8638
Fax: 785-233-5222
E-mail: troberts@echo.sound.net
Web Site: http://www.nursingworld.org/
   snas/ks
Office Hours: 8:00 AM-4:30 PM central time

Kentucky Nurses Association
Maureen Keenen, JD, Interim Executive
   Director
1400 South First Street
P.O. Box 2616
Louisville, KY 40201-2616
Phone: 502-637-2546/2547
Fax: 502-637-8236
E-mail: mkeenan@kentucky-nurses.org
Web Site: http://www.kentucky-nurses.org
Office Hours: 8:00 AM-4:30 PM eastern time

Louisiana State Nurses Association
Tawna Pounders, MNSc, RN, Executive
  Director
5700 Florida Boulevard, Suite 720
Baton Rouge, LA 70806
Phone: 225-201-0993 / 800-457-6378
Fax: 225-201-0971
E-mail: lsna@lsna.org or tpounders@lsna.org
Web Site: http://www.lsna.org
Office Hours: 9:00 AM-4:00 PM central time

ANA-MAINE
P.O. Box 254
Auburn, ME 04212-0254
Phone: 207-667-0260
E-mail: josephn@acadia.net
Web Site: http://www.anamaine.org

Maryland Nurses Association
Kathryn V. Hall, MS, RN, CNAA, Executive
  Director
849 International Drive
Airport Square 21, Suite 255
Linthicum, MD 21090
Phone: 410-859-3000
Fax: 410-859-3001
E-mail: marylandnursesassociation@erols.
  com
Web Site: http://www.nursingworld.org/snas/
  md
Office Hours: 8:30 AM-4:30 PM eastern time

**Massachusetts Association of Registered
  Nurses**
P.O. Box 70668
Quinsigamond Village Station
345 Greenwood Street
Worcester, MA 01607
Phone: 781-344-6926
Fax: 781-341-8495 Please call first-
E-mail: info@marnonline.org
Web Site: http://www.nursingworld.org/
  snas/ma

Michigan Nurses Association
Tom Renkes, MS, RN, Executive Director
2310 Jolly Oak Road
Okemos, MI 48864-4599
Phone: 517-349-5640, ext. 14
Fax: 517-349-5818
E-mail: tom.renkes@minurses.org
Web Site: http://www.minurses.org
Office Hours: 9:00 AM-5:00 PM eastern time

Minnesota Nurses Association
Erin Murphy, RN, Executive Director
1625 Energy Park Drive
St. Paul, MN 55108
Phone: 800-536-4662 / 651-646-4807, ext. 152
Fax: 651-647-5301
E-mail: emurphy@mnnurses.org
Web Site: http://www.mnnurses.org
Office Hours: 8:15 AM-4:30 PM central time

Mississippi Nurses Association
Betty R. Dickson, Executive Director
31 Woodgreen Place
Madison, MS 39110
Phone: 601-898-0670
Fax: 601-898-0190
E-mail: mna@msnurses.org or bdickson@
  netdoor.com
Web Site: http://www.msnurses.org
Office Hours: 8:00 AM-4:30 PM central time

Missouri Nurses Association
Belinda Heimericks, MSN, RN, Executive
  Director
1904 Bubba Lane, P.O. Box 105228
Jefferson City, MO 65110-5228
Phone: 888-662-MONA / 573-636-4623
Fax: 573-636-9576
E-mail: belinda@missourinurses.org
Web Site: http://www.missourinurses.org
Office Hours: 8:00 AM-5:00 PM central time

Montana Nurses Association
Sami Butler, RN, Executive Director
104 Broadway, Suite G-2
Helena, MT 59601
Phone: 406-442-6710
Fax: 406-442-1841
E-mail: info@mtnurses.org or sbutler@
mtnurses.org
Web Site: http://www.nursingworld.org/snas/
mt/
Office Hours: 8:30 AM-4:30 PM mountain
time

Nebraska Nurses Association
Chuck Stepanek, BS, Executive Director
715 South 14th Street
Lincoln, NE 68508
Phone: 800-201-3625 / 402-475-3859
Fax: 402-475-3961
E-mail: ne.nurses@prodigy.net
Web Site: http://www.nursingworld.org/snas/
ne/index.htm
Office Hours: 8:00 AM-4:30 PM central time

Nevada Nurses Association
Richard Schlegel, CAE, Executive Director
P.O. Box 530399
Henderson, NV 89053-0399
Phone: 702-260-7886
Fax: 702-260-7052
E-Mail: nvnurses@aol.com or schlegelra@
aol.com
Web Site: http://www.nvnurses.org
Office Hours: 9:00 AM-5:00 PM pacific time

New Hampshire Nurses Association
Robert Best, BSE, MPA, Executive Director
48 West Street
Concord, NH 03301-3595
Phone: 603-225-3783
Fax: 603-228-6672
E-mail: nh_nurses@compuserve.com
Web Site: http://www.nhnurses.org
Office Hours: 9:00 AM-5:00 PM eastern time

New Jersey State Nurses Association
Andrea Aughenbaugh, RN, CS, CAE, Chief
Executive Officer
1479 Pennington Road
Trenton, NJ 08618-2661
Phone: 609-883-5335, ext. 10
Fax: 609-883-5343
E-mail: njsna@njsna.org or andrea@njsna.org
Web Site: http://www.njsna.org
Office Hours: 8:30 AM-4:30 PM eastern time

New Mexico Nurses Association
Carrie Roberts, MSN, RN, CNP, Executive
Director
P.O. Box 29658
Santa Fe, NM 87592-9658
Phone: 505-471-3324
Fax: 505-471-3326
E-mail: nmnurses@hotmail.com
Web Site: http://www.nursingworld.org/snas/
nm
Federal Express Delivery Only:
3018 Cielo Court, Suite B
Santa Fe, NM 87507
Office Hours: 8:00 AM-5:00 PM mountain
time

New York State Nurses Association
Martha L. Orr, MN, RN, CAE, Executive
Director
11 Cornell Road
Latham, NY 12110
Phone: 518-782-9400 ext. 279
Fax: 518-782-9530
E-mail: martha.orr@nysna.org
Web Site: http://www.nysna.org
Office Hours: 8:30 AM-5:00 PM eastern time

North Carolina Nurses Association
Sindy Barker, CAE, Executive Director
103 Enterprise Street
Box 12025
Raleigh, NC 27605
Phone: 919-821-4250
Fax: 919-829-5807
E-mail: rns@ncnurses.org or sindybarker@ncnurses.org
Web Site: http://www.ncnurses.org
Office Hours: 8:30 AM-4:30 PM eastern time

North Dakota Nurses Association
Sharon Moos, MBA, RN, Executive Administrator
531 Airport Road, Suite D
Bismarck, ND 58504-6107
Phone: 701-223-1385
Fax: 701-223-0575
E-mail: ndna@prodigy.net
Office Hours: 8:30 AM-4:30 PM central time

Ohio Nurses Association
Gingy Harshey-Meade, MSN, RN, CNAA, Chief Executive Officer
4000 East Main Street
Columbus, OH 43213-2983
Phone: 614-237-5414 ext. 1020
Fax: 614-237-6081
E-mail: gharsheymeade@ohnurses.org or gingy@insight.rr.com
Office Hours: 8:30 AM-4:30 PM eastern time

Oklahoma Nurses Association
6414 North Santa Fe, Suite A
Oklahoma City, OK 73116
Phone: 405-840-3476
Fax: 405-840-3013
Web Site: http://www.oknurses.com
Office Hours: 8:30 AM-5:00 PM central time

Oregon Nurses Association
Susan E. King, MS, RN, Administrator for Professional Services
Ken Fitzsimon, JD, Administrator of Labor Relations
Sandy Marron, MBA, Administrator of Business Services
9600 S.W. Oak, Suite 550
Portland, OR 97223
Phone: 503-293-0011
Fax: 503-293-0013
E-mail: ona@oregonrn.org
Web Site: http://www.oregonrn.org
Office Hours: 8:30 AM-5:00 PM pacific time

Pennsylvania State Nurses Association
Michele P. Campbell, MSN, RN, Executive Administrator
P.O. Box 68525
Harrisburg, PA 17106-8525
Phone: 888-707-7762 / 717-657-1222
Fax: 717-657-3796
E-mail: psna@psna.org
Web Site: http://www.psna.org
Office Hours: 8:30 AM-4:30 PM eastern time

Rhode Island State Nurses Association
Pamela L. McCue, MSN, RN, Executive Director
550 S. Water Street, Unit 540B
Providence, RI 02903-4344
Phone: 401-421-9703
Fax: 401-421-6793
E-mail: risna@prodigy.net
Web Site: http://www.risnarn.org
Office Hours: Monday-Thursday 10:00 AM-3:30 PM eastern time

South Carolina Nurses' Association
Judith C. Thompson, Executive Director
1821 Gadsden Street
Columbia, SC 29201
Phone: 803-252-4781
Fax: 803-779-3870
E-mail: scna@prodigy.net or judith.thompson@
prodigy.net
Web Site: http://www.scnurses.org
Office Hours: 8:30 AM-4:30 PM eastern time

South Dakota Nurses Association
Ed Jacobson, Executive Director
P.O. Box 1015
Pierre, SD 57501-1015
Phone: 605-945-4265
Fax: 605-945-4266
E-mail: sdnurse1@dtgnet.com
Web Site: http://www.nursingworld.org/
snas/sd
Office Hours: 8:00 AM-3:00 PM central time

Tennessee Nurses Association
Louise Browning, CAE, Executive Director
545 Mainstream Drive, Suite 405
Nashville, TN 37228-1201
Phone: 615-254-0350
Fax: 615-254-0303
E-mail: lbrowntna@aol.com or lbrowning@
tnaonline.org
Web Site: http://www.tnaonline.org
Office Hours: 8:30 AM-5:00 PM central time

Texas Nurses Association
Clair B. Jordan, MSN, RN, Executive Director
7600 Burnet Road, Suite 440
Austin, TX 78757-1292
Phone: 512-452-0645
Fax: 512-452-0648
E-mail: memberinfo@texasnurses.org or
cjordan@texasnurses.org
Web Site: http://www.texasnurses.org
Office Hours: 8:00 AM-5:00 PM central time

Utah Nurses Association
3761 S. 700 East, #201
Salt Lake City, UT 84106
Phone: 801-293-8351
Fax: 801-293-8458
E-mail: una@xmission.com
Web Site: http://www.utahnurses.org
Office Hours: 9:00 AM-5:00 PM mountain
time

Vermont State Nurses Association
Margaret M. Sharpe, RN, BSN, Executive
Director
100 Dorset Street, Suite 13
South Burlington, VT 05403-6241
Phone: 802-651-8886
Fax: 802-651-8998
E-mail: vtnurse@prodigy.net
Web Site: http://www.uvm.edu/~vsna
Office Hours: Monday-Thursday 9:00 AM-
3:00 PM eastern time

Virgin Islands State Nurses Association
Verna Christian-Garcia, BSN, RN, Executive
Director
P.O. Box 583
Christiansted, St. Croix, VI 00821-0583
Phone: 809-773-1261
E-mail: vcgvina@viaccess.net

Virginia Nurses Association
Jan Marshall Johnson, MS, RN, Executive
Director
7113 Three Chopt Road, Suite 204
Richmond, VA 23226
Phone: 804-282-1808/2373
Fax: 804-282-4916
E-mail: vnajmj@aol.com
Web Site: http://www.virginianurses.com
Office Hours: 8:30 AM-5:00 PM eastern time

Washington State Nurses Association
Judith A. Huntington, MN, RN, Executive
  Director
575 Andover Park West, Suite 101
Seattle, WA 98188-3321
Phone: 206-575-7979, ext. 3002
Fax: 206-575-1908
E-mail: wsna@wsna.org or jhunting@wsna.org
Web Site: http://www.wsna.org
Office Hours: 8:30 AM-4:30 PM pacific time

West Virginia Nurses Association
Cheri Heflin, Executive Director
100 Capitol Street, Suite 1009
P.O. 1946
Charleston, WV 25301
Phone: 800-400-1226 / 304-342-1169
Fax: 304-346-1861
Phone: 304-346-0300 direct-
E-mail: centraloffice@wvnurses.org or Cheri@
  chandcompany.com
Web Site: http://www.wvnurses.org
Office Hours: 8:30 AM-4:30 PM eastern time

Wisconsin Nurses Association
Gina Dennik-Champion, MSN, MSH, RN,
  Executive Administrator
6117 Monona Drive
Madison, WI 53716
Phone: 608-221-0383
Fax: 608-221-2788
E-mail: wna@execpc.com or ginawna@execpc.
  com
Web Site: http://www.wisconsinnurses.org
Office Hours: 7:30 AM-4:00 PM central time

Wyoming Nurses Association
Beverly McDermott, MS, RN, Executive
  Director
Majestic Building, Room 305
1603 Capitol Avenue
Cheyenne, WY 82001
Phone: 307-635-3955
Fax: 307-635-2173
E-mail: wyonurse@aol.com or bjmcdermot@
  aol.com
Office Hours: Tuesday/Friday 9:00 AM-
  1:00 PM
Monday/Wednesday/Thursday 8:00 AM-
  1:00 PM mountain time

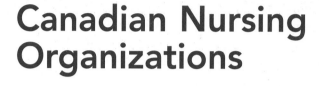

APPENDIX D

Canadian Nursing Organizations

Alberta Association of Registered Nurses
11620 - 168 Street
Edmonton, AB T5M 4A6
Phone: 780-451-0043
Fax: 780-452-3276
E-mail: aarn@nurses.ab.ca
Web Site: http://www.nurses.ab.ca

Association of Registered Nurses of Newfoundland and Labrador
55 Military Road, Box 6116
St. John's, NF A1C 5X8
Phone: 709-753-6040
Fax: 709-753-4940
E-mail: info@arnn.nf.ca
Web Site: http://www.arnn.nf.ca

Association of Registered Nurses of Prince Edward Island
17 Pownal Street
Charlottetown, PE C1A 3V7
Phone: 902-368-3764
Fax: 902-628-1430

College of Nurses of Ontario
101 Davenport Road
Toronto, ON M5R 3P1
Phone: 800-387-5526 / 416-928-0900
Fax: 416-928-5607
E-mail: mrisk@cnomail.org
Web Site: http://www.cno.org

College of Registered Nurses of Nova Scotia
Suite 600, Barrington Tower
Scotia Square, 1894 Barrington St.
Halifax, NS B3J 2A8
Phone: 902-491-9744
Fax: 902-491-9510
E-mail: info@rnans.ns.ca
Web Site: http://www.crnns.ca/index.html

Manitoba Association of Registered Nurses
647 Broadway Avenue
Winnipeg, MB R3C 0X2
Phone: 204-774-3477
Fax: 204-775-6052
E-mail: marn@marn.mb.ca
Web Site: http://www.marn.mb.ca

Northwest Territories Registered Nurses Association
Box 2757
Yellowknife, NT X1A 2R1
Phone: 867-873-2745
Fax: 867-873-2336
E-mail: nwtrna@internorth.com
Web Site: http://www.nwtrna.com

Nurses Association of New Brunswick/ Association des infirmières et infirmiers du Nouveau-Brunswick
165 Regent Street
Fredericton, NB E3B 7B4
Phone: 506-458-8731
Fax: 506-459-2838
E-mail: nanb@nanb.nb.ca
Web Site: http://www.nanb.nb.ca

Ordre des infirmières et infirmiers du Québec
4200, boul. Dorchester Ouest
Montreal, QC H3Z 1V4
Phone: 514-935-2501 / 1-800-363-6048
Fax: 514-935-1799
E-mail: inf@oiiq.org
Web Site: http://www.oiiq.org

Registered Nurses Association of British Columbia
2855 Arbutus Street
Vancouver, BC V6J 3Y8
Phone: 604-736-7331
Fax: 604-738-2272
E-mail: info@rnabc.bc.ca
Web Site: http://www.rnabc.bc.ca

Saskatchewan Registered Nurses' Association
2066 Retallack Street
Regina, SK S4T 7X5
Phone: 306-359-4200
Fax: 306-525-0849
E-mail: srna@srna.org
Web Site: http://www.srna.org

Yukon Registered Nurses Association
204 - 4133 - 4th Avenue
Whitehorse, YT Y1A 3T3
Phone: 867-667-4062
Fax: 867-668-5123
E-mail: yrna@yknet.ca

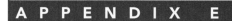

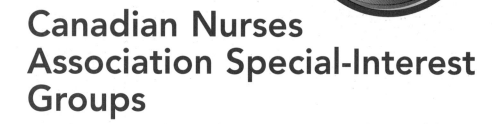

Canadian Nurses Association Special-Interest Groups

Aboriginal Nurses Association of Canada (ANAC)
ODAWA Native Friendship Centre
12 Stirling Avenue, 3rd Floor
Ottawa, ON K1Y 1P8
Web Site: http://www.anac.on.ca

Academy of Chief Executive Nurses (ACEN)
Victoria Hospital
800 Commissioners Road E
London, ON N6A 4G5

Alberta Occupational Health Nurses Association (AOHNA)
c/o Alberta Association of Registered Nurses
11620 - 168 Street
Edmonton, AB T5M 4A6
Web Site: http://www.aohna.ab.ca

Canadian Association for Enterostomal Therapy (CAET)
P.O. Box 48069
60 Dundas Street East
Mississauga, ON L5A 1W4
Web Site: http://www.caet.ca

Canadian Association for the History of Nursing (CAHN)
130 Caruthers Avenue
Kingston, ON K7L 1M7
Web Site: http://www.ualberta.ca/~jhibberd/CAHN_ACHN

Canadian Association of Burn Nurses (CABN)
1150 Glenridge Drive
Oakville, ON L6M 2K7

Canadian Association of Critical Care Nurses (CACCN)
P.O. Box 25322
London, ON N6C 6B1
Web Site: http://www.caccn.ca

Canadian Association of Nephrology Nurses and Technologists (CANNT)
336 Yonge Street, Suite 322
Barrie, ON, L4N 4C8
Web Site: http://www.cannt.ca

Canadian Association of Neuroscience Nurses (CANN)
71 Inch Bay
Winnipeg, MB R2Y 0X2
Web Site: http://www.cann.ca

Canadian Association of Nurses in AIDS Care (CANAC)
Casey House Hospice
9 Huntley Street
Toronto, ON M4Y 2K8
Web Site: http://www.canac.org

Canadian Association of Nurses in Independent Practice (CANIP)
55 McCaul Street
Toronto, ON M5T 2W7

Canadian Association of Nurses in Oncology (CANO)
R.R. #2, P.O. Box 51
Lisle, ON L0M 1M0
Web Site: http://www.cos.ca/cano/cano.htm

Canadian Association of Pediatric Nurses (CAPN)
PICU
Montreal Children's Hospital
2300 Tupper
Montreal, QC H3H 1P3

Canadian Clinical Nurse Specialist Interest Group (CCNSIG)
2 East - AAC
1763 Robie Street
Halifax, NS B3H 3C2

Canadian Council of Cardiovascular Nurses (CCCN)
222 Queen Street, Suite 1402
Ottawa, ON K1P 5V9
Web Site: http://www.cardiovascularnurse.com

Canadian Federation of Mental Health Nurses (CFMHN)
Faculty of Nursing
3rd Floor
Clinical Sciences Building
University of Alberta
Edmonton, AB T6G 2G3
Web Site: http://www.cfmhn.org

Canadian Gerontological Nursing Association (CGNA)
3223 Kenmarc Crescent SW
Calgary, AB T3E 4R4
Web Site: http://www.cgna.net

Canadian Holistic Nurses Association (CHNA)
50 Driveway
Ottawa, ON K2P 1E2
Web Site: http://mypage.direct.ca/h/hutchings/chna.html

Canadian Nurse Educators Association (CNEA)
400 Waterloo Street
Winnipeg, MB R3N 0S6

Canadian Nurses' Respiratory Society (CNRS)
Head Office
300 - 3 Raymond Street
Ottawa, ON K1R 1A3
Web Site: http://www.lung.ca/resp/etitle.html

Canadian Nursing Research Group (CNRG)
Faculty of Nursing
University of New Brunswick
P.O. Box 4400
Fredericton, NB E3B 5A3

Canadian Obstetric, Gynecologic and Neonatal Nurses (COGNN)
315 Oakwood Avenue
Winnipeg, MB R3L 1E8

Canadian Orthopaedic Nurses Association (CONA)
1515 Lareau
Chambly, QC J3L 5M7

Community Health Nurses Association of Canada (CHNAC)
21-1331 Commissioners Road West
London, ON N6K 1E2

National Emergency Nurses Affiliation Inc (NENA)
20 Jasper Street
St John's, NF A1A 4E2
Web Site: http://www.nena.ca

Operating Room Nurses Association of Canada (ORNAC)
1195 Richmond Rd, Suite 607
Ottawa, ON K2B 8E4
Web Site: http://www.ornac.ca

Index